The Handbook of Touch

Matthew J. Hertenstein, PhD, is Associate Professor of Psychology and Director of the Touch and Emotion Lab at DePauw University. Dr. Hertenstein has conducted research on touch from both a developmental perspective (focusing on infant development), as well as a social perspective (focusing on the communication of distinct emotions by adults). In addition to private funding sources, his empirical work has been funded by the *National Institute of Child Health and Human Development*, as well as the *National Institute of Mental Health* of the *National Institutes of Health*. His work has been featured nationally and internationally via a number of media outlets, including *National Public Radio, The New York Times, Psychology Today,* and the documentary entitled *Touch: The Essential Sense* produced by the *Canadian Broadcasting Corporation*. Conjointly with his empirical work, Dr. Hertenstein is the author of two comprehensive and peer-reviewed literature reviews in the area of touch, one of which addresses the literature on human, non-human primates, as well as rats. Finally, Dr. Hertenstein regularly reviews for a number of journals including *Child Development, Infancy,* and *Psychological Science.*

Sandra J. Weiss, PhD, DNSc, RN, FAAN, is a Professor in the Department of Community Health Systems and the Robert C. & Delphine Wentland Eschbach Endowed Chair at the University of California, San Francisco. Dr. Weiss has studied the phenomenon of touch as her primary area of research for 30 years. During this time, she has identified specific neurophysiologic and affective properties of touch and has developed measures of both touch behavior and tactile reactivity that have been used in research internationally. Her major research has focused on parental touch and its impact on the neuropsychological development and mental health of infants and children. She has also studied different properties of touch used by health professionals in hospital environments and their impact on the physiologic stability and health outcomes of medically compromised children and adults. Dr. Weiss is currently studying the ways in which genetic, neuroendocrine, and autonomic nervous system factors interact with environmental stressors to influence the tactile reactivity and neurobehavioral regulation of preterm infants. She is also testing the effects of various comforting interventions by parents on infant stress reactivity and response to pain in the neonatal intensive care unit. Her research has been funded by the National Institutes of Health, the Bureau of Health Services Administration, the State of California, and a variety of private foundations. Her work on touch has been covered by CNN, CBS, and ABC as part of programs on "The Senses," "Discoveries in Medical Science," and "Medical Advances." Dr. Weiss serves as a reviewer and is on the editorial boards of numerous journals that address a broad multidisciplinary audience. She has also served on varied NIH study sections throughout her career. She has been Director of both the Center for Family Health Studies and the Robert Wood Johnson, Postdoctoral Scholars Program at UCSF, and has been Associate Provost for Research at the University of California, Office of the President.

The Handbook of Touch

Neuroscience, Behavioral, and Health Perspectives

Editors

Matthew J. Hertenstein, PhD
DePauw University
Greencastle, Indiana

&

Sandra J. Weiss, PhD, DNSc, RN, FAAN
University of California
San Francisco, California

SPRINGER PUBLISHING COMPANY
NEW YORK

Copyright © 2011 Springer Publishing Company, LLC

All rights reserved.

No part of this publication may be reproduced, stored in a retrieval system, or transmitted in any form or by any means, electronic, mechanical, photocopying, recording, or otherwise, without the prior permission of Springer Publishing Company, LLC, or authorization through payment of the appropriate fees to the Copyright Clearance Center, Inc., 222 Rosewood Drive, Danvers, MA 01923, 978-750-8400, fax 978-646-8600, info@copyright.com or on the web at www.copyright.com.

Springer Publishing Company, LLC
11 West 42nd Street
New York, NY 10036
www.springerpub.com

Acquisitions Editor: Sheri W. Sussman
Production Editor: Dana Bigelow
Cover Design: David Levy
Composition: Newgen Imaging

ISBN: 978-0-8261-2191-2
E-book ISBN: 978-0-8261-2192-9

The author and the publisher of this Work have made every effort to use sources believed to be reliable to provide information that is accurate and compatible with the standards generally accepted at the time of publication. Because medical science is continually advancing, our knowledge base continues to expand. Therefore, as new information becomes available, changes in procedures become necessary. We recommend that the reader always consult current research and specific institutional policies before performing any clinical procedure. The author and publisher shall not be liable for any special, consequential, or exemplary damages resulting, in whole or in part, from the readers' use of, or reliance on, the information contained in this book. The publisher has no responsibility for the persistence or accuracy of URLs for external or third-party Internet Web sites referred to in this publication and does not guarantee that any content on such Web sites is, or will remain, accurate or appropriate.

Library of Congress Cataloging-in-Publication Data

The handbook of touch : neuroscience, behavioral, and health perspectives / editors, Matthew J. Hertenstein, Sandra J. Weiss.
   p. ; cm.
Includes bibliographical references and index.
ISBN 978-0-8261-2191-2 — ISBN 978-0-8261-2192-9 (e-book)
1. Touch.   I. Hertenstein, Matthew J.   II. Weiss, Sandra Jean, 1947–
[DNLM: 1. Touch—physiology. 2. Neurophysiology. 3. Touch Perception.   WR 102]
QP451.H153 2011
612.8'8—dc22   2011005047

Special discounts on bulk quantities of our books are available to corporations, professional associations, pharmaceutical companies, health care organization, and other qualifying groups.

If you are interested in a custom book, including chapters from more than one of our titles, we can provide that service as well.

For details, please contact:
Special Sales Department, Springer Publishing Company, LLC
11 West 42nd Street, 15th Floor, New York, NY 10036-8002
Phone: 877-687-7476 or 212-431-4370; Fax: 212-941-7842
Email: sales@springerpub.com

---

11 12 13 14 / 5 4 3 2 1

Printed in the United States of America by Hamilton Printing

Contents

Contributors *vii*
Preface *xi*

SECTION I THE NEUROBIOLOGY OF TOUCH

1. The Anatomy and Physiology of the Skin 3
   Desmond John Tobin

2. Sensory Processes of Touch 33
   Aislyn M. Nelson and Ellen A. Lumpkin

3. The Molecular and Genetic Basis of Touch 59
   Kate Poole, Stefan G. Lechner, and Gary R. Lewin

4. Brain Plasticity and Touch 85
   Hubert R. Dinse

SECTION II PERCEIVING THE PHYSICAL WORLD VIA TOUCH

5. Biomechanical and Neurophysiological Basis of the Processing of Tactile Stimuli 123
   Steven S. Hsiao

6. Hierarchical Neural Pathways of Haptic Object Processing 143
   Sunah Kim and Thomas W. James

7. The Organization and Function of Somatosensory Cortex 161
   Sliman J. Bensmaia and Jeffrey M. Yau

8. Crossmodal Interactions in Tactile Perception 189
   Charles Spence and Andrew J. Bremner

SECTION III MEASUREMENT OF TOUCH

9. Measurement of Tactile Response and Tactile Perception 219
   Catana Brown, Diane L. Filion, and Sandra J. Weiss

10. Measurement of Touch Behavior 245
    Sandra J. Weiss and Sandra K. Niemann

SECTION IV COMMUNICATION VIA TOUCH

11. Communicating Through Touch: Touching During Parent–Infant Interactions   273
    Dale M. Stack and Amelie D. L. Jean

12. The Communicative Functions of Touch in Adulthood   299
    Matthew J. Hertenstein

13. Gender and Status Patterns in Social Touch   329
    Judith A. Hall

14. Tactile Traditions: Cultural Differences and Similarities in Haptic Communication   351
    Peter A. Andersen

SECTION V THE RELEVANCE OF TOUCH FOR DEVELOPMENT AND HEALTH

15. Maternal Touch and the Developing Infant   373
    Ruth Feldman

16. Tactile Dysfunction in Neurodevelopmental Disorders   409
    Carissa J. Cascio

17. Touch in People Who Are Visually Impaired   435
    Morton A. Heller and Anne McClure Walk

18. Massage Therapy: A Review of Recent Research   455
    Tiffany Field

19. Haptic Feedback: Technology and Medical Applications   469
    Allison M. Okamura

Index   499

Contributors

Peter A. Andersen, PhD
Professor of Communication, San Diego State University, San Diego, California

Sliman J. Bensmaia, PhD
Assistant Professor of Organismal Biology and Anatomy, University of Chicago, Chicago, Illinois

Andrew J. Bremner, PhD
Senior Lecturer in Psychology, University of London, London, United Kingdom

Catana Brown, PhD, OTR
Associate Professor, Department of Occupational Therapy, Midwestern University, Glendale, Arizona

Carissa J. Cascio, PhD
Assistant Professor, Department of Psychiatry, Vanderbilt University, Nashville, Tennessee

Hubert R. Dinse, PhD
Associate Professor, Institut fur Neuroinformatik, Neural Plasticity Lab, Ruhr University, Bochum, Germany

Ruth Feldman, PhD
Professor, Department of Psychology and the Gonda Brain Sciences Center, Bar-Ilan University, Ramat-Gan, Israel

Tiffany Field, PhD
Director of the Touch Research Institute, University of Miami Medical School, Miami, Florida

Diane L. Filion, PhD
Professor, Department of Psychology, Associate Dean, College of Arts & Sciences, University of Missouri, Kansas City, Missouri

Judith A. Hall, PhD
Professor of Psychology, Northeastern University, Boston, Massachusetts

Morton A. Heller, PhD
Professor of Psychology, Eastern Illinois University, Charleston, Illinois

Matthew J. Hertenstein, PhD
Associate Professor and Director of the Touch and Emotion Lab, DePauw University, Greencastle, Indiana

Steven S. Hsiao, PhD
Professor, Krieger Mind/Brain Institute and the Solomon Snyder Department of Neuroscience, The Johns Hopkins University, Baltimore, Maryland

Thomas W. James, PhD
Assistant Professor, Department of Psychological and Brain Sciences, Cognitive Science Program and Program in Neuroscience, Indiana University, Bloomington, Indiana

Amelie D. L. Jean, MA
PhD Candidate in Psychology, Department of Psychology, Concordia University & Centre for Research in Human Development, Montreal, Quebec, Canada

Sunah Kim, PhD
Postdoctoral Fellow, Vision Science Program, School of Optometry, University of California, Berkeley, California

Associate Instructor, Cognitive Science Program and Program in Neuroscience, Indiana University, Bloomington, Indiana

Stefan G. Lechner, PhD
Postdoctoral Fellow, Department of Neuroscience, Max Delbruck Center for Molecular Medicine, Berlin, Germany

Gary R. Lewin, PhD
Professor, Charite Universitatsmedizin and Department of Neuroscience, Max Delbruck Center for Molecular Medicine, Berlin, Germany

Ellen A. Lumpkin, PhD
Associate Professor of Dermatology and of Physiology and Cellular Biophysics, Columbia University College of Physicians and Surgeons, New York, New York

Aislyn M. Nelson, BA
MD/PhD Candidate in Neuroscience, Baylor College of Medicine, Houston, Texas

Sandra K. Niemann, RN, PhD
Postdoctoral Fellow, Department of Community Health Systems, University of California, San Francisco, California

Allison M. Okamura, PhD
Professor of Mechanical Engineering, The Johns Hopkins University, Baltimore, Maryland

Kate Poole, PhD
Postdoctoral Fellow, Department of Neuroscience, Max Delbruck Center for Molecular Medicine, Berlin, Germany

Charles Spence, PhD
Professor of Experimental Psychology, Oxford University, Oxford, United Kingdom

Dale M. Stack, PhD
Professor of Psychology, Department of Psychology, Concordia University & Centre for Research in Human Development, Montreal, Quebec, Canada

Desmond John Tobin, BSc, PhD, FRCPath, FSB
Professor, Center for Skin Sciences, School of Life Sciences, University of Bradford, West Yorkshire, Great Britain

Anne McClure Walk, MA
PhD Candidate in Cognitive Neuroscience, Department of Psychology, Saint Louis University, Saint Louis, Missouri

Sandra J. Weiss, PhD, DNSc, RN, FAAN
Professor, Department of Community Health Systems, the Robert C. & Delphine Wentland Eschbach Endowed Chair, University of California, San Francisco, California

Jeffrey M. Yau, PhD
Postdoctoral Fellow in the Department of Neurology, Johns Hopkins University, Baltimore, Maryland

Preface

The study of touch has faced strong headwinds since its inception. In the face of such forces, *The Handbook of Touch* is a significant achievement for the field. Foremost among these forces has been the domination of Western philosophy by metaphors and examples that privilege vision over other sensory modalities. Historically, many philosophers believed that vision offered the most veridical perception of the world. Descartes' (1637/1965) view is representative: "All the management of our lives depends on the senses, and since that of sight is the most comprehensive and the noblest of these, there is no doubt that the inventions which serve to augment its power are among the most useful that there can be" (p. 65). This view is responsible, at least in part, for denigrating the role of other nonvisual modalities, including touch. Concurrently, there has been a tendency to devalue touch-related research as pseudoscience in some scientific arenas. Underlying such views are assumptions that touch has minimal implications for human development, health and disease, or effective social functioning. Without doubt, the research compiled within this handbook demonstrates the erroneous nature of such assumptions.

A number of other relevant factors have provided challenges to the study of touch. Societal proscriptions against touch abound in most parts of the world and across domains of society (e.g., in schools, the workplace, and the health care system). As described in this handbook, historical, religious, and cultural variables may explain why touch is verboten in so many facets of our communication. Research about touch has also been hampered for reasons of money and infrastructure. Although many major universities have an entire department dedicated to the study of vision, it is rare to find teams of faculty hired to study tactile processes and mechanisms. In addition, methodological challenges have impeded touch research. Much of tactile interaction takes place in privacy, making it difficult and, sometimes, inaccessible for researchers to study. Multiple complexities also exist within both the characteristics of a specific touch and larger patterns of tactile behavior. These create many degrees of freedom that must be either managed or examined.

Despite these headwinds, research regarding touch has continued to evolve and flourish, with a diversity that is both theoretically

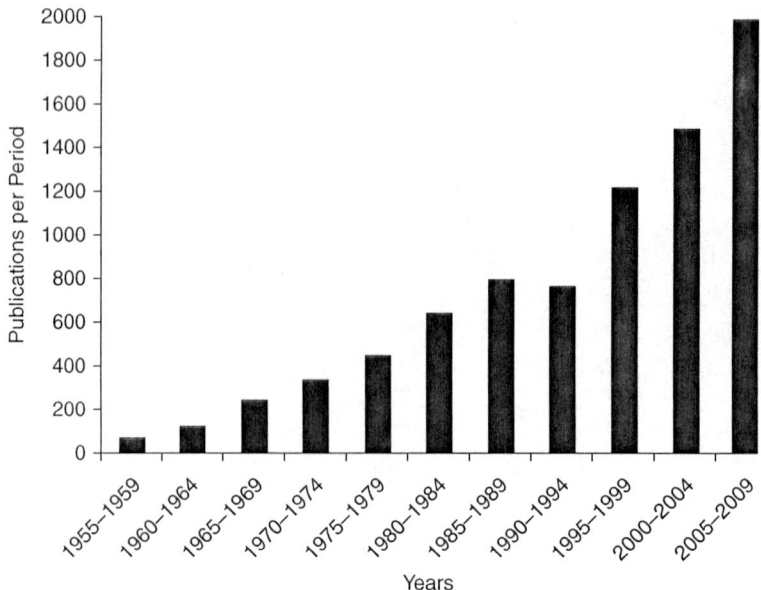

Citations for "touch" or "tactile" in Web of Science index (comprised of Science citation index and social sciences citation index). The same trend is apparent with other databases (e.g., PsychInfo).

and empirically rich. The field of touch has come into its own and *The Handbook of Touch* symbolizes this accomplishment. Evidence of the increasing interest in touch can be seen in citation trends over the years. As indicated in the above figure, the study of touch has grown exponentially. The current volume is a testament to the vitality of the field and the critical mass of knowledge that has been gathered on the topic.

The goals of this handbook are (1) to provide an authoritative and state-of-the-art resource for the field of touch; (2) to present a cross-disciplinary perspective on touch that will further dialogue and collaboration among related subfields; (3) to reflect and organize the broad diversity of scholarship within the field; and (4) to serve an expansive readership, including scholars, students, and applied professionals.

Five primary sections with 19 chapters comprise the current handbook. The first two sections integrate the latest research on the biological underpinnings of touch, with the second section emphasizing how we perceive the physical world via touch. The third section of the handbook includes two chapters which address the measurement of touch perception and touch behavior. The fourth section examines how touch is used in both child and adult communication and reviews the literature on touch in terms of gender and culture. Finally, the last section of the handbook covers a variety of ways in which touch plays an important role in development and health across the life span.

We would like to thank all of our authors for their superb contributions to *The Handbook of Touch* as well as our colleagues who encouraged us to undertake this project. We also acknowledge the support and guidance of Neil Salkind who helped to shape the project in its beginning stages.

Matthew J. Hertenstein
Greencastle, Indiana

Sandra J. Weiss
San Francisco, California

I

The Neurobiology of Touch

1

The Anatomy and Physiology of the Skin

DESMOND JOHN TOBIN

The skin, our body's largest organ, is located at the interface between our external and internal worlds. Given this location, it is strategically placed to provide not only a barrier against a range of noxious stressors (UV radiation, and mechanical, chemical, and biological insults) but also to act as the periphery's "sensing" system. Both roles have a critical influence on our sense of touch. While the structure or form of skin (particularly human skin) is well understood at the anatomic level, recent advances in disciplines such as molecular and cellular biology, signal transduction, proteomics, and genomics, amongst others, have been invaluable in aiding our attempts to unravel the complexities of skin function and have fuelled much of the enormous development in cutaneous research over the last couple of decades. Recent developments suggest that this organ is much more critical to maintaining total body homeostasis than previously thought. As an organ, the skin is invested with enormous functionality, incorporating all major support systems of blood, muscle, and innervation, and has prominent roles in immunocompetence, psycho-emotion, UV radiation (UVR) sensing, and endocrine function.

Regardless of all the high-tech molecular analyses available to today's biomedical scientist, structural examination of the skin remains key to a full appreciation of its function—or as the Nobel Prize laureate Albert Szent-Györgyi aptly put it, "If structure does not tell us anything about function, it means we have not looked at it correctly." Still, the past 30 years has seen enormous growth in our knowledge of skin function, with several new subspecialities of cutaneous science emerging, not least of which is cutaneous neuroendocrinology. In the context of any study of touch, the latter positions the skin as an important sensor of the periphery and has prompted some to call the skin our "brain on the outside" (Slominski, 2005; Tobin, 2006). It has been estimated that approximately 3,000 varieties of skin diseases can afflict us, causing untold human suffering (Lewin Group, 2004). With symptoms ranging from simple burning and itch to severe emotional and social effects—even physical disfigurement or death—the burden of skin disease extends into all aspects of our lives.

This chapter will focus on the anatomy and physiology of human skin with reference to its highly variable forms, especially between different body sites (intraindividual variations) and, where possible, between individuals of different race, gender, and age. The relationship of the skin's structure to its enormous multifunctionality will also be examined, including its association with the sense of touch.

OVERALL COMPOSITION OF HUMAN SKIN

Human skin represents a very heterogeneous covering for our bodies characterized by significant regional variations in structure, with resultant functional variations that can differ by several orders of magnitude (e.g., permeability). Adult human skin has a surface area of approximately 2 m^2 in area, is around 2.5 mm thick on average, and has an average density of 1.1 kg/m^3. The skin organ at 5–6 kg constitutes an impressive 6% of our total body weight. Excluding the muscle, bone, adipose, and blood systems, the skin exceeds all other organs in total mass (Goldsmith, 1990). As with all terrestrial mammals, the skin provides a vast physical barrier at the interface with the external environment and is designed to protect us against a range of insults, including desiccant (temperature, fluid, and electrolyte balance), mechanical, chemical, and microbial insults. Further protection is provided by the UVR-absorbing pigmentation system and the complex immunoregulatory sentinel networks, which sense tissue microenvironments for foreign or abnormally expressed components. One of the most apparent differences between humans and other mammals is the lack of a thick coat of hair—hence our moniker "naked ape." Likely related to this significant difference is the much greater permeability of the stratum corneum (S. corneum; upper epidermis layer) of furry mammals like rodents and lagomorphs (e.g., rabbits) than of human skin. Similarly, the sensation of touch will be very different on nonhairy (glabrous) versus "hairy" (nonglabrous) human skin. In general, glabrous skin is thicker and less permeable than "hairy" skin and is restricted to palms of the hands, soles of the feet, lips, labia minora, and part of penis—sites where features reflect functional adaptation.

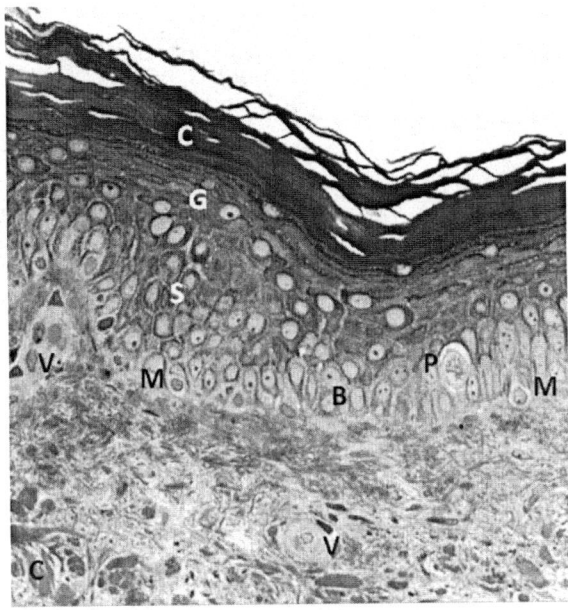

FIGURE 1.1 High-resolution light microscopy view of normal adult human skin (male, 62 years) showing epidermis (upper) and dermis (lower). S. corneum (C); S. granulosum (G); S. spinosum (S); S. basale (B); blood vessel (V); proliferating keratinocyte (P); melanocyte (M); collagen (C).

As shown in Figure 1.1, the skin consists of two broad tissue types, the epidermis (an external stratified, nonvascularized, epithelium) and the dermis (an underlying connective tissue consisting of fibroblasts). These fibroblasts produce dense, fibrous/elastic components called extracellular matrix (ECM). The dermis houses many of the skin's "business centers," including its vascular, neural, and lymphatic systems and its multiple accessory appendages. These include its excretory and secretory glands (sebaceous, eccrine, and apocrine glands), keratinizing structures (hair follicles and nails), sensory nerve receptors (Meissner's and Pacinian corpuscles that are important for sensing touch and pressure), mechanoreceptors (Pilo-Ruffini corpuscles), free terminals, and hair follicle endings. There is considerable variation in the presence and density of skin appendages and in epidermis and dermis thickness between different body sites (see Table 1.1). The epidermis comprises about 5% of the combined thickness of the epidermis and dermis except in those areas exposed to significant physical stress (palms and soles) where the epidermis may be as much as 60% of the total thickness of the epidermis and dermis. In addition, anatomists include a third skin layer, the subcutis or hypodermis, consisting of fatty connective tissue that connects the dermis to underlying skeletal components. Interested readers keen on learning more about the cell biology and physiology of skin can consult specialized texts (e.g., Freinkel & Woodley, 2001).

TABLE 1.1 Characteristics of Human Skin

Body Site	Thickness (μm)		Appendages (cm⁻²)		Temperature (°C)	Surface Lipid (μg/cm⁻²)
	Epidermis	Dermis	Sweat Glands	Hair Follicles		
Face	52	2,271		700		12
Cheek			320	880		
Forehead	82	1,500	350	750	34	24
Scalp				200–350		
Palm	575	1,100	400	0		
Fingers	547	1,207	0–50	Site specific		
Forearm	53	1,118	220	100	32	6
Axilla	44	1,186		65		
Thorax	51	1,676		75	33	10
Abdomen	42	2,163	210	70	33	
Thigh	61	1,298	125	55	31	5
Back	71	2,326		65		7
Pubis	45	1,014				
Sole	1,159	1,534				

Table contains data reprinted with permission from "The regional frequency and distribution of hair follicles in human skin", by G. Szabo, in *The Biology of Hair Growth* (pp. 33–38) by W. Montagna and R. A. Ellis (Eds.), 1958, New York: Academic Press. Copyright by Academic Press. Table contains data reprinted with permission from "Cutaneous anatomy and function," by R. P. Chilcott, in *Principles and Practice of Skin Toxicology* (pp. 4–16) by R. P. Chilcott and S. Price (Eds.), 2008, West Sussex, England. Copyright by John Wiley & Sons, Inc.

EPIDERMIS

Our skin is present to some extent from the beginning or very soon after conception. A distinct epidermis (ectoderm) and dermis (mesoderm) can be recognized as early as the first 1–2 weeks of estimated gestational age of human life. From a period of cellular reorganization called gastrulation (at the end of Week 1 postimplantation), the main germ layers (ectoderm, endoderm, and mesoderm) emerge. Of these, the (neuro)ectoderm goes on to yield both the epithelium (epidermis and epithelium of the cornea, nose, vagina, and part of the mouth) and the neuroderm, which contributes cells of the central nervous system and neural crest. It is noteworthy that our brain and skin form as part of the same primitive ectoderm that separates only during neurogenesis. Interestingly, the skin becomes populated with neuroectodermal cells again, not least in the form of the neural crest-derived melanocyte (pigment cells). This first epidermal layer, the single-layered periderm, is a transient self-proliferative layer restricted to fetal life. It consists of cells rich in apical surface microvilli (hair-like projections) and glycogen (starch) and is coated with mucopolysaccharides. This periderm ultrastructure, together with their numerous intercellular junctions, suggests it is important in the exchange of substances between mother and developing child (our first "touch") as well as in forming a protective layer.

The epidermis is a continually keratinizing or cornifying (hardening) stratified epithelium that terminates at mucocutaneous junctions (e.g., in the mouth). This surface is interrupted by the pores of glands and hair follicles. The outer layer consists of four major "strata" composed principally of keratin-producing cells called keratinocytes. The outermost S. corneum is a cornified layer of 15–30 sheets of nonviable, but biochemically active cells called corneocytes (see Figure 1.2). The next inner layer is the S. granulosum, a 3–5 sheet granular layer of nondividing keratinocytes producing granules of a protein called keratohyalin. These cells flatten as dividing cells below progressively push them to the skin surface.

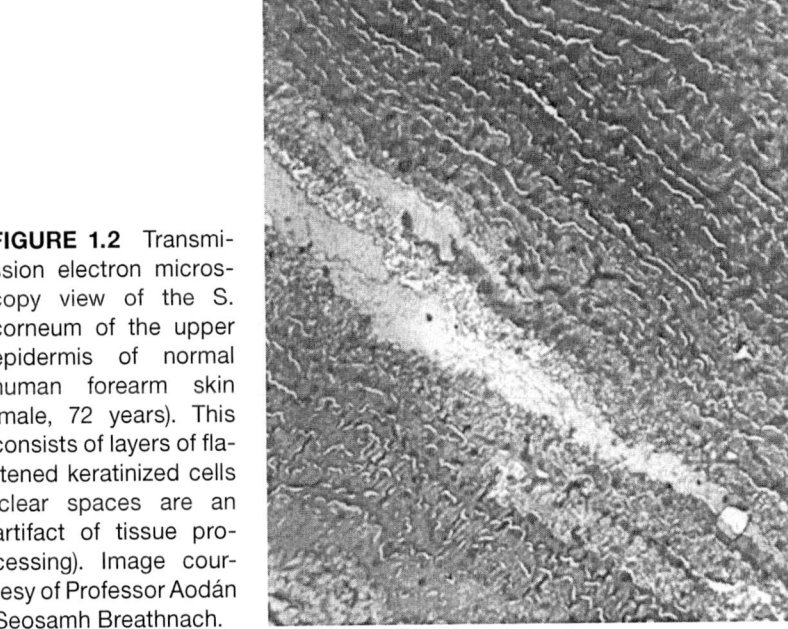

FIGURE 1.2 Transmission electron microscopy view of the S. corneum of the upper epidermis of normal human forearm skin (male, 72 years). This consists of layers of flattened keratinized cells (clear spaces are an artifact of tissue processing). Image courtesy of Professor Aodán Seosamh Breathnach.

At the same time, their cell organelles and nuclei break down, and their cell membranes become increasingly impermeable. This layer is followed by the S. spinosum, containing 8–10 sheets of keratinocytes with some limited capacity for cell division. Also found here are bone marrow-derived sentinel cells of the immune system called Langerhans cells, which scour the skin for evidence of breach by foreign entities. The basal or dividing layer of the epidermis is called the S. basale or S. germinativum. These cells are attached to a noncellular basement membrane that separates the epidermis from dermis below.

The transition from intrauterine to extrauterine life is not immediate as far as skin function is concerned. While a newborn baby's skin already has a 10-µm-thick S. corneum (with > 15 layers of corneocytes), full barrier function is achieved only after approximately 3 weeks of age. In addition to differentiating (i.e., maturing) keratinocytes, the S. basale also houses other keratinocytes with stem cell–like properties, the enigmatic Merkel cell (with sensory functions) and melanocytes. The latter are important pigment (melanin)–producing cells that help protect us against the damaging effects of UVR (Plonka et al., 2009). All epidermal cells (keratinocytes, melanocytes, Langerhans cells, and Merkel cells) express sensor proteins (e.g., transient receptor potential family of peptides) and neuropeptides and so participate in the skin's sensory system.

Merkel Cells

The Merkel Cell is probably the skin's most enigmatic cell type. It is a large, pale-staining cell located in the basal layer of mammalian epidermis, where it functions as a slow-adapting mechanoreceptor via synapse-like contacts with enlarged terminal endings of myelinated nerve fibers. Their function is more obvious in some mammals, where they cluster around whisker follicles. In humans, they are found in highest density in eccrine glandular ridges of glabrous (nonhairy) skin, within belt-like clusters of hair follicles and recently also in so-called touch-domes (described in the later section on hair follicles). Recent data indicate that these skin cells are derived from the neural crest in birds but from epidermal progenitors in mammals (Morrison et al., 2009). Other characteristic features of Merkel cells include the presence of numerous dense core, cytoplasmic granules containing neuropeptides, some of which are likely to act as neurotransmitters.

Epidermal Keratins

The strength of the skin is derived in large part from the production by keratinocytes of intermediate filaments called cytokeratin (8–15 nm) that contribute to the cells' cytoskeleton (Lane & McLean, 2004).The different layers of the epidermis contain varying amounts of keratin, ranging from approximately 30% in the S. basale to 80% in the S. corneum. High-resolution transmission electron microscopy has revealed how these filaments are organized into 3D arrays within the cell as tonofilament bundles and also between neighboring cells via docking at dynamic intercellular "spot-welds" called desmosomes (Figure 1.3).

Epidermal Cell Differentiation and Turnover

Basal keratinocytes are transformed to corneocytes in approximately 25 days, though this rate can vary by body site: 30 days on palms but

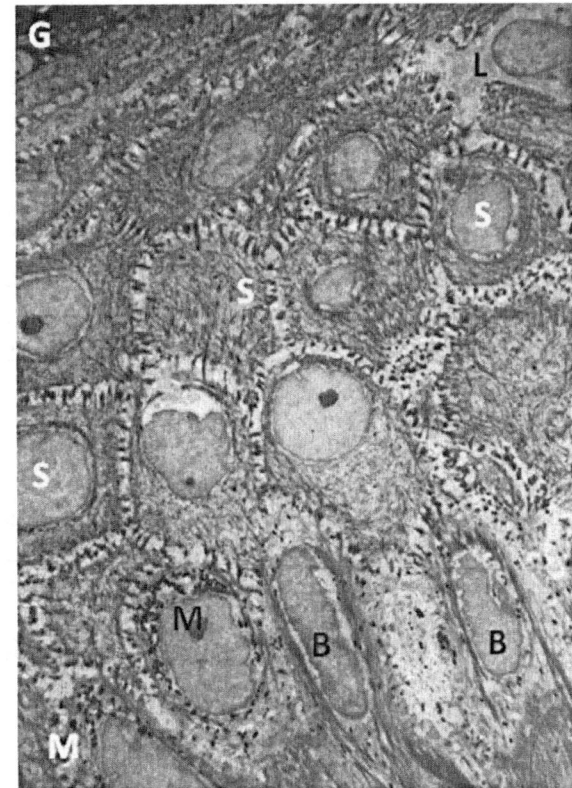

FIGURE 1.3 Transmission electron microscopy view of the epidermis of normal human forearm skin (male, 40 years) showing keratinocytes of the S. granulosum (G) and S. spinosum (S) with Langerhans cells (L) interspersed. Keratinocytes of the S. basale (B) are also shown, some of which contain melanin granules (M) transferred from melanocytes. Note melanin clustering over and around keratinocytes nuclei (M). Image courtesy of Professor Aodán Seosamh Breathnach.

only 10 days on scalp and 15 days on the back. Only recently has the mechanism emerged of how an epidermal basal cell transits through a relatively immature (i.e., undifferentiated) but proliferative S. basale cell on its way to becoming a nonviable, but metabolically active, corneocyte (Tu et al., 2004). It appears that each layer of the epidermis expresses, in a time-resolved manner, specific gene products (proteins) necessary to take the keratinocyte to the next stage. However, this is not the only fate for our epidermal keratinocytes. One would have perhaps expected that a damaged keratinocyte (e.g., after high sun-exposure) would eventually be removed by normal desquamation. However, this is not fail safe, so some keratinocytes undergo programmed cell death (apoptosis). To avoid this, the skin tries to protect keratinocytes by increasing melanin production and then concentrating transferred melanin over the vulnerable keratinocyte nucleus (see Figure 1.3).

One of the great recent advances in cutaneous science has been the identification of keratinocyte stem cells. It now appears that pluripotent stem cells (cells that are so immature that they have the potential to give rise to keratinocytes of the hair follicle, sebaceous gland, and epidermis) reside principally in the hair follicle rather than in the epidermis (Bickenbach & Grinnell, 2004; Sarin et al., 2005; Watt & Jensen, 2009). Calcium appears to play an important role in determining the controls for moving epidermal cells from the stem compartment to the so-called transit-amplifying compartment. This pivotal role for calcium in epidermal differentiation is reflected by its fourfold increase in concentration from the basal layer to the S. corneum. In addition, keratinocyte differentiation can be modulated by hormones and vitamins, such as retinoic acid (vitamin A from diet), vitamin D_3, thyroid hormone, and steroid hormones. The skin has nuclear receptors for several steroid hormones—including glucocorticoids, estrogen, androgen, and progesterone—and can metabolize active sex steroids from adrenal C19 precursor steroid in the skin itself (Gingras et al., 2003).

A plethora of interacting signaling systems finely tune and regulate keratinocyte function, particularly their intercellular adhesion and the communication that results from such intimate cell–cell contacts. Calcium is again a key factor here, and it controls the expression of several keratinocyte intercellular connections, including desmosome, adherens, gap, and tight junctions. These junctions are more than "spot welds" or "belts" that hold cells in close apposition. They are also important conduits for intercellular communication, and the increase in calcium from basal to upper layers facilitates an increase in desmosome size and number. A myriad of other proteins emerge onto the scene as the keratinocyte embarks on its differentiation-led journey—the interested reader will find several excellent recent reviews on this topic (Liu et al., 2009; Proksch et al., 2006).

The Permeability Barrier

Every basal keratinocyte eventually matures and differentiates into a keratinized cell to contribute to a tough external skin surface layer. The S. corneum requires particular specializations to cope with the continual onslaught of external insults. For example, application of solvents to the skin will remove lipids from the S. corneum and increase transepidermal water loss. However, such disruption induces a rapid repair of the barrier via epidermal metabolic changes. Under normal conditions, barrier function is amply provided for by an S. corneum organized into "bricks-and-mortar" arrays (Elias & Menon, 1991). This process represents the terminal stage of epidermal keratinocyte differentiation and these cells are afforded extra protection via a highly cross-linked layer—the cornified envelope (CE). The flattened epidermis sheets (squames) are packed with keratin filaments embedded within a matrix of fillagrin and interconnected via junctions termed corneodesmosomes. Human S. corneum contains approximately 15–26 layers of corneocytes, although ethnic differences exist (Rawlings, 2006; Weigand, Haygood, & Gaylor, 1974). The lipid-rich CE that surrounds individual corneocytes is itself organized into lipid-rich lamellar bilayers derived from the lipolytic enzyme-mediated fusion of granules (lamellar bodies) secreted by the corneocytes. Although essentially impervious to aqueous solutions, aqueous pores interrupt the hydrophobic nature of the S. corneum's lipid-rich matrix and so represent potential routes of entry for therapeutics. Barrier function in human epidermis depends on transglutaminase-mediated cross-linking of structural proteins and lipids during the terminal stages of keratinocyte differentiation (Griffin, Casadio, & Bergamini, 2002). During this process, these so-called "biological glues" catalyze the posttranslational modification of proteins by forming isopeptide bonds.

The quality of the S. corneum barrier depends on the presence of equimolar amounts of ceramides, cholesterol, and free fatty acids. Changes to the concentrations of any of these can affect barrier quality. For instance, aged and photo-aged skin exhibits a cholesterol-dominant barrier, while atopic dermatitis is associated with ceramide dominance and a predominance of free fatty acids is associated with psoriasis (Chuong et al., 2002). Endogenously produced fatty acids can be found in the lipid located between the layers of corneocytes in the S. corneum and in the so-called hydro lipid film at the skin surface. These biomolecules are crucial contributors to the structure–function relationship of the skin epidermis (Coderch, Lopez, de la Maza, & Parra, 2003), and perturbation in skin fatty acid status can cause disease. For example, atopic dermatitis is associated with abnormally reduced omega-6 fatty acid levels (and decreased ceramide content) and the hallmark of perturbed barrier function (i.e., increased water loss) from the skin surface. There is evidence that UVR increases lipid levels in the S. corneum, and this has been associated with improved barrier performance. Conversely, both photo-aged and chronologically aged epidermis exhibit abnormal barrier homeostasis and an overall reduction in S. corneum lipids, including cholesterol synthesis (Bouwstra, Thewalt, Gooris, & Kitson, 1997).

It appears that acid pH is required for maintenance of epidermal permeability barrier homeostasis, perhaps by providing optimal pH for the enzymes involved in extracellular processing of bilayer lipids. The precise origin of acidic pH in this system is still unclear, but may derive from exogenous sources, such as lactic acid in sweat, free fatty acids in sebum, and metabolites of skin microflora. "Friendly" skin microbes (e.g., micrococci) tend to like acidic pH while "enemy" microbes (e.g., staphylococci) prefer neutral or basic conditions.

Given its strategic location, the skin (and especially its epidermis) is constantly exposed to a battery of pharmaceutical and toxic agents via occupational, environmental, therapeutic, and systemic exposures. Adverse implications of these insults range from allergic contact dermatitis through hyperplasia (increased cellular proliferation) to skin cancer. Included here are xenobiotics (chemical substances foreign to the body, such as naturally occurring compounds, drugs, and environmental agents) that can be transported across the S. corneum in a rate-controlled manner on the basis of their physico-chemical traits (Du, Hoffman, & Keeney, 2004). Like the liver, human skin (especially its epidermis and sebaceous glands) expresses a wide variety of cytochrome P450 (CYP) enzymes, some specific to skin keratinocytes (Swanson, 2004). Dermatologic practice today has many drugs that are substrates, inducers, or inhibitors of the CYP enzyme family. Moreover, components in cosmetics, toiletries, and health care products commonly serve as substrates for CYP (Storm, Collier, Stewart, & Bronaugh, 1990), while retinoids used as potent therapeutic agents in skin disease are also metabolized in skin via a CYP-dependent hydroxylation (Swanson, 2004).

Epidermal thickness is the principal determinant of skin permeability variations by body site, though regional variation in lipid content and S. corneum morphology also contribute. Epidermal thickness as a function of skin permeability has been measured. For the nerve agent VX, scrotal skin is over 100-fold more permeable than ventral forearm skin, while cheek skin is 25-fold more permeable (Chilcott, 2008). Diffusion of penetrants can occur via the tortuous route between individual corneocytes (intercellular route), resulting in reduced absorption rates, or may be absorbed through individual cells (transcellular route), with faster rates of absorption. A third route is by diffusion down hair follicles and sweat ducts—the so-called "shunt pathways."

Skin Surface Morphology

This feature of skin varies by body site in association with variations in epidermal thickness, hair follicles (with associated sebaceous gland ducts) and eccrine sweat gland density, ridges/furrows/sulci (also known as dermatoglyphs), flexure lines, and Langer's lines. Indeed, these latter structures may contribute a capillary action for dispersal of surface oils, water, and other substances. The skin also sports an "acid mantle"—a thin film composed of body site-specific variable levels of sebum (triglycerides, wax esters, squalene), corneocytes debris, and sweat residues. Together, they give the skin surface an acid pH due to the presence of free fatty acids. Sebum may additionally contribute via its antimicrobial and waterproofing capabilities (Porter, 2001), or even as a vehicle for delivery via excretion of the powerful antioxidant vitamin E to the skin surface (Thiele, Weber, & Packer, 1999). Clearly, age-associated skin wrinkling also causes dramatic alterations in skin relief due to structural changes in the dermis. There is evidence that wrinkling, particularly in the periauricular area, can exhibit ethnic variation.

THE DERMIS

Immediately below the stratified epidermis is the shock absorbing dermis, which can be divided into an upper papillary and a lower reticular portion, reflecting their respective composition of connective tissue (mesenchymal) components, cell number, blood vessels, and nerves. Despite its greater volume, the dermis contains far fewer cells than the epidermis. Much of its bulk consists instead of fibrous and amorphous ECM interspersed between the skin's appendages, nerves, vessels, receptors, and dermal cells. Development of the ectodermally derived dermis during embryogenesis is complex (Haake, Scott, & Holbrook, 2001). While the neural crest ectoderm supplies the dermal cells for the skin on the face and anterior scalp, dermal mesenchyme of the back originates from the dermomyotome of the embryonic somite. These regional differences may impact on variable touch sensitivity in different body sites.

The predominant cell to develop from the superficial dermatome segments of the somite mesenchyme is the fibroblast. These cells are initially highly plastic, if not pluripotent, and likely give rise to several other cell types, including adipocytes. Many of these cells synthesize and secrete abundant ECM, rich in (muco)polysaccharides and components of collagens and elastin, though not fully assembled fibers. The adult dermal fibroblast is a heterogeneous migratory cell that makes and degrades ECM components. There is significant interest in factors that control dermal fibroblast differentiation (Chang et al., 2002), particularly in the context of their increased synthetic and proliferative activity during wound healing. The dermis is also home to several cell types, including multifunctional immune system cells like macrophages and mast cells. The latter can trigger allergic reactions by secreting bioactive mediators such as histamine.

Much of dermis functionality is mediated via its ECM—a highly complex mixture of bioactive macromolecules produced by dermal cells and then either secreted intact or alternatively assembled later outside the cells. This noncollagen, nonelastin dermal material lies outside the cells is amorphous and hydroscopic, but biologically very active, and is highly diverse and highly organized. It consists of proteoglycans, glycoproteins, water, and hyaluronic acid. While on one level the ECM can be seen as complex webs of suprastructure providing a scaffold for dermal activity, the bioactivity of these macromolecules provides for exquisite regulation of numerous cellular functions. While collagens are the principal ECM component, other members include elastin, fibrillins, LTBPs, fibulins, laminins, proteoglycans, integrins, and associated enzymes (Uitto, 1989). About 90% of total dermal protein consists of collagen and accounts for about 75% of the skin's total dry weight. While at least 25 collagens exist, half are present in skin consisting predominantly of collagen type I (85–90%), III (8–11%), and V (2–4%) (Brucker-Tuderman, 2003). The relative contribution of different collagens varies under different circumstances—for example, collagen III increases during wound healing. Collagens are critical for epidermis adherence to the dermis. Collagen VII forms part of the so-called "anchoring fibrils" that attach the basement membrane to the ECM of the upper dermis, while collagen XVII contributes to the so-called "anchoring filaments" that link the basal keratinocytes with the basement membrane.

CHAPTER 1   ANATOMY AND PHYSIOLOGY OF THE SKIN   **15**

Elasticity of Skin

The biomechanical properties of the skin contribute much to the sensation of touch. As skin exhibits both viscous and elastic properties, several parameters can be measured, including extensibility, viscoelastic deformation, and capacity for immediate recovery in response to deformations. Components contributing to these biomechanical properties of skin include collagen, elastin, and the ECM. Elastin provides the skin with its elasticity. These fibers are stretchable by more than their full resting length. Recent biochemical analysis has clarified the composition of three different classes of elastin fiber (Ramirez, 2000). The elasticity of the fiber derives from the amorphous portion, which contains the highly cross-linked protein called elastin.

The dermis changes significantly during our lives. In the neonate, the dermis is still transitional between the fetal and adult forms. For example, the high fetal-associated levels of soluble collagen (approximate 25%) do not reduce to the typical adult levels (1%) until 6 months after birth and are approximately 60% of their adult thickness. In this context, the dermis is slower to develop fully than the epidermis. These changes with maturity have implications for elasticity. There is a global decrease in skin elasticity as a function of aging (Couturaud, Coutable, & Khaiat, 2006), in part due to the steady decline in skin epidermal cell proliferation rates with age (especially in sun-exposed areas) (Stamatas et al., 2006). While extensibility is lowered in sun-exposed skin (more marked for Caucasian than African skin types), variations in viscoelastic responses do not differ significantly between sun-exposed and protected body sites. It should be noted the variation in skin thickness will impact on these measurements, though the content of elastic fibers per unit area is greater in black than in white skin (cf. Couturaud, 2009; Rawlings, 2006). In a similar way, the value of Young's modulus (the ratio of stress to strain, a measure of stiffness) is higher on forehead skin than on forearm. Data suggest little difference between sexes for the above parameters.

Vascularization

Development of a vascularized dermis is a crucial part of skin development and subsequent function in the adult. Vessels are formed initially as capillaries via vasculogenesis from precursors (angioblasts), and then from these preexisting vessels by angiogenesis. The regulatory control of the vasculature is complex and involves many regulatory molecules, such as vascular endothelial growth factor (Ribatti, Nico, & Crivellato, 2009). See Ryan (1976) for more details.

Innervation

The skin of mammals is highly innervated, mostly with sensory nerve fibers. This innervation develops segmentally (i.e., from dermatomes) out of the cutaneous branches of spinal nerves. Cutaneous nerves can be detected as early as 15 weeks EGA in humans, where they extend from the subcutaneous trunk and branch to form the subepidermal nerve plexus. Innervation of skin will also follow the development of its appendages, such as hair follicles and sweat glands, which are particularly highly innervated. Three tiers of nerve fiber bundles carry autonomic and peptidergic nerve fibers to their cutaneous targets. The epidermis, dermal blood vessels, glands (excluding hair follicles), and smooth muscles receive rather simple innervation consisting of individual nerve fibers that terminate on, or intermingle with, their target cell populations. Their functions include sensory perception, blood flow regulation, glandular secretion, and smooth muscle contraction. Occasional single nerve fibers terminate freely in the dermis or subcutis. It is conceivable that these fibers contact individual mesenchymal and especially immune cells there, since nearly every skin cell population, including fibroblasts and mast cells, have been shown to entertain such contacts (Peters et al., 2006).

Whereas the epidermal Merkel cell–axon complex functions as a slow-adapting mechanoreceptor with enlarged terminal endings of myelinated nerve fibers, the large onion-like Pacinian corpuscle (up to 4 mm in length) has a centrally located, single, unmyelinated axon located in the dermis and subcutis and functions as a rapidly adapting mechanoreceptor. These are most commonly found on the palms of the hands and soles of the feet, as well as less commonly on the nipples and genital skin. The Pacinian corpuscle remains the only skin receptor for which we have strong evidence of mechanical perceptions and transmission (Loewenstein & Skalak, 1966).

Another prominent neural end organ located in the skin's dermis is the Meissner corpuscle. This elongated structure is oriented perpendicular to the skin surface at the junction of the epidermis and dermis between the rete ridges of the epidermis. As with Pacinian receptors, the Meissner corpuscles are also concentrated in hairless skin of the extremities, especially the fingertips, and are thought to be responsible in part for the high degree of tactile precision in these skin areas. This structure consists of expanded nerve terminals surrounded by laminar cells (i.e., modified Schwann cells) with flattened processes (Figure 1.4).

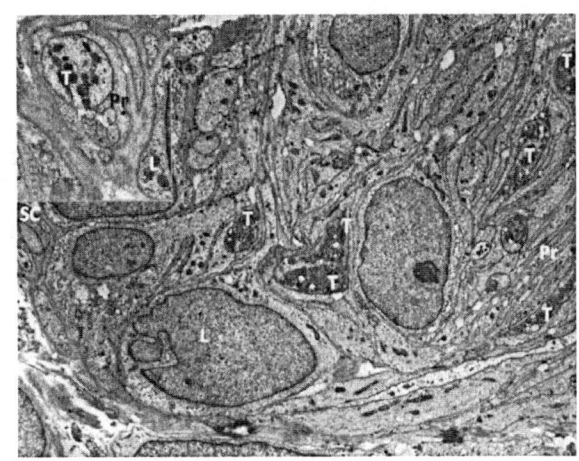

FIGURE 1.4 Meissner corpuscle of normal human digital skin (female, 8 years) located in the upper dermis close to the epidermis. This structure consists of expanded nerve terminal (T) surrounded by laminar cells (L) which are modified Schwann cells with flattened processes. Inset on upper left: Axonal terminal (T) just after entering a Meissner corpuscle. Image courtesy of Professor Aodán Seosamh Breathnach.

The nerves that supply this corpuscle are branches of thick myelinated axons, but this myelin sheath is lost close to entering the structure and becomes invested by the laminar cells. However, these structures are lacking in skin of the lips and tongue, both of which still exhibit very sensitive two-point discrimination.

Thus, in human skin, mechanoreceptors can be defined as slow adapting (e.g., the Merkel cell–axon complex and Ruffini corpuscles) or rapid adapting (e.g., Meissner and Pacinian corpuscles). The former continues to respond for some time during stimulation (i.e., to changing and static conditions) and can be categorized as either type 1 or type 2 slow-adapting mechanoreceptors. Type 1 (e.g., Merkel cell–axon complexes) discharge impulses irregularly over several minutes and are insensitive to lateral stretch, while type 2 (e.g., Ruffini corpuscles) exhibit a steady state of continuous impulses and are sensitive to lateral stretch. By contrast, rapid-adapting mechanoreceptors (e.g., Meissner and Pacinian corpuscles) discharge action potentials when the skin is indented in order to rapidly adapt to static conditions and respond to stimuli that deform the skin.

Cutaneous Neuroendocrinology

There has been much excitement recently about the discovery of the skin's capacity to act as a neuroendocrine organ in the periphery, and to do so in a manner largely independent of the body's traditional and central stress system (Chuong et al., 2002; Slominski, 2005). The cutaneous neuroendocrine system provides an overarching capacity for stress sensing. Particular importance lies in its having an equivalent of the central hypothalamic–pituitary–adrenal axis. While the structure of this stress system in skin may not be similarly organized, it is still organized with functionalities residing in the same tissue and sometimes even within the same cell type. Its principal constituent activities include the production of a number of important hormones and neurotransmitters. It produces corticotrophin-releasing hormone (and downstream proopiomelanocortin peptides, including endorphins; Bigliardi, Tobin, Gaveriaux-Ruff, & Bigliardi-Qi, 2009), steroids (e.g., androgens, estrogens), secosteroids (e.g., UVB-induced splitting of 7-dehydrocholesterol to produce vitamin D_3), serotonin (proinflammatory, pro-edema, vasodilatory, pro-pruritogenic), and melatonin (hair growth and pigmentation). A hypothalamic–pituitary–thyroid equivalent also appears to be expressed in skin (Gáspár et al., 2009; Slominski, Wortsman, Tuckey, & Paus, 2007). Much of these functionalities come from the skin appendages.

SKIN APPENDAGES

As befits its crucial role in body homeostasis, the skin is well-equipped with secretory (the release of chemicals for physiologic function) and excretory (the elimination of waste products) capabilities. These are conducted by sweat glands, sebaceous glands, ceruminous glands in the external ear canal, and mammary glands in the breast. Other skin appendages include nail and tooth. The development of skin appendages in utero follows the initial developmental processes that generate the epidermis and dermis, in that appendages are composed of epithelial and mesenchymal components. While the molecular regulation of appendage morphogenesis is hugely complex, to set the scene at its simplest, the dermal tissue establishes the growth of the particular appendage and the epithelial component generates the appendage's differentiated product (e.g., hair fiber, nail, feather, sweat, or milk). The genetic events that drive the early stages of appendage development, regardless of its final form, are actually very similar and are not only highly conserved across species but also across the different appendages themselves within the same species (Pispa & Thesleff, 2003).

Eccrine Sweat Glands

Humans are warm-blooded animals (homeotherms) and sport 3–4 million eccrine glands in their skin (see Figure 1.5), each producing a watery perspiration that serves principally to cool us and maintain our core temperature (at 37.5°C). At maximal output, the eccrine glands of an adult human can excrete up to 4.2 liters per hour in hot and humid locations. This equates to a heat loss of more than 25 kcal/minute, making humans the best sweaters in the animal kingdom. Larger and most densely packed on the palms and soles (see Table 1.1), eccrine glands have long thin ducts opening directly onto the skin surface and a proximal secretory coiled section consisting of

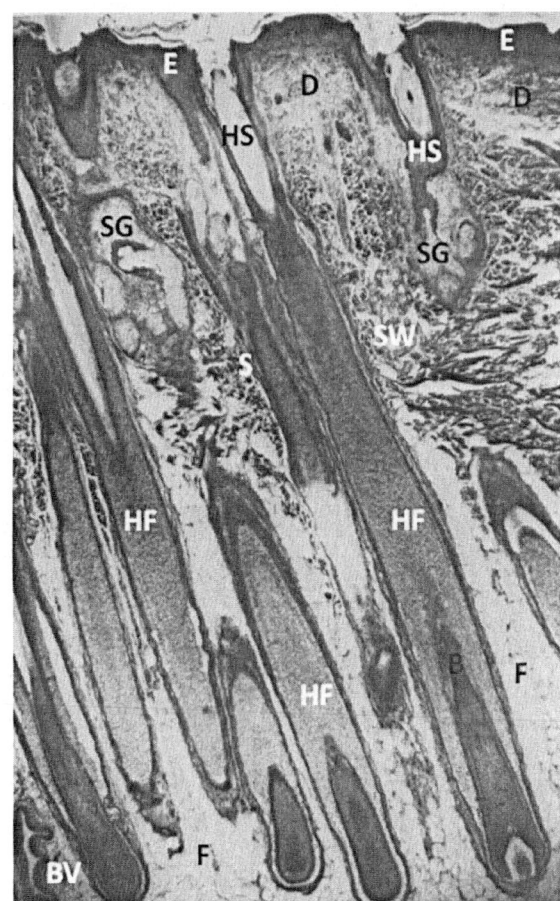

FIGURE 1.5 Longitudinal section of normal human scalp showing epidermis (E), dermis (D), subcutaneous fat layer (F), and skin appendages including hair follicle (HF) with hair shaft (HS), sebaceous gland (SG), eccrine sweat gland (SW), and blood vessel (BV).

secretory cells and contractile myoepthelial cells (Saga, 2002). Eccrine gland activity is regulated via neural stimulation using sympathetic nerve fibers distributed around the gland. These use the neurotransmitter acetylcholine and not the more usual adrenaline. Control of these nerves resides in so-called "sweat centers" in the hypothalamus of the brain. Sweating rate is directly proportional to skin temperature and is markedly reduced at temperatures below 30°C. While sweating can be induced by direct heating alone (39–46°C), generally physiologic sweating is due to a nervous reflex that can be emotional, thermoregulatory, or gustatory.

Sweat is a clear, odor-free, colorless, slightly acidic fluid that is almost fully water (99.0–99.5%), with the remainder consisting of the electrolytes NaCl, K^+ and HCO_3^-, and some inorganic compounds (such as lactate, urea, ammonia, calcium, heavy metals). Recently, the full functional power of sweat became more apparent with the detection of anti-malarial peptides, proteolytic enzymes, cytokines, and even antibody (immunoglobulin A). Importantly, there are significant regional variations in the composition of sweat. The composition of sweat from eccrine glands can be modulated by psycho-emotional and environmental factors such as being touched or one's perception of the touch received.

Apocrine Sweat/Scent Glands

Much less is known about the larger apocrine glands. In lower mammals, these glands secrete pheromones/hormones that trigger sexual and territorial responses but are not thought to play a significant role in humans. They are prominent only after puberty and then only in the groin, anal region, axilla, areola of the breast, and beard. Furthermore, there may be ethnic variations in their presence. For example, they are reported to be reduced in the axillae of Koreans and Japanese (Jun-Yul & Inn-Ki, 1982). Unlike eccrine glands, apocrine ducts exit to the surface indirectly via the hair follicle. However, like eccrine glands, they secrete their sterile, odor-free, weakly acidic product via extrusion from secretory cells. Apocrine gland sweat is thicker, more viscous than eccrine gland sweat and has a milky consistency due to its higher content of fatty acids. Some of these are odoriferous, especially so after decomposition on the skin surface by bacteria. Apocrine glands do not respond to heat, although psycho-emotional stimuli are implicated in stimulating secretory activity.

Sebaceous Glands

The manner of secretion by these sebum-producing glands is unique whereby their product, sebum, is released via disintegration of the sebocytes themselves. Sebaceous gland development is tightly related to the differentiation of the epidermis and hair follicle. Indeed with the exception of so-called "free" sebaceous glands of mucosa (e.g., in the lips), they are always associated with hair follicles to form pilosebaceous units (see Figure 1.5). Sebaceous glands are not found on palms, soles, or dorsum of feet. The nature of sebum's function in humans, the "naked ape" with no fur to protect, remains perplexing especially as significant evolutionary pressure must have driven the remarkable variation in the composition of human sebum. The first time humans really take notice of these glands is during puberty, when they become associated with acne. Up to 800 sebaceous glands/cm^2 can be found on the face, less elsewhere. In addition to sebum production, recent evidence also suggests other important roles for these glands (Zouboulis, 2004), including regulation of steroidogenesis, local androgen synthesis, skin barrier function, interaction with neuropeptides, potential production of both anti- and proinflammatory compounds, and synthesis of antimicrobial lipids. Indeed, normal bacterial flora, fungi, *P. acnes,* and even a mite called *Demodex folliculorum* richly colonize sebaceous follicles.

Sebaceous glands are part of the skin neuroendocrine system, and both produce and release corticotrophin-releasing factor, among others, in response to stress. They also express 5α-reductase (especially in the face and scalp), and so can convert testosterone to the more potent 5α-dihydro testosterone. Sebum is a yellowish viscous fluid containing triglycerides, free sterols and sterol esters, squalenes, wax, and free fatty acids (in a uniquely human form). The composition of sebaceous gland lipids appears to be under both genetic and hormonal control, and while significant interindividual and interethnic differences in sebum production exist, a rate of 0.3 mg sebum/10 cm^3/hour is normal (Plewig & Kligman, 2000).

The Hair Follicle

Hair follicles (and breasts) distinguish us among mammals. The hair follicle is our body's only permanently regenerating organ, as it transits through lifelong periods of growth (anagen), regression (catagen), and relative quiescence (telogen). Approximately 4–5 million hair follicles reside in our skin (see Figure 1.5), though only a paltry 2% of these are on our scalps! The most alabaster-skinned have just as many of these mini-organs as the hairiest of us, with hair visibility depending on hair size and distribution rather than number. Hairs, even the finest, emerge from highly innervated hair follicles and so respond to deflection, creating the sensation of touch. A deflection of less than 1° can be appreciated from impulses of slow-adapting mechanoreceptors (Biemesderfer et al., 1978). During soft brush stroking low-threshold unmyelinated mechanoreceptors (C-tactile), but not myelinated afferents, respond most vigorously at brush velocities of 1–10 cm/s^{-1}. These velocities were perceived by subjects as being the most pleasant (Löken, Wessberg, Morrison, McGlone, & Olausson, 2009). While it is clear that hair serves a critical role in thermoregulation in furry animals, its role in humans appears to be nonessential. It is interesting to note that not every hair is similarly sensitive to touch. For instance, hairs on the wrist and knee can be bent fully without arousing any sensation. Differential sensitivity may be linked to the stage of the hair growth cycle.

The hair follicle encapsulates all the important physiologic processes found in the human body, namely controlled cell growth and death, interactions between cells of different histologic type, cell differentiation and migration, and hormone responsivity. An important consideration for those interested in the chemistry of skin is that hair fiber growth occurs in a highly time-resolved manner and so "locks in" a snapshot of the individual's physiology and biochemistry at the time of hair fiber formation. This hair follicle mini-organ deserves further admiration for its ability to intersect with the body's systemic regulatory networks. Remarkably, the hair follicle can respond to most hormones known to biomedicine. Even more surprising is the hair follicle's capacity to produce for itself a wide range of hormones, such as sex steroid hormones, proopiomelanocortin peptides, corticotrophin-releasing hormone, and prolactin. Further, neuropeptides, neurotransmitters, and neurohormones are implicated in mediating hair follicle events, particularly those related to stress. Crucially, hair follicles in different regions of the body (e.g., beard and balding scalp) respond differently to different androgens.

Another big surprise to cutaneous scientists was the hair follicle's unique immunological status. Unlike the rest of the skin, the lower portion of the growing hair follicle is immunosilent due to its lack of tissue histocompatibility antigen expression. The hair follicle may enjoy immune "privilege" to prevent the inappropriate recognition of proteins that may result in immune system attack (Christoph et al., 2000). While hair canals contain a resident microflora of bacteria, including *Propionibacterium acnes, Staphylococcus aureus, Staphylococcus epidermidis, Demodex follicularum,* and *Malassezia species,* the hair follicle appears to have a very effective anti-infection capacity, as evidenced by the rarity of folliculitis in human scalp despite its approximately 100,000 individual hair follicles.

The hair follicle has long been recognized as the most densely and complexly innervated skin appendage (Hendrix, Picker, Liezmann, & Peters, 2008; Tobin & Peters, 2009). Nerve fibers that terminate on the hair follicle form two quite complex and distinct neuronal networks. While the complexity and elaboration of follicular innervations increase with size and function of the specific hair follicle type, the basic structure is common to virtually all hair follicles and species studied so far—whether they are tiny and pigment-free vellus hair follicles or large beard or scalp follicles. See Figure 1.5 for an example of large (so-called terminal) scalp hair follicles. One hair follicle neural network is located around the hair follicle ostium (opening) and innervates the hair follicle epithelium adjacent to the epidermis. Fibers constituting this network are fine and unmyelinated, and contain a wide range of neuronal markers from neurotransmitters to neuropeptides and neurotrophins. They outnumber epidermal innervations, and the wide range of nerve fiber subsets that are present suggests that they may have functions beyond obvious afferent and efferent ones. The close association of these fibers with immune cells in the hair follicle epithelium, such as dendritic Langerhans cells, clearly marks the hair follicle ostium as a high impact neuro-immune interaction site. Deeper into the skin, the second hair follicle neural network organizes itself around the isthmus and bulge region of the hair follicle. This location harbors hair follicle stem cells responsible for hair cycling and hair pigmentation as well as wound healing.

Supplied by a nerve fiber bundle of the deep dermal plexus, the flattened longitudinal axons stretch upward in a palisade manner along the basement membrane, which segregates the hair follicle epithelium from the surrounding mesenchyme. In the narrow space provided by the hooding sebaceous gland, these fibers terminate in a widening that contains many neuromediator-filled vesicles. Here they are free of their supporting Schwann cell lamellae and are ready to shed their content when stimulated. Around them, c-fibers closely intermingle with stabilizing collagen fibrils that encircle the hair follicle and associated longitudinal collagen fibers. Together they form a basket-like structure known variably as lanceolate, palisade, or Ruffini nerve ending. The function of this neural network is only partially elucidated and comprises high threshold mechanical nociception detecting, such as velocity detection. Its density and complexity may house many more functions. The nerve fiber bundle which supplies nerve fibers to both the isthmus and bulge cells is commonly accompanied by numerous mast cells. These innate immune system mast cells rapidly respond to environmental triggers relayed via the isthmus and bulge region. In this way acute, nonspecific neuro-inflammatory responses to endogenous and exogenous environmental challenges, such as neurogenic inflammation, can rapidly reach this control centre of the hair follicle (Tobin & Peters, 2009). The Ruffini (or Pilo-Ruffini) corpuscle is a specialized cylindrical, encapsulated nerve ending encircling the hair follicles (Biemesderfer et al., 1978). This type of slow-adapting mechanoreceptor is distinct from others that encircle the hair follicle in that it has branched terminal nerve fibers enclosed within a unique connective tissue compartment.

The skin can be divided very broadly into (a) hairy skin (general body surface) with free terminals in the skin between hair follicles and terminals around hair follicles (that turn these into tactile hairs) and (b) nonhairy or glabrous skin of the palmar–plantar surfaces and mucous membranes where these free terminals are enhanced with more defined corpuscular endings. Merkel cell–axon complexes (nonencapsulated) can also be found in the hair follicle outer root sheath or close to the entry site of the sweat glands duct and epidermis in palmar–plantar skin. These complexes have been referred to as Merkel's "touch spots." Recently, a distinct microanatomical structure called the "touch dome" or Haarscheibe was reported in the dermis of human hairy skin (Reinisch & Tschachler, 2005). This slowly adapting type 1 mechanoreceptor, which is the counterpart of the Merkel cell–axon complex in digital skin, contains dermal nerve fibers within laminin-5 positive dermal protrusions. In addition to A-beta fibers, these structures have fibers of the A-delta- and C- type. The epidermis overlying the touch domes is enriched in Merkel cells, by comparison with the rest of the epidermis in the nonglabrous skin.

The Hair Fiber

Irrespective of their caliber (diameter), length, color, or stage of growth, all hairs are constructed of a bulk cortex surrounded by a protective covering of flattened cuticle cells (Robbins, 2002; Tobin, 2005). А third component, the medulla, is commonly located in the center of the fiber surrounded by the cortex, especially of large terminal hair fibers (see Figure 1.5). The hair fiber is a highly integrated system of several components, including (in order of decreasing amount) "hard" keratins, water, lipids, pigment, and trace elements. Lipids on the hair fiber surface, such as the cuticle, provide a hydrophobic interface that protects the hair cortex from a hostile wet or dry environment and may aid alteration of the frictional quality of the fiber. Despite significant variability in hair form between humans of different ethnicities, the chemical composition of hair protein and the amino acid composition of hair shafts are very uniform across the ethnic groups.

Human hair is commonly grouped into just three main subtypes: Caucasian, Mongoloid Asian, and African. Differences between these groups are usually determined with respect to a range of parameters, including hair fiber diameter and its cross-sectional form, overall fiber shape, mechanical properties, combability, chemical make-up, and moisture level (Robbins, 2002; Tobin, 2005). For many of these parameters, Caucasian hair falls intermediate to the contrasting Asian and African ends of the spectrum. Recently, a systematic examination of the protein structure of hairs from Asian, Caucasian, and African individuals revealed no differences by x-ray analysis in the structure of the hair keratin. Asian and Caucasian hair fibers are more cylindric than those of Africans, and it has been shown that "breaking stress" and "breaking extension" values are lower in African hair fibers than in Caucasians or Asians. Despite these ethnic differences in the form of hair fibers, the chemistry of the hair keratin is remarkably similar throughout the human family. The compositional or structural features of hair fiber protein in these ethnicities thus do not provide immediate explanations for their behavioral differences (e.g., degree of curl or crimp).

The Nail

The nail is the least studied of the skin appendages. Apparently derived from the earlier claw, this hard, keratinized, appendage protects the distal end of the fingers and toes. When we speak of the nail, we are commonly referring just to the nail plate that overlays the highly vascularized nail bed and so appears pinkish. The cells that make up the nail plate are similar to those generating the corneocytes of the upper epidermis and the trichocytes that make up hair. So-called onychocytes in the nail are also filled with keratin. Up to 90% of nail keratins are of the hard "hair" keratin type; the remainder are soft "epidermal" keratins. Also present in nail are water, lipids, and trace elements, such as iron, zinc, and calcium. Overall, the nail contains much less lipid and water than the epidermis and becomes brittle at less than 7% water and soft at more than 30%. The nail's low lipid content contributes to its significantly greater water permeability than the epidermis. Clearly nails have an impact on the sense of touch from finger tips, especially when long, but also, in a qualitatively different way, when kept very short or even onychophagic.

SKIN PIGMENTATION

Of all our phenotypic traits, skin and hair color communicate more identity information to the observer than any other. Humans display a rich and varied palette of surface color that highlights striking, but superficial, variations between human subgroups. Skin color has traditionally (though rather crudely) been defined by the Fitzpatrick classification I–VI, based on susceptibility to burn rather than tan. While skin color and ethnicity are associated, ethnicity alone may not predict susceptibility to UV-related skin damage. Skin color depends principally on relative amounts of eumelanin (brown/black) and pheomelanin (red/yellow), and less on hemoglobin and carotenoids.

Meanwhile, the colors of our scalp hair can range from vivid red and sun-bleached blonde to sober brown, raven black, and with age, to steel gray and snow white. Despite such variation, all skin and hair color is derived from the pigment melanin, synthesized via melanogenesis—a phylogenetically ancient biochemical process (Slominski, Tobin, Shibahara, & Wortsman, 2004). Synthesis occurs within melanosomes—specialized organelles unique to highly dendritic, neural crest-derived cells called melanocytes. While follicular melanocytes are derived from epidermal melanocytes during hair follicle development, these subpopulations diverge in important ways. For example, melanin degrades almost completely in the mid to upper epidermis, whereas melanin granules (especially eumelanin) in hair remain minimally digested when transferred into hair cortical keratinocytes. Moreover, while hair bulb melanocytes are active only during the growth phase of the hair cycle, epidermal melanogenesis is continuous.

Pigment production in melanocytes of the skin and hair follicles is affected by numerous extrinsic and intrinsic factors, including body distribution, ethnicity and gender differences, variable hormone-responsiveness, genetic defects, hair-cycle dependent changes, age, UVR, climate and season, toxins, pollutants, chemical exposure, and infestations. In contrast to its direct regulatory role in epidermal pigmentation, UVR does not penetrate to the anagen hair bulb because of its depth in skin. The process of melanogenesis can be divided into

(a) the formation of the melanosome in which melanogenesis occurs and (b) the biochemical pathway that converts L-tyrosine into melanin. Unlike brown/black melanins, the red/yellow pheomelanins are photolabile. Interested readers are encouraged to read recent reviews on the topic (e.g., Slominski et al., 2004).

THE SKIN IMMUNE SYSTEM

It is appropriate that immune function should be strongly represented in the organ that is most directly responsible for separating physically the self from the non-self. However, the skin not only provides immune protection for itself but also helps protect the whole body. Greater stimulation of the immune system is likely to occur at this biological interface with the external environment than any other area of the body. This is particularly important during close human contact, where the risks of potential spread of infection are greater. Biological aggressors like bacteria, viruses, mold, yeast, fungi, and chemical insults that threaten our health can gain entry to our bodies via the skin and its numerous ports of entry (e.g., hair follicle canals or sweat gland pores). However, unless the skin itself is damaged or the host is compromised (e.g., immunosuppressed), most of these threats are repelled by our skin (Bos, 2004). The makeup of the SIS can be most simply described by its components, such as cellular and humoral components, or by when the immunity is acquired—that is, whether the immunity is innate (preexisting) or adaptive (subsequent to prior exposure to an immune response generating stimulus). In the last few years it has become clear that practically all cell types residing in and transiting through skin can exhibit immune functionality. The better characterized cellular components include keratinocytes, lymphocytes (various subpopulations in skin), Langerhans cells (and other skin dendritic cells), monocytes and macrophages, endothelial cells of blood and lymphatic vessels, mast cells (mediators of both immune and neuroendocrine responses), neutrophils, eosinophils, and basophils. Innate components include free radicals, antimicrobial peptides including defensins and cathelicidins, cytokines, chemokines, neuropeptides, adhesion molecules, and a wide range of pro- and anti-inflammatory mediators. Immunoglobulins (antibodies) are additional potent proteins secreted from B-lymphocytes that can neutralize threats to the body.

Given the surface location of skin, it is not surprising that the physiology and pathology of skin can be affected by ultraviolet sunlight. There is a general immunosuppressive effect of sunlight, with associated alteration of Langerhans cell function. Our increasing longevity will require us to depend even more on the skin immunosurveillance function to prevent and limit threats such as tumor growth.

IMPLICATIONS FOR PERCEPTION OF TOUCH

Touch, the fifth human sense, is located in our body's largest organ (the skin)—an organ which serves myriad functions in addition to general sensation. While sensation may also emit from structures deeper than the skin (e.g., joints and viscera), the skin's highly complex anatomy transduces tactile information through a multiplicity of open compartments, appendages, and receptors. Through its many mechanisms, the skin is capable of an extraordinarily broad range of sensory discrimination. Skin is involved in perception of temperature, pain, and itch, as well as so-called sensory blends such as wetness, pressure, vibration, tickle, and tingling. The skin's anatomy is critical for such perceptions. For example, the experience of pressure itself may not be perceptible without feeling deformation of the skin. Hair follicles (even the finest vellus hairs) also play a role in sensing tension from pull in or on the skin.

The importance of hair to touch cannot be overestimated. Many view haired skin as having only free nerve endings and innervated "collars" (rapidly adapting mechanoreceptors) around many hair follicles. The upper hair follicle in particular (close to emergence of the hair through the surface of the skin) is hugely invested with nerve fibers. However, as noted earlier, recent data suggest that haired skin also contains discrete touch-domes that are slowly adapting mechanoreceptors. Hairy skin is capable of perceiving all forms of sensation, despite having potentially fewer corpuscular receptors. But these latter receptor types may not be essential for the perception of sensation; instead, they may compensate for the absence of hairs on glabrous skin. This view may seem curious, given that glabrous skin also has free receptors that are quite identical to those in haired skin. The nature of the contribution to touch that is made by corpuscular receptors is difficult to determine because it would require isolating and stimulating the receptor, followed by gauging the resulting response in a conscious individual. It should also be noted that removal of hair follicles from skin only slightly raises the threshold for touch in nonglabrous skin. This finding suggests that hairs *per se* are not essential for the appreciation of touch or pressure and that free receptors are sufficient, as is found when eliciting the tickle response.

Finally, consider the fact that skin is not simply a group of anatomical components. The enormous morphological difference in skin across different regions of the body actually results in having many skins, even at a single age in our lives. These skins vary in the presence or absence of hair (of fine vellus or large terminal hair), sweat glands, sebaceous glands, and elastic fibers in the dermis. They also differ in hair density, whether hair follicles have associated arrector pili muscles, in levels of subcutaneous fat, in the prominence and density of sweat glands, in the density of elastic fibers in the dermis, and in the thickness of epidermis, among other features. All of these characteristics influence the sensation of touch across our bodies, even excluding the conscious implications of touch in any particular body site. In addition, this wonderful and complex tapestry that drapes our bodies provides for ongoing reassurance that we remain linked to the here-and-now.

REFERENCES

Bickenbach, J. R., & Grinnell, K. L. (2004). Epidermal stem cells: Interactions in developmental environments. *Differentiation, 72,* 371–380.

Biemesderfer, D., Munger, B. L., Binck, J., & Dubner, R. (1978). The pilo-Ruffini complex: A non-sinus hair and associated slowly-adapting mechanoreceptor in primate facial skin. *Brain Research, 142*(2), 197–222.

Bigliardi, P. L., Tobin, D. J., Gaveriaux-Ruff, C., & Bigliardi-Qi, M. (2009). Opioids and the skin—Where do we stand? *Experimental Dermatology, 18,* 424–430.

Bos, J. D. (2004). Skin immune system: Cutaneous immunology and clinical immunodermatology (3rd ed.). Boca Raton, FL: CRC Press.

Bouwstra, J. A., Thewalt, J., Gooris, G. S., & Kitson, N. (1997). A model membrane approach to the epidermal permeability barrier: An X-ray diffraction study. *Biochemistry, 36,* 7717–7725.

Brucker-Tuderman, L. (2003). Biology of the extracellular matrix. In J. L. Bolognia, J. L. Jorizzo, & R. P. Rapini (Eds.), *Dermatology* (pp. 1483–1495). Edinburgh, Scotland: Mosby.

Chang, H. Y., Chi, J. T., Dudoit, S., Bondre, C., van de Rijn, M., Botstein, D., & Brown, P. O. (2002). Diversity, topographic differentiation, and positional memory in human fibroblasts. *Proceedings of the National Academy of Sciences of the United States of America, 99,* 12877–12882.

Chilcott, R. P. (2008). Cutaneous anatomy and function. In R. P. Chilcott & S. Price (Eds.). *Principles and practice of skin toxicology* (pp. 4–16). Chichester, UK: John Wiley.

Christoph, T., Muller-Rover, S., Audring, H., Tobin, D. J., Hermes, B., Cotsarelis, G., ... Paus, R. (2000). The human hair follicle immune system: Cellular composition and immune privilege. *British Journal of Dermatology, 142,* 862–873.

Chuong, C. M., Nickoloff, B. J., Elias, P. M., Goldsmith, L. A., Macher, E., Maderson, P. A.,...Christophers, E. (2002). What is the "true" function of skin? *Experimental Dermatolology, 11,* 159–187.

Coderch, L., Lopez, O., de la Maza, A., & Parra, J. L. (2003). Ceramides and skin function. *American Journal of Clinical Dermatology, 4,* 107–129.

Couturaud, V. (2009). Biophysical characteristics of the skin in relation to race, sex, age, and site. In A. O. Barel, M. Paye, H. I. Maibach (Eds.), *Handbook of cosmetic sciences and technology* (pp. 5–24). New York: Informa Healthcare.

Couturaud, V., Coutable, J., & Khaiat, A. (2006). Skin biomechanical properties: In vivo evaluation of influence of age and body site by a non-invasive method. *Skin Research and Technology, 1,* 68–73.

Du, L., Hoffman, S. M., & Keeney, D. S. (2004). Epidermal CYP2 family cytochromes P450 during percutaneous penetration: Role of absorption rate and cutaneous enzyme activity. *Toxicology and Applied Pharmacology, 195,* 278–287.

Elias, P. M., & Menon, G. K. (1991). Structural and lipid biochemical correlates of the epidermal permeability barrier. *Advances in Lipid Research, 24,* 1–26.

Freinkel, R. K., & Woodley, D. T. (2001). *The biology of skin.* New York: Parthenon.

Gáspár, E., Hardenbicker, C., Bodó, E., Wenzel, B., Ramot, Y., Funk, W.,...Paus, R. (2009). Thyrotropin releasing hormone (TRH): A new player in human hair-growth control. *The FASEB Journal, 24,* 393–403.

Gingras, S., Turgeon, C., Brochu, N., Soucy, P., Labrie, F., & Simard, J. (2003). Characterization and modulation of sex steroid metabolizing activity in normal human keratinocytes in primary culture and HaCaT cells. *Journal of Steroid Biochemistry and Molecular Biology, 87,* 167–179.

Goldsmith, L. A. (1990). My organ is bigger than your organ. *Archives of Dermatology, 126,* 301–302.

Griffin, M., Casadio, R., & Bergamini, C. M. (2002). Transglutaminases: Nature's biological glues. *Biochemistry Journal, 368,* 377–396.

Haake, A., Scott, G. A., & Holbrook, K. A. (2001). Structure and function of the skin: Overview of the epidermis and dermis. In R. K. Freinkel & D. T. Woodley (Eds.), *The biology of skin* (pp. 19–45). New York: Parthenon.

Hendrix, S., Picker, B., Liezmann, C., & Peters, E. M. (2008). Skin and hair follicle innervation in experimental models: A guide for the exact and reproducible evaluation of neuronal plasticity. *Experimental Dermatology, 17,* 214–227.

Jun-Yul, C., & Inn-Ki, C. (1982). The distribution of the patterns of pubic hair and axillary hair. *Journal of Korean Dermatology, 20,* 231–237.

Lane, E. B., & McLean, W. H. (2004). Keratins and skin disorders. *The Journal of Pathology, 204,* 355–366.

Liu, B., Zhu, F., Xia, X., Park, E., & Hu, Y. (2009). A tale of terminal differentiation: IKK-alpha, the master keratinocyte regulator. *Cell Cycle, 8*(4), 527–531.

Lewin Group. (2004). *The burden of skin disease.* Retrieved from The Society for Investigative Dermatology Web site: http://www.sidnet.org/pdfs/Burden%20 of%20Skin%20Diseases%202004.pdf

Loewenstein, W. R., & Skalak, R. (1966). Mechanical transmission in a Pacinian corpuscle: An analysis and a theory. *Journal of Physiology, 182*(2), 346–378.

Löken, L. S., Wessberg, J., Morrison, I., McGlone, F., & Olausson, H. (2009). Coding of pleasant touch by unmyelinated afferents in humans. *Nature Neuroscience, 12,* 547–548.

Morrison, K. M., Miesegaes, G. R., Lumpkin, E. A., & Maricich, S. M. (2009). Mammalian Merkel cells are descended from the epidermal lineage. *Developmental Biology, 336*(1), 76–83.
Peters, E. M., Ericson, M. E., Hosoi, J., Seiffert, K., Hordinsky, M. K., Ansel, J. C.,…Scholzen, T. E. (2006). Neuropeptide control mechanisms in cutaneous biology: Physiological and clinical significance. *Journal of Investigative Dermatology, 26*(9), 1937–1947.
Pispa, J., & Thesleff, I. (2003). Mechanisms of ectodermal organogenesis. *Developmental Biology, 262*, 195–205.
Plewig, G., & Kligman, A. M. (2000). *Acne and rosacea* (3rd ed.). Berlin, Germany: Springer.
Plonka, P. M., Passeron, T., Brenner, M., Tobin, D. J., Shibahara, S., Thomas, A., …Schallreuter, K. U. (2009). What are melanocytes really doing all day long…? *Experimental Dermatology, 18*, 799–819.
Porter, A. M. (2001). Why do we have apocrine and sebaceous glands? *Journal of the Royal Society of Medicine, 94*(S), 236–237.
Proksch, E., Fölster-Holst, R., & Jensen, J. M. (2006). Skin barrier function, epidermal proliferation and differentiation in eczema. *Journal of Dermatological Sciences, 43*(3), 159–169.
Ramirez, F. (2000). Pathophysiology of the microfibril/elastic fiber system: Introduction. *Matrix Biology, 19*(6), 455–456.
Rawlings, A. V. (2006). Ethnic skin types: Are there differences in skin structure and function? *International Journal of Cosmetic Science, 28*, 79–93.
Reinisch, C. M., & Tschachler, E. (2005). The touch dome in human skin is supplied by different types of nerve fibers. *Annals of Neurology, 58*(1), 88–95.
Ribatti, D., Nico, B., & Crivellato, E. (2009). Morphological and molecular aspects of physiological vascular morphogenesis. *Angiogenesis, 12*, 101–111.
Robbins, C. R. (2002). *Chemical and physical behavior of human hair*. New York: Springer.
Ryan, T. J. (1976). The blood vessels of the skin. *Journal of Investigative Dermatology, 67*, 110–108.
Saga, K. (2002). Structure and function of human sweat glands studied with histochemistry and cytochemistry. *Progress in Histochemistry and Cytochemistry, 37*, 323–386.
Sarin, K. Y., Cheung, P., Gilison, D., Lee, E., Tennen, R.I., Wang, E.,…Artandi, S. E. (2005). Conditional telomerase induction causes proliferation of hair follicle stem cells. *Nature, 436*, 1048–1052.
Slominski, A. (2005). Neuroendocrine system of the skin. *Dermatology, 211*, 199–208.
Slominski, A., Tobin, D. J., Shibahara, S., & Wortsman, J. (2004). Melanin pigmentation in mammalian skin and its hormonal regulation. *Physiological Reviews, 84*, 1155–1228.
Slominski, A., Wortsman, J., Tuckey, R. C., & Paus, R. (2007). Differential expression of HPA axis homolog in the skin. *Molecular and Cellular Endocrinology, 265–266*, 143–149.
Stamatas, G. N., Estanislao, R. B., Suero, M., Rivera, Z. S., Li, J., Khaiat, A., & Kollias, N. (2006). Facial skin fluorescence as a marker of the skin's response to chronic environmental insults and its dependence on age. *British Journal of Dermatology, 154*, 125–132.

Storm, J. E., Collier, S. W., Stewart, R. F., & Bronaugh, R. L. (1990). Metabolism of xenobiotics. *Fundamentals of Applied Toxicology, 15,* 132–141.

Swanson, H. I. (2004). Cytochrome P450 expression in human keratinocytes: An arylhydrocarbon receptor perspective. *Chemico-Biological Interactions, 149,* 69–79.

Szabo, G. (1958). The regional frequency and distribution of hair follicles in human skin. In W. Montagna & R. A. Ellis (Eds.), *The biology of hair growth* (pp. 33–38). New York: Academic Press.

Thiele, J. J., Weber, S. U., & Packer, L. (1999). Sebaceous gland secretion is a major physiologic route of vitamin E delivery to skin. *Journal of Investigative Dermatology, 113,* 1006–1010.

Tobin, D. J. (2005). Human hair fiber. In D. J. Tobin (Ed.), *Hair in toxicology: An important biomonitor* (pp. 34–54). London: Royal Society of Chemistry.

Tobin, D. J. (2006). Biochemistry of human skin—Our brain on the outside. *Chemical Society Reviews, 35,* 52–67.

Tobin, D. J., & Peters, E. M. J. (2009). Neurobiology of hair. In R. D. Granstein & T. Luger (Eds.), *Neuroimmunology of the skin* (pp. 139–158). Berlin, Germany: Springer-Verlag.

Tu, C. L., Oda, Y., Komuves, L., & Bikle, D. D. (2004). The role of the calcium-sensing receptor in epidermal differentiation. *Cell Calcium, 35*(3), 265–273.

Uitto, J. (1989). Connective tissue biochemistry of the aging dermis. Age-associated alterations in collagen and elastin. *Clinics in Geriatric Medicine, 5,* 127–147.

Watt, F. M., & Jensen, K. B. (2009). Epidermal stem cell diversity and quiescence. *EMBO Molecular Medicine, 1,* 260–267.

Weigand, D. A., Haygood, C., & Gaylor, J. R. (1974). Cell layers and density of Negro and Caucasian stratum corneum. *Journal of Investigative Dermatology, 62,* 563–568.

Zouboulis, C. C. (2004). Acne and sebaceous gland function. *Clinical Dermatology, 22,* 360–366.

2

Sensory Processes of Touch

AISLYN M. NELSON AND ELLEN A. LUMPKIN

Touch is an ability we often take for granted; imagine what it would be like if we could not feel our environment. For instance, although we may not be consciously aware of the clothing that we wear throughout the day, we do know when a piece of clothing is added or removed. Imagine if something as benign as wearing clothes turned into an unbearable physical pain. This is a reality for many patients with chronic pain. In fact, touch hypersensitivity, also known as allodynia, is one of the most common complaints of chronic pain patients. Chronic pain manifests as a consequence of a number of frequently encountered diseases, including diabetes, HIV, neuropathies, and infections.

The peripheral biological processes that underlie normal touch sensation along with touch hypersensitivity are largely unknown and are currently under investigation. A great promise of this research rests on the therapeutic benefits it might provide for chronic pain patients. If science can target a specific cellular pathway or protein, patients can be relieved of their constant pain with minimal side effects.

AN OVERVIEW OF SOMATOSENSORY RECEPTION

Historical Perspective

As early as 300 BC, the sense of touch has captured the fascination of scientists. Aristotle was the first to recognize touch as one of the five primal senses that dictates how we perceive the world.

In subsequent centuries, scientists debated whether the body's sensory systems conveyed an accurate portrayal of the physical environment. The 4th century philosopher St. Augustine firmly believed that sensory information should be viewed with skepticism, whereas Rene Descartes, a 16th century French scientist, postulated that sensory input provided a faithful representation of the real world. In the late 16th century, Thomas Hobbes suggested that sensory experience is the foundation of all knowledge and memories, and thus fathered the idea of *empiricism*. John Locke expanded on this theory by stating that all ideas came from sensations. By the 18th century, the idea that humans are blank slates colored by sensory experience did not sit well with many scholars. Indeed, Immanuel Kant hypothesized that sensory inputs merely activated an innate network of knowledge.

The 20th century saw the advent of sophisticated experimental methods that allowed neurophysiologists to directly investigate nervous system mechanisms. Among the pioneers of neurophysiology was Lord Edgar Douglas Adrian, who won the 1932 Nobel Prize in Physiology or Medicine for discovering the physical basis of sensation (Adrian & Zotterman, 1926). By using radio amplifiers to magnify nerve impulses several thousandfold, Adrian was able to record action potentials from single somatosensory afferent fibers. With this preparation, he discovered the all-or-none basis of the action potential. His work was also the first to demonstrate the sensory rate-code—large stimuli elicit more impulses from a neuron than do small stimuli.

Informed by a century of experimental progress, most scientists have now come to the conclusion that perception of our environment is governed by a fusion of the two aforementioned schools of thought (Figure 2.1). The peripheral nervous system is composed of the sensory neurons that innervate our body and that obtain an enormous amount of information from the environment. The central nervous system receives and interprets these data. Thus, the world that we perceive is constructed by our sensory systems; however, there must be an intrinsic network equipped to process this vast amount of data.

Somatosensory Pathways

A prominent model for how the brain handles sensory input was formulated by Boring in 1942 as a *labeled-line* system (Boring, 1942). The model postulates that sensory neurons are dedicated to encode information about one sensory modality, which is a distinct aspect of sensory perception. Many of our senses adhere to the labeled lined model. For example, two separate neuronal networks subserve vision and taste. Moreover, we can appreciate that each of our senses have many

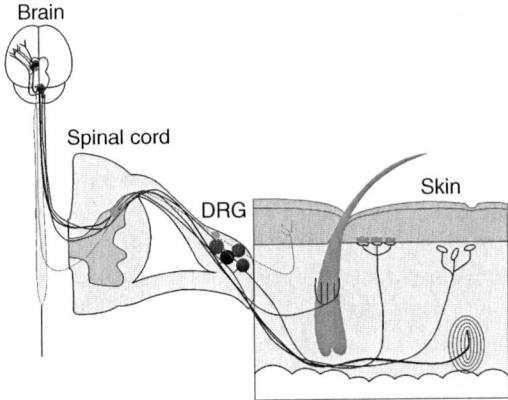

FIGURE 2.1 Somatosensory pathways. Nociception (small gray) is initiated by free nerve endings of unmyelinated or thinly myelinated afferents. The cell bodies of these sensory afferents are located in the dorsal root ganglia (DRG). Nociceptive neurons synapse in the dorsal horn of the spinal cord in laminae I/II and then cross the midline. Secondary nociceptive afferents travel up the spinal thalamic tract and synapse in the thalamus. Finally, the tertiary neurons make their way to cortical areas. Discriminative touch (large black) is initiated by the end organs of large myelinated neurons. The cell bodies of these peripheral sensory afferents are located in the DRG. Most discriminative touch afferents travel up the spinal cord in the dorsal column pathway and synapse in the brainstem. They also send collaterals into the dorsal horn. The secondary neurons then cross the midline and synapse in the thalamus. These tertiary neurons project to cortical areas.

characteristics. Boring recognized this and postulated that each sense had a subset of modalities, which are also processed by distinct sets of neurons. The labeled line model for encoding information allows for distinct sets of information to be handled and processed by unique areas of the central nervous system.

At first pass, the somatic senses, including touch, uphold Boring's hypothesis. Somatosensation can be divided into several subclasses: touch, pain, temperature, and proprioception (Figure 2.1). Discriminative touch, which reflects texture, shape, movement, and noxious touch are likewise encoded and processed by separate neuronal pathways. Discriminative touch is encoded by large myelinated peripheral sensory neurons that innervate the skin and travel along the spinal cord in what is known as the dorsal columns (Figure 2.1). These primary neurons travel up ipsilaterally, on the same side of the body, to their nuclei in the brainstem and synapse with secondary neurons. These primary neurons also send collaterals, or small projections, to neurons in the spinal cord, where they provide sensory feedback information, mainly for proprioception. The secondary neurons then cross over the midline of the brain on their way to the ventrolateral posterior (VPL) nucleus, a sensory relay nucleus in the thalamus. Finally, the relay neurons from the thalamic VPL travel to the primary somatosensory cortex. This dorsal column pathway keeps touch information segregated from other neuronal networks, like motor pathways.

The sensation of pain is also carried in its own labeled-line pathway. Noxious, or tissue damaging, mechanical stimuli activate unmyelinated peripheral sensory neurons, which travel back to the spinal cord and synapse ipsilaterally in areas of the dorsal horns known as laminae I and II (Figure 2.1). The secondary neurons from laminae I/II cross the midline and travel up the spinal cord contralaterally in the spinothalamic track. These secondary neurons synapse in the VPL and the relay neurons then travel to the primary somatosensory cortex, the cingulate gyrus, and the insula. The latter two cortical brain areas are involved in the affective, or emotional, components of pain.

Interestingly, and contrary to Boring's hypothesis, these nociceptive neurons can carry information on multiple sensory modalities, both painful touch and temperature. This apparent lack of specialization found in nociceptors lead Melzack and Wall (1965) to propose a patterned model in opposition to the labeled-line model. They hypothesized that the pattern of activation, rather than the specific neurons that carry the information, determines how the brain interprets distinct sensory modalities. This remains a highly debated subject, which will continue until the resources are available to identify and label specialized classes of sensory neurons. Then and only then will we be able to conclusively elucidate the principles of somatosensory processing.

PERIPHERAL SOMATOSENSORY RECEPTORS

Discriminative touch, like nociception, comprises several distinct modalities. Light touch is a perceptual combination of pressure, vibration, stretch, and hair movements; however, evidence from several model systems suggests that a labeled-line code does exist for discriminative touch. Light touch receptors can be segregated into groups based on their firing properties, including conduction velocity and adaptation properties (Figure 2.2). The different modalities of touch are important to appreciate because together they generate tactile perception, such as the feeling of the paper of this book.

Our understanding of the sensory processes of touch comes from both human studies and animal models. Microneurography in human

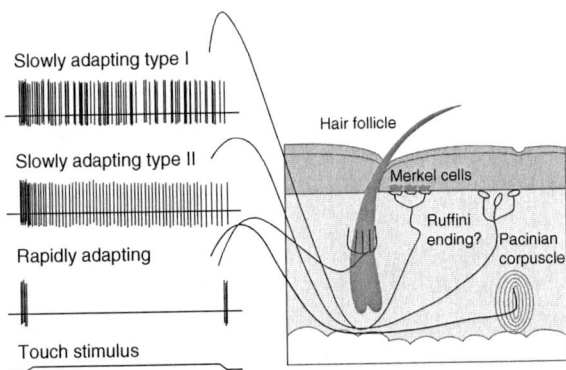

FIGURE 2.2 Light touch receptive Aβ afferents. Slowly adapting type I (SAI) afferents innervate Merkel cells at the epidermal/dermal border. The SAI has a sustained firing pattern that becomes very irregular throughout the stimulus. SAII afferents are correlated with Ruffini-ending organs. SAII responses are sustained throughout the stimulus and have a very regular firing pattern. Hair follicles, Pacinian corpuscles and Meissner's corpuscles (not pictured) are the end organs of rapidly adapting (RA) afferents. These RA neurons have robust onset and offset responses.

subjects can provide important information about touch sensation; however, these data are largely correlative. Microneurography is a procedure in which thin electrodes are used to record responses from cutaneous neurons in an alert human. Mechanical stimuli are applied to the skin, and the neurons activated by the stimulation are identified. Once the responses from a single neuron are isolated, the electrode is used to stimulate the sensory fiber and the person reports the perceived sensation. The area typically studied is the hand because of its high sensitivity to tactile stimulation. Microneurography allows scientists to match human percepts with neurophysiological data.

To complement human perceptual studies, animal models allow scientists to modify specific groups of cells and then to assay how that modification affects nervous system function. Fundamental insights into the principles of somatosensory signaling have come from studies of rodents, amphibians, fruit flies, and nematodes. One powerful approach is reverse genetics, in which a known genetic locus is modified and abnormal phenotypes are assessed through behavioral, physiological, and morphological studies. To measure the neurophysiological outputs of somatosensory afferents in rodent models, ex vivo skin–nerve recording preparations are particularly useful. The hind-paw skin and its innervating nerve are dissected out of the animal while remaining connected to each other. The skin can be stimulated with mechanical, thermal, or chemical stimuli, and the responses from individual somatosensory neurons are recorded (Reeh, 1986). This method corresponds nicely with the in vivo human microneurography studies. Together, these approaches allow scientists to elucidate how a cell type or molecule contributes to sensory responses and complex behaviors.

To understand the outcomes of the scientific endeavors described in this chapter, it may be helpful to summarize the basic steps of touch transduction (Figure 2.3). First, forces, such as pressure, stretch or hair movements, impinge upon touch-sensitive cells in the skin. Second, by opening mechanotransduction channels, these forces are transduced into electrical signals, called generator potentials, which depolarize the cell's plasma membrane. Third, when threshold is reached, action potentials are triggered to transmit sensory information along sensory afferent fibers to the central nervous system. Each peripheral somatosensory receptor differs from the others in the details of this cascade, and those nuances will be discussed in the following sections.

C- and Aδ-Somatosensory Afferents Primarily Encode Noxious Sensory Information

The somatosensory afferents that transmit noxious inputs can be divided into subgroups based on their physiological properties. C-fibers are unmyelinated afferents that conduct action potentials at less than 2 m/second in humans and less than 1 m/second in mice (Gasser, 1941). C-fibers terminate as free nerve endings in the epidermis of the skin (Figure 2.1). The vast majority of these C-fibers, which are discussed in more detail later, are nociceptors that carry information about noxious mechanical, chemical, and thermal inputs.

In addition to nociceptors, a small population of C-afferents that express vesicular glutamate transporter 3 have been identified as

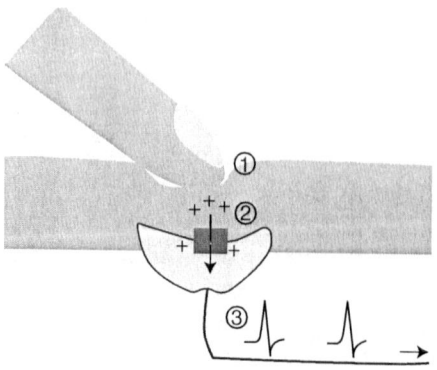

FIGURE 2.3 Mechanotransduction model. (1) Force, such as compression illustrated here, impinges upon touch-sensitive cells in the skin. (2) This force is transduced into a generator potential (+) via the opening of mechanotransduction channels. (3) The generator potential depolarized the cell, which triggers action potential firing, transmitting sensory information toward the central nervous system.

low-threshold mechanoreceptors (Seal et al., 2009). In healthy skin, these afferents can be activated by light touch. Interestingly, during inflammation, these C-fibers are key contributors to touch hypersensitivity. Thus, along with providing our sense of acute pain, C-fibers play an important role in pathological touch sensation.

Thinly myelinated neurons also encode information about painful stimuli. Aδ afferents are thinly myelinated neuronal fibers that conduct action potentials in the range of 2–9 m/second (Gasser, 1941). Thus, the information they convey reaches the brain more quickly than C-fiber information. Aδ-afferents can be further subdivided based on mechanical threshold and adaptation properties into high-threshold mechanoreceptors (HTM) and Down hair afferents (D-hair). HTM afferents display sustained firing throughout a stimulus and respond to noxious forces. By contrast, D-hairs have among the lowest mechanical thresholds of any light touch receptor and they respond most robustly at the onset and offset of touch.

Nociceptors. Painful touch comes in two flavors. First, acute pain, which is the type of pain you feel when you stub your toe or touch a sharp object, is a normal physiological response that warns you of potentially harmful objects or situations in the environment. Second, pathological pain, or hyperalgesia, occurs when a patient has increased sensitivity to touch. A subtype of hyperalgesia, allodynia, is a pathological state in which nonpainful stimuli are perceived as painful. These pathological pain sensations do not serve a survival propose, instead they decrease the patients' quality of life. To treat pathological pain sensations, we must understand how touch activates nociceptors, and how these mechanisms change in pathological states.

Nociceptive neurons express specific membrane proteins that mediate distinct aspects of pain. For example, capsaicin, a pungent ingredient in chili peppers, activates a receptor known as transient receptor potential vanilloid 1 (TRPV1), which is highly expressed in nociceptors (Lumpkin & Caterina, 2007). Mice lacking the TRPV1 receptor have several behavioral defects, including unresponsiveness to capsaicin, a moderate deficit in response to acute heat, and dramatically impaired sensitivity to inflammatory-evoked thermal hyperalgesia (Lumpkin & Caterina, 2007). These animals have no change in behavioral thresholds to noxious mechanical stimuli. Several groups have used resiniferatoxin (RTX), a TRPV1 agonist, to cause excitotoxicity and death in nociceptive neurons that express TRPV1. RTX-ablation eliminates both thermal hyperalgesia and inflammatory pain, whereas the motor system and discriminative touch remain intact (Tender et al., 2005). The specific expression of this receptor in a subset of nociceptive neurons is extremely useful because therapeutics targeted for TRPV1 may eliminate hyperalgesia while leaving other somatosensory functions, such as acute touch, intact.

Nociceptors also express specific subtypes of voltage-gated Na$^+$ (Na$_V$) channels. Na$_V$ channels are activated by generator potentials to initiate action potentials. Several mouse models have illustrated the importance of these channels in nociception. Mutations in Na$_V$1.7, a Na$^+$ channel preferentially expressed in nociceptors, have been shown to cause congenital insensitivity to pain in both mice and in humans. Mice lacking Na$_V$1.7 show increased mechanical and thermal pain thresholds, and when subjected to inflammatory pain models, hyperalgesia was not observed (Momin & Wood, 2008). Genetic analysis in humans corroborates the mouse data. Indeed a small group of individuals lacking Na$_V$1.7 have no perception of pain and traumatic events, such as breaking a bone, often go unnoticed. Conversely, a gain of function mutation in the Na$_V$1.7 in humans produces disabling hypersensitivity to pain.

Other voltage-gated Na$^+$ channels have also been linked to the cellular processes of pain. Na$_V$1.8-deficient mice demonstrated a slight enhancement of their pain thresholds to acute noxious stimuli and inflammatory-induced hyperalgesia; however, their maximal response was equal to that of the control mice (Momin & Wood, 2008). The Na$_V$1.9 channel does not appear to be directly involved in sensing noxious stimuli in a healthy adult, yet it seems to play a large role in the hypersensitivity people experience when they have an injury or chronic pain condition. Studies of these voltage-gated Na$^+$ channels showcase the utility of identifying specific molecules that are expressed in a distinct population of sensory neurons; one can determine the role those neurons play in the processing of sensory information.

Nociceptive neurons are interesting sensory fibers because they can sense both mechanical and chemical stimuli produced by a noxious mechanical force. For example, nociceptors highly express ATP receptors of the P2X and P2Y families (Benarroch, 2010). P2X receptors are ion channels that allow cations to flow into the cell causing a depolarization. P2Y receptors are G-protein-coupled receptors, most of which are linked to G$_q$ and activate phospholipase C. Animal behavior studies of P2X and P2Y knockout mice have shown these receptors to be important for injury/inflammatory-mediated pain.

How can ATP, the cell's intracellular energy source, serve as an extracellular ligand for P2X and P2Y receptors? In addition to ATP's metabolic role, tissue damage, sympathetic stimulation, and other processes can trigger the ATP release extracellularly (Benarroch, 2010). Thus, ATP receptors are not intrinsically mechanosensitive, yet, activation of these receptors can signal an intense, tissue-damaging mechanical stimulus.

In summary, although we try to avoid activating nociceptive neurons, they play an essential role in our processing of tactile sensory information in both normal and disease states.

Aβ Somatosensory Afferents Include Light Touch Receptors

In addition to C-fibers and Aδ afferents, the skin is abundantly innervated by thickly myelinated somatosensory neurons, or Aβ afferents, that conduct action potentials ≥10 m/second (Gasser, 1941). Aβ afferents can be subdivided by their adaptation properties into rapidly adapting (RA) and slowly adapting (SA) afferents.

RA Afferents

RA-Aβ neurons are characterized by brief bursts of action potentials at the onset and offset of touch stimuli (Figure 2.2; Adrian & Zotterman, 1926). Examining other neuronal properties, such as size of receptive field and modality of the activating stimulus, can further differentiate RA-Aβ fibers. RA-type I (RAI) Aβ neurons have small receptive fields and respond most robustly to bending of hair follicles (Johnson, 2001). Human microneurography studies have illustrated that RAI Aβ-fibers are responsible for sensing object slip (Blake et al., 1997). Other RA afferents have very large receptive fields and are correlated to two specific sensory end organs, Pacinian and Meissner's corpuscles, which along with the sensory neurons themselves, are neural crest derivatives (Hachisuka et al., 1984). Let us consider these specialized sensory end organs.

Pacinian corpuscles. The unique encapsulated structure of the Pacinian corpuscle is essential to its function as a vibration detector. Pacinian corpuscles are found deep in the dermis, hypodermis, and internal organs. One of the many functions governed by the Pacinian corpuscle is the ability to perceive with high fidelity, the position and movement of objects or tools that we grip in our hands. These neurons are incredibly sensitive and can detect vibrations in the range of 100–300 Hz (Johnson, 2001).

Interestingly, the morphological structure of the Pacinian corpuscle is responsible for this frequency tuning. The Pacinian corpuscle consists of many concentric lamellae of modified Schwann cells surrounding the RA-Aβ afferent terminal (Figures 2.1 and 2.2). Deformation of the lamellae causes a change in the corpuscle's pressure, opening cationic transduction channels allowing Na^+ influx into the terminal, which depolarizes the membrane (Loewenstein & Rathkamp, 1958). This lamellar capsule acts as a procession of high-pass mechanical filters, which cancels out the surrounding noise while tuning the vibration detection range. Acute removal of the capsule results in hyperactivity of the neuron to mechanical stimuli (Loewenstein & Mendelson, 1965). Thus, although the capsule is essential for frequency tuning of the afferent, it is not necessary for mechanosensitivity.

Many sensory fibers require growth factors from the surrounding environment. Pacinian-RA fibers are dependent upon several neurotrophin growth factors and their Trk receptors for survival (Sedy et al., 2004). Recent work has just begun to identify growth factor genes that are specifically expressed in RA fibers (Luo et al., 2009). A tyrosine kinase receptor, Ret, much like the neurotrophin receptors, is necessary for the development of the entire structure of the Pacinian corpuscle. Ret knockout mice may therefore allow studies that will define the role of Pacinian corpuscles in encoding tactile information.

Meissner's corpuscles. Meissner's corpuscles are found in the dermis of glabrous skin and are composed of an RA-Aβ afferent surrounded by enfoldings of specialized Schwann cells (Johnson et al., 2000). These corpuscles have large receptive fields and are extremely sensitive to acute skin deformation. Meissner's corpuscles are in fact the best touch receptor for encoding a sudden force applied to the skin surface (Macefield et al., 1996). The development of Meissner's corpuscles relies on the neurotrophin growth factor, brain-derived neurotrophic factor (BDNF), and its receptor, TrkB. Mice lacking the TrkB receptor have a complete loss of Meissner's corpuscles (Gonzalez-Martinez et al., 2005). Furthermore, overexpression of BDNF produces an increase in the size and innervation density of the corpuscles (LeMaster et al., 1999).

RA-corpuscle complexes are very important for touch sensation. The sensitivity to changes in dynamic force encoded by Meissner's corpuscles and the Pacinian afferents's ability to report vibration illustrate a possible unifying role of RA sensory neurons in the feedback control of grip (Johnson, 2001). These two corpuscles are model examples of how the structure of touch receptors directly impacts their sensory function. Furthermore, the importance of accessory cells in the sensory processing of mechanical force can be fully appreciated.

SA Afferents

Let us turn our attention to the other type of Aβ fibers, the SA afferents. The hallmark of SA afferents is that they produce responses throughout the length of a sustained stimulus (Figure 2.2). During an initial dynamic phase, the neuron fires action potentials very rapidly. During the static phase of the stimulus, the firing rate relaxes, or adapts, to a plateau level. The firing pattern during this static period, along with receptive field size and modality of activating stimulus, can be used to further subdivide SA-Aβ fibers into type I (SAI) and type II (SAII) afferents (Iggo & Muir, 1969).

SAI afferents. The hallmark of the SAI afferent is its markedly irregular firing pattern during the static phase of a touch-evoked response (Figure 2.2). The time between action potentials, known as the interspike interval, calculated from SAI afferents is distributed over a broad range of values (Iggo & Muir, 1969). It is unclear what causes the irregularity in the firing of these SAI Aβ fibers during the static phase. Other distinctive characteristics include punctate receptive fields, robust responses to low-force compressive stimuli, and very low spontaneous firing rates in the absence of touch.

Human microneurography studies have demonstrated that SAI afferents encode shape and texture of objects. Importantly, these afferents are necessary for fine tactile discrimination such as reading Braille characters (Johnson, 2001). Human subjects report the sensation of a "soft painting brush held tangentially against the skin" during SAI afferent stimulation (Haeberle & Lumpkin, 2008).

Merkel cell–neurite complexes. The sensory end organs of SAI afferents are Merkel cell–neurite complexes (Iggo & Muir, 1969). These comprise specialized epidermal cells, called Merkel cells, in contact with branches of the SAI afferent (Figures 2.1 and 2.2).

The role of Merkel cells in touch reception has been debated for over a century. Merkel cells may be secondary sensory receptors cells, much like hair cells of the vertebrate inner ear, which mediate mechanotransduction and then signal to SAI afferents via neurotransmitter release. Alternatively, Merkel cells may serve as accessory cells that provide metabolic support or release neuromodulators to modify the output of intrinsically mechanosensitive SAI afferents. Several lines of investigation support each hypothesis.

Consistent with both potential functions, histological and molecular evidence indicates that Merkel cells are presynaptic cells that are poised to release glutamate and neuropeptides on SAI afferent terminals. Although Merkel cells are epidermally derived (Morrison et al., 2009; Van Keymeulen et al., 2009), they express many neuronal molecules, including machinery necessary for synaptic transmission (Haeberle & Lumpkin, 2004). Moreover, electron micrographs have illustrated that Merkel cells form synaptic-like contacts with SAI afferents, and dense-core vesicles are concentrated in the Merkel cell's cytoplasm at these sites.

To determine whether SAI afferents are intrinsically mechanosensitive in the absence of Merkel cells, scientists have attempted to remove Merkel cells from rodent skin and then to record responses from SAI afferents. Two groups have done so using photoablation; however, these studies have produced conflicting results. One group found no change in mechanical sensitivity of SAI afferents after photoablation of Merkel cells, whereas another group found SAI responses to be greatly diminished (Haeberle & Lumpkin, 2008). Two technical caveats limit interpretation of these results. First, photoablation may not eliminate all of the Merkel cells. Second, photoablation might also damage the SAI afferent, compromising any intrinsic mechanosensitivity or the ability to propagate action potentials. These acute ablation studies have not provided a satisfactory answer our question.

Thus, several groups have investigated the role of neurotrophins in the Merkel cell–neurite complex. Cutaneous overexpression of NT-3, the neurotrophin whose receptor is TrkC, results in increased numbers Merkel cells and somatosensory afferents in the skin (Albers et al., 1996). NT-3 knockout mice lose Merkel cells and SAI afferents in the first two weeks of life (Airaksinen et al., 1996). Whether the loss of Merkel cells is secondary to the loss of SAI afferents or due to a direct requirement of NT-3 is currently under investigation. BDNF and its receptor, TrkB, are also important for SAI afferent function (Carroll et al., 1998). Like NT-3 mutants, mice engineered to lack the low-affinity neurotrophin receptor p75 lose Merkel cells postnatally (Kinkelin et al., 1999). Interestingly, their SA responses were reported to be comparable to control mice; however the authors did not distinguish between subtypes of SA afferents. Although genetically manipulating neurotrophin pathways has provided substantial insights into the maintenance of Merkel cell–neurite complexes, the lack of specific and complete ablation of these complexes leaves the field still questioning which pathways distinguish Merkel cell–neurite complexes from other touch receptors.

Let us now consider the hypothesis that Merkel cells are secondary mechanosensory cells necessary for encoding light touch responses. If this were the case, animals without Merkel cells should completely lack SAI responses. To test this prediction, a conditional knockout mouse was generated to disrupt expression of *Atoh1* (Maricich et al.,

2009). This transcription factor is expressed specifically in Merkel cells in the skin (Ben-Arie et al., 2000). In other cell types of the *Atoh1* lineage, including mechanosensory hair cells, *Atoh1* disruption prevents cell development (Bermingham et al., 1999). Histochemical experiments confirmed that Merkel cells also failed to develop in the absence of *Atoh1* expression. To determine the status of SAI responses in these mutant mice, electrophysiological recordings were preformed using the mouse ex vivo skin–nerve preparation. In *Atoh1* knockout mice lacking Merkel cells, no SAI firing patterns were observed, demonstrating that Merkel cells are necessary to produce canonical SAI responses (Maricich et al., 2009). Interestingly, the afferent hyperinnervates (i.e., has many more branches) the portion of skin where Merkel cells fail to develop. Are these aberrant neurons capable of firing action potentials? Are they mechanically sensitive? We now have the tools to answer these questions.

In addition to these in vivo studies, several groups have turned to in vitro experiments with cultured Merkel cells to assess their intrinsic mechanosensitivity. Although some reports indicate that Merkel cells fail to respond to direct touch, these cells are activated by other mechanical stimulus paradigms (Haeberle & Lumpkin, 2008). Merkel cells represent only about 0.1% of the cells in the epidermis; therefore to purify them, a transgenic mouse was developed to express green fluorescent protein in skin Merkel cells (Lumpkin et al., 2003). Dissociated Merkel cells are responsive to hypotonic-induced cellular swelling (Haeberle et al., 2008). By measuring the intracellular calcium levels, one can visualize dynamic cellular changes in calcium in response to stimuli. These techniques revealed that calcium-permeable ion channels mediate the Merkel cell's response to hypotonic-induced cell swelling (Haeberle et al., 2008). These cation channels are distinct from voltage-gated Ca^{2+} channels and the endoplasmic reticulum Ca^{2+} channels found in Merkel cells (Piskorowski et al., 2008; Yamashita et al., 1992). Merkel cells also express stretch-activated ion channels (Boulais et al., 2009). The molecular identity of these mechanosensitive channels, and whether they are required for touch sensitivity in vivo remain open questions.

As with the RA afferents, it will be important to dissect the relationship between the anatomical structure of the Merkel cell–neurite complex and how its morphology affects the processing of touch sensation. Furthermore, the properties of the aberrant SAI neuron in Merkel-cell knockout mice will shed light on the debate of whether the SAI neuron itself is mechanosensitive.

SAII afferents. Aβ afferents also contain a SAII population (Figure 2.2). SAII afferents are similar to SAI neurons in that they fire throughout the entire length of the stimulus. Unlike SAI afferents, SAII afferents have an exceedingly regular firing pattern, or a narrow range of interspike intervals, during the static phase of stimulation (Chambers & Iggo, 1967). They are also spontaneously active and respond robustly to skin stretch in many species. SAII receptive field size is also considerably larger than an SAI receptive field. It is critical to be able to physiologically distinguish SAII from SAI afferents in order to assess behavioral phenotypes in mutant mice.

The mechanical modality that most effectively activates SAII neurons appears to be stretch. Human reports from microneurography studies found that SAII afferent stimulation produces a feeling of skin stretch, suggesting that SAII neurons are important for determining the direction of object motion and hand or finger position (Johnson, 2001). Secondary sensory receptor cells have not been associated with SAII afferents; therefore, these afferents are likely to be intrinsically mechanosensitive.

Ruffini endings. Ruffini endings have been proposed as the end organ of SAII afferents (Figures 2.1 and 2.2). Ruffini endings exist only in the dermis of glabrous, or nonhairy, skin. Behavioral studies have implicated Ruffini endings in the kinesthetic sense of the hand and finger positioning (Edin & Johansson, 1995). Although correlative studies have localized Ruffini endings to the receptive fields of SAII afferents, definitive evidence of SAII innervation is lacking due to the scarcity of Ruffini endings and molecular markers of SAII afferents.

Keratinocytes

Keratinocytes, which compose our body's largest organ, the skin, act as a physical and chemical barrier to the outside world, but do they function somatosensory cells? These cells make up 99% of the epidermis, where they are ideally positioned to participate in the senses of touch and pain. Morphological studies have illustrated that keratinocytes directly couple with Merkel cells at desmosomes, which are cell–cell contacts stabilized by specialized proteins and intermediate filaments (Mihara et al., 1979). Peripheral sensory afferents also invade the epidermis and terminate in specific layers (Lumpkin & Caterina, 2007). Although synaptic-like contacts have not been described between keratinocytes and these afferent endings, their proximity suggests potential interaction.

Keratinocytes also secrete several chemicals that are capable of altering neuronal discharges. As discussed above, ATP is well-established to activate nociceptors. A second example is interleukins, which are involved in inflammation. Third, keratinocytes express β-endorphins, a ligand for opioid receptors, which are expressed in nociceptive sensory neurons (Lumpkin & Caterina, 2007). These molecules are likely to participate in inflammatory pain states, but could they play a role in normal touch sensation?

Finally, keratinocytes express several proteins implicated in cutaneous sensation (Lumpkin & Caterina, 2007). Expression of TRPV1, the capsaicin receptor, has been reported in keratinocytes. In cell culture studies, capsaicin stimulation causes the release of interleukin-8 from keratinocytes. Keratinocytes also express TRPV3 and TRPV4, which have both been implicated in warmth sensing. Several groups have demonstrated that TRPV4 responds to hypotonic-induced cell swelling and thus may function as a mechanosensor (Alessandri-Haber et al., 2003; Liedtke, 2005). Finally, ATP receptors of the P2Y subfamily, such as P2Y2, are found in keratinocytes. These receptors are involved in inflammatory hyperalgesia, and thus may contribute to mechanical hypersensitivity. Activation of P2Y2 causes intracellular Ca^{2+} to increase, resulting in more ATP release.

Although these studies are suggestive, direct interaction between keratinocytes and epidermal neuronal axons remains elusive. Coculture systems with these cells may prove to be very informative and shed light on the sensory potential of keratinocytes.

MOLECULAR PROCESSES OF TOUCH

Mechanical forces initiate touch sensation. Typically, chemical ligands are not involved in activating mechanosensory receptors unless there is significant tissue injury caused by the force. Thus, many scientists hypothesize that specialized molecular pathways respond to mechanical stimuli. Hence, the term mechanotransduction: the ability of a mechanical force applied to a cell to generate an electrical signal. Despite numerous efforts to identify mechanotransduction proteins, the molecules underlying mechanotransduction in mammals are still largely unknown.

There are several hypotheses for how mechanotransduction occurs in a sensory cell (Figure 2.4; Lumpkin & Caterina, 2007). One of the most notable features of mechanotransduction is its remarkable speed, which has led to two direct gating models (Figure 2.4A and 2.4B). The advantage of a direct mechanotransduction channel is that it allows for fine temporal resolution. Anecdotally, we know that our ability to perceive touch is incredibly fast. Furthermore, other sensory cells that transduce mechanical forces, like auditory and vestibular hair cells, respond to stimuli within 40 μs (Corey & Hudspeth, 1979). This fine

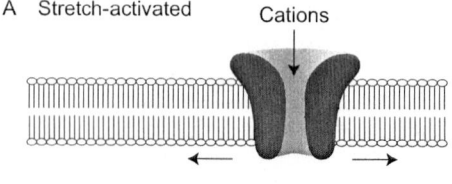
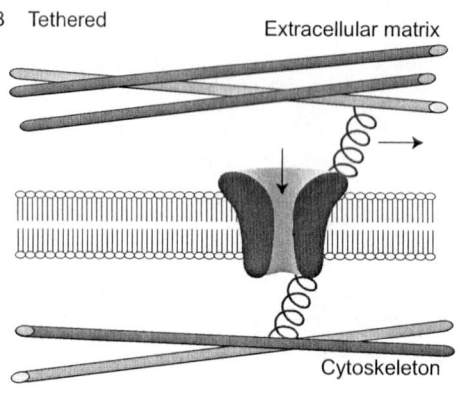
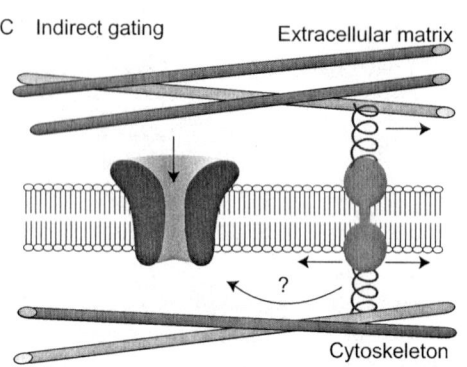

FIGURE 2.4 Molecular models of mechanotransduction. (A) The stretch-activated model predicts that force-sensitive ion channels in the plasma membrane of mechanosensory cells are activated by changes in membrane tension. (B) The tethered model predicts that mechanotransduction channels are linked to extracellular and/or intracellular proteins. Forces on these tethering proteins cause a conformational change in the mechanotransduction channel allowing ions to flow through the channel. (C) The indirect gating model predicts that second messengers are involved in the opening of mechanotransduction channels.

temporal resolution should thus be reflected in the molecular mechanism employed to transmit that stimulus.

One direct-gating model postulates that plasma membrane stretch-sensitive ion channels transduce mechanical inputs (Figure 2.4A). Such channels are sensitive to changes in tension or curvature of the plasma membrane. In bacteria and numerous eukaryotic cell types, stretch-sensitive ion channels have been identified; however, it is unknown whether these channels play a role in mammalian touch reception.

An exciting recent report describes the Piezo family, a new class of large, transmembrane proteins that might function as stretch-sensitive channels in touch receptors (Figure 2.5A; Coste et al., 2010). Although they lack homology to known ion channels, Piezo expression is sufficient to induce stretch-sensitive currents in heterologous cells. Notably, Piezo2 is required for touch- and stretch-evoked currents in a subset of cultured somatosensory neurons; however, future studies are needed to determine whether Piezo proteins are important for touch sensation in vivo.

A second model predicts that extracellular and intracellular connections, or tethers, are required for mechanosensitivity (Figure 2.4B). In this model, a transduction channel contacts extracellular or cytoskeletal proteins, which are capable of activating the ion channel. The tethers focus the force on the channel's gate, which allows activation to occur under minute forces.

Strong support for the tether model comes from studies of vertebrate hair cells, which underlie our sense of hearing. Hair cells have tiered stereocilia on their apical surface. Each stereocilium is connected via a tip link to its taller neighbor. These tip links are necessary for efficient gating of mechanotransduction channels (Assad et al., 1991). Recent studies of deafness mutations in humans and other vertebrates have identified protocadherin-15 and cadherin-23 as components of the tip link (Kazmierczak et al., 2007). Interestingly, electron micrographs illustrate contacts between somatosensory neurons and the extracellular matrix (Hu et al., 2010). Are homologs to these tip link proteins required for mechanotransduction in touch?

In cases where mechanosensory signaling is relatively slow it is possible that mechanotransduction, like phototransduction or chemotransduction, is mediated through second messenger-signaling pathway (Figure 2.4C). This model predicts that the mechanosensitive membrane protein is not itself an ion channel, but rather is linked by secondary intermediates to ion-channel opening. Second messenger pathways are intrinsically slower than a direct-gating model; however, there is greater potential for amplification of the signal. Consistent with an indirect gating model, a subset of polymodal sensory neurons in *Caenorhabditis elegans* requires lipid metabolites for osmotic somatosensation (Lumpkin & Caterina, 2007).

Which model of mechanotransduction describes touch reception in mammalian somatosensory neurons is actively under investigation. Different modalities of touch may be processed by distinct mechanisms. Model systems have identified several candidate proteins that have the potential to encode mechanical stimuli. Each family of proteins will be discussed next (Figure 2.5).

Transient Receptor Potential Channels

TRP channels are capable of supporting all of the mechanotransduction models mentioned above (Christensen & Corey, 2007). TRP channels can

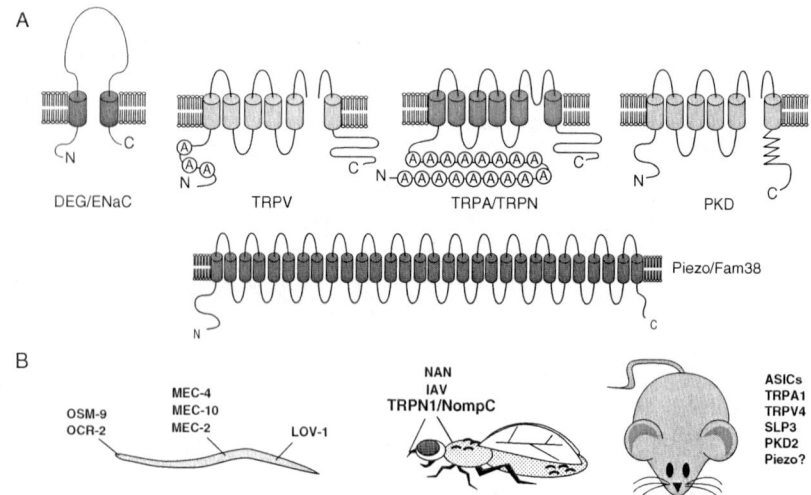

FIGURE 2.5 Mechanotransduction channels. (A) DEG/ENaC, TRPV, TRPN/TRPA, and PKD are implicated in mechanotransduction. DEG/ENaC have two transmembrane domains. TRPV, TRPN/TRPA, and PKD channels all have six transmembrane domains with a pore-loop region. TRPV and TRPN/TRPA channels also have ankyrin (A) repeats. Piezo proteins are predicted to have ~30 transmembrane domains but no pore-loops have been identified. (B) Each ion-channel family described in A has been linked to mechanotransduction in one or more of the illustrated animal models: *C. elegans* (worm), *Drosophila* (fly) and mouse. Reprinted with permission from "Feeling the pressure in mammalian somatosensation," by E.A. Lumpkin and D.A. Bautista, 2005, *Current Opinion in Neurobiology, 15*, 382–388. Copyright 2005 by Elsevier.

be divided into seven subfamilies based on their amino acid sequences: ankryin (TRPA), canonical (TRPC), vanilloid (TRPV), melastatin (TRPM), no mechanoreceptor potential (TRPN), polycystic kidney disease (PKD), and musolipin (TRPML). Many of these proteins form ion channels capable of passing monovalent and divalent cations. Furthermore, multiple TRP channels have extensive extracellular and intracellular domains that mediate interactions with accessory proteins.

TRPV channels have well-established roles in somatosensory signaling (Figure 2.5; Mutai & Heller, 2003). Besides their involvement in pain, several TRPV receptors have been implicated in mechanotransduction. OSM-9 and OCR-2, TRPV homologs found in *C. elegans*, localize to sensory cilia in polymodal sensory neurons (Figure 2.5B; Lumpkin & Caterina, 2007). Disruption of these proteins in *C. elegans* causes touch and osmotic sensation dysfunction. Studies in *Drosophila* have also pointed to TRPV channels as important for mechanosensory signaling. TRPV isoforms, nanchung (Nan) and inactive (Iav), are essential for several mechanical-mediated processes, including proprioception (balance and body position), hearing and touch (Figure 2.5B; Lumpkin & Caterina, 2007). Furthermore, when NAN or IAV are heterologously expressed, they are responsive to hypotonic-evoked cell swelling indicating they can transduce mechanical force. Here, TRPVs appear to be intrinsically mechanosensitive and support the stretch-gating model.

Interestingly, TRPV4 is expressed in mammalian mechanosensory cells, such as hair cells, Merkel cells and somatosensory neurons (Liedtke, 2008). TRPV4 is responsive to hypotonic stimuli and is the mammalian ortholog of OSM-9: in *C. elegans* TRPV4 rescues, or ameliorates, the mechanosensory and osmosensory defects of OSM-9 mutants (Figure 2.5B; Liedtke et al., 2000, 2003). Disappointingly, mice lacking TRPV4 have only slight changes in acute mechanical thresholds (Liedtke & Friedman, 2003; Suzuki et al., 2003). More significantly, the mechanosensitivity of visceral somatosensory afferents is dramatically reduced in TRPV4 knockout mice (Brierley et al., 2008). Thus although TRPV4 may not play a major role in touch, it is important in transmitting mechanosensory information in visceral organs.

TRPN1 and TRPA1 are two additional TRP channels that have been implicated in mechanosensory transduction. A notable feature both of these subunits is that they each express numerous ankryin repeats. TRPN1 has 29 ankryin repeats, whereas TRPA1 has 17 repeats (Figure 2.5A; Lumpkin & Bautista, 2005). Ankryin repeats have been proposed to act as a spring, which has the potential for converting a mechanical force into a cellular signal (Howard & Bechstedt, 2004). Accordingly, *Drosophila* TRPN1 (NOMPC) mutants have touch, hearing and proprioceptive defects (Figure 2.5B; Lumpkin & Caterina, 2007). The *C. elegans* homolog of TRPN1, *trp-4*, is expressed in mechanosensory neurons and mutants have locomotion phenotypes consistent with proprioceptive defects. In zebrafish, interfering with *trpn1* demolishes mechanically evoked potentials in hair cells (Lumpkin & Caterina, 2007). Thus, TRPN1 appears to have a role in mechanotransduction conserved throughout many species.

Although the mammalian genome does not contain a TRPN homolog, TRPA1 is expressed in hair cells, nociceptors and other somatosensory neurons. Alas, TRPA1 knockout mice have few touch deficits (Bautista et al., 2006), and normal auditory function (Kwan et al., 2006). Interestingly, TRPA1 appears to be important for mechanical and thermal hypersensitivity. Indeed, the *Drosophila* TRPA homolog, *painless*, is necessary for pain withdrawal behaviors (Tracey et al., 2003). Thus, while TRPA1 may not play a major role in transducing touch perception, it does play a role in pathological touch states.

Finally, the PKD subfamily of TRP receptors has surfaced as candidate mechanotransduction channels (Figure 2.5A). PKD1 and PKD2 were discovered as the major genetic cause of PKD. PKD causes large fluid-filled cysts in the kidneys, as well as cysts in the liver and other organs, aneurysms and premature death. Physiological studies have found that PKD1 and PKD2 form a complex that localizes to the primary cilia of kidney epithelial cells (Nauli et al., 2003; Qian et al., 1997). This complex is proposed to form a calcium-permeable cation channel that is sensitive to fluid flow. The absence of either PKD1 or PKD2 prohibits the proper localization and assembly of the complex, thus causing cyst formation due to lack of correct fluid flow signaling (Figure 2.5B; Yoder, 2007). As demonstrated by the many people who suffer from this disease, the PKD protein complex is an essential molecule in the kidney.

PKD1 and PKD2 are also expressed in endothelial cells that line capillaries and in vascular smooth muscle cells (Sharif-Naeini et al., 2009). In endothelial cells, the complex is again proposed to sense fluid flow, whereas in the vascular smooth muscle cells, PKD1/PKD2 may act as a sensor of arterial pressure (Sharif-Naeini et al., 2009). Thus, PKD1 and PKD2 can convey both shear force, like fluid flow, and pressure. The *C. elegans* PKD homolog, LOV-1, is expressed in mechanosensory neurons required for male mating behavior (Figure 2.5B; Barr & Sternberg, 1999). Recently, PKD proteins have been found in several other mechanosensory cells, including Merkel cells (Haeberle et al., 2008). Do PKD1 and PKD2 act as mechanotransduction channels in these cells types?

Degenerin/Epithelial Na$^+$ Channels (DEG/ENaC)

DEG/ENaC channels have also been implicated in mechanosensation in several model systems (Figure 2.5A). In *C. elegans*, touch neurons located in the body express the mechanotransduction channels MEC-4 and MEC-10, which have large extracellular domains (Figure 2.5B; Goodman, 2006). These channels have accessory subunits MEC-2 and MEC-6. The loss of any of these components of the mechanotransduction complex results in deficits in touch-evoked behaviors. Although specialized microtubules, encoded by *mec-12* and *mec-7*, are required for touch-evoked behaviors, a recent study suggests that microtubules do not interact with channel complex itself. By contrast, extracellular matrix components, encoded by *mec-1*, *mec-5*, and *mec-9*, are required to properly localize the MEC transduction complex in these neurons (Goodman, 2006).

Mammalian isoforms of DEG/ENaC channels are known as acid-sensing ion channels (ASICs; Waldmann et al., 1997). There are three ASIC channels found in peripheral somatosensory neurons (Figure 2.5B). ASIC knockout mice have yielded somewhat subtle results. Recordings from cutaneous neurons demonstrated only modest changes in touch-evoked responses but the response thresholds to mechanical stimuli were not affected (Lumpkin & Caterina, 2007). Thus in mammals, ASIC channels do not appear to be principal mechanotransduction channels that sensory cells use to process touch, rather they play a role in modulating sensory processing.

Stomatin-Like Proteins

Along with pore-forming units, the MEC complex contains accessory proteins, like MEC-2, a stomatin-like protein (SLP; Goodman et al., 2002). This integral membrane protein interacts with specifically with MEC-4 and potentiates the conductivity of the channel. A mammalian homolog of SLP, SLP3, also points to this protein's involvement in mechanosensory signaling (Figure 2.5B; Wetzel et al., 2007). In mice lacking SLP3, a least one third of cutaneous mechanosensory neurons are unable to respond to mechanical stimuli. The subset of sensory neuron affected by the loss of SLP3 has yet to be clearly defined; however, the identification of these neurons has the potential to provide tremendous insight into the mechanisms of touch.

DIRECTION OF THE FIELD

As this chapter demonstrates, we are only beginning to understand the sensory processes of touch. Much remains to be accomplished. First, while sensory neurons can be categorized physiologically, genetic identification and visualization in the intact skin is paramount to resolving the mechanisms of different touch modalities. The recent discovery of genetic markers for Merkel cells, RA afferents and Aδ low-threshold mechanoreceptors will now allow scientists to selectively eliminate that subpopulation of sensory neurons and examine how behavior is affected. Furthermore, the identification of specific genes permits physicians to perform genomic analyses on patients and see if touch pathologies are correlated with genetic variants.

Second, behavioral touch paradigms must also become more sensitive and specific. It is difficult to test shape discrimination in a mouse because a mouse cannot describe what it is touching. Nevertheless, quantifying the latency for a mouse to raise its paw in response to a mechanical stimulus is far too crude. Although recently reported texture discrimination tasks are promising (Wetzel et al., 2007), future behavioral paradigms might benefit the most from mimicking natural environments and exploiting the fact that mice rely chiefly on their whiskers to gather tactile information.

Third, Pacinian corpuscles, Meissner's corpuscles and Merkel cells are specific touch receptors, yet they may only represent a minority of the touch receptors located in the skin. Furthermore, to date, only Merkel cells have been selectively manipulated in transgenic mice. We still lack markers that distinguish between Pacinian and Meissner's corpuscles, making it difficult to access the role each RA subtype plays in the animal's behavioral response to touch. We need specific markers to isolate each modality and see where in the puzzle of sensation it fits.

Finally, the field is heavily focusing on identifying mechanotransduction channels involved in touch. The importance of this objective is at least threefold. First, discovering mechanosensitive ion channels involved in touch will help us understand how the body processes tactile sensory information. Second, it may give us insight into the mechanotransduction channels underlying other mechanically mediated senses, like hearing. Third, targeting a specific protein with agonists or antagonists has great potential for therapeutic intervention in touch hypersensitivity.

After 23 centuries, the field of touch remains fascinating. We are still unraveling the basic mechanisms of how mammals encode arguably their most important sense. One day, tactile sensation will be understood at the same microscopic level as vision or vascularization, but that will not occur until many of the questions posed above are answered.

ACKNOWLEDGMENT

The authors are supported by NIAMS grants AR051219 and NS073119 (to EAL) and a McNair Scholar Award (to AMN).

REFERENCES

Adrian, E. D., & Zotterman, Y. (1926). The impulses produced by sensory nerve endings: Part 3. Impulses set up by Touch and Pressure. *Journal of Physiology,* 61, 465–483.

Airaksinen, M. S., Koltzenburg, M., Lewin, G. R., Masu, Y., Helbig, C., Wolf, E., ... Meyer M. (1996). Specific subtypes of cutaneous mechanoreceptors require neurotrophin-3 following peripheral target innervation. *Neuron, 16,* 287–295.

Albers, K. M., Perrone, T. N., Goodness, T. P., Jones, M. E., Green, M. A., & Davis, B. M. (1996). Cutaneous overexpression of NT-3 increases sensory and sympathetic neuron number and enhances touch dome and hair follicle innervation. *Journal of Cell Biology, 134,* 487–497.

Alessandri-Haber, N., Yeh, J. J., Boyd, A. E., Parada, C. A., Chen, X., Reichling, D. B., Levine JD. (2003). Hypotonicity induces TRPV4-mediated nociception in rat. *Neuron, 39,* 497–511.

Assad, J. A., Shepherd, G. M., & Corey, D. P. (1991). Tip-link integrity and mechanical transduction in vertebrate hair cells. *Neuron, 7,* 985–994.

Barr, M. M., & Sternberg, P. W. (1999). A polycystic kidney-disease gene homologue required for male mating behaviour in C. elegans. *Nature, 401,* 386–389.

Bautista, D. M., Jordt, S. E., Nikai, T., Tsuruda, P. R., Read, A. J., Poblete, J.,...Julius D. (2006). TRPA1 mediates the inflammatory actions of environmental irritants and proalgesic agents. *Cell, 124,* 1269–1282.

Ben-Arie, N., Hassan, B. A., Bermingham, N. A., Malicki, D. M., Armstrong, D., Matzuk, M.,...Zoghbi HY. (2000). Functional conservation of atonal and Math1 in the CNS and PNS. *Development, 127,* 1039–1048.

Benarroch, E. E. (2010). Adenosine triphosphate: a multifaceted chemical signal in the nervous system. *Neurology, 74,* 601–607.

Bermingham, N. A., Hassan, B. A., Price, S. D., Vollrath, M. A., Ben-Arie, N., Eatock, R. A.,...Zoghbi HY. (1999). Math1: An essential gene for the generation of inner ear hair cells. *Science, 284,* 1837–1841.

Blake, D. T., Hsiao, S. S., & Johnson, K. O. (1997). Neural coding mechanisms in tactile pattern recognition: the relative contributions of slowly and rapidly adapting mechanoreceptors to perceived roughness. *Journal of Neuroscience, 17,* 7480–7489.

Boring, E. G. (1942). *Sensation and perception in the history of experimental psychology.* New York: Appleton Century Crofts Inc.

Boulais, N., Pennec, J. P., Lebonvallet, N., Pereira, U., Rougier, N., Dorange, G.,...Misery L. (2009). Rat Merkel cells are mechanoreceptors and osmoreceptors. *Public Library of Science One, 4,* e7759.

Brierley, S. M., Page, A. J., Hughes, P. A., Adam, B., Liebregts, T., Cooper, N. J.,...Blackshaw LA. (2008). Selective role for TRPV4 ion channels in visceral sensory pathways. *Gastroenterology, 134,* 2059–2069.

Carroll, P., Lewin, G. R., Koltzenburg, M., Toyka, K. V., & Thoenen, H. (1998). A role for BDNF in mechanosensation. *Nature Neuroscience, 1,* 42–46.

Chambers, M. R., & Iggo, A. (1967). Slowly-adapting cutaneous mechanoreceptors. *Journal of Physiology, 192,* 26P–27P.

Christensen, A. P., & Corey, D. P. (2007). TRP channels in mechanosensation: direct or indirect activation? *Nature Reviews Neuroscience, 8,* 510–521.

Corey, D. P., & Hudspeth, A. J. (1979). Response latency of vertebrate hair cells. *Biophysical Journal, 26,* 499–506.

Coste, B., Mathur, J., Schmidt, M., Earley, T. J., Ranade, S., Petrus, M. J.,...Patapoutian, A. (2010). Piezo1 and Piezo2 are essential components of distinct mechanically activated cation channels. *Science, 330*(6000), 55–60.

Edin, B. B., & Johansson, N. (1995). Skin strain patterns provide kinaesthetic information to the human central nervous system. *Journal of Physiology, 487,* 243–251.

Gasser, H. (1941). The Classification of Nerve Fibers. *Ohio Journal of Science, XLI,* 145–159.

Gonzalez-Martinez, T., Farinas, I., Del Valle, M. E., Feito, J., Germana, G., Cobo, J., Vega JA. (2005). BDNF, but not NT-4, is necessary for normal development of Meissner corpuscles. *Neuroscience Letters, 377,* 12–15.

Goodman, M. B. (2006). Mechanosensation. *WormBook,* 1–14.

Goodman, M. B., Ernstrom, G. G., Chelur, D. S., O'Hagan, R., Yao, C. A., & Chalfie, M. (2002). MEC-2 regulates C. elegans DEG/ENaC channels needed for mechanosensation. *Nature, 415,* 1039–1042.

Hachisuka, H., Mori, O., Sakamoto, F., Sasai, Y., & Nomura, H. (1984). Immunohistological demonstration of S-100 protein in the cutaneous nervous system. *Anatomical Record, 210,* 639–646.

Haeberle, H., Bryan, L. A., Vadakkan, T. J., Dickinson, M. E., & Lumpkin, E. A. (2008). Swelling-activated Ca^{2+} channels trigger Ca^{2+} signals in Merkel cells. *Public Library of Science ONE, 3,* e1750.

Haeberle, H., Fujiwara, M., Chuang, J., Panditrao, M. V., Bechstedt, S., Howard, J., & Lumpkin, E. A. (2004). Molecular profiling reveals synaptic release machinery in Merkel cells. *Proc Natl Acad Sci U S A, 101*(40), 14503–14508.

Haeberle, H., & Lumpkin, E. A. (2008). Merkel cells in somatosensation. *Chemosensory Perception, 1,* 110–118.

Howard, J., & Bechstedt, S. (2004). Hypothesis: a helix of ankyrin repeats of the NOMPC-TRP ion channel is the gating spring of mechanoreceptors. *Current Biology, 14,* R224–226.

Hu, J., Chiang, L. Y., Koch, M., & Lewin, G. R. (2010). Evidence for a protein tether involved in somatic touch. *EMBO Journal, 29,* 855–867.

Iggo, A., & Muir, A. R. (1969). The structure and function of a slowly adapting touch corpuscle in hairy skin. *Journal of Physiology, 200,* 763–796.

Johnson, K. O. (2001). The roles and functions of cutaneous mechanoreceptors. *Current Opinion in Neurobiology, 11,* 455–461.

Johnson, K. O., Yoshioka, T., & Vega-Bermudez, F. (2000). Tactile functions of mechanoreceptive afferents innervating the hand. *Journal of Clinical Neurophysiology, 17,* 539–558.

Kazmierczak, P., Sakaguchi, H., Tokita, J., Wilson-Kubalek, E. M., Milligan, R. A., Muller, U., Kachar B. (2007). Cadherin 23 and protocadherin 15 interact to form tip-link filaments in sensory hair cells. *Nature, 449,* 87–91.

Kinkelin, I., Stucky, C. L., & Koltzenburg, M. (1999). Postnatal loss of Merkel cells, but not of slowly adapting mechanoreceptors in mice lacking the neurotrophin receptor p75. *European Journal of Neuroscience, 11,* 3963–3969.

Kwan, K. Y., Allchorne, A. J., Vollrath, M. A., Christensen, A. P., Zhang, D. S., Woolf, C. J., Corey DP. (2006). TRPA1 contributes to cold, mechanical, and chemical nociception but is not essential for hair-cell transduction. *Neuron, 50,* 277–289.

LeMaster, A. M., Krimm, R. F., Davis, B. M., Noel, T., Forbes, M. E., Johnson, J. E., Albers KM. (1999). Overexpression of brain-derived neurotrophic factor enhances sensory innervation and selectively increases neuron number. *Journal of Neuroscience, 19,* 5919–5931.

Liedtke, W. (2005). TRPV4 plays an evolutionary conserved role in the transduction of osmotic and mechanical stimuli in live animals. *Journal of Physiology, 567,* 53–58.

CHAPTER 2 SENSORY PROCESSES OF TOUCH   57

Liedtke, W. (2008). Molecular mechanisms of TRPV4-mediated neural signaling. *Annual New York Academy of Science, 1144*, 42–52.

Liedtke, W., & Friedman, J. M. (2003). Abnormal osmotic regulation in trpv4-/- mice. *Proceedings of the National Academy of Science U S A, 100*, 13698–13703.

Loewenstein, W. R., & Mendelson, M. (1965). Components of receptor adaptation in a Pacinian corpuscle. *Journal of Physiology, 177*, 377–397.

Loewenstein, W. R., & Rathkamp, R. (1958). The sites for mechano-electric conversion in a Pacinian corpuscle. *Journal of General Physiology, 41*, 1245–1265.

Lumpkin, E. A., & Bautista, D. M. (2005). Feeling the pressure in mammalian somatosensation. *Current Opinion in Neurobiology, 15*, 382–388.

Lumpkin, E. A., & Caterina, M. J. (2007). Mechanisms of sensory transduction in the skin. *Nature, 445*, 858–865.

Lumpkin, E. A., Collisson, T., Parab, P., Omer-Abdalla, A., Haeberle, H., Chen, P.,...Johnson JE. (2003). Math1-driven GFP expression in the developing nervous system of transgenic mice. *Gene Expression Patterns, 3*, 389–395.

Luo, W., Enomoto, H., Rice, F. L., Milbrandt, J., & Ginty, D. D. (2009). Molecular identification of rapidly adapting mechanoreceptors and their developmental dependence on ret signaling. *Neuron, 64*, 841–856.

Macefield, V. G., Hager-Ross, C., & Johansson, R. S. (1996). Control of grip force during restraint of an object held between finger and thumb: responses of cutaneous afferents from the digits. *Experimental Brain Research, 108*, 155–171.

Maricich, S. M., Wellnitz, S. A., Nelson, A. M., Lesniak, D. R., Gerling, G. J., Lumpkin, E. A., Zoghbi HY. (2009). Merkel cells are essential for light-touch responses. *Science, 324*, 1580–1582.

Melzack, R., & Wall, P. D. (1965). Pain mechanisms: a new theory. *Science, 150*, 971–979.

Mihara, M., Hashimoto, K., Ueda, K., & Kumakiri, M. (1979). The specialized junctions between Merkel cell and neurite: an electron microscopic study. *Journal of Investigative Dermatology, 73*, 325–334.

Momin, A., & Wood, J. N. (2008). Sensory neuron voltage-gated sodium channels as analgesic drug targets. *Current Opinion in Neurobiology, 18*, 383–388.

Morrison, K. M., Miesegaes, G. R., Lumpkin, E. A., & Maricich, S. M. (2009). Mammalian Merkel cells are descended from the epidermal lineage. *Developmental Biology, 336*, 76–83.

Mutai, H., & Heller, S. (2003). Vertebrate and invertebrate TRPV-like mechanoreceptors. *Cell Calcium, 33*, 471–478.

Nauli, S. M., Alenghat, F. J., Luo, Y., Williams, E., Vassilev, P., Li, X.,...Zhou J. (2003). Polycystins 1 and 2 mediate mechanosensation in the primary cilium of kidney cells. *Nature Genetics, 33*, 129–137.

Piskorowski, R. A., Haeberle, H., Panditrao, M., & Lumpkin, E. A. (2008). Voltage-activated ion channels and calcium-induced calcium release shape calcium signaling in Merkel cells. *Pflugers Archiv European Journal of Physiology, 457*, 197–209.

Qian, F., Germino, F. J., Cai, Y., Zhang, X., Somlo, S., & Germino, G. G. (1997). PKD1 interacts with PKD2 through a probable coiled-coil domain. *Nature Genetics, 16*, 179–183.

Reeh, P. W. (1986). Sensory receptors in mammalian skin in an in vitro preparation. *Neuroscience Letters, 66*, 141–146.

Seal, R. P., Wang, X., Guan, Y., Raja, S. N., Woodbury, C. J., Basbaum, A. I., Edwards RH. (2009). Injury-induced mechanical hypersensitivity requires C-low threshold mechanoreceptors. *Nature, 462*, 651–655.

Sedy, J., Szeder, V., Walro, J. M., Ren, Z. G., Nanka, O., Tessarollo, L.,...Kucera J. (2004). Pacinian corpuscle development involves multiple Trk signaling pathways. *Developmental Dynamics, 231*, 551–563.

Sharif-Naeini, R., Folgering, J. H., Bichet, D., Duprat, F., Lauritzen, I., Arhatte, M.,...Honoré E. (2009). Polycystin-1 and -2 dosage regulates pressure sensing. *Cell, 139*, 587–596.

Suzuki, M., Mizuno, A., Kodaira, K., & Imai, M. (2003). Impaired pressure sensation in mice lacking TRPV4. *Journal of Biological Chemistry, 278*, 22664–22668.

Tender, G. C., Walbridge, S., Olah, Z., Karai, L., Iadarola, M., Oldfield, E. H., Lonser RR. (2005). Selective ablation of nociceptive neurons for elimination of hyperalgesia and neurogenic inflammation. *Journal of Neurosurgery, 102*, 522–525.

Tracey, W. D., Jr., Wilson, R. I., Laurent, G., & Benzer, S. (2003). painless, a Drosophila gene essential for nociception. *Cell, 113*, 261–273.

Van Keymeulen, A., Mascre, G., Youseff, K. K., Harel, I., Michaux, C., De Geest, N.,...Blanpain C. (2009). Epidermal progenitors give rise to Merkel cells during embryonic development and adult homeostasis. *Journal of Cell Biology, 187*, 91–100.

Waldmann, R., Champigny, G., Bassilana, F., Heurteaux, C., & Lazdunski, M. (1997). A proton-gated cation channel involved in acid-sensing. *Nature, 386*, 173–177.

Wetzel, C., Hu, J., Riethmacher, D., Benckendorff, A., Harder, L., Eilers, A.,...Lewin G.R. (2007). A stomatin-domain protein essential for touch sensation in the mouse. *Nature, 445*, 206–209.

Yamashita, Y., Akaike, N., Wakamori, M., Ikeda, I., & Ogawa, H. (1992). Voltage-dependent currents in isolated single Merkel cells of rats. *Journal of Physiology, 450*, 143–162.

Yoder, B. K. (2007). Role of primary cilia in the pathogenesis of polycystic kidney disease. *Journal of the American Society of Nephrology, 18*, 1381–1388.

3

The Molecular and Genetic Basis of Touch

KATE POOLE, STEFAN G. LECHNER, AND GARY R. LEWIN

As we navigate the physical world, we rely on our senses to give us feedback about our environment. Specialized sensory systems transduce external stimuli into electrical impulses that are interpreted by the brain as specific modalities of sensory experience. The retina of the eye allows us to see; the cochlea of the ear detects compression waves within a given range, allowing us to hear; chemosensation by specialized epithelia is involved in gustation and olfaction; and the somatosensory system allows us to sense touch, temperature changes, and pain.

The somatosensory system is based on a network of specialized neurons that innervate glabrous and hairy skin. The somata of these cells are located in the dorsal root ganglia (DRG) and have a distinct pseudo-unipolar morphology. As shown in Figure 3.1, each cell has a single axon that bifurcates, with a distal process that innervates the skin and a proximal process that extends to the spinal cord and forms synapses in the dorsal horn. The population of the DRG neuronal cells is heterogeneous, with functional cell subsets of nociceptors (including high-threshold mechanoreceptors), thermoreceptors, and low-threshold mechanoreceptors. Specialized terminal endings of these neurons in the skin transduce mechanical stimuli into electrical signals above a certain threshold, leading to membrane depolarization, action potential initiation, and subsequent propagation to the spinal cord. Thus, our sense of touch requires a functional molecular mechanotransducer, proper innervation of the skin, action potential initiation and propagation, and ultimate integration of these signals. In terms of genetic disruption, then, there are many levels at which genetic mutation could perturb our sense of touch. As such, it is fascinating that there are no identified human genetic disorders that lead to a total attenuation of touch sensation from birth. Nor have any genetic

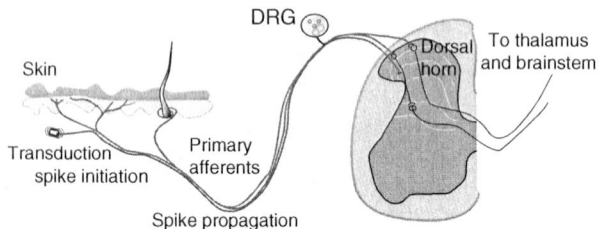

FIGURE 3.1 The cell bodies of mammalian somatosensory neurons lie in the DRG and have a single axonal process that bifurcates with the peripheral process innervating the skin and the proximal process forming synapses in the dorsal horn of the spinal cord. The transduction of touch stimuli by mechanoreceptive neurons occurs at the tips of the axonal processes in the skin, leading to spike initiation and propagation along the axonal process.

mutations that specifically affect touch been identified. However, genetic disorders with broader effects (including hypo- or hypersensitivity to touch), such as neurodegeneration or demyelination disorders, have been noted (for a recent review, see Tan & Katsanis, 2009). In comparison, genetic mutations that lead to deafness and blindness are well-known. In the somatosensory system, a SCN9A mutation causes a loss of function in $Na_v1.7$ (a voltage-gated sodium channel expressed in nociceptors) that results in a congenital insensitivity to pain (Cox et al., 2006). The fact that there are no congenital touch insensitivities known in newborns suggests that the sense of touch is so fundamental to our development and survival that a total, congenital loss of touch may be lethal before or around birth.

The lack of known mutations that specifically affect touch suggests that information on the molecules involved in mechanotransduction cannot be deduced easily from analysis of human disease mutations. However, there are various model organisms that are genetically manipulable and can be screened for defects in defined behavioral responses to touch stimuli, such as the nematode *Caenorhabditis elegans* and the fruit fly *Drosophila melanogaster*. Such an approach, starting with a phenotype (i.e., a behavioral response to touch) and then screening the progeny of mutagenized animals for changes in such behavior and subsequently isolating the gene responsible, is known as forward genetic screening. As a mammalian model, the mouse, *Mus musculus*, is not amenable to forward genetic screening, but using information derived from the other model organisms, genes in the mouse can be targeted for deletion or manipulation, an approach known as reverse genetics. Using these model organisms we can start to build a picture of molecules involved in the transduction of touch stimuli.

CHAPTER 3 THE MOLECULAR AND GENETIC BASIS OF TOUCH 61

In mammals, the structures of sensory endings that transduce mechanical stimuli have been well described, as has the nature of the nerves that transmit these signals to the central nervous system. However, the molecules responsible for the original transduction event have proved difficult to isolate and identify, in large part due to the inaccessibility of the relevant terminal endings of the sensory neurons and the presumed limited quantities of these molecules. This chapter will focus on knowledge that exists regarding the molecules of mechanotransduction, along with the genetic and molecular approaches used in their discovery. Research from model, multicellular organisms to mammals is examined.

MECHANOTRANSDUCTION: EXPERIMENTAL APPROACHES

When investigating touch sensation, there are many angles from which to study the problem. Touch sensation can be disrupted by mutations that affect the organism at different levels. Such perturbations can be experimentally addressed in three ways: (1) by monitoring transduction at the single-cell level, (2) by monitoring signal propagation along nerves, or (3) by monitoring touch-driven behavior at the organismal level. As touch sensation appears to be a fundamentally important process, there are likely multiple redundancies and, as such, an effect at the single-cell level may not be well reflected at the behavioral level.

To study mechanotransduction at the single-cell level, neuronal sensory cells are monitored by patch-clamp analysis during mechanical stimulation (see Figure 3.2). In the case of mammalian cells, this involves acute preparation of DRG neurons and the mechanical stimulation of either the soma or neurites in culture (Drew et al., 2004; Drew, Wood, & Cesare, 2002; Hu & Lewin, 2006) as both cell bodies and terminal endings of the sensory cells are largely inaccessible in situ.

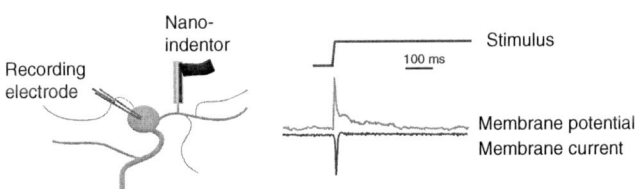

FIGURE 3.2 Whole-cell patch-clamp technique is used to investigate the transduction event in single DRG cells during fine mechanical stimulation. In mechanoreceptors, the stimulus leads to an RA membrane current and a concurrent change in membrane potential.

In the case of C. *elegans,* it is difficult to acutely prepare and culture cells, as the cells must be dissociated from the embryo and allowed to differentiate in culture (Bianchi & Driscoll, 2006). As an alternative, a technique has been developed in which the cuticle of the worm is slit open and the neuronal cell body patched in situ, while the side of the worm is mechanically stimulated (Goodman, Hall, Avery, & Lockery, 1998; O'Hagan, Chalfie, & Goodman, 2005). For *D. melanogaster,* the mechanoreceptor bristle is innervated by a single neuron which can be monitored with a recording electrode placed over the tip of a clipped hair shaft (Kernan, Cowan, & Zuker, 1994). Such single-cell studies allow direct detection of modulation of the transduction event, important for the identification of potential mechanosensitive channels.

In addition to studying mechanotransduction at the cellular level using patch-clamp recordings from cultured sensory neurons, extracellular recording techniques (such as ex-vivo skin-nerve preparation) are frequently used to study touch responses in mammals. Peripheral nerves (e.g., the saphenous nerve) are dissected together with their target tissue (hindlimb skin) and electrical activity in response to mechanical stimulation of the target tissue is recorded from single nerve fibers using extracellular electrodes (Figure 3.3). The skin-nerve technique can be used to study signal propagation along the nerve in mammals.

Finally, there are a number approaches to studying responses to touch stimuli at the behavioral level. In *C. elegans,* worms display distinct behavioral responses to mechanical stimulation, moving away from physical stimuli, with distinct responses to either harsh or gentle body touch. Adult *D. melanogaster* displays uncoordinated behavior when mechanotransduction is disrupted. Additionally, defined behavioral responses to touch have been used at the larval stage to identify touch-insensitive mutants (Kernan et al. 1994). Amongst mammals, mice have been shown to discriminate between differently sized grids

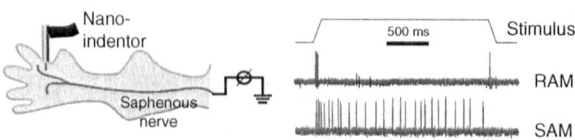

FIGURE 3.3 The in vitro skin-nerve technique can be used to monitor signal propagation in nerves in response to mechanical stimulation. RAM fibers respond during the dynamic phases of the stimulus, while SAM fibers continually fire spikes during the static phase of the stimulus.

CHAPTER 3 THE MOLECULAR AND GENETIC BASIS OF TOUCH

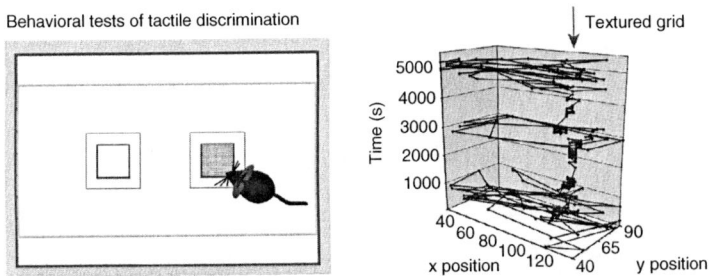

FIGURE 3.4 The grid test can be used to study tactile driven behavior in mice. The mouse is presented with two surfaces within a darkened box—smooth surface and textured grid. The movement of the mouse is monitored to analyze whether sensation of the textured grid leads to a longer, curiosity-driven dwell time. A representative trace of mouse movement over time is shown on the right, with the mouse spending more time on the textured test grid than in other regions of the box.

(Figure 3.4). When studying touch sensation in humans, psychophysical tests can be used to determine thresholds for vibration detection and discrimination of structures of different sizes. These defined behavioral responses allow one to determine whether a given gene is involved in touch sensation by screening mutants (whether generated by forward or reverse genetic techniques) and identifying those with an aberrant behavioral response to touch.

C. elegans AS A MODEL TO DEFINE TOUCH-RELATED GENES

Touch Responses in *C. elegans*

The nematode, *C. elegans*, displays well-defined responses to mechanical stimuli that can be described as four distinct behaviors: Response to nose touch, tap, harsh body touch, and gentle body touch. In addition to well-defined behavioral responses to touch, genes can be manipulated with mutagenic agents. Using these techniques, cell fate for all somatic cells has been described and a neural network map has been determined (White, Southgate, Thomson, & Brenner, 1986). These features have allowed comprehensive forward genetic screens to identify molecules involved in the mechanotransduction event underlying the gentle body-touch response, as well as gene products involved in regulating expression of these molecules and in the development of touch-responsive neurons (TRNs).

A set of six nonciliated TRNs (ALML, ALMR, AVM, PLML, PLMR, and PVM) that extend long processes, known as the microtubule cells, has been shown by laser ablation to be the gentle body-touch–sensitive neurons (Chalfie & Sulston, 1981). These cells display two unique features. The first is the presence of microtubules containing 15 protofilaments, as opposed to the 11 protofilament-containing microtubules found in other cell types (Chalfie & Thomson, 1982). The second is the presence of dense extracellular matrix structures between the TRN process and the cuticle (Chalfie et al., 1985). PVD neurons mediate harsh body touch and, as seen for the TRNs, extend long neurites. However, the neurons of the PVD cells branch to form an extensive dendritic network (Tsalik et al., 2003). Unlike the TRNs and PVD, the neurons responsible for response to nose touch (ASH, FLP, and OLQ) are ciliated (Way & Chalfie, 1989). These neurons innervate sensilla in the C. elegans nose. The ASH neuron has been shown to be polymodal, responding to mechanical stimuli, noxious chemicals (Kaplan & Horvitz, 1993), and high osmolarity (Bargmann, Thomas, & Horvitz, 1990).

Genes Involved in Response to Gentle Body Touch

Using multiple mutagenic methods, 421 touch-insensitive mutants have been generated, with the mutations falling into 18 complementation groups (Chalfie & Au, 1989; Chalfie & Sulston, 1981). These touch-insensitive mutants were selected on the basis of disruption of TRN-mediated behavioral responses to gentle body touch. Characterizing whether the mutations disrupted generation, specification, or only touch sensitivity allowed classification of these *mec* mutations into those required for development of the TRNs and those that do not disrupt the differentiation of touch cells but have a functional phenotype (Chalfie & Au, 1989). This latter phenotype would suggest that these mutations likely lie in genes required for the functional gentle body-touch response.

Genes Required for the Generation and Specification of Touch-Receptive Neurons

The initial screen for *mec* mutations identified *unc-86* as required for appropriate division of precursor cells leading to the generation of TRNs and *mec-3* as a transcription factor that specifies TRN cell fate after generation (Way & Chalfie, 1988, 1989). In *mec-3* mutants, the cells that would become the TRNs in the wild-type develop into neuronal cells, but lack features of wild-type touch-responsive cells, such as the 15-protofilament microtubules. The *unc-86* gene has an expression pattern broader than *mec-3* and is involved in both cell fate and the function of additional neuronal types, not just the TRNs. The finding that UNC-86 is present in both precursor cells and in TNRs in the adult worm (Finney & Ruvkun, 1990) suggested an additional function in touch sensation beyond the original generation of cells that develop into TRNs. In fact, UNC-86 is required for efficient expression of MEC-3-regulated genes. In the absence of UNC-86, MEC-3 binds only poorly and an UNC-86::MEC-3 heterooligomer has been shown to bind regulatory elements, controlling expression of various *mec* genes (Duggan, Ma, & Chalfie, 1998). The *mec-3* gene product is not restricted to the six TRNs required for response to gentle body touch but is also expressed in the FLP and PVD neurons (Way & Chalfie, 1989). In addition to being required for specification and maintenance of function of the TRNs, *mec-3* is also required for the FLP neuron to mediate the response to harsh body touch.

Genes Required for Transduction of Touch Stimuli

One fundamentally important observation about mechanotransduction in neurons is that the transduction event is extremely rapid (Hu & Lewin, 2006; Kernan et al., 1994), suggesting that the physical stimulus directly gates an ion channel rather than requiring a second messenger. This suggests that a mechanically gated ion channel, which opens in direct response to physical displacement of the transduction machinery, is most likely at the core of any mechanotransduction complex. The twelve *mec* genes that are downstream targets of *mec-3*, identified as those involved in the function of the touch-sensitive cells, indicate the existence of a complex transduction machinery, in which a channel may be necessary, but not sufficient, for the transduction of mechanical stimuli into an electrical signal. The *mec* genes include cytoskeletal components (*mec-7* and *mec-12*), extracellular proteins involved in mantle formation (*mec-1*, *mec-5*, and *mec-9*), membrane-associated proteins (*mec-2*), channel proteins from the Deg/ENaC family (*mec-4* and *mec-10*), and other *mec* genes of unknown function.

The *mec* genes have been identified on the basis of changed behavior in response to stimuli, but in order to determine whether a gene is required for mechanotransduction itself, responses to mechanical stimuli need to be studied at the level of transduction. In a heterologous system, *Xenopus laevis* oocytes, the constitutively active mutants of the MEC-4 protein mediated amiloride-sensitive sodium currents (Goodman et al., 2002). The MEC-10 protein can form a complex with MEC-4 in such a system but does not form channels on its own (Goodman et al., 2002). Studies indicate that the presence of either MEC-2 or MEC-6 in *X. laevis* oocytes lead to ~40-fold (Goodman et al., 2002) or ~30-fold increases (Chelur et al., 2002), respectively, in current mediated by the MEC-4/MEC-10 channel. While these findings suggest a complex with a Deg/ENaC channel at its core, modulated by interactions with MEC-2 and MEC-6, direct evidence for a role in mechanotransduction is still lacking.

By using a slit-worm preparation, cellular responses to mechanical stimuli can be monitored in vivo using the whole-cell patch-clamp technique. Null mutations in *mec-2*, *mec-4*, and *mec-6* all abolish mechanically responsive currents (MRCs; O'Hagan et al., 2005). In addition, a hypomorphic allele, *mec-4*(e1339), reduces but does not abolish the behavioral response to touch, leading to a reduction in peak current compared with the wild-type. Additional mutations in both *mec-4* and *mec-10* can change the ion selectivity of the channel (O'Hagan et al., 2005), supporting the hypothesis that MEC-4 and MEC-10 form the mechanosensitive channel complex.

The accessory proteins that are required for mechanotransduction, MEC-2 and MEC-6, are localized to puncta in the touch-sensitive cells that also contain MEC-4 (Zhang et al., 2004). Extracellular proteins, MEC-5 (the unique collagen found in the mantle of the microtubule cells), and MEC-1 (a protein with EGF and Kunitz-like domains) are also localized to these puncta, indicating that both extracellular and intracellular components are important for the formation of a functional mechanotransduction complex. The correct formation and localization of these puncta are dependent on multiple factors, including *mec-1*, *mec-5*, and *mec-9* (Emtage, Gu, Hartwieg, & Chalfie, 2004). Localization of MEC-4 and MEC-2 to such characteristic puncta is abolished by mutations in any one of *mec-1*, *mec-5*, or *mec-9*, and this localization of MEC-2 is also dependent on its conserved PHB domain and its ability to bind cholesterol (Huber et al., 2006).

Mutations in the *mec-7* and *mec-12* genes do not affect puncta formation, but can affect their distribution. Specifically, when the TRN-specific, 15-protofilament microtubules are disrupted, the localization of MEC-2 is more dispersed along the neuronal process (Bounoutas, O'Hagan, & Chalfie, 2009). Additionally, disruption of all microtubules in the TRNs leads to a stronger distribution phenotype with MEC-2 puncta found only in the proximal region of the neurite, as opposed to along its length. In a *mec-7* null mutation [*mec-7*(u142)], MEC-2 distribution is affected and MRCs are reduced but not abolished, suggesting that the 15-protofilament microtubules are not directly involved in channel gating (Bounoutas et al., 2009). The role of microtubules in mechanotransduction is not, however, merely due to an effect on the localization of the channel complex. A *mec-12* mutation, the *e1605* allele, did not affect the distribution of MEC-2, yet resulted in a significant reduction in MRC amplitude in these cells compared to the wild-type (Bounoutas et al., 2009). These data suggest multiple roles for microtubules in mechanotransduction (Bounoutas et al., 2009).

Lessons Learned From Identification of the *C. elegans mec* Genes

Clearly there is much information available, at the genetic level, about touch sensation in *C. elegans*. However, the precise role of all the components is still not clear. There is definitive evidence that a MEC-4/MEC-10 channel is the mechanosensitive channel (O'Hagan et al., 2005), but exactly how the additional MEC proteins interact and modulate the activity of this channel has not yet been described. Single-channel recordings have shown that the effect of MEC-6 and MEC-2 on the channel is to increase the number of channels in an active state, not the number of channels at the membrane or the open probability of these channels (Brown, Liao, & Goodman, 2008). How this effect is mediated, however, is unknown.

There are three basic models for the gating of mechanically responsive channels at cellular membranes: a membrane stretch model, a single-tether model, and a dual-tether model.

The first model suggests that stretch-induced rearrangements of negatively charged phosphate residues in the lipid bilayer cause conformational changes, and thus gating, of mechanotransduction ion channels. The latter models hypothesize that force is transduced via intracellular and/or extracellular protein tethers that directly link the channel to the cytoskeleton and/or the extracellular matrix, respectively. The bacterial mechanically sensitive channels, MscL and MscS, are activated by membrane stretch alone (Hase, Le Dain, & Martinac, 1995; Sukharev, Martinac, Arshavsky, & Kung, 1993). Such a gating mechanism is unlikely to underpin touch sensation in the worm, as the MEC-4/MEC-10 complex is not activated by membrane stretch in heterologous systems (Goodman et al., 2002), suggesting a reliance on accessory molecules. This is further supported by the fact that *mec* mutations occur in both intracellular and extracellular components. In a single-tether model, an extracellular tether transfers force from the extracellular matrix either to the membrane or to the channel itself. Finally, the dual-tether model proposes links not only between the cell and extracellular matrix, but also an additional intracellular tether that links the channel to the cytoskeleton. There is, as yet, no definitive evidence to describe whether touch in *C. elegans* follows a dual- or single-tether model, nor which of the *mec* genes specifically form any tether-like structures.

TOUCH SENSATION IN *D. melanogaster* AS A MODEL TO DEFINE TOUCH-RELATED GENES

The fruit fly, *D. melanogaster*, has been used in forward genetic screens to identify genes involved in mechanosensation, as this organism is also amenable to genetic manipulation (Kernan et al., 1994). In this case, the search for genes involved in mechanosensation is somewhat compounded by the fundamental reliance of this organism on the ability to detect mechanical stimuli, making most mutations in mechanosensation lethal in the adult (Kernan et al., 1994). Many behaviors displayed by *D. melanogaster* require mechanosensation, including walking, flight, a cleaning reflex in response to parasites, and behaviors that depend on auditory stimuli. Further, these behaviors are mediated by an array of different sensory organs.

Sensory Structures in *D. melanogaster*

There are two classes of neurons involved in mechanosensation in *D. melanogaster*: Type I, ciliated cells, and Type II, nonciliated cells. The Type II neurons are multidendritic neurons that are involved in sensing harsh touch and stretch of the muscles and viscera. The Type I ciliated cells are found in various sensory structures, such as the campaniform sensilla, the chordotonal organs, and the sensory bristles. The campaniform sensilla are flex sensors that detect indentation of the exoskeleton, whereas the chordotonal organs include a number of internal sensory structures that are involved in detection of stretch and of vibrations, including vibration from auditory stimuli.

The sensory bristles are involved in detecting touch and are the most abundant sensory structures on adult *D. melanogaster*. Each mechanoreceptive bristle shaft is innervated by a single Type I neuron, surrounded by four accessory cells. The endolymph in which these cells are bathed has characteristic high K^+, low Ca^{++} concentrations (Grunert & Gnatzy, 1987). When the bristle is displaced, there is an influx of K^+ ions, presumably from the opening of cation channels, leading to depolarization. Intracellular electrophysiological recordings have not been performed, but, as each bristle is innervated by an individual neuron single cell, depolarization can be monitored by placing an electrode over the clipped end of a bristle shaft and recording from the extracellular endolymph (Corfas & Dudai, 1990; Kernan et al., 1994; Walker, Willingham, & Zuker, 2000). The depolarization in response to mechanical stimulation of the bristle has a latency of around 200 μs, too fast to be explained by a second messenger cascade (Walker et al., 2000). Thus, in *D. melanogaster*, as in *C. elegans*, mechanotransduction likely involves direct mechanical gating of ion channels.

Genes Involved in Touch

As the *D. melanogaster* larvae also display defined behavioral responses to touch, they have been used to screen for mutations affecting this behavior, thus avoiding complications arising from lethality. In the research of Kernan et al. (1994), mutations identified in the larval stage that led to a severe uncoordinated phenotype in the adult, *uncoordinated* (*unc*) and *uncoordinated-like* (*uncl*), were identified, as well as *touch-insensitive larva A-D* (*tilA-D*) mutations. The uncoordinated phenotype of the *unc* and *uncl* mutants was lethal in the adult. To study the effect of these mutations on sensory transduction, the investigators created mosaic animals containing patches of marked, mutant tissue. These otherwise wild-type animals no longer exhibited lethal uncoordination. In patches containing mutations in *unc* or *uncl*, the morphology of the sensory bristles was normal; however, any legs included in a patch of mutant tissue displayed uncoordination. The direct measurement of mechanoreceptor potential (MRP) from mutant bristles showed that the MRP response was absent in *unc* mutants and reduced in *uncl* mutants. This correlation between an effect on mechanotransduction in the sensory bristle and severe uncoordination in the adult led to a second screen for mutations and identification of an adult uncoordinated phenotype. Mutants were then analyzed using electrophysiology to identify mutations that led to the reduction or abolition of the MRC in sensory bristles. This second screen identified three mutant loci, named *no mechanoreceptor potential A, B,* and *C* (*nompA, nompB,* and *nompC,* respectively), that showed almost complete loss of MRCs (Kernan et al., 1994). These findings regarding genetic mutations affecting touch in uncoordinated flies are consistent with knowledge that sensory feedback via mechanoreceptors is essential for the proper coordination of movement. The *nompA*, *nompB*, *nompC*, and *unc* mutants have all been molecularly characterized. Further investigation of different *nompC* mutants showed that three alleles (*nompC^1*, *nompC^2*, and *nompC^3*) led to severe uncoordination coupled with a loss of MRCs (Walker et al., 2000). A fourth allele (*nompC^4*) led to clumsiness in the adult. The *nompC^4* allele does not affect the amplitude of the MRC, but it significantly reduces the inactivation time constant, leading to a faster decay of the MRP and a subsequent decrease in the number of action potentials generated.

NOMPC and other TRP family channels. NOMPC is an ion channel with similarities to the TRPN family of ion channels. The NOMPC protein also contains 29 ankyrin (ANK) repeats that could indicate an interaction with the cytoskeleton and have been proposed to act as a gating spring (Howard & Bechstedt, 2004). The fact that *nompC* null mutations do not completely abolish the MRC (Walker et al., 2000) suggests that there are redundant channels that also transduce mechanical signals, that NOMPC is not itself a mechanotransducer but modulates the activity of such a channel, or that NOMPC forms heteromers with an additional channel subunit that retains some activity in the absence of NOMPC. NOMPC has also been shown to have a role in transducing auditory stimuli in Johnston's organ, but again in *nompC* mutants the response to auditory stimuli is reduced, not abolished, implicating an additional channel required for hearing in *D. melanogaster* (Eberl, Hardy, & Kernan, 2000). There are two additional transient receptor potential (TRP) channels, from the TRPV family, in *D. melanogaster*: Nanchung (NAN) and Inactive (IAV). Both *nan* and *iav* mutants display mild uncoordination and reduced locomotion, and both mutants are deaf (Gong et al., 2004; Kim et al., 2003). The NAN and IAV proteins form a complex, and correct localization to the cilia of these proteins is interdependent. In both *nan* and *iav* mutants, sound-evoked potentials are absent, which originally suggested a fundamental role in the mechanotransduction complex that mediates hearing in *D. melanogaster* (Gong et al., 2004; Kim et al., 2003). However, further studies have shown that in *nan* and *iav* mutants there are self-sustained oscillations of the antennae, presumably from excessive mechanical feedback, suggesting a role in controlling mechanical amplification rather than in the original transduction event (Gopfert, Albert, Nadrowski, & Kamikouchi, 2006).

The NOMPA and NOMPB proteins. In *nompA* mutants, the sensory endings of the Type I, ciliated neurons fail to attach to the dendritic cap. NOMPA is a large, extracellular protein produced by the support cells that surround the neuron. Using a GFP-NOMPA fusion protein, it was shown that the extracellular region of the protein localizes to the extracellular matrix of the dendritic cap that forms physical links to the sensory process (Chung, Zhu, Han, & Kernan, 2001). As seen in C. elegans, there seems to be a requirement for contacts between the extracellular matrix and touch-responsive cells for efficient mechanotransduction.

The NOMPB protein is required for proper assembly of cilia in both mechanosensory and olfactory neurons (Han, Kwok, & Kernan, 2003). Interestingly, *unc* also encodes a protein involved in the assembly of sensory cilia, but is required for flagella formation in sperm cells as well (Baker, Adhikarakunnathu, & Kernan, 2004). The expression pattern of *nompB* suggests that it is specifically involved in cilia formation in Type I neurons as it is not expressed in other cell types and that the protein localizes to sensory cilia and around basal bodies.

Common Features of Mechanotransduction in *C. elegans* and *D. melanogaster*

The screening of randomly generated mutants in *C. elegans* and *D. melanogaster* for mechanosensory defects has led to the description of putative components of mechanosensory complexes. The proteins identified as important for the transduction event in *C. elegans* are not homologous to those found in *D. melanogaster*. However, the proteins predicted to be involved do share some properties. Firstly, transduction latencies suggest a channel complex that is directly gated by mechanical forces, not a reliance on a second messenger. There is also a requirement in both systems for contacts between the neuronal cells that respond to touch and elements of the extracellular matrix. In *C. elegans*, there are membrane-associated factors and cytoskeletal factors which modulate transduction. In *D. melanogaster*, it is not yet clear if NOMPC is the mechanosensitive channel or an accessory protein, but the presence of 29 ANK repeats suggests an interaction with the cytoskeleton. As mammals are not suited to use in forward genetic screens, the information derived from such model organisms provides a starting point to use direct mutagenesis in mice to search for homologous genes that are involved in mechanotransduction in mammals.

TOUCH SENSATION IN MICE: A MODEL FOR UNDERSTANDING MAMMALIAN TOUCH

Mice have a somatosensory system which is almost identical to that of humans and so the identification of transduction molecules in this species will have a direct impact on our understanding of human touch. In vertebrates, the sensation of touch is mediated by sensory neurons that reside in the trigeminal ganglia and the DRG, which extend peripheral axons that innervate the skin. These sensory neurons can broadly be divided into low-threshold mechanoreceptors, specialized to detect touch modalities such as vibration or light indentation of the skin, and nociceptors, which detect noxious or potentially harmful stimuli. Touch perception is a multistep process that begins at the peripheral nerve terminals of sensory neurons, where indentation of the skin activates mechanically gated ion channels that convert mechanical forces into receptor potentials. The next step is action potential initiation and propagation to the spinal cord, shown earlier in Figure 3.1. The final step is the central processing in sensory cortices and higher brain regions. Thus, when studying the role of a given gene in touch perception, a combination of experimental techniques that complement one another and allow insights at all the different levels of information processing is employed.

A behavioral assay that is frequently used to investigate the effects of genetic manipulations on acute mechanosensitivity at the level of the whole organism is the von Frey test. For this test, a series of von Frey filaments (polyester fibers of varying stiffness which deliver a fixed amount of force) are presented perpendicular to the paw to determine the minimal force required to elicit a paw withdrawal reflex. However, all subsets of mechanoreceptors are potentially activated using this method, and so caution is necessary when interpreting results with respect to touch receptor sensitivity. Another test that is used to assess tactile acuity is the so-called grid test, which has only recently been developed (Wetzel et al., 2007). In this test, mice are presented with a smooth and a textured surface cue placed in the floor of a completely darkened arena and the time spent on either of the surfaces is measured. As noted earlier (see Figure 3.4), wild-type mice spend significantly more time on a textured surface than on a smooth surface. However, mice with impaired tactile acuity show no preference for either surface (Wetzel et al., 2007).

A more direct approach to study the functionality of different subsets of mechanoreceptors is to use the in vitro skin-nerve technique. Here, the saphenous nerve and the hind limb skin are placed in an organ bath and action potentials, evoked by mechanical stimulation of the skin, are recorded from single-nerve fibers teased apart from the nerve bundle (Koltzenburg, Stucky, & Lewin, 1997). With this technique a qualitative and quantitative characterization of mechanoreceptors is possible and different subtypes, such as rapidly adapting (RA) mechanoreceptors (RAMs), slowly adapting (SA) mechanoreceptors

CHAPTER 3   THE MOLECULAR AND GENETIC BASIS OF TOUCH

(SAMs), and D-hair mechanoreceptors, can easily be distinguished by means of their firing patterns, force sensitivities, and fiber conduction velocities. However, despite the many advantages of this technique, one major drawback is that the actual mechanotransduction current that triggers action potential generation is not recorded. Thus, altered response properties of primary afferents observed in genetically modified mice can either result from changes in the overall excitability or from altered mechanotransduction currents.

Consequently, researchers have used cultures of dissociated DRG neurons as a model system to measure these currents. Mechanical stimulation of neurites (Hu, Chiang, Koch, & Lewin, 2010; Hu & Lewin, 2006) and the cell somata (Drew et al., 2002; Lechner, Frenzel, Wang, & Lewin, 2009; Lechner & Lewin, 2009) of cultured sensory neurons evokes different types of mechanically gated currents in different subsets of neurons. Putative low-threshold mechanoreceptive neurons (large diameter cells with narrow action potentials) typically respond with a so-called RA current that activates within less than a millisecond after the onset of the mechanical stimulus. This current is also found in a subpopulation of nociceptors. Other nociceptors, however, exhibit intermediately adapting (IA) and SA currents. There is now compelling evidence, both genetic and pharmacological, that these currents are required for normal mechanotransduction in vivo (Drew et al., 2007; Lechner et al., 2009; Wetzel et al., 2007), and thus identifying the ion channels that mediate mechanically gated currents has become a focus in attempts to unravel the molecular nature of the mammalian mechanotransducer.

Genes Involved in Mechanotransduction

Despite the wealth of information available on touch genes in model organisms discussed earlier in this chapter (*C. elegans* and *D. melanogaster*), little is known about the molecular mechanisms underlying mechanotransduction at the nerve endings of mouse sensory neurons. One reason is that high-throughput genetic approaches that would allow the screening for genes involved in mechanotransduction are not available for mice. Moreover, most naturally occurring mutations that alter touch perception affect processes downstream from the initial transduction event and thus do not provide an indication of which proteins may be involved in mechanotransduction in mammals (Tan & Katsanis, 2009). As a result, most studies have focused on the role of mammalian homologs of genes shown to be involved in mechanotransduction in model organisms. This approach seems warranted based on physiological similarities between touch responses in *C. elegans* and those in the mouse. An example of these similarities is shown in the recordings of stimulus response at the bottom of Figure 3.5 although methods for obtaining these responses differ. In *C. elegans* the TRNs are monitored in situ, using the slit worm preparation. Inward sodium currents are observed on both the application and removal of a mechanical stimulus. These currents lead to a change in membrane potential. Mechanosensitive neurons from the mouse cannot be accessed in situ. However, acutely dissociated cells cultured on laminin retain a mechanosensitive response. Low-threshold mechanoreceptors from the mouse will also respond to both application and removal of physical stimuli with a sodium current.

MEC gene homologs. The ASIC family of ion channels appeared promising candidates as mechanotransduction ion channels, since they are widely expressed in sensory neurons and are members of the Deg/ENaC sodium channel superfamily (Waldmann & Lazdunski, 1998). This family includes the putative pore-forming subunits of the *C. elegans* mechanotransduction complex, MEC-4 and MEC-10 (Chelur et al.,

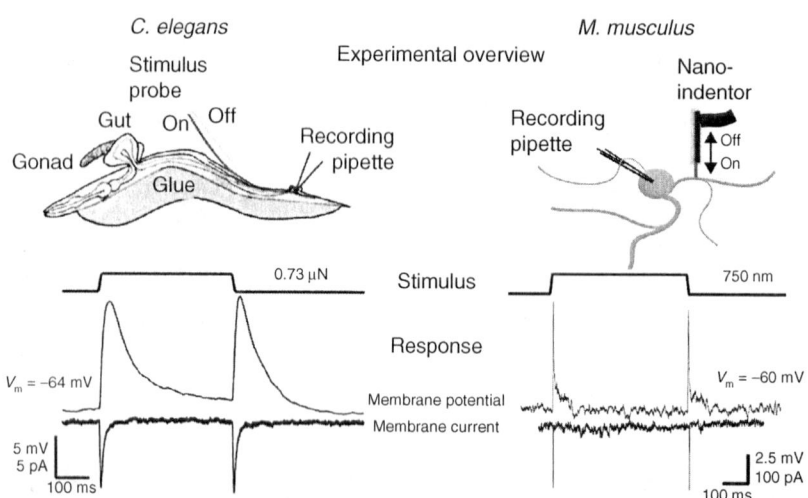

FIGURE 3.5 A comparison of responses to mechanical stimuli in *C. elegans* (left panel) and *M. musculus* (mouse, right panel). Left panel adapted with permission from "The MEC-4 DEG/ENaC channel of *Caenorhabditis elegans* touch receptor neurons tranduces mechanical signals," by R. O'Hagan, M. Chalfie, & M. Goodman, 2005, *Nature Neuroscience*, 8, 43–50. Copyright 2004 by Nature Publishing Group.

2002; Lai, Hong, Kinnell, Chalfie, & Driscoll, 1996). In mouse DRGs, expression of ASIC2 is enriched in large-diameter neurons (i.e., in putative low-threshold mechanoreceptors). In accordance with this, electrophysiological recordings from single primary afferents indicate that the sensitivity of RAMs, but not that of other cutaneous mechanoreceptors, is substantially reduced in mice lacking ASIC2 (Price et al., 2000). By contrast, deletion of ASIC3 resulted in increased sensitivity of RAMs and in reduced mechanosensitivity of thinly myelinated Aδ nociceptors (Price et al., 2001). Subsequent studies have focused on the effect of ASIC gene deletion on mechanically gated transduction currents recorded from dissociated sensory neurons using the patch-clamp technique. Interestingly, neither single mutants of ASIC2 or ASIC3 nor double mutants of ASIC2 or ASIC3 displayed changes in their mechanotransduction currents (Drew et al., 2004; Lechner et al., 2009). These results indicate that ASIC channels are not part of the primary mechanotransduction complex but rather play a modulatory role. This is supported by electrophysiology data that show that benzamil, which blocks Deg/ENaC currents underlying touch sensation, does not inhibit the RA current in low-threshold mechanoreceptors in acute culture, but it does increase the latency of current activation (Hu & Lewin, 2006). Benzamil will block mechanosensation in an ASIC2- or ASIC3-dependent manner in certain visceral afferents, suggesting that these channels do play a role in mechanotransduction in mammals, not just in mechanotransduction underlying touch sensation (Page, Brierley, Martin, Hughes, & Blackshaw, 2007).

Another *mec* gene whose homologs have been studied in great detail is *mec-2*. The *mec-2* gene encodes a membrane protein with a stomatin homology domain which is also found in a large family of mammalian genes (Green & Young, 2008). Mice lacking the founding member of this gene family—stomatin—show significantly reduced mechanical sensitivity in D-hair low-threshold mechanoreceptors (Martinez-Salgado et al., 2007). However, a more striking phenotype has been observed in mice lacking stomatin-like protein 3 (*slp3*). A complete loss of mechanosensitivity in ~40% of all Aβ and Aδ fibers is observed in *slp3* mutants, as shown using single fiber recordings from the skin-nerve preparation. Consistent with this observation, 40% of all sensory neurons lack a mechanically gated current in patch-clamp recordings made from acutely cultured DRG neurons (Wetzel et al., 2007). Furthermore, *slp3* mutant mice lose the ability to recognize fine textured floor gratings (<500 μm) in the grid test for tactile acuity. Together, these findings strongly suggest that SLP3 is an essential component of the mechanotransduction complex in a subset of cutaneous mechanoreceptors.

Transient receptor potential channels. In addition to *mec* genes, members of the TRP ion channel family have been consistently found to play crucial roles in invertebrate mechanotransduction (Christensen & Corey, 2007). As previously described, NOMPC has been identified as a candidate mechanotransducer in the *D. melanogaster* sensory bristles (Kernan et al., 1994). A NOMPC homolog (TRPA1) has also been identified in the vertebrate zebrafish and was originally reported to be involved in mechanotransduction in sensory hair cells (Sidi, Friedrich, & Nicolson, 2003) based on studies in morpholinos. However, subsequent analysis of *trpa1* zebrafish mutants revealed that such channels are required for chemosensation but are not involved in mechanotransduction (Prober et al., 2008). Several mammalian TRPs were shown to be directly gated by membrane stretch or cell swelling (Clapham, Julius, Montell, & Schultz, 2005), but there is still only little evidence for a possible role of these channels in mechanotransduction events that underlie touch sensation.

At first glance, TRPA1 seemed to be a good candidate as a mechanotransducer for several reasons. First, TRPA1 is a homolog of the Drosophila TRPA channel PAINLESS, which is required for the detection of painful mechanical stimuli in *D. melanogaster* (Tracey, Wilson, Laurent, & Benzer, 2003). It is also the only mammalian TRP channel that contains N-terminal ANK repeats, which have been proposed to act as gating springs in the mechanotransduction channel NOMPC (Howard & Bechstedt, 2004). Moreover, TRPA1 is widely expressed in the DRG in nociceptors. However, initial behavioral studies assessing acute mechanosensitivity in TRPA1-deficient mice using von Frey filaments gave rather conflicting results. While one study showed no differences in paw withdrawal thresholds (Bautista et al., 2006), two other studies reported reduced von Frey thresholds in TRPA1 mutant mice (Kwan et al., 2006; Petrus et al., 2007). Recently, Stucky and colleagues directly investigated the possible role of TRPA1 in mechanotransduction using the in vitro skin-nerve preparation (Kwan, Glazer, Corey, Rice, & Stucky, 2009). They showed that the response properties of both nociceptors and mechanoreceptors are altered in TRPA1-deficient mice, though in contrary ways; while nociceptors and SAMs are less sensitive to mechanical stimulation, RAMs display increased mechanosensitivity. However, researchers also found TRPA1 to be expressed in cells that are in close contact with the sensory nerve endings such as epidermal and hair follicle keratinocytes, indicating a possible modulatory role of TRPA1. Further studies using cell-type-specific *trpA1* knockout mice will be necessary to reveal the exact function of TRPA1 in touch sensation.

Another TRP channel that was originally proposed to function in mechanotransduction is TRPV4. Mouse TRPV4 is activated by cell swelling and can restore mechanoreceptor function in *C. elegans osm-9* mutants (Liedtke & Friedman, 2003). However, disrupting TRPV4 expression in mice has only modest effects on acute mechanosensation as measured with behavioral assays (Liedtke & Friedman, 2003; Suzuki, Mizuno, Kodaira, & Imai, 2003). Additionally, available data show that there is no change in the baseline mechanical threshold of sensory afferent fibers in TRPV4 knockout mice as measured with the skin-nerve technique (Chen, Alessandri-Haber, & Levine, 2007).

In summary, there is some evidence that links individual TRP genes with pain and mechanosensory behavior, but there remains very little direct evidence that TRP channels directly participate in the transduction of mechanical stimuli by any mammalian sensory cells. TRPs are commonly activated by intracellular signaling pathways like phosphorylation and intracellular ions like Ca^{2+}, and many of the phenotypes may be explained by this type of mechanism.

Alternative Approaches for the Identification of Mammalian Genes Involved in Touch

The studies discussed so far clearly show that trying to unravel the molecular basis of mechanotransduction by simply looking at mammalian homologs of invertebrate mechanotransduction genes has hardly been crowned with success. Moreover, these studies suggest that we should move beyond focusing on Deg/ENaCs and TRP channels in the pursuit of the mechanotransduction channel. But what should be the focus of future research in the field if we are to fully understand the genes and molecules required for mechanosensory transduction and touch sensation in mammals?

Lessons Learned From Development

An approach that has the potential to provide insights into the molecular mechanisms underlying mammalian mechanotransduction is to study developmental mutants that lack specific subsets of sensory neurons or that lack a specific functional property, such as mechanosensitivity. To generate such mutants, one requires a detailed knowledge of the timing and the genetic control of the developmental acquisition of mechanosensitivity.

Electrophysiological studies in rat and chick embryos indicate that functional mechanoreceptors are already present shortly before birth or hatching (Fitzgerald, 1987). However, because of methodological limitations, only late embryonic stages could be tested in these studies. Until recently, it was still unclear precisely when functional maturation of mechanoreceptors occurs. We have addressed this fundamental question by investigating the developmental emergence of mechanically gated currents, using the patch-clamp technique, in DRG neurons isolated from different embryonic stages (Lechner et al., 2009). We have shown that mechanosensitivity emerges in three distinct waves during embryonic and postnatal development. First, low-threshold mechanoreceptors, characterized by the expression of the neurotrophin receptors TrkB and/or TrkC, become mechanosensitive, acquiring an RA current (E13.5). Second, nociceptors express the nerve growth factor (NGF) receptor TrkA, in which RA currents emerge around E15.5. Interestingly, nociceptor-specific SA currents only emerge after birth in a significant proportion of neurons (P0). The first wave of mechanosensitivity acquisition occurs independent of neurotrophic support, but the acquisition of RA currents in nociceptors is strictly dependent on target-derived NGF. E12.5 sensory neurons that lack the proapoptotic regulator BAX (these cells survive in the absence of neurotrophic factors) never acquire an RA current when cultured in the absence of NGF but become mechanosensitive within 24 hours when the growth medium is supplemented with NGF.

Thus, ion channels that are required for mechanotransduction should be expressed in DRG neurons taken from E13.5 or older embryos and in E12.5 Bax–/– cultures treated with NGF, but should be absent in sensory neurons from E11.5 to E12.5 DRGs and in E12.5 Bax–/– cultures treated with anti-NGF. Interestingly, only a few members of the TRP– and Deg/ENaC channel families, including ASIC2b, ASIC3, TRPV1, TRPM8, and TRPC4, showed expression profiles that correlated with the presence or absence of mechanotransduction. However, mice lacking these genes have a normal mechanotransduction current. These findings strongly suggest that we should extend our search for transduction ion channels beyond TRP- and Deg/ENaC-channels.

Mammalian Touch Requires a Tether

As mentioned earlier in this review, it has been proposed that mechanosensitive channels may be opened either by membrane stretch or by a tether protein (Gillespie & Walker, 2001). We have recently tested whether mammalian mechanoreceptors that mediate touch

CHAPTER 3 THE MOLECULAR AND GENETIC BASIS OF TOUCH

require an extracellular tether. Our research indicates that the RA mechanosensitive current in touch sensory neurons from mice is only observed when a highly distinctive extracellular protein is present. This tether protein, visualized with transmission electron microscopy, forms characteristic protein filaments with a length of 100 nm. These tethers attach sensory neuronal membranes to a laminin-containing matrix (Hu et al., 2010). By ablating this link with specific enzymes that cut only a limited set of amino acid sequences, mechanosensitive currents were immediately abolished. The mechanosensitive current always reappeared when the tether was resynthesized by sensory neurons. Using similar site-specific enzymes, in vivo mechanoreceptor responses were completely abolished without affecting the electrical excitability of sensory receptors (Hu et al., 2010). We postulate that the large protein tether that we have visualized is required to transfer force directly from the extracellular matrix, around the mechanoreceptor ending in the skin, to the channel complex (see Figure 3.6). Major efforts are being made in our lab to identify the molecular nature of this tether, which may represent a molecular target to directly manipulate touch in mammals, including humans. Moreover, if the "touch tether" is attached directly to the channel, then molecular characterization of the complex may be facilitated by its identification.

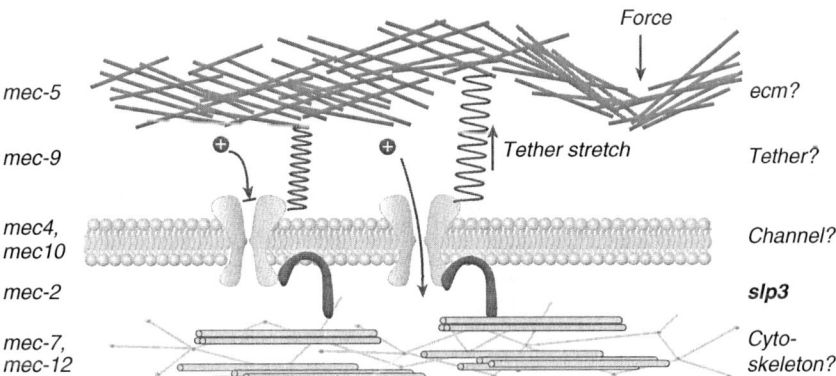

FIGURE 3.6 Model of the mechanotransduction protein complex. The pore-forming channel subunits (*mec-4* and *mec-10* in C. elegans, currently unidentified in mammals) are connected to components of the extracellular matrix (*mec-5*) by a molecular tether. On the intracellular side, the channel subunits interact with *mec-2* and *slp3*, respectively, which may link the channel to the cytoskeleton. It is thought that compression of the skin causes stretch of the tether, which leads to the opening of the mechanosensitive ion channel.

Implications for Human Touch

There are exciting times ahead in the molecular dissection of touch since, for the first time, researchers are beginning to identify directly the molecular players for transduction in mammals. The field of mechanosensation has been marked by a constant exchange of ideas and has identified molecules between different model organisms as varied as *D. melanogaster*, *C. elegans*, and *M. musculus*. It is clear that without the genetic information from these classical model systems the identification of molecules involved in human touch would be much more difficult. Any or all of the human genes that encode proteins involved in mechanosensory transduction may carry mutations or sequence variations that have quantitative influence on touch traits in humans.

As noted in this review, some proteins, like SLP3, appear to be necessary for touch receptor function in mice. However, mice lacking this protein are viable, presumably because not all touch receptors require the protein. Nevertheless, mice lacking SLP3 show severe behavioral deficits in their ability to discriminate tactile surfaces. Thus, it is conceivable that some people may carry severe mutations in the human *slp3* gene but do not present clinically relevant symptoms. Bearing in mind that fruit flies with mild deficits in touch receptors are uncoordinated, it is plausible that human individuals with similar genetic deficits are simply an order of magnitude clumsier than the average individual. We believe that ablation of genes that are even more central to the mechanotransduction process, for example, genes that encode the as-yet undiscovered ion channel, might not be compatible with survival until term in humans. It is striking in this regard that the mechanotransduction process in touch receptors has been shown by our research team to mature very early during embryonic development. Therefore, a complete loss of function in these touch neurons may have dire consequences for normal in utero development of human preterm infants. Research in the next few years will surely reveal the degree to which these speculations are true regarding the relevance of our molecular discoveries to human touch.

REFERENCES

Baker, J. D., Adhikarakunnathu, S., & Kernan, M. J. (2004). Mechanosensory-defective, male-sterile unc mutants identify a novel basal body protein required for ciliogenesis in Drosophila. *Development, 131,* 3411–3422.

Bargmann, C. I., Thomas, J. H., & Horvitz, H. R. (1990). Chemosensory cell function in the behavior and development of *Caenorhabditis elegans*. *Cold Spring Harbor Symposia on Quantitative Biology, 55,* 529–538.

Bautista, D. M., Jordt, S. E., Nikai, T., Tsuruda, P. R., Read, A. J., Poblete, J., ... Julius, D. (2006). TRPA1 mediates the inflammatory actions of environmental irritants and proalgesic agents. *Cell, 124,* 1269–1282.

Bianchi, L., & Driscoll, M. (2006). Culture of embryonic *C. elegans* cells for electrophysiological and pharmacological analyses. *WormBook,* 1–15.

Bounoutas, A., O'Hagan, R., & Chalfie, M. (2009). The multipurpose 15-protofilament microtubules in *C. elegans* have specific roles in mechanosensation. *Current Biology, 19,* 1362–1367.

Brown, A. L., Liao, Z., & Goodman, M. B. (2008). MEC-2 and MEC-6 in the *Caenorhabditis elegans* sensory mechanotransduction complex: Auxiliary subunits that enable channel activity. *Journal of General Physiology, 131,* 605–616.

Chalfie, M., & Au, M. (1989). Genetic control of differentiation of the *Caenorhabditis elegans* touch receptor neurons. *Science, 243,* 1027–1033.

Chalfie, M., & Sulston, J. (1981). Developmental genetics of the mechanosensory neurons of *Caenorhabditis elegans*. *Developmental Biology, 82,* 358–370.

Chalfie, M., Sulston, J. E., White, J. G., Southgate, E., Thomson, J. N., & Brenner, S. (1985). The neural circuit for touch sensitivity in *Caenorhabditis elegans*. *The Journal of Neuroscience, 5,* 956–964.

Chalfie, M., & Thomson, J. N. (1982). Structural and functional diversity in the neuronal microtubules of *Caenorhabditis elegans*. *Journal of Cell Biology, 93,* 15–23.

Chelur, D. S., Ernstrom, G. G., Goodman, M. B., Yao, C. A., Chen, L., O'Hagen, R., & Chalfie, M. (2002). The mechanosensory protein MEC-6 is a subunit of the *C. elegans* touch-cell degenerin channel. *Nature, 420,* 669–673.

Chen, X., Alessandri-Haber, N., & Levine, J. D. (2007). Marked attenuation of inflammatory mediator-induced C-fiber sensitization for mechanical and hypotonic stimuli in TRPV4−/− mice. *Molecular Pain, 3,* 31.

Christensen, A. P., & Corey, D. P. (2007). TRP channels in mechanosensation: Direct or indirect activation? *Nature Reviews, Neuroscience, 8,* 510–521.

Chung, Y. D., Zhu, J., Han, Y., & Kernan, M. J. (2001). nompA encodes a PNS-specific, ZP domain protein required to connect mechanosensory dendrites to sensory structures. *Neuron, 29,* 415–428.

Clapham, D. E., Julius, D., Montell, C., & Schultz, G. (2005). International Union of Pharmacology. XLIX. Nomenclature and structure-function relationships of transient receptor potential channels. *Pharmacological Reviews, 57,* 427–450.

Corfas, G., & Dudai, Y. (1990). Adaptation and fatigue of a mechanosensory neuron in wild-type Drosophila and in memory mutants. *The Journal of Neuroscience, 10,* 491–499.

Cox, J. J., Reimann, F., Nicholas, A. K., Thornton, G., Roberts, E., Springell, K., ... Woods, C. G. (2006). An SCN9A channelopathy causes congenital inability to experience pain. *Nature, 444,* 894–898.

Drew, L. J., Rohrer, D. K., Price, M. P., Blaver, K. E., Cockayne, D. A., Cesare, P., ... Wood, J. N. (2004). Acid-sensing ion channels ASIC2 and ASIC3 do not contribute to mechanically activated currents in mammalian sensory neurones. *The Journal of Physiology, 556,* 691–710.

Drew, L. J., Rugiero, F., Cesare, P., Gale, J. E., Abrahamsen, B., Bowden, S.,... Wood, J. N. (2007). High-threshold mechanosensitive ion channels blocked by a novel conopeptide mediate pressure-evoked pain. *PLoS One, 2*, e515.

Drew, L. J., Wood, J. N., & Cesare, P. (2002). Distinct mechanosensitive properties of capsaicin-sensitive and -insensitive sensory neurons. *The Journal of Neuroscience, 22*, RC228.

Duggan, A., Ma, C., & Chalfie, M. (1998). Regulation of touch receptor differentiation by the *Caenorhabditis elegans* mec-3 and unc-86 genes. *Development, 125*, 4107–4119.

Eberl, D. F., Hardy, R. W., & Kernan, M. J. (2000). Genetically similar transduction mechanisms for touch and hearing in Drosophila. *The Journal of Neuroscience, 20*, 5981–5988.

Emtage, L., Gu, G., Hartwieg, E., & Chalfie, M. (2004). Extracellular proteins organize the mechanosensory channel complex in *C. elegans* touch receptor neurons. *Neuron, 44*, 795–807.

Finney, M., & Ruvkun, G. (1990). The unc-86 gene product couples cell lineage and cell identity in *C. elegans*. *Cell, 63*, 895–905.

Fitzgerald, M. (1987). Spontaneous and evoked activity of fetal primary afferents in vivo. *Nature, 326*, 603–605.

Gillespie, P. G., & Walker, R. G. (2001). Molecular basis of mechanosensory transduction. *Nature, 413*, 194–202.

Gong, Z., Son, W., Chung, Y. D., Kim, J., Shin, D. W., McClung, C. A.,... Kim C. (2004). Two interdependent TRPV channel subunits, inactive and Nanchung, mediate hearing in Drosophila. *The Journal of Neuroscience, 24*, 9059–9066.

Goodman, M. B., Ernstrom, G. G., Chelur, D. S., O'Hagan, R., Yao, C. A., & Chalfie, M. (2002). MEC-2 regulates *C. elegans* DEG/ENaC channels needed for mechanosensation. *Nature, 415*, 1039–1042.

Goodman, M. B., Hall, D. H., Avery, L., & Lockery, S. R. (1998). Active currents regulate sensitivity and dynamic range in *C. elegans* neurons. *Neuron, 20*, 763–772.

Gopfert, M. C., Albert, J. T., Nadrowski, B., & Kamikouchi, A. (2006). Specification of auditory sensitivity by Drosophila TRP channels. *Nature Neuroscience, 9*, 999–1000.

Green, J. B., & Young, J. P. (2008). Slipins: Ancient origin, duplication and diversification of the stomatin protein family. *BMC Evolutionary Biology, 8*, 44.

Grunert, U., & Gnatzy, W. (1987). K^+ and Ca^{++} in the receptor lymph of arthropod cuticular mechanoreceptors. *Journal of Comparative Physiology, A, 161*, 329–333.

Han, Y. G., Kwok, B. H., & Kernan, M. J. (2003). Intraflagellar transport is required in Drosophila to differentiate sensory cilia but not sperm. *Current Biology, 13*, 1679–1686.

Hase, C. C., Le Dain, A. C., & Martinac, B. (1995). Purification and functional reconstitution of the recombinant large mechanosensitive ion channel (MscL) of *Escherichia coli*. *Journal of Biological Chemistry, 270*, 18329–18334.

Howard, J., & Bechstedt, S. (2004). Hypothesis: A helix of ankyrin repeats of the NOMPC-TRP ion channel is the gating spring of mechanoreceptors. *Current Biology, 14*, R224–226.

Hu, J., Chiang, L. Y., Koch, M., & Lewin, G. R. (2010). Evidence for a protein tether involved in somatic touch. *EMBO Journal, 29*, 855–867.

Hu, J., & Lewin, G. R. (2006). Mechanosensitive currents in the neurites of cultured mouse sensory neurones. *The Journal of Physiology, 577*, 815–828.

Huber, T. B., Schermer, B., Muller, R. U., Hohne, M., Bartram, M., Calixto, A., ... Benzing, T. (2006). Podocin and MEC-2 bind cholesterol to regulate the activity of associated ion channels. *Proceedings of the National Academy of Sciences of the United States of America, 103*, 17079–17086.

Kaplan, J. M., & Horvitz, H. R. (1993). A dual mechanosensory and chemosensory neuron in *Caenorhabditis elegans*. *Proceedings of the National Academy of Sciences of the United States of America, 90*, 2227–2231.

Kernan, M., Cowan, D., & Zuker, C. (1994). Genetic dissection of mechanosensory transduction: Mechanoreception-defective mutations of Drosophila. *Neuron, 12*, 1195–1206.

Kim, J., Chung, Y. D., Park, D. Y., Choi, S., Shin, D. W., Soh, H., ... Kim, C. (2003). A TRPV family ion channel required for hearing in Drosophila. *Nature, 424*, 81–84.

Koltzenburg, M., Stucky, C. L., & Lewin, G. R. (1997). Receptive properties of mouse sensory neurons innervating hairy skin. *Journal of Neurophysiology, 78*, 1841–1850.

Kwan, K. Y., Allchorne, A. J., Vollrath, M. A., Christensen, A. P., Zhang, D. S., Woolf, C. J., ... Corey, D. P. (2006). TRPA1 contributes to cold, mechanical, and chemical nociception but is not essential for hair-cell transduction. *Neuron, 50*, 277–289.

Kwan, K. Y., Glazer, J. M., Corey, D. P., Rice, F. L., & Stucky, C. L. (2009). TRPA1 modulates mechanotransduction in cutaneous sensory neurons. *The Journal of Neuroscience, 29*, 4808–4819.

Lai, C. C., Hong, K., Kinnell, M., Chalfie, M., & Driscoll, M. (1996). Sequence and transmembrane topology of MEC-4, an ion channel subunit required for mechanotransduction in *Caenorhabditis elegans*. *Journal of Cell Biology, 133*, 1071–1081.

Lechner, S. G., Frenzel, H., Wang, R., & Lewin, G. R. (2009). Developmental waves of mechanosensitivity acquisition in sensory neuron subtypes during embryonic development. *EMBO Journal, 28*, 1479–1491.

Lechner, S. G., & Lewin, G. R. (2009). Peripheral sensitisation of nociceptors via G-protein-dependent potentiation of mechanotransduction currents. *The Journal of Physiology, 587*, 3493–3503.

Liedtke, W., & Friedman, J. M. (2003). Abnormal osmotic regulation in trpv4–/– mice. *Proceedings of the National Academy of Sciences of the United States of America, 100*, 13698–13703.

Martinez-Salgado, C., Benckendorff, A. G., Chiang, L. Y., Wang, R., Milenkovic, N., Wetzel, C., ... Lewin, G. R. (2007). Stomatin and sensory neuron mechanotransduction. *Journal of Neurophysiology, 98*, 3802–3808.

O'Hagan, R., Chalfie, M., & Goodman, M. B. (2005). The MEC-4 DEG/ENaC channel of *Caenorhabditis elegans* touch receptor neurons transduces mechanical signals. *Nature Neuroscience, 8*, 43–50.

Page, A. J., Brierley, S. M., Martin, C. M., Hughes, P. A., & Blackshaw, L. A. (2007). Acid sensing ion channels 2 and 3 are required for inhibition of visceral nociceptors by benzamil. *Pain, 133*, 150–160.

Petrus, M., Peier, A. M., Bandell, M., Hwang, S. W., Huynh, T., Olney, N., ... Patapoutian, A. (2007). A role of TRPA1 in mechanical hyperalgesia is revealed by pharmacological inhibition. *Molecular Pain, 3*, 40.

Price, M. P., Lewin, G. R., McIlwrath, S. L., Cheng, C., Xie, J., Heppenstall, P. A., ... Welsh, M. J. (2000). The mammalian sodium channel BNC1 is required for normal touch sensation. *Nature, 407*, 1007–1011.

Price, M. P., McIlwrath, S. L., Xie, J., Cheng, C., Qiao, J., Tarr, D. E., ... Welsh, M. J. (2001). The DRASIC cation channel contributes to the detection of cutaneous touch and acid stimuli in mice. *Neuron, 32*, 1071–1083.

Prober, D. A., Zimmerman, S., Myers, B. R., McDermott, B. M., Jr., Kim, S. H., Caron, S., ... Schier, A. F. (2008). Zebrafish TRPA1 channels are required for chemosensation but not for thermosensation or mechanosensory hair cell function. *The Journal of Neuroscience, 28*, 10102–10110.

Sidi, S., Friedrich, R. W., & Nicolson, T. (2003). NompC TRP channel required for vertebrate sensory hair cell mechanotransduction. *Science, 301*, 96–99.

Sukharev, S. I., Martinac, B., Arshavsky, V. Y., & Kung, C. (1993). Two types of mechanosensitive channels in the *Escherichia coli* cell envelope: Solubilization and functional reconstitution. *Biophysical Journal, 65*, 177–183.

Suzuki, M., Mizuno, A., Kodaira, K., & Imai, M. (2003). Impaired pressure sensation in mice lacking TRPV4. *Journal of Biological Chemistry, 278*, 22664–22668.

Tan, P. L., & Katsanis, N. (2009). Thermosensory and mechanosensory perception in human genetic disease. *Human Molecular Genetics, 18*, R146–155.

Tracey, W. D., Jr., Wilson, R. I., Laurent, G., & Benzer, S. (2003). painless, a Drosophila gene essential for nociception. *Cell, 11*, 261–273.

Tsalik, E. L., Niacaris, T., Wenick, A. S., Pau, K., Avery, L., & Hobert, O. (2003). LIM homeobox gene-dependent expression of biogenic amine receptors in restricted regions of the *C. elegans* nervous system. *Developmental Biology, 263*, 81–102.

Waldmann, R., & Lazdunski, M. (1998). H(+)-gated cation channels: Neuronal acid sensors in the NaC/DEG family of ion channels. *Current Opinion in Neurobiology, 8*, 418–424.

Walker, R. G., Willingham, A. T., & Zuker, C. S. (2000). A Drosophila mechanosensory transduction channel. *Science, 287*, 2229–2234.

Way, J. C., & Chalfie, M. (1988). mec-3, a homeobox-containing gene that specifies differentiation of the touch receptor neurons in *C. elegans*. *Cell, 54*, 5–16.

Way, J. C., & Chalfie, M. (1989). The mec-3 gene of *Caenorhabditis elegans* requires its own product for maintained expression and is expressed in three neuronal cell types. *Genes and Development, 3*, 1823–1833.

Wetzel, C., Hu, J., Riethmacher, D., Benckendorff, A., Harder, L., Eilers, A., & Lewin, G. R. (2007). A stomatin-domain protein essential for touch sensation in the mouse. *Nature, 445*, 206–209.

White, J. G., Southgate, E., Thomson, J. N., & Brenner, S. (1986). The structure of the nervous system of the nematode *Caenhorabditis elegans*. *Philosophical Transactions of the Royal Society of London, 314*, 1–340.

Zhang, S., Arnadottir, J., Keller, C., Caldwell, G. A., Yao, C. A., & Chalfie, M. (2004). MEC-2 is recruited to the putative mechanosensory complex in *C. elegans* touch receptor neurons through its stomatin-like domain. *Current Biology, 14*, 1888–1896.

4

Brain Plasticity and Touch

HUBERT R. DINSE

During the last decades, both functional and structural brain plasticity has been identified as the major determinant of perceptual and motor abilities. There is now agreement that alterations of tactile perception result from use-dependent or experience-dependent neuroplasticity mechanisms. While plasticity of the sense of touch can develop over long periods of training, significant alteration can occur almost instantly under conditions of task switching. While the former is most likely based on learning processes occurring in brain areas devoted to the processing of tactile information, the latter reflects the shifting of processing between different available modes that have been implemented before. Because structural modification in the periphery, such as changes in density and properties of mechanoreceptors, appear unlikely to follow these temporal patterns, it has been suggested that most of the adaptational capacity underlying the sense of touch must be cortical in nature.

This chapter summarizes recent work describing the many different facets that modify and alter the sense of touch (for reviews covering the sense of touch, see Dinse & Merzenich, 2002; Feldman & Brecht, 2005). First, factors influencing tactile performance are discussed to enhance an understanding of the context within which plasticity occurs. Then, developmental studies related to maturation and aging, as well as injury-related modifications associated with touch, are surveyed. Next, the effects of losing a body part are noted, followed by a discussion of the effects of training, physical exercise, and use, along with recent studies on perceptual tactile learning. Evidence for crossmodal plasticity is reviewed and findings about tool use, brain–machine interface, and virtual body ownership are summarized. The efficacy of repetitive sensory stimulation and transcranial magnetic stimulation (TMS) in altering the sense of touch is then examined. Finally, the role of touch in rehabilitation and possible modality-specific effects involved in altering the sense of touch are discussed.

FACTORS INFLUENCING TACTILE PERFORMANCE AND PLASTICITY

Hierarchy of Tactile-Haptic Task Performance

The sense of touch is not a uniform entity, but comprises quite diverse features. From an operational point of view, investigation of the sense of touch requires breaking down performance and functions related to touch into measurable variables. In our studies on the plasticity of the sense of touch, we have referred to a hierarchy of tasks and task complexities, which differ in the involvement of proprioception and motor functions, as well as the amount of cognitive demand. Accordingly, the underlying neural substrates differentially involve, in a graded way, contribution from the periphery and from various cortical areas, including so-called primary, input-receiving areas as well as higher-order, associative, and often multimodal areas.

Mechanoreceptor Density and Tactile Performance

The distribution of mechanoreceptors across the skin of the body is not uniform, but highest in fingers and face (particularly in the lips and the tongue) and lowest in the upper legs and the back. These regional differences are reflected in manifold differences in tactile performance as quantified by measuring gap detection (Stevens & Choo, 1996), suggesting a simple relation between mechanoreceptor density and tactile performance. While this relationship may be valid for comparison across different body parts, the association is far more complex when considering a finer spatial scale, such as a comparison across fingers. Questions have arisen regarding the extent to which plastic alterations reported in the hand and fingers are due to changes of central somatosensory cortical processing, with a minor role played by the tactile periphery in the determination of tactile behavior and performance.

An early study found evidence of a poor relationship between histology and tactile performance when comparing touch detection and two-point discrimination thresholds at three sites on the distal phalanx of the little finger with the histology of the same three sites in amputated fingers (Bruce & Sinclair, 1980). In addition, according to postmortem analysis, the density of Meissner's corpuscles in the index and ring fingers differs (Dillon, Haynes, & Henneberg, 2001), while functionally assessed tactile acuity does not (Vega-Bermudez & Johnson, 2001). On the other hand, females have higher densities of Meissner's corpuscles compared with males (Dillon et al., 2001), and their tactile acuity is superior (see Figure 4.1; Peters, Hackeman, & Goldreich, 2009). As discussed in the section on Aging and Tactile Performance, an age-associated reduction in the number of Meissner's corpuscles has been observed, but this is not necessarily related to a decrease in tactile sensitivity (Bruce, 1980).

Combined, these findings create controversy about the role of peripheral versus central aspects of processing that determine perception. The reason for the lack of a simple relation between receptor density and perceptual outcome is that central somatosensory

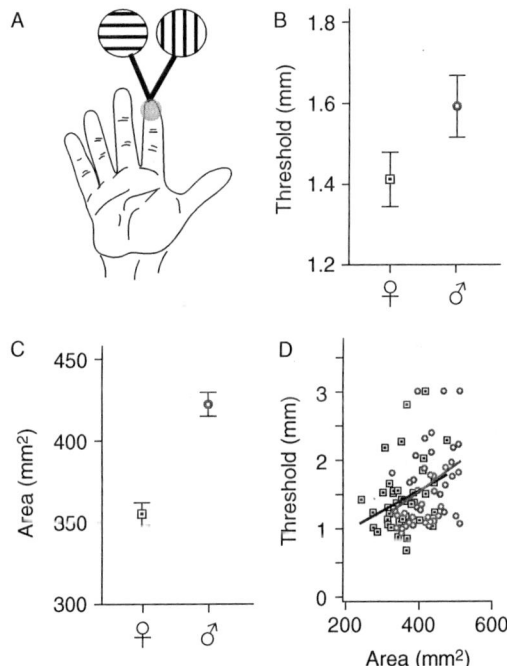

FIGURE 4.1 Tactile acuity in men and women varies due to differences in finger size. (A) Two-interval forced choice grating orientation task (GOT). An adaptive procedure estimated the width of grooves whose orientation the participant could distinguish with 76% probability (GOT threshold). (B) Mean GOT thresholds by gender. Lower thresholds correspond to better acuity. (C) Mean IF distal phalanx surface area by gender. (D) Scatterplot of threshold versus phalanx surface area, with female (light) and male (dark) regression lines. Reprinted with permission from "Diminuitive Digits Discern Delicate Details: Fingertip Size and the Sex Differences in Tactile Spatial Acuity" by R. M. Peters, E. Hackeman, & D. Goldreich, 2009, *Journal of Neuroscience*, 29, 15756–15761. Copyright 2009 by the Society for Neuroscience.

representations are not a mere mirror of the afferent input signals, but extract additional information through active computation based on the interaction of inhibitory and excitatory processes. This issue will be taken up in the subsequent discussion of developmental and age-related alterations of the sense of touch.

Dependence of Tactile Perception and Learning on Skin Accessibility

The crucial role of skin coverage of the fingertips on tactile/haptic sensations and motor execution has been demonstrated in many studies. Local anesthesia studies have demonstrated that the suppression of cutaneous inputs affects complex motor tests more than simple tests (Ebied, 2004). For example, recording of finger movement in expert touch typists under anesthesia of the right index fingertip increased typing errors of that finger sevenfold (Rabin & Gordon, 2004). A comparison of different tactile and sensorimotor tasks performed in young adults and healthy elderly demonstrated that skin coverage severely impaired tactile function, but in a highly task-dependent way (Dinse, Wilimzig, & Kalisch, 2008). Moreover, the susceptibility was age dependent. In elderly individuals, some tasks such as two-point discrimination suffered little as compared to young adults, while haptic object recognition was dramatically impaired. These studies emphasize that maximal tactile–haptic performance requires unrestricted skin access. Little is known regarding the ways in which prolonged skin coverage and training under coverage conditions (as is the case in surgeons wearing gloves) alter dependence of haptic performance on coverage.

DEVELOPMENTAL CONTRIBUTIONS TO TACTILE PERFORMANCE

Tactile Performance of Children and Adolescents

During development the perception of touch is refined due to maturation and experience. Data regarding early development are scarce, however, because of apparent difficulties in studying very young children using quantitative, psychophysical assessment tools. For example, in a study exploring two-point discrimination thresholds in children aged 2–13 years, only those older than 6 years were able to reliably perform the required tests (Cope & Antony, 1992). In a more recent study, tactile acuity and digital dexterity were tested in children and adolescents aged 4–17 years (Bleyenheuft, Wilmotte, & Thonnard, 2010). As shown in Figure 4.2, an exponential improvement with age was observed for both tests, with a rapid gain in tactile performance between 4 and 10 years. In contrast, performance in children and adolescents aged 10–17 years appeared to reach a plateau. These data demonstrate a developmental gradient of tactile and haptic performance. Remarkably, no correlation was found between the scores for both tests, indicating independent development of specific processing qualities. Further experiments are needed to clarify whether the poor performance often found for very young children is due to immature tactile and haptic processing, or instead may reflect problems in task understanding and task execution.

Data about mechanoreceptor density in children in relation to their tactile performance are not available, and data from animal research are not conclusive (Casserly, Thambipillai, Macken, & Fitzgerald, 1994; Fitzgerald 1961). Finger size of children aged 10–12 years is ~50% that of adults, but tactile acuity is comparable (Bleyenheuft et al., 2010; Bockelmann & Dinse, 2009). At least three explanations for these findings are possible. If the number of receptors is comparable to that in adults, then the density must be much higher in children because of

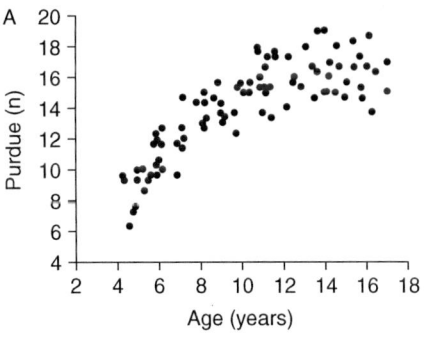
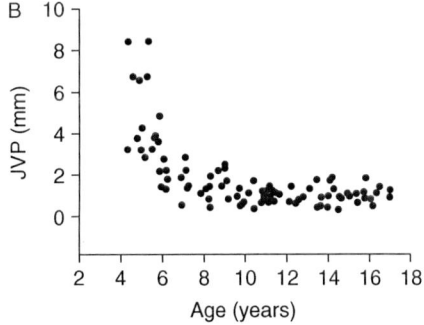

FIGURE 4.2 Development of tactile acuity and sensorimotor abilities in children and adolescents. The evolution of rough scores with age for (A) the purdue peg-board test and (B) the GOT. Each dot represents one child. Reprinted with permission from "Relationship between tactile spatial resolution and digital dexterity during childhood," by Y. Bleyenheuft, P. Wilmotte, & J.L. Thonnard, 2010, *Somatosensory and Motor Research*, 27, 9–14. Copyright 2010 by Informa Healthcare.

their smaller fingers. This density, however, should predict better acuity, and this is not the case. Alternatively, under the assumption that density and acuity are strictly correlated, the comparable acuity in children should predict comparable density, which translates into a substantially smaller number of receptors. This scenario requires that the number of receptors increases with age. A third, alternative explanation for these contradictory data could be that in children the cortical processing machinery is not fully developed, which, despite the higher receptor density, would limit superior performance.

Touch and vision are closely interconnected (see the section Crossmodal Plasticity later in this chapter). Accordingly, many studies focus on the development of crossmodal transfer and integration. Several studies have shown that adults integrate visual and haptic information in a statistically optimal fashion, weighting each sense according to its reliability (Ernst & Banks, 2002). In children younger than 8 years, integration of visual and haptic spatial information is far from optimal. For size discrimination, haptic information dominates in determining both perceived size and discrimination thresholds, whereas for orientation discrimination, vision dominates. Only later, in children 8–10 years, does the integration become statistically adult-like (Gori, Del Viva, Sandini, & Burr, 2008). Similarly, a developmental gradient was found in a delayed matching-to-sample paradigm to test children's tactual, visual, and crossmodal transfer abilities for texture (Picard, 2007). Transfer performance from vision to touch was found to increase between 5 and 8 years of age, whereas transfer performance from touch to vision did not vary with age and matched touch-to-touch performance. At the age of 8 years, asymmetrical crossmodal abilities were observed, where vision-to-touch transfer was higher than touch-to-vision transfer.

Aging and Tactile Performance

Aging exerts major reorganization and remodeling at all levels of brain structure and function, which is paralleled by a progressive decline of mental and physical abilities (Hoff & Mobbs, 2001). On the other hand, it is now well-documented that age-related changes are not a simple reflection of degenerative processes, but rather a complex mix of plastic, adaptive, and compensatory mechanisms, suggesting that brain plasticity is operational into old age (Dinse, 2006; Godde, Berkefeld, David-Jürgens, & Dinse, 2002; Mahncke, Bronstone, & Merzenich, 2006). Considering the current demographic changes in many civilizations, there is an urgent need for measures permitting an independent lifestyle into old age. Therefore, strategies such as training, exercising, practicing, and stimulation that make use of neuroplasticity principles are essential to maintain health and functional independence throughout lifespan.

While sensory processes gradually emerge during development, they lose efficiency in old age. Glasses and hearing aids are a standard aid for elderly people. Yet, in contrast to vision and hearing, the dramatic age-related deterioration of the sense of touch goes mostly unnoticed because there are no conditions such as reading newspapers or obtaining a driver's licence which might reveal this impairment. As a result, the sense of touch and its vital role for coping with activities of daily living is widely underestimated. Elderly individuals progressively adapt to the loss of high-level tactile performance and learn to compensate by developing behavioral strategies, such as relying more on visual control to overcome the decrement in the sense of touch.

Aging affects sensing through receptors, transmission through neurons at various stations along the sensory pathway, and central processing by the brain. Therefore, multiple factors are involved in the age-related decline of the sense of touch. At a peripheral level, skin conformance undergoes alterations in old age (Vega-Bermudez & Johnson, 2004; Woodward, 1993), with a loss of dermal receptors and a change in the morphology of Meissner's and Pacinian corpuscles (Bolton, Winkelmann, & Dyck, 1966; Bruce, 1980). Transmission of touch information is affected by slowing of nerve conduction with increasing age and reduction of action-potential amplitude (Peters, 2002). In contrast to eyes and ears, which are close to the brain, the distances of skin receptors from the brain vary greatly across the body. Skin receptors located on the feet are particularly vulnerable to a slowing down of conduction—by up to 20 or 30% (Reinke & Dinse, 1996). It is believed that the slower conduction emerging during aging results in greater temporal dispersion of incoming afferent information. This harms central processing and thus contributes to perceptual impairment. At a central level, there is now agreement that neuron loss is a rare event (Hof & Mobbs, 2001). However, at a subcellular level, cortical sensory processing is affected through manifold age-related alterations of ion channels and receptor composition. In longitudinal studies in healthy elderly, regional brain volumes and gray matter density were substantially reduced; however, changes were very regional so that the time course of aging effects varied considerably over cortical areas (Raz et al., 1997; Sowell et al., 2003).

At a perceptual level, a simple measure of tactile perceptual performance is tactile acuity, which describes the ability to resolve fine

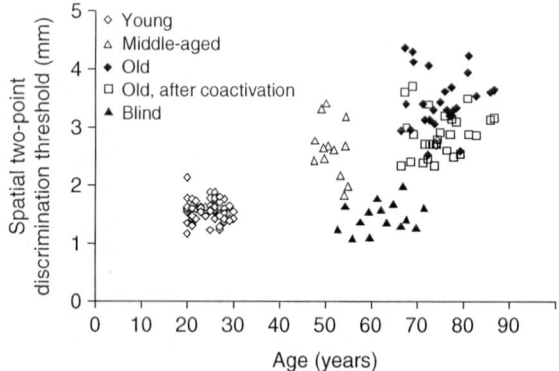

FIGURE 4.3 The impact of age, training, and sensory stimulation on tactile acuity as measured by spatial discrimination thresholds. Each symbol represents an individual subject. Modified from "Tactile co-activation resets age-related decline of human tactile discrimination," by H. Dinse et al., 2006, *Annals of Neurology*, 60, 88–94. Copyright by American Neurological Association. Adapted with permission from "Tactile and learning abilities in early-and late-blind subjects," by C. Heinisch, T. Kalisch & H.R. Dinse, 2006, Society for Neuroscience Annual Meeting, Atlanta, Georgia (Abstract 52.4/N2).

spatial details. Usually, measures of tactile acuity are obtained by testing two-point discrimination, gap detection, or grating orientation. Whatever technique is used, there is agreement that tactile acuity is significantly reduced during aging (Dinse et al., 2006; Stevens, 1992; Woodward, 1993). Figure 4.3 shows this decline in spatial discrimination with aging. However, tactile acuity declines much more vigorously for some body regions than for others. According to one study (Stevens & Choo, 1996), deterioration of acuity in the great toe averaged ~400% between young and elderly subjects (aged 65–87 years) as compared to an average decline of 130% observed on the fingertip.

To acquire insight into changes of cortical maps that parallel degradation of tactile performance, somatosensory evoked potential mapping has been employed in combination with electric source localization. One study has shown that the distance between the dipoles of the index and the little fingers increased in elderly subjects, indicating a cortical map expansion that paralleled a decline of tactile acuity (Kalisch, Ragert, Schwenkreis, Dinse, & Tegenthoff, 2009). In adults, map expansion is typically associated with a gain in perceptual performance (Elbert, Pantev, Wienbruch, Rockstroh, & Taub, 1995; Pleger, et al., 2003). This atypical relation between map expansion and perceptual performance could be explained by an age-related reduction of intracortical inhibition mechanisms leading to disintegration of cortical maps, a process that is different from learning-related map changes that are assumed to result from Hebbian learning and strengthening of connections.

Studies in blind adult individuals have shown that their tactile performance is superior to those in age-matched sighted persons (Goldreich & Kanics, 2003; Van Boven, Hamilton, Kauffman, Keenan, & Pascual-Leone, 2000). Their enhanced tactile abilities have been assumed to arise from the unusual and extensive use of the reading fingers to gather fine-scale spatial tactile information. Interestingly, as shown in Figure 4.3, elderly blind Braille readers do not show typical age-related changes, suggesting that maintained use of the fingers might play a role in preserving intact acuity (Dinse, Tegenthoff, Heinisch, & Kalisch, 2009; Legge, Madison, Vaughn, Cheong, & Miller, 2008). These observations are in line with the view that use-dependent plastic capacities are operational into old age (Dinse, 2006; Mahncke et al., 2006).

We have used tactile coactivation (a form of repetitive sensory stimulation that will be described in more detail in an upcoming section) as an alternative intervention to interfere with the age-related impairment of tactile perception (Dinse et al., 2006). When the same coactivation protocol used in previous studies with young individuals was applied to aged participants, we found that they responded differently. Prior to coactivation, the discrimination threshold of individuals under 60 years of age was better than those who were 60 years and older. After coactivation, this difference disappeared and the tactile acuity of the older individuals matched the average performance of participants aged 47–59 years (see Figure 4.3). These results demonstrate that age-related decline of perception is not irreversible and can be improved by specific stimulation protocols (Dinse et al., 2006). Interestingly, participants who had the highest thresholds before the start of the study showed the largest improvement, while participants with low thresholds (better acuity) had only limited improvement. This finding suggests that elderly individuals with the largest tactile impairment benefited most from the treatment.

Sensory stimulation in elderly individuals also restores to a considerable extent haptic and sensorimotor performance (Kalisch, Tegenthoff, & Dinse, 2008). Of particular interest are recent data in which repeated application of repetitive stimulation over several weeks resulted in a stabilization of tactile improvement (Kalisch, Tegenthoff, & Dinse, 2010). Many other attempts to interfere with the age-related decline of sensory capacities have been described (see the section The Effects of Physical Activity and Exercise). For example, adding noise to a transmitted signal can improve the ability to reliably transfer information, a phenomenon known as stochastic resonance. Electrical noise stimulation applied to the hand of elderly individuals lowers touch thresholds (Dhruv, Niemi, Harry, Lipsitz, & Collins, 2002), and noise stimulation to the foot can improve postural stability in young and elderly individuals (Priplata, Niemi, Harry, Lipsitz, & Collins, 2003).

Despite the accumulation of degenerative processes during aging, these findings demonstrate that the typical decline in tactile performance is not inevitable; rather, it is preventable and subject to restoration by training and stimulation. Preservation of sufficient tactile acuity in old age is an important prerequisite for the maintenance of independent living, so these approaches may be beneficial in preserving everyday sensorimotor competence in the elderly.

PLASTICITY ASSOCIATED WITH LOSS OF A BODY PART

Loss of a body part leads to major brain reorganization, which includes both functional and structural changes (Kaas, 2000). Immediate alterations are assumed to be due to up–down regulation of excitatory and inhibitory transmitter systems such as glutamate and GABA (Qü, Mittmann, Luhmann, Schleicher, & Zilles, 1998). In addition, delayed alterations include sprouting of connections that occur at many levels from brain stem to cortex (Florence, Taub, & Kaas, 1998). The main effect of amputation or deafferentation consists of an expansion of cortical territories representing intact skin portions into cortical regions that formerly represented the deafferented areas (Merzenich et al., 1984; Yang et al., 1994). As a result, the deafferented regions are not silenced, but come to represent neighboring areas. In the loss of a hand, neurons of the hand representation develop representations of the face and upper arm, both of which are adjacent in the map of the somatosensory homunculus.

Conceivably, at a perceptual level, these major restructurings could result in major disturbances in perception. The so-called phantom limb sensation describes the phenomenon that an amputated body part is still sensed when neighboring skin portions are touched. So, in the example of the hand amputation, touching either the face or the upper arm results in a double sensation where both the touched and the missing body parts are sensed (Ramachandran, Rogers-Ramachandran, & Stewart, 1992).

CHAPTER 4   BRAIN PLASTICITY AND TOUCH   95

PLASTICITY ASSOCIATED WITH ACTIVE STIMULATION

The Effects of Intensified or Reduced Use

Consequences of the use or disuse of a body area on cortical map topography and performance are captured in the concept of use-dependent plasticity and are intensively investigated. Animal studies first demonstrated that cortical maps are enlarged as a result of modified use. For example, a major natural source of differential tactile input is the stimulation of the rat ventrum in nursing behavior. In lactating rats, the primary somatosensory cortex (SI) representation of the ventral trunk skin was found to be significantly larger than in matched postpartum nonlactating or virgin controls (Xerri, Stern, & Merzenich, 1994). These data, indicating the critical role of use of a body part or region, were confirmed and extended by imaging studies in humans that revealed enlarged cortical representations of the hand and fingers in musicians or blind Braille readers who used these body parts extensively (Elbert et al., 1995; Pascual-Leone & Torres, 1993; Sterr et al., 1998).

The final outcome of any reorganizational process is not necessarily beneficial. There is increasing evidence that abnormal perceptual experiences arise from maladaptive plastic reorganization. The so-called hand-arm vibration syndrome (HAVS) has been associated with prolonged exposure to vibrations transmitted to the human hand-arm system from handheld power tools and handheld vibrating work pieces. Patients suffering from HAVS report the development of paresthesia or tingling in digits, pain or tenderness in the wrist and hand, digital blanching, and cold intolerance—in addition to a deteriorated tactile performance such as impairment of frequency and two-point discrimination (Coughlin, Bonser, Turton, Kent, & Kester, 2001).

Regardless of outcomes, there is now agreement that use is a major factor driving plasticity of cortical processing and cortical maps, driving either the development of outstanding sensorimotor skills or the problems associated with overuse. However, little is known about how periods of disuse affect cortical representations and parallel perceptual performance in humans. In humans, enforced disuse resulting from wearing a cast for several weeks (following a hand or arm fracture in an individual with an otherwise intact nervous system) impaired perceptual performance and resulted in a shrinkage of somatosensory cortical maps of the hand (Lissek et al., 2009). As shown in Figure 4.4, hemodynamic responses in SI correlated positively with hand-use frequency and negatively with discrimination thresholds, indicating

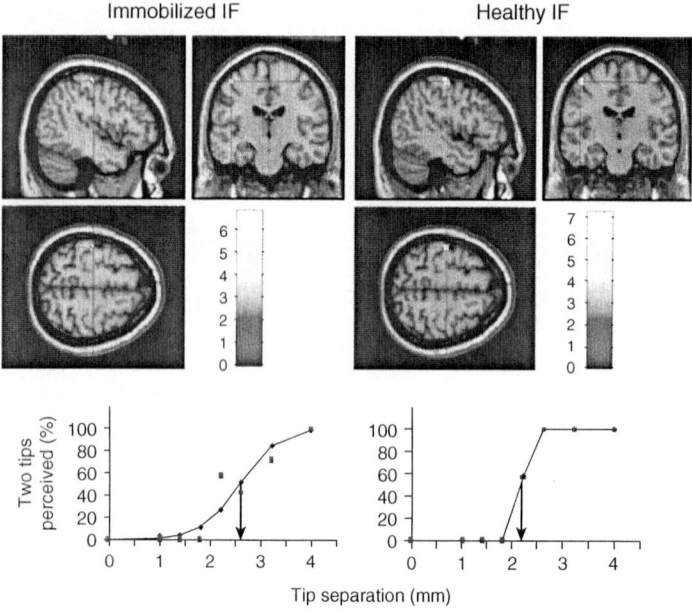

FIGURE 4.4 Blood-oxygen-level-dependent (BOLD) signals recorded in SI of a single subject, showing the effects of 2 weeks of right-side immobilization on the cortical IF representation of the immobilized (top left) and healthy hand (top right). Activations are projected on the left hemisphere on an axial, sagittal, and coronal T1-weighted, normalized magnetic resonance imaging (MRI) slice. At the bottom, psychometric functions illustrate the impact of 2 weeks of immobilization on tactile discrimination thresholds for the subject shown above. Correct responses in percentages are plotted as a function of separation distance together with the results of a logistic regression line. Fifty percent levels of correct responses as well as tactile discrimination thresholds are shown. Reprinted with permission from "Immobilization impairs tactile perception and shrinks somatosensory cortical maps," by S. Lissek et al., 2009, *Current Biology*, 19, 837–842. Copyright 2009 by Cell Press.

that reduced activation was most prominent in subjects with severe perceptual impairment. Two to three weeks after cast removal, perceptual and cortical changes recovered. These findings suggest that brief periods of reduced use of a body part have overt, measurable consequences and thus must be regarded as a significant driving force of brain organization equivalent to enhancement of use. According to these data, whatever one is doing or not doing leaves measurable traces in brain organization, either beneficial or harmful. Doing nothing does have negative consequences, suggesting that a continuous stream of sensory input may be necessary to keep brain organization and perceptual abilities intact (Lissek et al., 2009).

The Effects of Physical Activity and Exercise

Numerous lines of evidence converge regarding the beneficial influence of physical activity engendered through aerobic exercise on selective aspects of brain function (Hillman, Erickson, & Kramer, 2008). In particular, in elderly individuals, there is a close association between physical fitness and enhanced cognitive performance (Colcombe et al., 2006). We have recently studied the impact of multiyear regular ballroom dancing in a group of neurologically healthy elderly subjects in comparison to a passive control group (Kattenstroth, Kolankowska, Kalisch, & Dinse, 2010). Besides recording posture and balance parameters, we extended the assessment to measurements of cognitive, attentional, intellectual, perceptual, and sensorimotor performance. Surprisingly, at each of these different levels, the dancer group showed a superior performance, indicating the far-reaching beneficial effects of dancing beyond aspects of balance and posture. While high-level performance in posture and balance can be linked to the requirements imposed by dancing, tactile abilities appear rather unrelated to dancing.

For example, enhanced tactile discrimination abilities found in blind Braille readers have been associated with the unusual and extensive use of the fingers to gather fine-scale spatial tactile information (Van Boven et al., 2000). Similarly, tactile acuity in professional pianists is significantly higher as compared to nonmusicians, which has been attributed to the extreme usage of the fingers during piano playing (Ragert, Ragert, Schmid, Altenmueller, & Dinse, 2004). Therefore, the superior tactile discrimination found in the dance group might reflect factors that are independent of dancing activities and differential use but rather some more overarching effects of activity on the brain.

Animal research on the effects of physical exercise suggests a crucial involvement of brain-derived neurotrophin factors and other nerve growth factors (Neeper, Gomez-Pinilla, Choi, & Cotman, 1995), which play a fundamental role in control and maintenance of synaptic connections and brain plasticity. More generally, mild stress response in cells has been advocated as a major driving force that upregulates stress resistance genes and growth factors (Mattson, 2008). Among the factors inducing mild stress are sensory stimulation, physical activity, and cognitive challenges; all of them involved in dancing. In a recent study of experienced adult Tai Chi practitioners, superior spatial tactile acuity in comparison to matched controls has been reported (Kerr et al., 2008). This has been explained by assuming that individuals with a high fitness level are drawn to Tai Chi or that Tai Chi itself drives cortical changes which lead to superior tactile acuity. It is also possible that enhanced performance in tactile discrimination may arise as a consequence of increased levels of neurotrophins, which are upregulated during dancing and which might also be upregulated in Tai Chi practitioners.

Perceptual Learning and the Effects of Training

Perceptual learning is a form of implicit learning where perceptual abilities improve through practice, training, or pure exposure to stimulation. Perceptual learning involves relatively long-lasting changes to an organism's perceptual system that improve its ability to respond to its environment and are caused by this environment. Perceptual learning is not achieved by a unitary process (Fahle & Poggio, 2002; Goldstone, 1998). Changes involve peripheral, specific adaptations; general, strategic adaptations; mechanisms driven by feedback and reward; and mechanisms that operate on the statistical structure of the stimuli.

Recent studies have shown that skill acquisition is associated with selective plastic reorganizational changes in the cortical representations of those body parts that receive stimuli during perceptual learning. Recanzone and coworkers were the first to demonstrate that alterations of cortical sensory processing developed during perceptual learning (Recanzone, Merzenich, Jenkins, Grajski, & Dinse, 1992). They showed that tactile frequency discrimination training in monkeys over many sessions leads to a reduction of the perceived discrimination threshold and to an expansion of the maps in somatosensory cortex that represent the used finger. Most importantly, this study showed that there was a linear correlation between the individual amount of perceptual improvement induced by the training and the individual amount of cortical map expansion. These data imply that cortical map size is a reliable predictor of individual performance.

However, the outcome of cortical reorganization can be highly task specific. When subjects received passive tactile stimulation of thumb and little finger over a period of 4 weeks, the representations of the fingers in primary somatosensory cortex were closer together after training. However, when subjects had to discriminate stimuli, magnetoencephalography imaging revealed that the digital representations were further apart than before. Thus, the same prolonged repetitive stimulation produced two opposite effects, suggesting that activation in the same region of cortex is specific to different tasks (Braun, Schweizer, Elbert, Birbaumer, & Taub, 2000).

Perceptual learning is often characterized by high specificity to stimulus parameters such as location or orientation, with little generalization of what is learned to other locations or to other stimulus configurations. Limited generalization is taken as evidence for high locality of effects in early representations, while transfer is taken as evidence for the involvement of higher processing levels (Fahle, 1997). In addition, transfer and generalization are task and modality specific. In the tactile domain, Sathian and Zangaladze (1997) provided evidence that practice-related improvement is specific for properties of the stimulus used in training. They reported substantial interdigital transfer of practice effects for discrimination of gratings varying in either groove width or ridge width and also for spatial acuity-dependent discrimination of grating orientation. Although tactile learning was task specific, there was generalization across fingers. In another, so-called tactile hyperacuity task, subjects had to discriminate a row of three dots in which the central dot was offset laterally from a row without such offset. Performance at the right index finger pad improved with practice, which transferred completely to the left index finger (IF), demonstrating intermanual transfer (Sathian & Zangaladze, 1998).

In a study of tactile interval discrimination, subjects were trained for 900 trials per day for 10–15 days (Nagarajan, Blake, Wright, Byl, & Merzenich, 1998). Learning at the trained base interval generalized completely across untrained skin locations on the trained hand and to the corresponding untrained skin location in the contralateral hand. There was partial generalization to untrained base intervals similar to the trained one, but not to more distant base intervals. Interestingly, learning with somatosensory stimuli generalized to auditory stimuli presented at comparable base intervals. These results demonstrate temporal specificity in learning somatosensory interval discrimination that generalizes across skin location, hemisphere, and modality.

Time Scales of Tactile Plasticity

Improvements in the sense of touch can occur on many different time scales. For example, in some tasks, a few trials are sufficient to drive improvement. In other situations, performance improves even after weeks or months of practicing. What remains to be clarified are conditions that require either short- or long-term training as well as those in which improvements saturate. It has been suggested that one notable source of human inefficiency is that, unlike the ideal observer, human learning relies more heavily on previous decisions, resulting in a lack of learning in trials that follow a previously incorrect decision (Eckstein, Abbey, Pham, & Shimozaki, 2004).

In studies of long-term training over weeks and months, one typically finds an early phase of rapid improvement followed by a second phase of much slower learning. It has been suggested that the early phase represents task understanding and the development of an appropriate strategy, while the second phase of improvement is due to selective and specific changes in cortical processing of tactile changes (Recanzone, Jenkins, Hradek, & Merzenich, 1992). This view is consistent with the observation that gain obtained during the first phase is unspecific and transfers easily to other sites, whereas the gain accumulated during the second phase is highly specific to the trained condition.

EFFECTS OF PASSIVE STIMULATION

Exposure Through Repetitive Stimulation

In addition to use, experience, training, and practice, perceptual performance can also be persistently altered by passive stimulation, that is, through systematic variation of the statistics of the inputs. Currently, different forms of so-called repetitive sensory stimulation procedures are widely investigated by different groups as a means to drive learning and plasticity processes, using different terms such as "peripheral nerve stimulation" (Sawaki, Wu, Kaelin-Lang, & Cohen, 2006), "exposure-based learning" (Gutnisky, Hansen, Iliescu, & Dragoi, 2009), "co-activation" (Godde, Stauffenberg, Spengler, & Dinse, 2000; Pleger et al., 2001, 2003), "unattended activation-based learning" (Dinse et al., 2005), and "repetitive sensory stimulation" (Kalisch, Tegenthoff, & Dinse, 2009).

For several years, we have been developing tactile learning protocols that use repetitive sensory stimulation as a measure to induce plastic processes. The basic idea is to utilize the broad knowledge we now have about brain plasticity to design specific stimulation protocols through which it becomes feasible to purposefully change brain organization and thus perception and behavior. We have introduced new forms of repetitive sensory stimulation protocols—for example, "co-activation"—that have been shown to induce learning processes that improve tactile and sensorimotor performance in human subjects in a very short time scale of hours to minutes. Notably, the overall gain in performance is comparable to the effects induced by several days or months of training (Dinse et al., 2005).

Using neuroimaging and electrical source localization, we demonstrated that coactivation led to a selective increase in the size of the cortical representation of the fingers used (Dinse, Ragert, Pleger, Schwenkreis, & Tegenthoff, 2003; Pleger et al., 2001, 2003). Under the assumption that changes of cortical maps representing the coactivated finger reflect changes in cortical processing causally related to the processing of tactile information, we hypothesized that cortical alterations should correlate with the changes in individual performance. Linear correlation analysis revealed significant relations between the coactivation-induced cortical map changes within SI on the postcentral gyrus (see magnified detail in Figure 4.5A) and a parallel perceptual improvement in two-point discrimination abilities (Figure 4.5B). No activated clusters were found within secondary somatosensory cortex (SII). Accordingly, little gain in spatial discrimination abilities was only associated with small changes in cortical maps. On the other hand, those subjects who showed a large cortical reorganization also

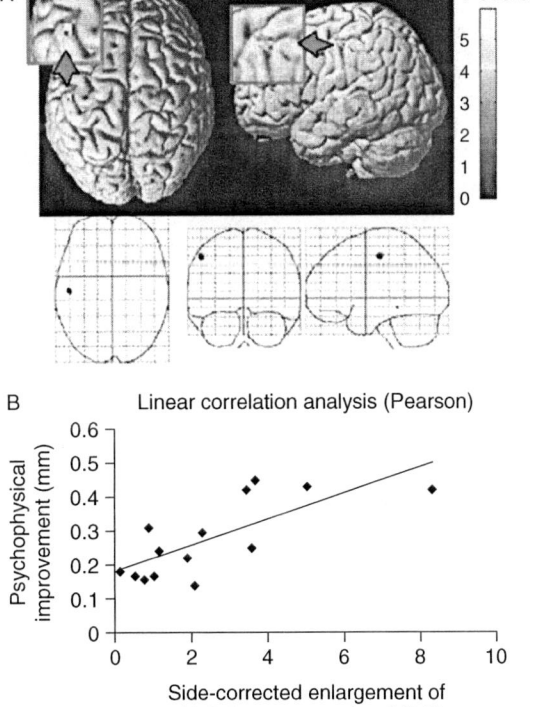

FIGURE 4.5 (A) Coactivation-induced changes in two-point tactile discrimination thresholds were associated with activation in SI as indicated by BOLD signals. (B) The corresponding number of activated voxels per cluster ($K = ((\text{rightpost} - \text{rightpre}) - (\text{leftpost} - \text{leftpre}))/\text{rightpre}$) in SI was positively correlated with coactivation-induced changes in psychophysical thresholds for tactile acuity. Reprinted with permission from "Functional imaging of perceptual learning in human primary and secondary somatosensory cortex," by S. B. Pleger et al., 2003, *Neuron, 40*, 643–653. Copyright 2003 by Cell Press.

had better tactile acuity as evidenced by the lowest thresholds, that is, they benefited most from coactivation (Dinse et al., 2003; Pleger et al., 2001, 2003). A similar result has been obtained for changes of cortical excitability. Following coactivation, paired-pulse suppression was reduced, and the amount of suppression was positively correlated with the individual gain in performance (Höffken et al., 2007).

To test the hypothesis that coactivation is mediated by plasticity mechanisms requiring NMDA receptor activation, we used memantine, a selective NMDA receptor blocker, which eliminated coactivation-induced changes both psychophysically and cortically. On the other hand, application of single doses of amphetamine doubled the effectiveness of coactivation (Dinse et al., 2003), implying the involvement of neuromodulatory systems.

The potential of repetitive stimulation is not limited to young adult subjects, but has been applied in musicians whose tactile performance is already enhanced. Therefore, the question with these musicians was whether there is room for further improvement. Despite their better baseline performance, coactivation resulted in an even higher gain of tactile acuity. While baseline performance correlated well with the duration of daily piano practicing, the coactivation-induced improvement was correlated with the number of years of extensive piano playing (Ragert et al., 2004). These findings imply stronger capacities for plastic reorganization in pianists and point to enhanced learning abilities, which have been discussed in respect to meta-plasticity. Support for enhanced learning capabilities in musicians comes from a recent study employing paired associative stimulation, which showed a wider modification range of synaptic plasticity for musicians than nonmusician controls (Rosenkranz, Williamon, & Rothwell, 2007).

According to cellular studies, long-term potentiation (LTP) and long-term depression (LTD) of synaptic transmission are the leading candidates for activity-dependent changes in the strength of synaptic connections. Typically, to induce LTP in brain slices, high-frequency stimulation is used, while LTD can be reliably evoked by low-frequency stimulation in the range of 1 Hz. We, therefore, explored the potential efficacy of stimulation protocols that are used in these studies in driving tactile perceptual changes. We found that short periods of peripheral high-frequency stimulation induced a lowering of tactile discrimination thresholds, indicated by improved tactile acuity, whereas low-frequency stimulation resulted in an impaired performance on the stimulated finger (Ragert, Franzkowiak, Schwenkreis, Tegenthoff, & Dinse, 2008). These results indicate that brief stimulation protocols resembling those used in cellular LTP and LTD studies for only 30 minutes can induce meaningful and persistent frequency-dependent, bidirectional alterations of tactile discrimination behavior.

Repetitive stimulation does not require training of particular tasks, which makes repetitive, stimulation-induced alterations task independent. We have, therefore, proposed that repetitive stimulation alters the entire neural processing of tactile and haptic information. Consequently, one could expect that repetitive stimulation not only affects two-point discrimination thresholds but essentially all tasks related to tactile, haptic, and sensorimotor processing. The available data are consistent with this hypothesis, as repetitive stimulation leads to remodeling of a wide range of tactile, haptic, and even sensorimotor tasks. We found improved performance for tactile acuity (as measured by two-point or grating discrimination), frequency discrimination, localization, dot-pattern discrimination, haptic object recognition, decision making (multiple choice reaction times), and sensorimotor performance (Peg-Board). Interestingly, localization tasks (within finger or across fingers) became impaired, which is in line with data from blind Braille readers, who improve acuity at the cost of localization (Sterr et al., 1998). These findings imply a general trade-off between discrimination and localization performance (see the section Plasticity in One Area at the Cost of Another below). The only parameter not affected by repetitive stimulation was touch threshold, which supports the argument that tactile acuity relies on changes of synaptic efficacy and synaptic connections and therefore is subject to neuroplasticity mechanisms. In contrast, touch thresholds seem to reflect predominantly peripheral factors such as mechanoreceptor density and mechanoreceptor composition, which remain unaffected by cortical plasticity processes.

Our current view is that coactivation drives synaptic plasticity processes in the cortical areas representing the stimulated sites. The observed expansion of the cortical maps can be regarded as a recruitment of processing resources. In an attempt to unify these observations, we used computational mean field approaches which revealed that perceptual impairment depends on changes of amplitude and width of lateral interaction processes (Dinse, Wilimzig, et al., 2008).

The effectiveness of passive repetitive stimulation and TMS (see the next section) appears to result from a similar process—namely, that sensory stimulation must be sufficient to drive the neural system past the point of a learning threshold (Seitz & Dinse, 2007). Factors such as reinforcement or motivation appear to play a permissive role, but optimizing sensory inputs by implementing specific high-frequency or burst-like stimulations, which are known to induce synaptic plasticity in brain-slice preparations, can also serve to boost responses that normally are insufficient to drive learning past this learning threshold.

Transcranial Magnetic Stimulation

Repetitive sensory stimulation is not the only form of passive learning. Under the assumption that simultaneously applied sensory stimuli induce synchronous neural activity at a cortical site representing the location of tactile stimulation, one could shortcut the sensory pathway in examining plasticity. An approach is to apply so-called high-frequency TMS from outside the scull directly to somatosensory cortex to induce synchronous activity. During a typical TMS experiment, an electromagnetic coil is placed above the scalp. The coil produces magnetic pulses that pass through the skull and induce electric currents within the brain that alter the activity of the underlying neurons. Repetitive TMS (rTMS) is increasingly used both as a tool to explore the mechanisms and consequences of cortical plasticity in the human brain and as a new therapeutic strategy.

In our research, applying 20 minutes of 5 Hz TMS over the finger representation of SI has led to similar changes as those observed after repetitive stimulation. As shown in Figure 4.6, these changes were paralleled by an expansion of the cortical finger representation and an increase of cortical excitability in SI that returned to baseline after ~2–3 hours (Ragert, Becker, Tegenthoff, Pleger, & Dinse, 2004; Tegenthoff et al., 2005).

We then asked whether enhancement of tactile acuity induced by repetitive stimulation could be further improved by a combination of repetitive stimulation (coac) and 5 Hz rTMS (coac + rTMS). In fact, following coac + rTMS, the gain in acuity was further enhanced. However, further improvement after coac + rTMS depended on the effectiveness of the repetitive stimulation protocol when applied alone. Subjects who showed little gain in tactile performance after coactivation alone showed the largest improvement after coac + rTMS, implying that the combined application was selective for poor learners (Ragert et al., 2003).

Similar to repetitive stimulation, TMS techniques allow for easy adoption of the wide range of stimulation protocols used in brain slice experiments to explore synaptic plasticity mechanisms. The theta burst stimulation (TBS) protocol employs short bursts of high-frequency (50 Hz) TMS for only a few minutes. Applying intermittent TBS (iTBS) over left SI for only 3 minutes increased cortical excitability within the stimulated brain area and resulted in improvement of tactile discrimination behavior that persisted for at least 30 minutes (Ragert, Kalisch, Bliem, Franzkowiak, & Dinse, 2008). Similarly, the transcranial direct current stimulation, which has been shown to induce polarity-specific excitability changes in the brain, improves tactile acuity when applied (anodal) over S1 (Ragert, Vandermeeren, Camus, & Cohen, 2008).

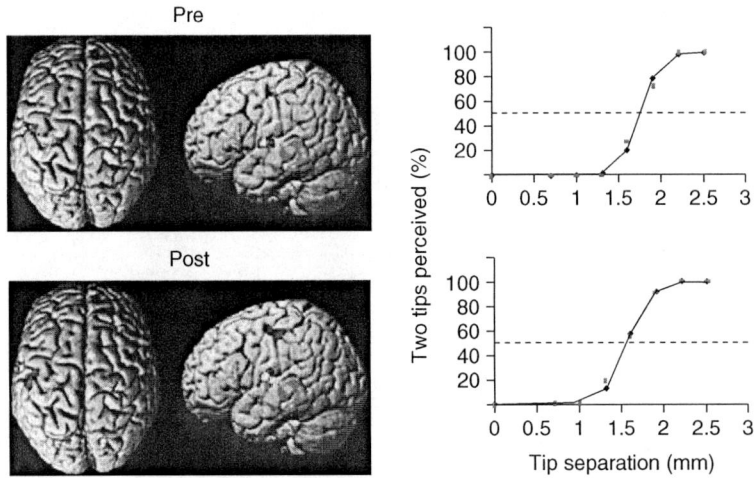

FIGURE 4.6 Single repetitive TMS (rTMS) effects on BOLD signals detected-pre-rTMS and post-rTMS are shown (on the left) for both the left SI ipsilateral to the rTMS site in the postcentralgyrus and the contralateral SII in the parietaloperculum above the Sylvian fissure. Activations are projected on a rendered T1-weighted MRI dataset. Graphs on the right illustrate the rTMS-induced improvement of tactile discrimination threshold for the individual from pre-rTMS on the top to post-rTMS on the bottom. Correct responses in percent (squares) are plotted as a function of separation distance together with the results of a logistic regression line. From "Persistent improvement of tactile discrimination performance and enlargement of cortical somatosensory maps after 5 Hz rTMS" by M. Tegenthoff et al., 2005, *PloS Biology*, 3, e362. Copyright 2005 by Public Library of Science. Open access article.

These findings all demonstrate that meaningful improvement of perceptual performance can be obtained even by specific stimulation of brain areas from outside the scull. Most notably, this intervention does not leave the cortical processing in a disorganized state but, on the contrary, leads to the emergence of different, yet organized and meaningful behavior, as indicated by the improvement of discrimination performance (Tegenthoff et al., 2005).

Plasticity in One Area at the Cost of Another

A frequently asked question in plasticity and learning is whether the enhancement of a particular ability occurs at the cost of others. In other words, is there a simultaneous trade-off between abilities we gain and those we lose? When subjects improve their tactile discrimination abilities (i.e., perceive two closely spaced stimuli as two), this develops at the cost of localization performance (i.e., accurately telling the position of a stimulus on the skin; Kalisch et al., 2008; Sterr et al., 1998, 2003). Interestingly, both types of changes evolve without altering touch thresholds, which implies a trade-off between localization and discrimination on the one hand, but independence of both parameters from touch threshold on the other hand. Another example comes from haptic exploration, where haptic recognition is poorly associated with tactile acuity but correlated with measures of nonverbal intelligence (Kalisch & Dinse, 2009). In the earlier developmental discussion regarding children, it was also noted that a lack of correlation was observed between acuity and dexterity performance (Bleyenheuft, Wilmotte, & Thonnard, 2010).

These findings imply that cortical processing modes that are independent from each other and that cannot be optimized in parallel exist. In this view, the average individual performance most likely reflects a sort of a trade-off where one may achieve optimal versus maximal performance. Through perceptual learning or other plasticity-enforcing conditions, it is possible to further enhance certain skills but not all skills, resulting in an improvement of some skills at the cost of impairing others.

To understand tactile spatial discrimination performance and its alterations during learning, we have provided a computational model using a mean field approach (Wilimzig & Dinse, 2007). Cortical population activity within cortical maps is modelled with a Mexican hat interaction of short-range excitation and longer-range inhibition (Wilson & Cowan, 1973). In the model, stimulation at a single site evokes single peaks of activation coding for the subjective experience of a single point, while simultaneous stimulation at two sites (like in two-point discrimination experiments) evokes two peaks, which are read out for perceiving two points. In contrast, localization refers to the ability to precisely read out the location of monomodal distributions of population activation. Spatial discrimination and localization are affected oppositely by lateral interaction (Dinse, Wilimzig, et al., 2008; Wilimzig & Dinse, 2007). Lateral inhibition reduces coexisting, ongoing activation present at other locations of the cortical population. As coexisting activation is necessary for bimodal activation profiles coding for the perception of two points, strong lateral inhibition deteriorates discrimination performance. On the other hand, lateral inhibition suppresses the influence of noisy fluctuations of activation, leading to a subsequent reduction in the variance of the read out peak position. Thus, lateral inhibition improves localization performance but decreases discrimination performance.

Rehabilitation Using Passive Stimulation

Sensorimotor impairment resulting from stroke can have extensive physical, psychological, financial, and social implications despite available neurorehabilitative treatments. Intact somatosensory input is not only crucial for tactile perception but also for sensorimotor performance. Loss of sensory abilities of the more involved upper extremity, particularly the hand, further complicates the individual's ability to use the hand for functional tasks in spite of possible recovery of motor functions.

Generally, rehabilitation following stroke based on neuroplasticity mechanisms utilizes task-specific training and massed practice to drive reorganization and improve sensorimotor function (Taub, Uswatte, & Elbert, 2002). However, since many patients suffer from restricted mobility, development of additional and alternative approaches that could supplement, enhance, or even replace conventional training procedures would be advantageous. Therefore, in the last years, many attempts have been made to search for additional rehabilitative approaches (Koesler, Dafotakis, Ameli, Fink, & Nowak, 2008; Sawaki et al., 2006; Wu, Seo, & Cohen, 2006). As noted earlier, the particular advantage of repetitive stimulation is its passive nature, which does not require active participation or attention of the subjects. Therefore, repetitive stimulation can be applied in parallel to other occupations, making the intervention substantially easier to implement and more acceptable to the individual.

In studies exploring the efficacy of repetitive stimulation as therapeutic intervention, stimulation was applied using quite different protocols. The duration of stimulation varied between 20 minutes and 2 hours per day, whereas the duration of the whole intervention ranged from a single application to 8 weeks of repeated application. The stimulation sequences in most cases used repetitive square pulses in a frequency range of 1–100 Hz, with higher frequencies applied more often. In chronic stroke patients, individuals were treated with repetitive stimulation for 4 days a week for 6 weeks, which led to a significant improvement of sensory and motor performance of the affected hand. Remarkably, after a follow-up of 6 weeks, the same magnitude of improved sensorimotor performance could be observed (Smith, Dinse, Kalisch, Johnson, & Walker-Batson, 2009). In another study on subacute stroke patients, daily application of repetitive stimulation over 4 weeks induced improvement on basic tactile tasks, such as touch threshold and tactile acuity, and on sensorimotor performance, improvements which were preserved even after 3 months of follow-up (Dinse, Bohland, et al., 2008). Accordingly, there is converging evidence that repetitive stimulation-induced effects can be quite long lasting.

It has been suggested that possible mechanisms underlying repetitive sensory stimulation include facilitation of sensorimotor integration in the relevant brain networks by increasing cortical excitability and neural activity (Calautti & Baron, 2003). Additional interpretations refer to interhemispheric competition models for sensory and motor processing, utilizing upregulation of excitability within the stroke-affected hemisphere, or downregulation of excitability within the unaffected hemisphere (Hummel & Cohen, 2006).

Combined, the effectiveness of repetitive sensory stimulation in improving tactile and sensorimotor performance, together with the advantage of using it under everyday conditions by laypeople at their homes, make repetitive sensory stimulation-based principles prime candidates for interventions in impaired populations (Dinse et al., 2005; Kalisch, Tegenthoff, et al., 2009).

THE RELATIONSHIP OF SOMATOSENSORY PLASTICITY TO OTHER CORTICAL AREAS

Crossmodal Plasticity

The role of visual cortex for touch perception. Crossmodal plasticity involves reorganization of neurons to integrate the function of two or more sensory systems. Crossmodal plasticity is a type of neuroplasticity and often occurs after sensory deprivation such as blindness or deafness. In these instances, crossmodal plasticity can strengthen other sensory systems to compensate for the lack of vision or hearing (Sathian & Stilla, 2010; Théoret, Merabet, & Pascual-Leone, 2004).

To identify differences in crossmodal reorganization depending on the onset of blindness, blind subjects have been studied by means of positron emission tomography to identify cerebral regions activated in association with Braille reading. In the congenitally blind and early-onset blind groups, the occipital cortex was strongly activated, but not in the late-onset blind group. These results indicate that there is a sensitive period for this form of functionally relevant crossmodal plasticity (Cohen et al., 1999).

To determine whether the visual cortex can process somatosensory information in a functionally relevant way, TMS has been used to disrupt the function of different cortical areas in people who were blind from an early age as they identified Braille or embossed Roman letters (Cohen et al., 1997). Transient stimulation of the visual cortex induced errors in both tasks and distorted the tactile perceptions of blind subjects. These data suggest that blindness from an early age can cause the visual cortex to be recruited to a role in somatosensory processing, and it has been suggested that this crossmodal plasticity may account in part for the superior tactile perceptual abilities of blind subjects.

A prominent feature of visual cortex is the orientation sensitivity of its neurons, making it a prime stage for processing of oriented stimuli. For oriented tactile stimuli, specific forms of crossmodal activation and crossmodal plasticity also appear to be present in normal, sighted individuals. For example, the use of focal TMS to disrupt function of the occipital cortex has been shown to interfere with the tactile discrimination of grating orientation (Zangaladze, Epstein, Grafton, & Sathian, 1999). The specificity of this effect was illustrated by its time course and spatial restriction over the scalp and by the failure of occipital TMS to affect either detection of an electrical stimulus applied to the finger pad or tactile discrimination of grating texture. The findings indicate that visual cortex is closely involved in tactile discrimination of orientation. The extent to which visual imagery is implicated in these processes remains to be clarified. A critical role of vision has been corroborated by a study in which subjects were kept for 90 minutes in the complete dark. Immediately after deprivation, subjects displayed a transient improvement of tactile spatial acuity in a grating orientation task (Facchini & Aglioti, 2003).

Modification of touch perception by viewing touch. These and other studies on crossmodal and multisensory integration indicate an intimate relationship between vision and touch. Because of this relationship, many studies have addressed how the sense of touch is modified under defined viewing conditions.

In one study, participants watched videos showing a hand being touched by a stick and a second video showing the stick touching the space beneath the hand. Touch thresholds of the IFs were tested with von Frey filaments. There was a significant enhancement of the touch threshold after showing the video with the touched hand but not after showing the video with no touch of the hand (Schaefer, Heinze, & Rotte, 2005).

To clarify the role of somatosensory cortex in the modulation of tactile perception through vision information, subjects were asked to look at a hand in a video being touched on the first digit (D1) in synchrony with felt touches on their real hidden hand, as compared with watching a video with asynchronous touches. During synchronous stimulation, subjects reported feeling the tactile sensation on the video hand, thus indicating that in this condition the subjects regarded the video hand as their own touched hand. This feeling disappeared in the asynchronous condition. The results using neuromagnetic source imaging revealed that the cortical representation of D1 moved to a more inferior location during synchronous in comparison to asynchronous stimulation and rest (Schaefer, Flor, Heinze, & Rotte, 2006).

It is well documented that observing the actions of others activates the premotor cortex normally involved in the execution of the same actions (Rizzolatti, Fadiga, Gallese, & Fogassi, 1996). A similar mechanism appears to apply to the sight of touch. In an fMRI study, participants were touched on their legs while viewing movies of other people or objects being touched. It was found that the secondary somatosensory cortex was activated both when the participants were touched and when they observed someone or something else getting touched by objects. The primary somatosensory cortex showed no significant activation during the observation of touch, although it showed a trend in that direction (Keysers et al., 2004).

These findings support the idea that human subjects possess a shared brain circuitry dealing both with personal experience of touch and with the corresponding event occurring to other living beings and inanimate objects. Consequently, when we witness touch, we do not just see touch but also understand touch through an automatic link with our own experience of touch (Keysers et al., 2004).

SOMATOSENSORY CHANGES IN THE CONTEXT OF BODY SCHEMA AND BODY OWNERSHIP

When we touch something with a tool, we feel the touch at the tip of the tool, rather than in the larger hand that holds the tool. Accordingly, when an object is used as a tool, it is felt as a part or an extension of an arm or the fingers, indicating that the tool is incorporated into our body image. Thus, alterations of body schemata have been hypothesized as the basis of the behavioral and perceptual assimilation of tool and hand.

In an elegant and simple experiment, it was shown that the judgment of the temporal order of two successive stimuli, delivered to the tips of sticks held in each hand, was dramatically altered by crossing the sticks without changing the positions of the hands (where the actual mechanoreceptors are located). This suggested that the somatosensory signals evoked at the hands were referred to the spatial locations of the tips of the sticks before the cutaneous signals were ordered in time (Yamamoto & Kitazawa, 2001). Comparing the functional organization of SI during tool use and when executing the task with the fingers revealed that the cortical representations of D1 and D5 were further apart during tool use than during non-tool use and rest (Schaefer, Rothemund, Heinze, & Rotte, 2004). These data suggest that somatosensory maps in early cortical areas are part of the neural network representing the modified schema of the hand in which the tool was incorporated.

It is generally believed that cortical plasticity mechanisms allow signals from implanted prostheses to be handled by the brain like natural sensors or actuators. Brain–computer interfaces (BCIs) are direct communication pathways between a brain and an external device, where electrical brain signals are analyzed in real time for control of external devices. BCIs are often aimed at assisting, augmenting, or repairing human cognitive or sensory-motor functions. In a series of pioneering studies, it was demonstrated that primates can learn to reach and grasp virtual objects by controlling a robot arm through a closed-loop BMI (Carmena et al., 2003, O'Doherty, Lebedev, Hanson, Fitzsimmons, & Nicolelis, 2009). Continuous BMI operation by monkeys led to significant improvements in both model predictions and behavioral performance, implicating the involvement of behavioral and perceptual learning. BMI-related functional reorganization in multiple cortical areas suggested that the dynamic properties of the BMI were incorporated into motor and sensory cortical representations, thereby modifying the homuncular structure.

How virtual limbs and bodies can come to feel like real limbs and bodies is a question of great interest, addressing how body ownership is established and can be manipulated. The starting point for studying this question was the so-called rubber hand illusion (Botvinick & Cohen, 1998). Synchronous tapping on a hidden real arm and on an aligned visible rubber arm placed in front of an individual resulted in a feeling of ownership of the fake rubber arm. These data indicated that visuotactile correlations are prerequisites for inducing an illusion of ownership. Using virtual environments, researchers are currently investigating the conditions in which virtual ownership of the entire body can be achieved—an ownership requiring recalibration of visual, tactile, and proprioceptive representations (Slater, Perez-Marcos, Ehrsson, & Sanchez-Vives, 2009).

Modality Specificity of Touch Plasticity

Massive and enduring plastic changes have been described for all modalities, confirming the contemporary view that all cortical areas are modifiable beyond the critical sensitive periods during development. These findings demonstrate that the sensorimotor cortical representations in adults are not hardwired but retain a self-organizing capacity operational throughout life. On the other hand, somatosensory cortex appears to differ from visual cortex in the readiness of inducibility and in the magnitude, stability, and time course of changes (Leonhard & Dinse, 2009; Smirnakis et al., 2005).

Generally, different forms and magnitudes of plastic changes might be due to differences in cellular, pharmacological, and histochemical properties that reflect area-specific constraints of the molecular equipment available in that area. While this can explain existing differences in the outcome of plastic changes, the reasons for the emergence of such differences in cellular properties remain a question. In the plasticity of the sense of touch, the concepts of "use" and "no-use" allow an easy and intuitive description and classification of plastic changes. Given the obvious lack of conditions reflecting "use-dependent" plasticity in the visual or auditory domain, it is very possible that the scheme of differential use is an inappropriate concept that does not fit the specific constraints of other sensory systems. Furthermore, the visual cortex is characterized by a number of so-called functional maps that are overlaid across the retinotopic gradient, thereby generating a highly complicated form of topological structure (Swindale, Shoham, Grinvald, Bonhoeffer, & Hubener, 2000). Up to now, comparable topological features have not been described for the somatosensory cortex. It has been suggested that these global topological constraints may impose forces that stabilize the underlying cortical networks (Wolf & Geisel, 1998), thereby limiting and restricting plastic changes.

As an alternative explanation, we have suggested that although VI and SI are regarded as primary cortical areas, the type of preprocessing occurring subcortically and at the level of the retina renders VI and SI areas dissimilar in terms of their position within a hierarchy of bottom–up and top–down processing, thereby affecting the readiness and susceptibility for plastic reorganization (Leonhard & Dinse, 2009). As a result, it is possible that part of the observed dissimilarities reflect genuine modality-specific differences, building on important constraints associated with the processing of modality-specific sensory information. Comparative studies focusing on modality-specific features of cortical plasticity will reveal further insight into principles governing neocortical organization.

REFERENCES

Bleyenheuft, Y., Wilmotte, P., & Thonnard, J. L. (2010). Relationship between tactile spatial resolution and digital dexterity during childhood. *Somatosensory and Motor Research, 27*, 9–14.

Bockelmann, A., & Dinse, H. R. (2009). [Tactile acuity in children]. Unpublished raw data.

Bolton, C. F., Winkelmann, R. K., & Dyck, P. J. (1966). A quantitative study of Meissner's corpuscles in man. *Neurology, 16,* 1–9.

Botvinick, M., & Cohen, J. (1998). Rubber hands 'feel' touch that eyes see. *Nature, 391,* 756–756.

Braun, C., Schweizer, R., Elbert, T., Birbaumer, N., & Taub, E. (2000). Differential activation in somatosensory cortex for different discrimination tasks. *Journal of Neuroscience, 20,* 446–450.

Bruce, M. F. (1980). The relation of tactile thresholds to histology in the fingers of elderly people. *Journal of Neurology, Neurosurgery, and Psychiatry, 43,* 730–734.

Bruce, M. F., & Sinclair, D. C. (1980). The relationship between tactile thresholds and histology in the human finger. *Journal of Neurology, Neurosurgery, and Psychiatry, 43,* 235–242.

Calautti, C., & Baron, J. C. (2003). Functional neuroimaging studies of motor recovery after stroke in adults: A review. *Stroke, 34,* 1553–1566.

Carmena, J. M., Lebedev, M. A., Crist, R. E., O'Doherty J. E., Santucci, D. M., Dimitrov, D. F.,...Nicolelis, M. A. (2003). Learning to control a brain-machine interface for reaching and grasping by primates. *PLoS Biology, 1,* E42.

Casserly, I., Thambipillai, T., Macken, M., & Fitzgerald, M. J. (1994). Innervation of the tylotrich-touch dome complexes in rat skin: Changing patterns during postnatal development. *Journal of Anatomy, 185,* 553–563.

Cohen, L. G., Celnik, P., Pascual-Leone, A., Corwell, B., Falz, L., Dambrosia, J.,...Hallett, M. (1997). Functional relevance of cross-modal plasticity in blind humans. *Nature, 389,* 180–183.

Cohen, L. G., Weeks, R. A., Sadato, N., Celnik, P., Ishii, K., & Hallett, M. (1999). Period of susceptibility for cross-modal plasticity in the blind. *Annals of Neurology, 45,* 451–460.

Colcombe, S., Kramer, A., Erickson, K., Scalf, P., McAuley, E., Cohen, N., Elavsky, S. (2006). Cardiovascular fitness, cortical plasticity, and aging. *Proceedings of the National Academy of Sciences of the United States of America, 101,* 3316–3321.

Cope, E. B., & Antony, J. H. (1992). Normal values for the two-point discrimination test. *Pediatric Neurology, 8,* 251–254.

Coughlin, P. A., Bonser, R., Turton, E. P., Kent, P. J., & Kester, R. C. (2001). A comparison between two methods of aesthesiometric assessment in patients with hand-arm vibration syndrome. *Occupational Medicine, 51,* 272–277.

Dhruv, N. T., Niemi, J. B., Harry, J. D., Lipsitz, L. A., & Collins, J. J. (2002). Enhancing tactile sensation in older adults with electrical noise stimulation. *Neuroreport, 13,* 597–600.

Dillon, Y. K., Haynes, J., & Henneberg, M. (2001). The relationship of the number of Meissner's corpuscles to dermatoglyphic characters and finger size. *Journal of Anatomy, 199,* 577–584.

Dinse, H. R. (2006). Cortical reorganization in the aging brain. *Progress in Brain Research, 157,* 57–80.

Dinse, H. R., Bohland, J., Kalisch, T., Kraemer, M., Freund, E., Beeser, E., ... Stephan, K. M. (2008). Repetitive sensory stimulation training in stroke. *European Journal of Neurology, 15(S-3),* 400.

Dinse, H. R., Kalisch, T., Ragert, P., Pleger, B., Schwenkreis, P., & Tegenthoff, M. (2005). Improving human haptic performance in normal and impaired human populations through unattended activation-based learning. *ACM Transactions on Applied Perception, 2,* 71–88.

Dinse, H. R., Kleibel, N., Kalisch, T., Ragert, P., Wilimzig, C., & Tegenthoff, M. (2006). Tactile co-activation resets age-related decline of human tactile discrimination. *Annals of Neurology, 60,* 88–94.

Dinse, H. R., & Merzenich, M. M. (2002). Adaptation of inputs in the somatosensory system. In M. Fahle and T. Poggio (Eds.), *Perceptual learning* (pp. 19–42). Cambridge: MIT Press.

Dinse, H. R., Ragert, P., Pleger, B., Schwenkreis, P., & Tegenthoff, M. (2003). Pharmacological modulation of perceptual learning and associated cortical reorganization. *Science, 301,* 91–94.

Dinse, H. R., Tegenthoff, M., Heinisch, C., & Kalisch, T. (2009). Ageing and touch. In B. Goldstein (Ed.), *The Sage encyclopedia of perception* (pp. 21–24). Thousand Oaks, CA: Sage.

Dinse, H. R., Wilimzig, C., & Kalisch, T. (2008). Learning effects in haptic perception. In M. Grunwald (Ed.), *Human haptic perception: Basics and applications* (pp. 165–182). Basel, Switzerland: Birkhäuser.

Ebied, A. M., Kemp, G. J., & Frostick, S. P. (2004). The role of cutaneous sensation in the motor function of the hand. *Journal of Orthopaedic Research, 22,* 862–866.

Eckstein, M. P., Abbey, C. K., Pham, B. T., & Shimozaki, S. S. (2004). Perceptual learning through optimization of attentional weighting: Human versus optimal Bayesian learner. *Journal of Vision, 4,* 1006–1019.

Elbert, T., Pantev, C., Wienbruch, C., Rockstroh, B., & Taub, E. (1995). Increased cortical representation of the fingers of the left hand in string players. *Science, 270,* 305–307.

Ernst, M. O., & Banks, M, S. (2002). Humans integrate visual and haptic information in a statistically optimal fashion. *Nature, 415,* 429–433.

Facchini, S., & Aglioti, S. M. (2003). Short term light deprivation increases tactile spatial acuity in humans. *Neurology, 60,* 1998–1999.

Fahle, M. (1997). Specificity of learning curvature, orientation, and vernier discriminations. *Vision Research, 37,* 1885–1895.

Fahle, M., & Poggio, T. (2002). *Perceptual learning.* Cambridge: MIT Press.

Feldman, D. E., & Brecht, M. (2005). Map plasticity in somatosensory cortex. *Science, 310,* 810–815.

Fitzgerald, M. J. (1961). Developmental changes in epidermal innervation. *Journal of Anatomy, 95,* 495–514.

Florence, S. L., Taub, H. B., & Kaas, J. H. (1998). Large-scale sprouting of cortical connections after peripheral injury in adult macaque monkeys. *Science, 282,* 1117–1121.

Godde, B., Berkefeld, T., David-Jürgens, M., & Dinse, H. R. (2002). Age-related changes in primary somatosensory cortex of rats: evidence for parallel degenerative and plastic-adaptive processes. *Neuroscience and Biobehavioral Reviews, 26,* 743–752.

Godde, B., Stauffenberg, B., Spengler, F., & Dinse, H. R. (2000). Tactile co-activation induced changes in spatial discrimination performance. *Journal of Neuroscience, 20*, 1597–1604.

Goldstone, R. L. (1998). Perceptual learning. *Annual Review of Psychology, 49*, 585–612.

Gori, M., Del Viva, M., Sandini, G., & Burr, D. C. (2008). Young children do not integrate visual and haptic form information. *Current Biology, 18*, 694–698.

Gutnisky, D. A., Hansen, B. J., Iliescu, B. F., & Dragoi, V. (2009). Attention alters visual plasticity during exposure-based learning. *Current Biology, 19*, 555–560.

Heinisch, C., Kalisch, T., & Dinse, H. R. (2006, October). *Tactile and learning abilities in early-and late-blind subjects.* Poster session presented at the annual meeting of the Society for Neuroscience, Atlanta, Georgia.

Hillman, C., Erickson, K., & Kramer, A. (2008). Be smart, exercise your heart: Exercise effects on brain and cognition. *Nature Reviews, Neuroscience, 9*, 58–65.

Hof, P. R., & Mobbs, C. V. (2001). *Functional neurobiology of aging.* San Diego: Academic Press.

Höffken, O., Veit, M., Knossalla, F., Lissek, S., Bliem, B., Ragert, P., ... Tegenthoff, M. (2007). Sustained increase of somatosensory cortex excitability by tactile co-activation studied by paired median nerve stimulation in humans correlates with perceptual gain. *Journal of Physiology, 584*, 463–471.

Hummel, F. C., & Cohen, L. G. (2006). Non-invasive brain stimulation: A new strategy to improve neurorehabilitation after stroke? *Lancet Neurology, 5*, 708–712.

Kaas, J. H. (2000). The reorganization of somatosensory and motor cortex after peripheral nerve or spinal cord injury in primates. *Progress in Brain Research, 128*, 173–179.

Kalisch, T., & Dinse, H. R. (2009). [Correlation between tactile acuity and haptic object recognition]. Unpublished raw data.

Kalisch, T., Ragert, P., Schwenkreis, P., Dinse, H. R., & Tegenthoff, M. (2009). Human age-related decline in tactile perception is accompanied by enlargement of the hand representation in somatosensory cortex. *Cerebral Cortex, 19*, 1530–1538.

Kalisch, T., Tegenthoff, M., & Dinse, H. R. (2008). Improvement of sensorimotor functions in old age by passive sensory stimulation. *Clinical Interventions in Aging, 3*, 673–690.

Kalisch, T., Tegenthoff, M., & Dinse, H. R. (2009). Sensory stimulation therapy. *Frontiers in Neuroscience, 3*, 96–97.

Kalisch, T., Tegenthoff, M., & Dinse, H. R. (2010). Repetitive electric stimulation for several weeks elicits enduring improvement of sensorimotor performance in seniors. *Neural Plasticity, 2010*;690531 (Epub 2010 Apr. 14).

Kattenstroth, J. C., Kolankowska, I., Kalisch, T., & Dinse, H. R. (2010). Superior sensory, motor, and cognitive performance in elderly individuals with multi-year dancing activities. *Frontiers in Aging Neuroscience, 2*, 31. doi:10.3389/fnagi.2010.00031.

Kerr, C., Shaw, J., Wasserman, R., Chen, V., Kanojia, A., Bayer, T., & Kelley, J. (2008), Tactile acuity in experienced Tai Chi practitioners: Evidence for use dependent plasticity as an effect of sensory-attentional training. *Experimental Brain Research, 188*, 317–322.

Keysers, C., Wicker, B., Gazzola, V., Anton, J. L., Fogassi, L., & Gallese, V. (2004). A touching sight: SII/PV activation during the observation of touch. *Neuron, 42*, 395–346.

Koesler, I. B., Dafotakis, M., Ameli, M., Fink, G. R., & Nowak, D. A. (2008). Electrical somatosensory stimulation modulates hand motor function in healthy humans. *Journal of Neurology, 255,* 1567–1573.

Legge, G. E., Madison, C., Vaughn, B. N., Cheong, A. M., & Miller, J. C. (2008). Retention of high tactile acuity throughout the life span in blindness. *Perception and Psychophysics, 70,* 1471–1488.

Leonhard, R., & Dinse, H. R. (2009). Receptive field plasticity of area 17 visual cortical neurons of adult rats. *Experimental Brain Research, 199,* 401–410.

Lissek, S., Wilimzig, C., Stude, P., Pleger, B., Kalisch, T., Maier, C., … Dinse, H. R. (2009). Immobilization impairs tactile perception and shrinks somatosensory cortical maps. *Current Biology, 19,* 837–842.

Mahncke, H. W., Bronstone, A., & Merzenich, M. M. (2006). Brain plasticity and functional losses in the aged: Scientific bases for a novel intervention. *Progress in Brain Research, 157,* 81–109.

Mattson, M. (2008). Hormesis defined. *Aging Research Reviews, 7,* 1–7.

Merzenich, M. M., Nelson, R. J., Stryker, M. P., Cynader, M. S., Schoppmann, A., & Zook, J. M. (1984). Somatosensory cortical map changes following digit amputation in adult monkeys. *Journal of Comparative Neurology, 224,* 591–605.

Nagarajan, S. S., Blake, D. T., Wright, B. A., Byl, N., & Merzenich, M. M. (1998). Practice-related improvements in somatosensory interval discrimination are temporally specific but generalize across skin location, hemisphere, and modality. *Journal of Neuroscience, 18,* 1559–1570.

Neeper, S. A., Gomez-Pinilla, F., Choi, J., & Cotman, C. (1995). Exercise and brain neurotrophins. *Nature, 373,* 109.

O'Doherty, J. E., Lebedev, M. A., Hanson, T. L., Fitzsimmons, N. A., & Nicolelis, M. A. (2009). A brain-machine interface instructed by direct intracortical microstimulation. *Frontiers in Integrative Neuroscience, 3,* 20.

Pascual-Leone, A., & Torres, F. (1993). Plasticity of the sensorimotor cortex representation of the reading finger in Braille readers. *Brain, 116,* 39–52.

Peters, A. 2002. The effects of normal aging on myelin and nerve fibers: A review. *Journal of Neurocytology, 31,* 581–593.

Peters, R. M., Hackeman, E., & Goldreich, D. (2009). Diminutive digits discern delicate details: Fingertip size and the sex difference in tactile spatial acuity. *Journal of Neuroscience, 29,* 15756–1561.

Picard, D. (2007). Tactual, visual, and cross-modal transfer of texture in 5- and 8-year-old children. *Perception, 36,* 722–736.

Pleger, B., Dinse, H. R., Ragert, P., Schwenkreis, P., Malin, J. P., & Tegenthoff, M. (2003). Shifts in cortical representations predict human discrimination improvement. *Proceedings of the National Academy of Sciences of the United States of America, 98,* 12255–12260.

Pleger, B., Foerster, A. F., Ragert, P., Dinse, H. R., Schwenkreis, P., Nicolas, V., & Tegenthoff, M. (2003). Functional imaging of perceptual learning in human primary and secondary somatosensory cortex. *Neuron, 40,* 643–653.

Priplata, A. A., Niemi, J. B., Harry, J. D., Lipsitz, L. A., & Collins, J. J. (2003). Vibrating insoles and balance control in elderly people. *Lancet, 362,* 1123–1124.

Qü, M., Mittmann, T., Luhmann, H. J., Schleicher, A., & Zilles, K. (1998). Long-term changes of ionotropic glutamate and GABA receptors after unilateral permanent focal cerebral ischemia in the mouse brain. *Neuroscience, 85,* 29–43.

CHAPTER 4   BRAIN PLASTICITY AND TOUCH   117

Rabin, E., & Gordon, A. M. (2004). Tactile feedback contributes to consistency of finger movements during typing. *Experimental Brain Research, 155,* 362–369.

Ragert, P., Becker, M., Tegenthoff, M., Pleger, B., & Dinse, H. R. (2004). Sustained increase of somatosensory cortex (SI) excitability by 5Hz repetitive transcranial magnetic stimulation (rTMS) studied by paired median nerve stimulation. *Neuroscience Letters, 356,* 91–94.

Ragert, P., Dinse, H. R., Pleger, B., Wilimzig, C., Frombach, E., Schwenkreis, P., & Tegenthoff, M. (2003). Combination of 5 Hz repetitive transcranial magnetic stimulation (rTMS) and tactile co-activation boosts tactile discrimination in humans. *Neuroscience Letters, 348,* 105–108.

Ragert, P., Franzkowiak, S., Schwenkreis, P., Tegenthoff, M., & Dinse, H. R. (2008). Improvement of tactile perception and enhancement of cortical excitability through intermittent theta burst rTMS over human primary somatosensory cortex. *Experimental Brain Research, 184,* 1–11.

Ragert, P., Kalisch, T., Bliem, B., Franzkowiak, S., & Dinse, H. R. (2008). Differential effects in human tactile discrimination behavior evoked by tactile high- and low-frequency stimulation. *BMC Neuroscience, 9,* 9.

Ragert, P., Schmid, A., Altenmueller, E., & Dinse, H. R. (2004). Superior tactile performance and learning in professional pianists: Evidence for meta-plasticity in musicians. *European Journal of Neuroscience, 19,* 473–478.

Ragert, P., Vandermeeren, Y., Camus, M., & Cohen, L. G. (2008). Improvement of spatial tactile acuity by transcranial direct current stimulation. *Clinical Neurophysiology, 119,* 805–811.

Ramachandran, V. S., Rogers-Ramachandran, D., & Stewart, M. (1992). Perceptual correlates of massive cortical reorganization. *Science, 258,* 1159–1160.

Raz, N., Gunning, F. M., Head, D., Dupuis, J. H., McQuain, J., Briggs, S. D.,...Acker, J. D. (1997). Selective aging of the human cerebral cortex observed in vivo: differential vulnerability of the prefrontal gray matter. *Cerebral Cortex, 7,* 268–282.

Recanzone, G. H., Jenkins, W. M., Hradek, G. T., & Merzenich, M. M. (1992). Progressive improvement in discriminative abilities in adult owl monkeys performing a tactile frequency discrimination task. *Journal of Neurophysiology, 67,* 1015–1030.

Recanzone, G. H., Merzenich, M. M., Jenkins, W. M., Grajski, K., & Dinse, H. R. (1992). Topographic reorganization of the hand representation in cortical area 3b of owl monkeys trained in a frequency discrimination task. *Journal of Neurophysiology, 67,* 1031–1056.

Reinke, H., & Dinse, H. R. (1996). Functional characterization of cutaneous mechanoreceptor properties in aged rats. *Neuroscience Letters, 216,* 171–174.

Rizzolatti, G., Fadiga, L., Gallese, V., & Fogassi, L. (1996). Premotor cortex and the recognition of motor actions, *Cognitive Brain Research, 3,* 131–141.

Rosenkranz, K., Williamon, A., & Rothwell, J. C. (2007). Motorcortical excitability and synaptic plasticity is enhanced in professional musicians. *Journal of Neuroscience, 27,* 5200–5206.

Sathian K., & Stilla, R. (2010). Cross-modal plasticity of tactile perception in blindness. *Restorative Neurology and Neuroscience, 28,* 271–281.

Sathian, K., & Zangaladze, A. (1997). Tactile learning is task specific but transfers between fingers. *Perception and Psychophysics, 59,* 119–128.

Sathian, K., & Zangaladze, A. (1998). Perceptual learning in tactile hyperacuity: Complete intermanual transfer but limited retention. *Experimental Brain Research, 118*, 131–234.

Sawaki, L., Wu, C. W., Kaelin-Lang, A., & Cohen, L. G. (2006). Effects of somatosensory stimulation on use-dependent plasticity in chronic stroke. *Stroke, 37*, 246–247.

Schaefer, M., Heinze, H. J., & Rotte, M. (2005). Viewing touch improves tactile sensory threshold. *Neuroreport, 16*, 367–370.

Schaefer, M., Rothemund, Y., Heinze, H. J., & Rotte, M. (2004). Short-term plasticity of the primary somatosensory cortex during tool use. *Neuroreport, 15*, 1293–1297.

Schaefer, S., Huxhold, O., & Lindenberger, U. (2006). Healthy mind in healthy body? A review of sensorimotor–cognitive interdependencies in old age. *European Review of Aging and Physical Activity, 3*, 45–54.

Seitz, A. R., & Dinse, H. R. (2007). A common framework for perceptual learning. *Current Opinion in Neurobiology, 17*, 148–153.

Slater, M., Pérez-Marcos, D., Ehrsson, H., & Sanchez-Vives, M. V. (2009). Inducing illusory ownership of a virtual body. *Frontiers in Neuroscience, 3*, 214–220.

Smirnakis, S. M., Brewer, A. A., Schmid, M. C., Tolias, A. S., Schüz, A., Augath, M.,...Logothetis, N. K. (2005). Lack of long-term cortical reorganization after macaque retinal lesions. *Nature, 453*, 300–307.

Smith, P. S., Dinse, H. R., Kalisch, T., Johnson, M., & Walker-Batson, D. (2009). Effects of repetitive electrical stimulation to treat sensory loss in persons poststroke. *Archives of Physical Medicine and Rehabilitation, 90*, 2108–2111.

Sowell, E. R., Peterson, B. S., Thompson, P. M., Welcome, S. E., Henkenius, A. L., & Toga, A. W. (2003). Mapping cortical change across the human life span. *Nature Neuroscience, 6*, 309–315.

Sterr, A., Muller, M. M., Elbert, T., Rockstroh, B., Pantev, C., & Taub, E. (1998). Changed perceptions in Braille readers. *Nature, 391*, 134–135.

Stevens, J. C. (1992). Aging and spatial acuity of touch. *Journal of Gerontology, 47*, P35–40.

Stevens, J. C., & Choo, K. K. (1996). Spatial Acuity of the Body Surface over the Life Span. *Somatosensory and Motor Research, 13*,153–166.

Swindale, N. V., Shoham, D., Grinvald, A., Bonhoeffer, T., & Hubener, M. (2000). Visual cortex maps are optimized for uniform coverage. *Nature Neuroscience, 3*, 822–826.

Taub, E., Uswatte, G., & Elbert, T. (2002). New treatments in neurorehabilitation founded on basic research. *Nature Reviews, Neuroscience, 3*, 228–236.

Tegenthoff, M., Ragert, P., Pleger, B., Schwenkreis, P., Förster, A. F., Nicolas, V., & Dinse, H. R. (2005). Persistent improvement of tactile discrimination performance and enlargement of cortical somatosensory maps after 5 Hz rTMS. *PloS Biol, 3*, e362.

Théoret, H., Merabet, L., & Pascual-Leone, A. (2004). Behavioral and neuroplastic changes in the blind: Evidence for functionally relevant cross-modal interactions. *Journal of Physiology, Paris, 98*, 221–233.

Van Boven, R. W., Hamilton, R. H., Kauffman, T., Keenan, J. P., & Pascual-Leone, A. (2000). Tactile spatial resolution in blind Braille readers. *Neurology, 54*, 2230–2236.

Vega-Bermudez, F., & Johnson, K. O. (2004). Fingertip skin conformance accounts, in part, for differences in tactile spatial acuity in young subjects, but not for the decline in spatial acuity with aging. *Perception and Psychophysics, 66,* 60–67.

Vega-Bermudez, F., & Johnson, K. O. (2001). Differences in spatial acuity between digits. *Neurology, 56,* 1389–1391.

Wilimzig, C., & Dinse, H. R. (2007). The role of cortical interaction for spatial discrimination, localization and its learning-induced changes. *Computational and Systems Neuroscience Abstracts,* p. 248.

Wilson, H. R., & Cowan, J. D. (1973). A mathematical theory of the functional dynamics of cortical and thalamic nervous tissue. *Kybernetik, 13,* 55–80.

Wolf, F., & Geisel, T. (1998). Spontaneous pinwheel annihilation during visual development. *Nature, 395,* 73–78.

Woodward, K. L. (1993). The relationship between skin compliance, age, gender, and tactile discriminative thresholds in humans. *Somatosensory and Motor Research, 10,* 63–67.

Wu, C. W., Seo, H. J., & Cohen, L. G. (2006). Influence of electric somatosensory stimulation on paretic-hand function in chronic stroke. *Archives of Physical Medicine and Rehabilitation, 87,* 351–357.

Xerri, C., Stern, J. M., & Merzenich, M. M. (1994). Alterations of the cortical representation of the rat ventrum induced by nursing behavior. *Journal of Neuroscience, 14,* 1710–1721.

Yamamoto, S., & Kitazawa, S. (2001). Sensation at the tips of invisible tools. *Nature Neuroscience, 4,* 979–980.

Yang, T. T., Gallen, C. C., Ramachandran, V. S., Cobb, S., Schwartz, B. J., & Bloom, F. E. (1994). Noninvasive detection of cerebral plasticity in adult human somatosensory cortex. *Neuroreport, 5,* 701–704.

Zangaladze, A., Epstein, C. M., Grafton, S. T., & Sathian, K. (1999). Involvement of visual cortex in tactile discrimination of orientation. *Nature, 401,* 587–590.

II
Perceiving the Physical World via Touch

5

Biomechanical and Neurophysiological Basis of the Processing of Tactile Stimuli

STEVEN S. HSIAO

Our ability to interact with our environment depends on the diverse set of afferent fibers that provide inputs to the somatosensory system. These afferent fibers derive their inputs from receptors located in the skin, muscles, tendons, and joints and play a key role in determining the information that humans perceive about their environment. Moreover, the afferent fibers provide important feedback that lets us move about and interact with objects that we grasp and manipulate with our hands. There are four classes of afferent fiber types. The first class, thermoreceptive afferents, tells us whether objects we are touching are cold or warm. The second class of fibers indicates whether we are in contact with skin irritants or if we are in pain. The third class of fibers provides information about cutaneous and hairy inputs to the skin and encodes information about both the shape of two-dimensional form and the texture of objects that we grasp and explore, either directly with our hands or indirectly through tools that we hold in our hands. The fourth class of fibers, which are called proprioceptive afferents, provides information about the internal state of our bodies, such as its spatial position, forces, and movements. This set of afferents plays a dual role and provides sensory feedback to the motor system.

The neural basis for the rich sensations that we perceive with our hands comes from the diverse set of sensory afferents which have specialized receptor endings. These endings are selective to different forms of environmental energy—classically called the adequate stimulus (the sensory input that most effectively evokes action potentials in the afferent fiber). Thus, the adequate stimulus for a warm thermoreceptive afferent is a stimulus that increases the temperature of the skin above room temperature but does not cause a burn. The afferents can also be divided into different classes based on their conduction velocity, which is determined solely by the diameter of the fiber and whether the fiber is myelinated. Conduction velocity is important since it defines the speed at which the information is carried to the spinal cord and central nervous system and is one of the factors that limit the rate at which information is processed in the nervous system.

The diversity and importance of the somatic inputs to behavior is captured by the simple act of grasping and throwing a snowball. When the snowball is held in the hand, practically all of the peripheral afferents that innervate the hand are activated. Thermal receptors provide information about the temperature. Simultaneously, the cutaneous receptors provide information about the texture and local curvature of the ball on the skin, and proprioceptive afferents in conjunction with the cutaneous receptors provide information about the global size and shape of the ball. These sensory inputs encode in their patterns of action potentials an initial or peripheral neural representation of the snowball which is then sent to the central nervous system, where the inputs are integrated and transformed to produce central representations that allow us to recognize the snowball. Furthermore, after the snowball is perceived, inputs from these sensory afferents are then used by the motor system in a highly coordinated fashion to release and throw the ball. The neural mechanisms underlying the simple act of grasping and throwing a ball are not well understood.

In this chapter, the biomechanical and neurophysiological basis of tactile perception is reviewed. The focus is on the tactile perceptual functions mediated by the cutaneous afferents that innervate the glabrous skin. Different kinds of cutaneous afferents that innervate the skin are reviewed first. For each afferent type, the anatomical and transduction mechanisms that provide the mechanoreceptive afferents with modality-specific responses are identified. Then the sensory afferent systems related to proprioception are discussed briefly. Throughout the chapter, we will concentrate on the responses of receptors of the glabrous skin of the hand as a paradigm for understanding the basic mechanisms underlying perception. Much less is known about the receptors innervating hairy skin and their associated afferent systems and as such these systems will not be reviewed.

CUTANEOUS MECHANORECEPTIVE AFFERENTS

The neural basis of cutaneous perception involves four types of mechanoreceptive afferents that show selectivity to different aspects of mechanical stimuli. Two of the four afferent types, namely the rapidly adapting

(RA) and Pacinian corpuscle (PC) afferents, respond to dynamic motion on the skin. Both these afferent types are classified as RA because they respond to transient indentation and are silent to steady pressure. The other two afferent types, the slowly adapting type 1 (SA1) and slowly adapting type 2 (SA2) afferents, are classified as such because they show a sustained response to a sustained stimulation of the skin. They are called slowly adapting because the firing rates show a mild or slow decline in discharge rate with the sustained input. Although the SA1 afferents respond well to static stimuli, they are significantly more sensitive to moving stimuli. The neural responses of these afferent fiber types have been studied in humans, nonhuman primates, and rodents. The data show that while RA, PC, and SA1 afferent fibers are commonly found in the different species, the SA2 afferents that are reported in humans are absent in nonhuman primates (Pare, Behets, & Cornu, 2003).

SA1 Afferents Are the Spatial System

SA1 afferents are A-β fibers with conduction velocities ranging from ~40 to 60 m/sec. Like all the afferent fibers, the SA1 afferents have their cell bodies located in the dorsal root ganglia. These myelinated afferent fibers branch repeatedly (~5–20 times) as they reach the skin and terminate in the basal layer of the epidermis where they lose their myelin sheaths and become enveloped by a specialized set of epidermal cells called Merkel cell neurite complex. The Merkel cells are located at the base of the primary epidural ridges, which are also referred to as the intermediate ridges. The tops of these ridges are where the sweat ducts exit the finger pads (see Figure 5.1).

Until recently, the evidence that Merkel cells play a role in SA1 function has been mainly circumstantial. However, recent evidence shows that the Merkel cell/neurite complex plays a critical role in giving the SA1 afferents their unique response properties. In those studies (Maricich et al., 2009), the investigators produced mice that lack the gene *Atoh1*, which is a transcription factor necessary for the production of normal Merkel cells, and found that animals without Merkel cells do not have normal SA1-like responses. The results strongly suggest that Merkel cells play a critical role in encoding mechanical stimuli by the SA1 afferents. While the physiological mechanisms are not understood, data from electron micrographs reveal that there are synapse-like junctions between the Merkel cells and the axon terminals. One possibility is that the Merkel cells, not the neurite ending, sense the mechanical stimuli. Another is that the Merkel cells function as active modulators of the mechanoreceptive inputs to the

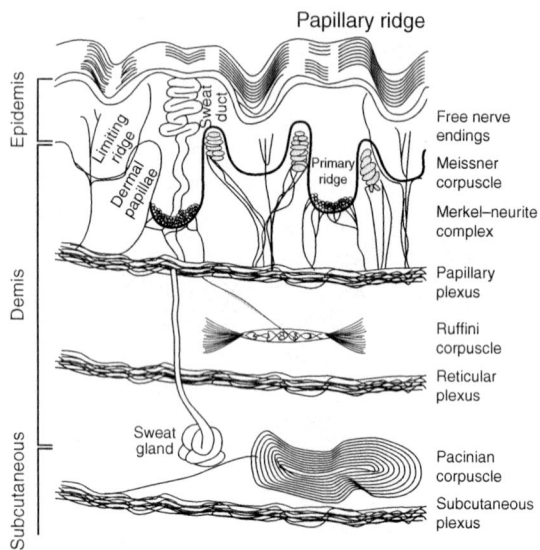

FIGURE 5.1 Anatomical illustration of the glabrous skin of a human finger pad, showing the Papillary ridges that form the fingerprints. These ridges are also the outlets for the sweat ducts. Merkel cells lie in the epidermis at the base of the ridge which is deeper than the Meissner's corpuscles which lie between the ridges. The figure shows a PC and the hypothetical location for the Ruffini corpuscle which was originally thought to be the end organ for the SA2 afferent. Adapted with permission from "The somatosensory system," by S. Hendry & S. S. Hsiao, 2008, *Fundamental neuroscience* (pp. 581–608). San Diego: Academic Press. Copyright 2008 by Academic Press.

afferent ending. Further studies are needed to determine how action potentials are generated in the SA1 afferents following a mechanical stimulus (Ogawa, 1996).

While the detailed mechanisms that underlie the activation of the SA1 afferents have yet to be worked out, there is significant evidence to suggest that the mechanisms involve the close interplay between the stimulus patterns on the skin and the stresses and strains at the receptor site. At a macroscopic level the skin can be subdivided into the epidermis, dermis, and the subcutaneous tissue (Figure 5.1). On the surface lie the papillary ridges, which are the structures that form the fingerprints and are the sites where the sweat ducts emerge from the skin. These papillary ridges lie immediately above an anatomical structure called the intermediate ridge which protrudes into the dermal layer. As stated earlier, the Merkel cell/neurite complex resides at the base of these intermediate ridges. Cauna (1954) initially proposed that this papillary/intermediate ridge structure functions like a lever arm whereby movements on the skin surface cause the lever arm to move which then leads to mechanical deformations of the Merkel cell–neurite complex. However, recent studies (Gerling & Thomas, 2008) used a finite-element model to show that the papillary and intermediate ridges do not move as a single lever arm and that stresses at the papillary ridge appear to play a minimal role in producing the stresses and strains at the Merkel cell/neurite complex. Instead, they propose that the epidermis/dermis interface functions like a stiff deformable shell covering an elastic bending support, with the Merkel cell/neurite complex embedded at the base of this support.

In a landmark study, Phillips and Johnson (1981) used a continuum mechanics model to determine the mechanisms that activate the mechanoreceptive channels in the SA1 afferent endings. While it is clear that the receptors must ultimately respond to mechanical stresses that produce strains at the receptor channels, the details of what aspect of strain drives the responses were not known. Phillips and Johnson assumed that the skin was a homogeneous, elastic isotropic medium and that superimposing the effects of multiple line loads on the skin could approximate the effect of a complex spatial pattern indented into the skin. Using this continuum mechanics model, they then estimated the stresses and strains produced by edges and gratings at different depths below the skin. To infer which strains were being encoded by the peripheral afferents, they compared the strains produced by the model with the responses of the peripheral afferents recorded from the primary afferents of nonhuman primates to edges and gratings. They found that the neural responses of the SA1 afferents to the indented gratings closely matched a specific component of the tissue strain near the nerve ending (i.e., strain energy density or a closely related component like the maximum compressive strain or maximum tensile strain). In subsequent studies, Srinivasan and Dandekar (1996) used a finite-element model to show that the stresses and strains that most closely matched the neural responses of the SA1 afferents to indented gratings were produced by a waterbed model of the skin, in which the finger pad is treated as a bendable membrane enclosing an incompressible fluid. This model closely resembles the model that has recently been proposed by Gerling and Thomas. More recently, Sripati, Bensmaia, and Johnson (2006) expanded Phillips and Johnson's model to use point loads rather than line loads. Using this expanded model, they found that they could produce close approximations of the neural responses of the SA1 afferents to arbitrary statically indented patterns that spanned two dimensions.

A consequence of the afferents encoding strain patterns in the skin is the effect of surround suppression, whereby the responses to edges are greatly enhanced relative to the immediate surround. This mechanism is conceptually similar to surround inhibition effects that are observed in the retina. But while surround suppression in the retina is the result of neurogenic lateral inhibitory networks among neighboring cells, the suppression that is observed in the SA1 afferents is the result of skin mechanics. In regions where a uniform flat stimulus is indented, the stresses are uniformly shared across the skin and the rates evoked in the SA1 afferents are correspondingly low. However, the stresses increase dramatically at the edge and, because the SA1 afferents are sensitive to the maximum compressive strain, afferents located just under the edge have high firing rates while afferents located beyond the edge have low firing rates. The result is that SA1 afferents have enhanced response to edges.

Anatomical studies in both humans and nonhuman primates report that the SA1 afferents innervate the finger pad densely: ~100 afferents/cm^2 at the fingertip (see Hsiao, 2003, for a review). This translates to an innervation density of ~1 afferent per mm which is approximately the spatial resolution of the tactile system. The receptive field (RF) for a typical SA1 afferent is circular with a diameter of ~2.5 mm. The three-dimensional response profile of the RF is hill shaped which allows for the receptor to be differentially sensitive to where patterns are indented within the RF. A consequence of these afferents having high innervation densities and small RFs is that the representation of spatial form at the peripheral afferent level is a high-resolution isomorphic spatial neural image of stimuli contacting the finger pad. An example of an isomorphic response of a SA1 afferent to scanned embossed dot patterns is provided in Figure 5.2. It is for this reason that the SA1 system is considered to be the tactile spatial system. Combined psychophysical and neurophysiological experiments, reviewed below, show that this system is responsible for fine form and texture perception.

RA Afferents Are Specialized to Detect Motion

Like the SA1 afferents, the RA afferent fibers are A-β fibers. The conduction velocities for these afferents range from 20 to 65 m/sec which shows that that there is a greater temporal spread of information from these afferents as the information is relayed to the central nervous system. Although both SA1 and RA afferents branch repeatedly as they approach the skin, RA afferents tend to branch more; a single afferent branches ~30–80 times. Each branch projects to the border between the epidermal and dermal layers of the skin and ends in a specialized

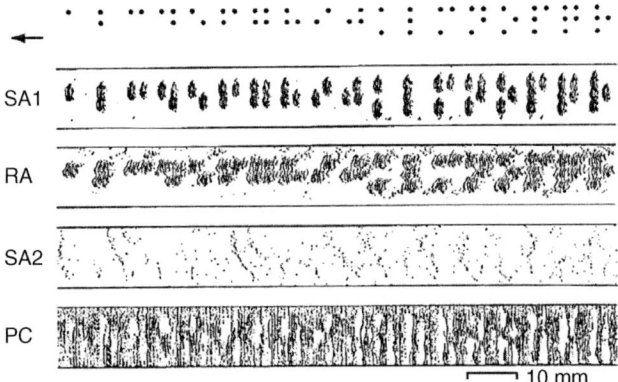

FIGURE 5.2 SEPs recorded from a human peripheral nerve. The stimuli were embossed Braille-like dot patterns (top row). The bottom four rows are the responses of different afferents to the dot pattern scanned across the afferent's RF: SA1, RA, SA2, and PCs. Note that the SA1 afferents are the spatial system and have responses that are crisper than the other three afferent types. Adapted with permission from "Representation of Braille characters in human nerve fibers," by J. Phillips, R. Johansson, & K. Johnson, 1990, *Experimental Brain Research, 81*, 589–592. Copyright 1990 by Springer.

anatomical structure called a Meissner's corpuscle. Meissner's corpuscles are located in the dermis between the sweat ducts and the limiting ridges which are the ridges adjacent to the intermediate ridges (Guinard, Usson, Guillermet, & Saxod, 2000). Like Merkel cells, Meissner's corpuscles lie very close to the skin surface and, as such, are only sensitive to deformations of the skin directly above the corpuscle. The corpuscles that innervate a single RA afferent are tightly clustered; as a result, RAs have RFs that are slightly larger (~3–4 mm in diameter) than the receptive fields of the SA1 afferents. RA afferents, by definition, do not respond to sustained input but instead respond vigorously to stimulus transients. The mechanisms that cause the RA afferents to fire are not known; however, the interaction between the Meissner's corpuscle and the neurite ending, which meanders back and forth as it ascends through the corpuscle, must play a role in giving these afferents their unique properties. Figure 5.1 shows a typical Meissner's corpuscle; it is clear from this figure that it is a complicated structure. It consists of a series of flattened supportive cells that form a vertical stack of lamellae surrounded by a connective tissue capsule. A typical capsule is ~100 µm in length and has a girth of ~50 µm. From electron micrographs it appears that each corpuscle is tethered into the adjacent dermal papillae by strands of connective tissue. One hypothesis is that the RA property of this afferent comes from the way that these connective tissue strands move to relieve the stress following an indentation of the skin. Recent studies reveal that the Meissner's corpuscle is not exclusively devoted to the A-β fiber afferent but is also associated with a C-fiber afferent (Pare, Smith, & Rice, 2002). The role that this particular C-fiber input plays in perception is not known. The two afferent fibers can be seen entering the corpuscle in Figure 5.1.

RA afferents are much less sensitive to the spatial details of scanned embossed patterns than the SA1 afferents. While SA1 afferents can resolve details of dot patterns and gratings which have spacing that are less than 1.0 mm, RA afferents only poorly resolve details of spatial patterns. Biomechanical models like the ones described earlier suggest that these afferents respond to horizontal tensile strain or to some strain measure that is affected by changes in the receptor surface area.

RA afferents innervate the skin of the fingertip with a density that is slightly higher than what is reported for the SA1 afferents (~150 afferents/cm^2). The high innervation density suggests that these afferents must play an important role in processing local information from the skin. The RF shape for these afferents differs from the hill-shaped RF of SA1 afferents and instead is relatively uniform. As stated earlier, compared with the SA1 afferents, the RA afferents poorly discriminate the fine spatial features of stimuli (see Figure 5.2). RAs begin to respond to embossed stimuli that are as small as 4 μm in height and RA firing rates plateau when stimulus height is ~400 μm. This sensitivity range for stimulus height is significantly smaller than what is seen in SA1 afferents; SA1s are much more sensitive to stimulus height and show peak firing rates for stimuli that are 1–2 mm in height.

While RA afferents provide a spatial representation of stimuli on the skin, Figure 5.2 illustrates that, because they have larger RFs, the representation is coarser than the SA1 response. What distinguishes the RA afferents from their peripheral counterparts is their exquisite sensitivity to small motions of the skin (Gardner & Palmer, 1989). Studies reviewed later provide evidence that RA afferents are sensitive to low-frequency vibrations and play a critical role in detecting when surfaces slip on the skin. This supports the notion that these afferents are velocity and motion detectors.

PC Afferents Are Specialized to Detect Vibration

PC afferents have a different organization than the SA1 and RA afferents; each afferent terminates in a single PC. The PCs lie deep in the dermis and heavily innervate deep body tissues in the gut. The PC afferent has been studied more extensively than the other cutaneous afferents with quantitative models that will not be discussed here (see Bell, Bolanowski, & Holmes, 1994, for a review). The property that distinguishes this afferent is its extreme sensitivity to mechanical stimuli. Pacinian afferents respond to vibratory amplitudes as small as 10 nm applied to the skin (Brisben, Hsiao, & Johnson, 1999) and are readily activated by light blowing. Because of their extreme sensitivity, it is difficult to define their RF borders. Classical neurophysiological studies showed that the RF properties of these afferents are derived from the PC which comprises multiple layers of fluid-filled sacs. These sacs are thought to act as high-pass filters and function to protect the neurite ending that lies at the center of the corpuscle from low-frequency vibrations. Numerous studies have shown that these afferents are exquisitely sensitive to vibrations in the range of 150–250 Hz. Recent studies show that the glia that make up the lamina are not completely passive and that, in addition to being mechanoreceptive filters, they may also release GABA which activates receptors on the neurite ending. This mechanism may play a role in modulating the adaptive properties of these neurons (Pawson, Pack, & Bolanowski, 2007).

Individual PC afferents convey spatial information poorly. There are only ~350 afferents per finger and ~800 afferents in the palm (Brisben et al., 1999). The evidence points to the PC afferents as being the tactile temporal system and responsible for encoding information from vibrations that are transmitted through tools or probes to the hand (Johnson, Yoshioka, & Vega-Bermudez, 2000).

SA2 Afferents Detect Skin Stretch

There are significant controversies about the role and even the existence of the SA2 afferents. Like the PC afferents, the SA2 afferents are located deep in the dermis (Figure 5.1). Surprisingly, SA2 afferents have not been found in nonhuman primates, suggesting that there may be differences in the way that somatosensory information is processed in humans and monkeys. For years it was thought that the receptor ending of the afferent was a specialized structure called the Ruffini complex. However, recent anatomical studies (Pare et al., 2003) have been unable to confirm those findings, and for now the receptor ending for the SA2 afferents is unknown. Nonetheless, neurophysiological studies in humans report that there is a slowly adapting afferent that responds distinctly differently than SA1 afferents. Specifically, these studies show that there are slowly adapting afferents with extreme sensitivity to stretch and poor sensitivity to indentation (Edin, Westling, & Johansson, 1992). The interspike interval distribution for these afferents is highly uniform and regular (Chambers, Andres, von Duering, & Iggo, 1972). The afferent has large RFs with indistinct borders that span large regions of skin. Finally, as exemplified in Figure 5.2, the afferent responds poorly to scanned embossed spatial patterns. The results suggest that there is a different kind of slowly adapting afferent in the human with a receptor ending that is elongated (to give the afferent its orientation selectivity to the direction of stretch) and responds to changes in strain (since these afferents appear to be sensitive to velocity). Further studies are needed to uncover the anatomical and biomechanical mechanisms of these afferents.

The role that SA2 afferents play in perception is not well understood. One view, based on the adequate stimulus that drives these afferents, is that they provide information about skin stretch. For example, studies have shown that subjects have a clear sense of joint angle after the inputs from the muscle spindle afferents have been disconnected (Refshauge, Kilbreath, & Gandevia, 1998). Since joint afferents, which are located in the joint capsules, only respond at joint extremes, it is highly likely that the SA2 skin afferents play a role in signaling joint angle. The current prevailing view is that the primary role of the SA2 afferents is to provide information about joint angle and hand conformation.

Neural Coding: Role of the Afferent Systems in Perception

Much of what we know about the functional role of the peripheral mechanoreceptive afferents comes from psychophysical studies in humans combined with neurophysiological studies in nonhuman primates (Johnson & Hsiao, 1992). Those studies make the cross-species assumption that the neural mechanisms in the two species are similar. Therefore, experiments are designed whereby the same stimulus is used for human and monkey studies and the peripheral neural code is determined by investigating what aspect of the neural response tallies with the psychophysical behavior. In the next section, four of these studies are described.

RAs and PCs are responsible for the perception of flutter and vibration. In a classic study that was published in the mid-1960s, Vernon Mountcastle and his colleagues showed that the perception of vibration is a dual sense with low-frequency vibrations ("flutter") coded by the RA afferents and high-frequency vibrations (above ~100 Hz) coded by PC afferents (Talbot, Darian-Smith, Kornhuber, & Mountcastle, 1968). In psychophysical experiments in humans and monkeys, they found that the sensory detection threshold for vibratory stimuli ranged from 5 Hz to ~300 Hz in a U-shaped function with the minimal threshold being around 200 Hz. They then recorded the responses of SA1, RA, and PC afferents using the same vibrations and found that the thresholds for activating the RA afferents closely matched the lower limb of the detection threshold curve and that the response thresholds for the rest of the curve are matched well by the absolute thresholds needed to activate the PC afferents (Figure 5.3). These studies suggest that the RA and PC afferents play nonoverlapping roles in coding time-varying tactile stimuli, with the PC afferents being the tactile sensor that detects high-frequency vibration and the RA afferents the tactile sensor that detects low-frequency flutter.

RAs are responsible for detecting motion. Johannson and his colleagues performed a combined psychophysical and neurophysiological study in humans performing a grip task (see Johansson, 1996, for a review). In their study, humans grasped and lifted objects between their thumb and index finger while single unit afferents in the subject's arm were simultaneously recorded. Researchers found that the RA afferents responded to microslips of the object and faithfully encoded the rate of load force change. This change then resulted in an increase in grip force to prevent further slip of the object. In contrast the SA1 afferents

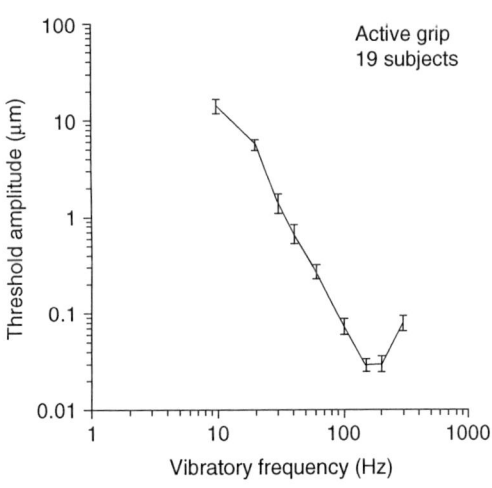

FIGURE 5.3 Detection thresholds for stimuli when subjects actively grasp a vibrating rod. Low-frequency vibrations below ~100 Hz are coded by the RA afferents and high frequencies are coded by the PC afferents. Adapted with permission from "Detection of vibration transmitted through an object grasped in the hand," by A. Brisben, S. S. Hsiao & K. Johnson, 1999, *Journal of Neurophysiology, 81*, 1548–1558. Copyright by the American Physiological Society.

were sensitive to the actual load and grip force but not to changes in these forces. These studies support the notion that the RA afferents are the motion-sensing system.

PCs are responsible for texture perception through tools. The question arises as to the utility of having a receptor system specialized for detecting high-frequency vibrations. One possibility is that this system is used to detect disturbances at a distance; for example, the PC would sense vibrations when someone approaches or when listening to loud music. A second possibility is that the PC system plays a critical role when sensing our environment through tools. Yoshioka, Bensmaia, Craig, and Hsiao (2007) recently showed that the dimensions of texture perception with the bare finger and tool are highly similar but not identical. These data suggest that the mechanisms for these percepts are different. The notion that textures can be sensed through tools is supported by seminal studies of Katz (1989) who found that texture perception through a tool is lost when the vibrations transmitted from the tool are dampened. More recently, Brisben et al. (1999) showed that subjects can detect minute vibrations that are transmitted through a tool; these vibrations can only be sensed by the PC afferent system. Yoshioka et al. (2007) further found that when using a tool, subjects have a clear sense of the roughness, hardness, and stickiness of a wide range of surfaces, which suggests that complex, multidimensional aspects of surface texture must be coded in the temporal firing patterns of the PC afferents.

SA1 afferents are responsible for cutaneous form and texture perception. There is now overwhelming evidence that the SA1 afferents are responsible for coding spatial form and texture with the bare finger. As stated earlier, the SA1 afferent system is the spatial processing system. The threshold for spatial acuity on the fingertip is ~1.0 mm which is close to the theoretical limit of spatial acuity based on the innervation densities of the SA1 afferents and is close to the spatial resolution capacity of the SA1 afferents. As shown previously in Figure 5.2, no other afferent fiber comes close to having this spatial resolution capacity.

Figure 5.4 shows the spatial event plots (SEPs) for a typical SA1 afferent and a corresponding confusion matrix from humans performing a letter discrimination task. Humans have a high capacity to do letter recognition tasks with their bare finger. When stimuli are scaled to the same receptor height in vision and touch, the corresponding confusion matrices in the two systems are nearly identical showing that form is processed similarly in vision and touch (Hsiao, 1998). An inspection

CHAPTER 5 PROCESSING OF TACTILE STIMULI 135

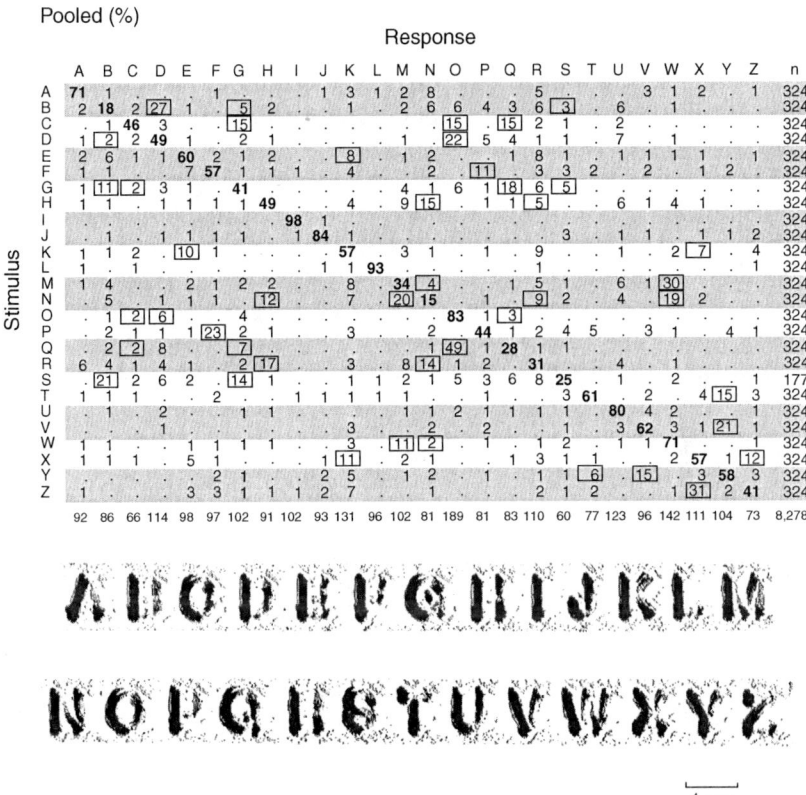

FIGURE 5.4 Top: Confusion matrix of subjects identifying embossed letters 6.0 mm in height. The diagonal represents correct responses and the off diagonal represents confusions. The patterns of confusions are highly predictable based on the visual shape of the letters suggesting that the mechanisms used by the two systems are similar. Bottom: SEP of a typical SA1 afferent to scanned letters. Each dot represents the occurrence of an action potential that was evoked as the letters were scanned across the neuron's RF. Many of the confusions shown at the top of the figure can be explained by the similarity in the neural representations of these letters at the bottom of the figure. Adapted with permission from "Human tactile pattern recognition: Active versus passive touch, velocity effects, and patterns of confusion," by F. Vega-Bermudez, K. Johnson, & S. S. Hsiao, 1991, *Journal of Neurophysiology*, 65, 531–546. Copyright by the American Physiological Society.

of the SEPs in Figure 5.4 suggests why this may be the case. The psychophysical errors that are observed in the confusion matrix are predictable based on the peripheral afferent discharge of the SA1 fibers. For example, the SA1 representation of the letter B is similar to the SA1 representation of the letter D, which explains the human behavior of Bs being confused with Ds (Vega-Bermudez, Johnson, & Hsiao, 1991). Similar studies of surface curvature also implicate the SA1 afferents as being critical for the perception of curvature (Goodwin, Browning, & Wheat, 1995; Goodwin & Wheat, 1992).

Combined psychophysical and neurophysiological studies also implicate the SA1 afferents in coding tactile roughness perception when surfaces are scanned by the bare finger. A large number of psychophysical studies show that the perception of roughness and smoothness is a unidimensional percept—suggesting that roughness is based on a single neural code. In a series of studies, Hsiao and Johnson and their colleagues asked subjects to give subjective magnitude estimates of roughness of a wide range of embossed dot patterns which varied in spacing, width, and height, as well as gratings with ridges spaced down to 100 µm. In the first study, dot spacing was varied with elements that were spaced close together to elements that sparsely contacted the skin (Connor, Hsiao, Phillips, & Johnson, 1990). In the second study, dot patterns varied in both spacing and temporal pattern and contacted the skin during scanning (Connor & Johnson, 1992). In the third study, dots varied in height and width; these stimulus parameters are known to differentially activate the RA and SA1 afferents (Blake, Hsiao, & Johnson, 1997) and allowed us to show that roughness is coded by the SA1 and not the RA system. In the fourth study, fine and coarse gratings were used with spatial periods that are below the spatial acuity range of the SA1 afferents (Yoshioka, Gibb, Dorsch, Hsiao, & Johnson, 2001). These studies found that a single neural coding mechanism, based on the spatial variation in firing rates between the SA1 afferents, accounted for subjects' perception of roughness in all four studies. The correlations between the psychophysical behavior and the SA1 spatial variation neural code was greater than 0.96 for the surfaces which span practically all surface textures (see Figure 5.5). The code has not been tested for smooth surfaces with element spacing below 100 µm.

While combined psychophysical and neurophysiological studies have yet to be performed for other aspects of texture, it is highly likely that some measure of the spatial response properties of the SA1 system is also responsible for softness perception (Srinivasan & LaMotte, 1996).

Intensity coding. Not all of tactile perception is based on the outputs of a single subset of peripheral afferents as suggested by the studies reviewed earlier. In a recent study, Muniak, Ray, Hsiao, Dammann, and Bensmaia (2007) performed a psychophysical study where humans

CHAPTER 5 PROCESSING OF TACTILE STIMULI 137

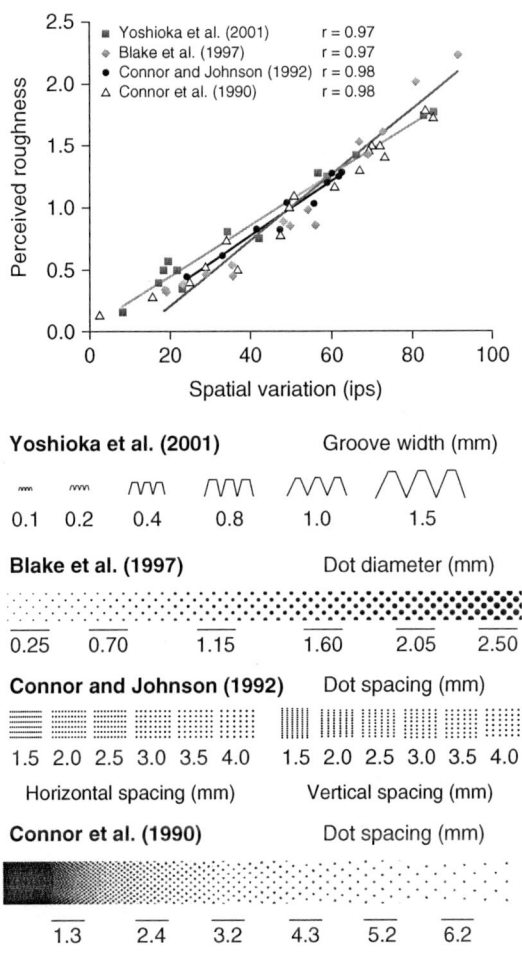

FIGURE 5.5 Summary results of four studies that investigate the neural mechanisms of roughness perception. The graph at the top shows the spatial variation measure of the neural response of the SA1 afferent versus the psychophysical subjective magnitude estimate of the roughness of the pattern. A total of 47 patterns were tested. The patterns that were used in each of the four studies are shown at the bottom. The neural code predicted closely the perceived magnitude estimates for all four studies. Adapted with permission from "Coding of object shape and texture," by S. S. Hsiao & S. Bensmaia, 2008, *Handbook of the senses: Vol. 6. Somatosensation* (6th ed., pp. 55–66). Oxford: Acadmic Press/Elsevier. Copyright by Academic Press.

made subjective magnitude estimates of the intensity of vibratory stimuli that varied from simple sinusoids to complex waveforms composed of multiple frequencies. The frequency range was chosen to activate all the peripheral mechanoreceptive afferent fibers. The authors wished to determine whether a simple perceptual parameter like intensity, which is not modality specific, is coded by a single afferent type or if it is coded by combined inputs from the different afferent fibers. They found that all three afferent types (SA1, RA, and PC) appear to contribute to the perceived intensity of complex vibratory stimuli. Thus, while previous studies show that tactile perception is modality selective when it comes to percepts like form, texture, and vibration, this study indicated that the inputs from these afferent systems are processed in parallel and contribute toward the percepts of simple tactile parameters like intensity.

PROPRIOCEPTION

Much less is known about the neural mechanisms underlying proprioception. There are four candidate afferent fiber types that are known to provide information about body position and forces. Two of those afferent types are muscle spindles, which are referred to as Type Ia and Type II. These muscle spindle afferents are imbedded in specialized spindle-like structures located in the intrafusal muscle fibers and are part of the feedback control system used to control muscles. Muscle spindles are ideally suited to provide information about muscle length and velocity since they are positioned in parallel to the extrafusal muscle fibers, and changes in muscle length are directly related to changes in joint angle. In fact, when muscle spindles are artificially activated by a vibrator placed on the belly of the muscle, subjects experience the illusion of the muscle changing length. An example of this is the "Pinocchio illusion," where subjects placing a finger on their nose perceive that it is growing if the spindle in the triceps' muscle is activated. A problem with these afferents being solely responsible for joint angle was described earlier—individuals can still detect joint angle when muscle spindle afferents are disconnected. Furthermore, evidence indicates that these afferents provide a poor representation of muscle length and velocity (Dimitriou & Edin, 2008), which suggests that they would give inaccurate estimates of joint angle.

The third type of proprioceptive afferent is the Golgi tendon organ. The receptor for this afferent type is located in the tendon of the muscle and as such these afferents cannot provide information about muscle length (Dimitriou & Edin, 2008) but provide information about muscle force.

The fourth type of proprioceptive afferent are the joint afferents which are bare nerve endings and paciform-like endings located in the joint capsules. While these afferents were originally thought to carry information about joint angle, neurophysiological studies show that they respond poorly to the mid-angles of joints and are driven most vigorously when the joints are at the limits of motion. A working hypothesis is that these afferents function as limit detectors and signal when the joint is about to be hyperextended. Patients with artificial joints have intact joint angle perception in spite of having joint afferents removed; this is further evidence that joint afferents are not critical for coding joint angle. Thus, current evidence points to the SA2 afferents, muscle spindles, or some combination of the two as being responsible for signaling joint angle.

CONCLUSIONS

In the last few decades, there has been significant progress in our understanding of the functional organization of the peripheral afferent systems. Those studies have shown that peripheral mechanoreceptive afferents are highly specialized to encode different aspects of tactile inputs. The SA1 system can be considered the spatial system. These afferents densely innervate the skin and provide the central nervous system with a crisp isomorphic representation of the two-dimensional spatial pattern of stimuli indented in the skin. This system is akin to the parvocellular system in the visual system and encodes information about the local form and texture of surfaces. The RA system can be considered the motion system. These afferents respond to minute motions on the skin and provide information about low-frequency vibrations. The peripheral representation of these afferents is also isomorphic and there is evidence that the central pathways can use these inputs to discriminate large spatial patterns. This pathway is akin to the magnocellular pathway in vision. The PC system is ideally suited for processing information about fast temporal events on the skin. These afferents are highly sensitive to vibrations and encode detailed temporal patterns about transient events. These afferents underlie our ability to discriminate surfaces when we use tools. Much less is known about the SA2 afferent system. Studies in human subjects suggest it underlies our ability to perceive joint angle and hand conformation. However, if this is so, then how do nonhuman primates, who do not have SA2 afferents, signal joint position? Further research is needed to understand this process. In addition, studies are needed to investigate and characterize the receptor endings for these afferents.

While the inputs from the different afferent systems are initially encoding information along modality-independent processing streams, it is clear that these parallel processes are ultimately integrated in the cortex to give gestalt percepts of objects. In particular, tactile object perception must involve the integration of cutaneous inputs, which provide information about the local form and texture, with proprioceptive inputs, which provide information about where the cutaneous inputs are relative to each other in three-dimensional space (Hsiao, 2008). How this is done in the central nervous system is currently under investigation.

REFERENCES

Bell, J., Bolanowski, S. J., & Holmes, M. H. (1994). The structure and function of Pacinian corpuscles: A review. *Progress in Neurobiology, 42*, 79–128.

Blake, D. T., Hsiao, S. S., & Johnson, K. O. (1997). Neural coding mechanisms in tactile pattern recognition: The relative contributions of slowly and rapidly adapting mechanoreceptors to perceived roughness. *Journal of Neuroscience, 17*, 7480–7489.

Brisben, A. J., Hsiao, S. S., & Johnson, K. O. (1999). Detection of vibration transmitted through an object grasped in the hand. *Journal of Neurophysiology, 81*, 1548–1558.

Cauna, N. (1954). Nature and functions of the papillary ridges of the digital skin. *Anatomical Record, 119*, 449–468.

Chambers, M. R., Andres, K. H., von Duering, M., & Iggo, A. (1972). The structure and function of the slowly adapting type II mechanoreceptor in hairy skin. *Quarterly Journal of Experimental Physiology, 57*, 417–445.

Connor, C. E., Hsiao, S. S., Phillips, J. R., & Johnson, K. O. (1990). Tactile roughness: Neural codes that account for psychophysical magnitude estimates. *Journal of Neuroscience, 10*, 3823–3836.

Connor, C. E., & Johnson, K. O. (1992). Neural coding of tactile texture: Comparison of spatial and temporal mechanisms for roughness perception. *Journal of Neuroscience, 12*, 3414–3426.

Dimitriou, M., & Edin, B. B. (2008). Discharges in human muscle receptor afferents during block grasping. *Journal of Neuroscience, 28*, 12632–12642.

Edin, B. B., Westling, G., & Johansson, R. S. (1992). Independent control of human finger-tip forces at individual digits during precision lifting. *Journal of Physiology, 450*, 547–564.

Gardner, E. P., & Palmer, C. I. (1989). Simulation of motion on the skin. II. Cutaneous mechanoreceptor coding of the width and texture of bar patterns displaced across the Optacon. *Journal of Neurophysiology, 62*, 1437–1460.

Gerling, G. J., & Thomas, G. W. (2008). Fingerprint lines may not directly affect SA-I mechanoreceptor response. *Somatosenssory Motor Research, 25*, 61–76.

Goodwin, A. W., Browning, A. S., & Wheat, H. E. (1995). Representation of curved surfaces in responses of mechanoreceptive afferent fibers innervating the monkey's fingerpad. *Journal of Neuroscience, 15*, 798–810.

Goodwin, A. W., & Wheat, H. E. (1992). Human tactile discrimination of curvature when contact area with the skin remains constant. *Experimental Brain Research, 88*, 447–450.

Guinard, D., Usson, Y., Guillermet, C., & Saxod, R. (2000). PS-100 and NF 70–200 double immunolabeling for human digital skin Meissner corpuscle 3D imaging. *Journal of Histochemistry and Cytochemistry, 48*, 295–302.

Hendry, S., & Hsiao, S. S. (2008). The somatosensory system. In L. R. Squire, F. E. Bloom, N. Spitzer, L. S. du, A. Ghosh, & D. Berg (Eds.), *Fundamental neuroscience* (pp. 581–608). San Diego, CA: Academic Press.

Hsiao, S. S. (1998). Similarities between touch and vision. In J. W. Morley (Ed.), *Neural aspects of tactile sensation* (pp. 131–165). Amsterdam, The Netherlands: Elsevier.

Hsiao, S. S. (2008). Central mechanisms of tactile shape perception. *Current Opinion in Neurobiology, 18*, 418–424.

Hsiao, S. S., & Bensmaia, S. (2008). Coding of object shape and texture. In A. I. Basbaum, A. G. Kaneko, M. Shepard, & G. Westheimer (Eds.), *Handbook of the senses*: Vol. 6. *Somatosensation* (6th ed., pp. 55–66). Oxford: Acadmic Press/Elsevier.

Hsiao, S. S., Johnson, K. O., & Yoshioka, T. (2003). Processing of tactile information in the primate brain. In M. Gallagher & R. J. Nelson (Eds.), *Comprehensive handbook of psychology*: Vol.3. *Biological psychology* (3rd ed., pp. 211–236). New York, NY: Wiley.

Johansson, R. S. (1996). Somatosensory signals and sensorimotor transformations in reactive control of grasp. In O. Franzén, R. S. Johansson, & L. Terenius (Eds.), *Somesthesis and the neurobiology of the somatosensory cortex* (pp. 271–282). Basel, Switzerland: Birkhäuser.

Johnson, K. O., & Hsiao, S. S. (1992). Neural mechanisms of tactual form and texture perception. *Annual Review of Neuroscience, 15*, 227–250.

Johnson, K. O., Yoshioka, T., & Vega-Bermudez, F. (2000). Tactile functions of mechanoreceptive afferents innervating the hand. *Journal of Clinical Neurophysiology, 17*, 539–558.

Katz, D. (1989). *The world of touch*. Hillsdale, NJ: Erlbaum (Krueger, L.E. translator; published originally in 1925).

Maricich, S. M., Wellnitz, S. A., Nelson, A. M., Lesniak, D. R., Gerling, G. J., Lumpkin, E. A., & Zoghbi, H. Y. (2009). Merkel cells are essential for light-touch responses. *Science, 324*, 1580–1582.

Muniak, M. A., Ray, S., Hsiao, S. S., Dammann, J. F., & Bensmaia, S. J. (2007). The neural coding of stimulus intensity: Linking the population response of mechanoreceptive afferents with psychophysical behavior. *Journal of Neuroscience, 27*, 11687–11699.

Ogawa, H. (1996). The Merkel cell as a possible mechanoreceptor cell. *Progress in Neurobiology, 49*, 317–334.

Pare, M., Behets, C., & Cornu, O. (2003). Paucity of presumptive ruffini corpuscles in the index finger pad of humans. *Journal of Comparative Neurology, 456*, 260–266.

Pare, M., Smith, A. M., & Rice, F. L. (2002). Distribution and terminal arborizations of cutaneous mechanoreceptors in the glabrous finger pads of the monkey. *Journal of Comparative Neurology, 445*, 347–359.

Pawson, L., Pack, A. K., & Bolanowski, S. J. (2007). Possible glutaminergic interaction between the capsule and neurite of Pacinian corpuscles. *Somatosensory and Motor Research, 24*, 85–95.

Phillips, J. R., Johansson, R. S., & Johnson, K. O. (1990). Representation of Braille characters in human nerve fibers. *Experimental Brain Research, 81*, 589–592.

Phillips, J. R., & Johnson, K. O. (1981). Tactile spatial resolution: III. A continuum mechanics model of skin predicting mechanoreceptor responses to bars, edges, and gratings. *Journal of Neurophysiology, 46*, 1204–1225.

Refshauge, K. M., Kilbreath, S. L., & Gandevia, S. C. (1998). Movement detection at the distal joint of the human thumb and fingers. *Experimental Brain Research, 122*, 85–92.

Srinivasan, M. A., & Dandekar, K. (1996). An investigation of the mechanics of tactile sense using two-dimensional models of the primate fingertip. *Journal of Biomechanical Engineering, 118*, 48–55.

Srinivasan, M. A., & LaMotte, R. H. (1996).Tactual discrimination of softness: Abilities and mechanisms. In O. Franzén, R. S. Johansson, & L. Terenius (Eds.),

Somesthesis and the neurobiology of the somatosensory cortex (pp. 123–135). Basel, Switzerland: Birkhäuser.

Sripati, A. P., Bensmaia, S. J., & Johnson, K. O. (2006). A continuum mechanical model of mechanoreceptive afferent responses to indented spatial patterns. *Journal of Neurophysiology, 95,* 3852–3864.

Talbot, W. H., Darian-Smith, I., Kornhuber, H. H., & Mountcastle, V. B. (1968). The sense of flutter-vibration: Comparison of the human capacity with response patterns of mechanoreceptive afferents from the monkey hand. *Journal of Neurophysiology, 31,* 301–334.

Vega-Bermudez, F., Johnson, K. O., & Hsiao, S. S. (1991). Human tactile pattern recognition: Active versus passive touch, velocity effects, and patterns of confusion. *Journal of Neurophysiology, 65,* 531–546.

Yoshioka, T., Bensmaia, S. J., Craig, J. C., & Hsiao, S. S. (2007). Texture perception through direct and indirect touch: An analysis of perceptual space for tactile textures in two modes of exploration. *Somatosensory and Motor Research, 24,* 53–70.

Yoshioka, T., Gibb, B., Dorsch, A. K., Hsiao, S. S., & Johnson, K. O. (2001). Neural coding mechanisms underlying perceived roughness of finely textured surfaces. *Journal of Neuroscience, 21,* 6905–6916.

6

Hierarchical Neural Pathways of Haptic Object Processing

SUNAH KIM AND THOMAS W. JAMES

Despite a great deal of investigation of the mechanisms of object perception in humans and other animals, a full understanding of how we perceive objects and recognize them still poses many challenges. In everyday life, our sensory systems constantly generate percepts of objects in the environment, and this includes percepts generated by our sense of touch. This chapter summarizes the neural mechanisms of haptic object processing and compares the neural pathways of haptic object processing with those of visual object processing. The haptic object processing system is shown to be hierarchically organized in the human and nonhuman primate brains and to converge with the visual object processing system at multiple neural sites.

HIERARCHICAL ORGANIZATION OF THE BRAIN IN HAPTIC OBJECT PROCESSING

Early Stages of Haptic Object Processing

The many properties of objects can be divided roughly into two classes for the purposes of haptic recognition: macrogeometric properties such as shape and size and microgeometric properties such as surface texture and hardness. During the early stages of sensory processing, these two classes of haptic recognition are processed by separate channels and are only integrated in final stages of processing. This section reviews findings of neurophysiological and neuroimaging studies of haptic recognition of macrogeometric and microgeometric properties and examines the evidence for a hierarchical organization of the haptic object processing system.

In the primate brain, the primary somatosensory cortex (SI) includes Brodmann Areas 3a, 3b, 1, and 2 and is located on the postcentral gyrus. It receives inputs from peripheral afferent neurons via thalamocortical projections (DiCarlo, Johnson, & Hsiao, 1998; Hsiao, Johnson, & Twombly, 1993; Krubitzer, Huffman, Disbrow, & Recanzone, 2004). Areas 3b and 1 in SI receive inputs primarily from cutaneous receptors, whereas Areas 3a and 2 receive inputs from deeper receptors, particularly from muscle and joints, respectively. Notably, neurons in Areas 1 and 2 not only receive inputs from peripheral afferent neurons, but also receive inputs from Areas 3a and 3b, suggesting a hierarchical flow of information processing at the earliest stages of cortical processing (Hyvärinen & Poranen, 1978; Iwamura & Tanaka, 1978). Some empirical findings suggest that separate "channels" for processing macrogeometric and microgeometric properties of objects may also exist at this stage. Neurons in Area 1 respond selectively to roughness (Hsiao et al., 1993; Randolph & Semmes, 1974), whereas neurons in Area 2 respond selectively to edges or curvature (Iwamura & Tanaka, 1978; Randolph & Semmes, 1974). This suggests that microgeometric properties of objects are processed in Area 1, whereas macrogeometric properties are processed at the same stage of hierarchy, but in Area 2. It is worth noting that receptive field size and complexity increase from Areas 3a and 3b to Areas 1 and 2 as information is pooled at higher levels of the hierarchical somatosensory system (Iwamura, 1998).

From these earliest stages of the somatosensory system in SI, information proceeds mainly to Brodmann Area 5, to the secondary somatosensory cortex (SII), and further to the insular cortex. Area 5 is located in the parietal cortex caudal to Area 2 (Duffy & Burchfiel, 1971; Iwamura, 2003; Murray & Mishkin, 1984) and superior to the lateral sulcus. A functionally defined SII has been proposed to reside in the upper bank of the lateral sulcus within the parietal operculum in monkeys (Burton, Fabri, & Alloway, 1995; Friedman, Jones, & Burton, 1980; Woolsey, 1943) as well as in humans (Disbrow, Roberts, & Krubitzer, 2000; Eickhoff, Amunts, Mohlberg, & Zilles, 2006; Maldjian et al., 1999). Despite the many recent studies investigating the anatomical location and function of SII, the details of the exact spatial extent of SII and the definition of subregions are not clear. For example, Disbrow and colleagues (2000) examined human somatosensory cortex in the Sylvian fissure using functional magnetic resonance imaging (fMRI); their somatic stimuli activated mostly the upper bank of the lateral sulcus but also rostrally and caudally adjacent areas to the region. The patterns and magnitude of activation were also not consistent across

CHAPTER 6 HAPTIC OBJECT PROCESSING 145

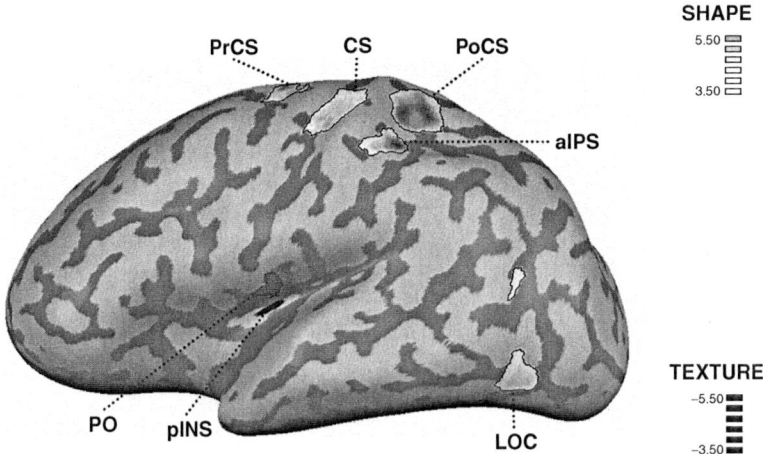

FIGURE 6.1 Human cortical regions involved in haptic shape and texture processing. A group-average statistical parametric map (SPM) derived by contrasting haptic shape processing with haptic texture processing in 18 healthy subjects is displayed on an inflated left hemisphere representation of a representative subject. CS, central sulcus; PrCS, precentral sulcus; PoCS, postcentral sulcus; aIPS, anterior part of intraparietal sulcus; PO, parietal operculum; pINS, posterior insula; LOC, lateral occipital complex.

subjects, and it is unclear whether or not SII extends into the posterior insular cortex (pINS). Location of this area is shown in Figure 6.1. Like the hierarchical progression from Areas 3a and 3b to Areas 1 and 2, hierarchical progression from SI to Area 5 and SII is demonstrated by an increase in receptive field size and complexity in the brains of both monkeys (Duffy & Burchfiel, 1971; Frackowiak et al., 2004; Iwamura, 2003; Sinclair & Burton, 1993) and humans (Duffy & Burchfiel, 1971; Frackowiak et al., 2004; Iwamura, 2003), suggesting that Area 5 and SII reside at higher stages of somatosensory processing than SI. Because of the increased receptive field size, it is possible that Area 5 and SII do not have somatotopic representations, but recent neuropsychological and neuroimaging evidence suggests that Area 5 and SII have at least four different somatotopic maps and that these maps correspond directly to maps in Areas 3a, 3b, 1, and 2 in SI (Bodegard, Geyer, Grefkes, Zilles, & Roland, 2001; Eickhoff, Amunts, et al., 2006; Eickhoff, Schleicher, Zilles, & Amunts, 2006). Although Area 5 and SII show somatotopic organization, the representations are less finegrained than those found in SI (Frackowiak et al., 2004; Ruben et al., 2001), which is consistent with those areas representing a higher stage of hierarchical processing. Unlike SI, SII responds to both contralateral and ipsilateral stimulations (Disbrow, Roberts, Poeppel, & Krubitzer, 2001; Kopietz et al., 2009; Ruben et al., 2001), which potentially facilitates the integration of information from right and left sides of the body. The removal of cortex in or adjacent to SII causes impairments of interhemispheric transfer of learning (Garcha & Ettlinger, 1978) as well as texture and shape discrimination (Murray & Mishkin, 1984). Taken together, these studies suggest that the early stages of somatosensory processing are organized hierarchically and are separated into macrogeometric and microgeometric channels.

Neural Pathways of Macrogeometric Properties: Shape

Shape and texture are two of the most effective properties for recognizing an object by touch, either actively (haptically) or passively. Shape is a macrogeometric property that is processed as early as the peripheral afferent neurons, specifically the slowly adapting type I (SA1) afferents (Johnson & Hsiao, 1992). SA1 afferents project mainly to Area 3b in SI through the dorsal column nuclei and the thalamus (DiCarlo et al., 1998), which then projects to Area 2.

There is evidence that selectivity for shape also persists in the higher-order cortical stages of haptic perception. The lateral occipital tactile visual area (LOtv; shown in Figure 6.2) is a subregion of the lateral occipital complex (LOC; shown earlier in Figure 6.1). The LOtv, an area once regarded as putatively visual, is known to be involved in haptic object processing as well as visual object processing (Amedi, Jacobson, Hendler, Malach, & Zohary, 2002; Kim & James, 2010; Pietrini et al., 2004; Stilla & Sathian, 2008). Stimuli used in several of these studies included objects that could be identified only by their shape, but not by their microgeometric properties, or vice versa. For instance, Stilla and Sathian (2008) presented participants with objects varying in shape but not texture, or texture but not shape, and contrasted these two conditions. LOtv was found to be one of the cortical regions that are selective for object shape, but not for object texture, suggesting that LOtv plays a role in processing the shape characteristics of objects.

These neuroimaging findings of haptic object processing in LOtv are supported by a clinical case study with a patient, D.F., who has visual agnosia (James, James, Humphrey, & Goodale, 2005). Patient D.F. has cortical damage in the LOC, which is assumed to be responsible for her visual object agnosia. Interestingly, she exhibits difficulty with haptic object recognition tasks as well as visual object recognition tasks, if the objects can be identified only by their shape, not by

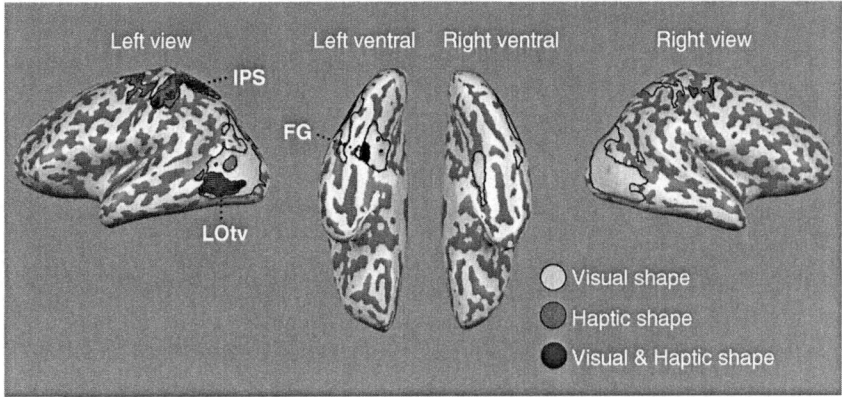

FIGURE 6.2 Visual and haptic shape-selective brain regions. Group-average SPMs derived by contrasting object shape processing with texture processing are displayed on lateral, posterior, and ventral views of an inflated cortical model of a representative brain. Visual shape-selective regions are shown in white-shaded areas with black outline, and haptic shape-selective regions are shown in gray-shaded areas with black outline. Black-shaded areas represent brain regions that respond to both visual and haptic shapes. Adapted with permission from "Enhanced effectiveness in visuo-haptic object-selective brain regions with increasing stimulus salience," by S. Kim and T. W. James, 2010, *Human Brain Mapping*, *31*, 678–693. Copyright 2010 by John Wiley and Sons.

their texture. Along with the case study of D.F., there are other clinical cases of patients with damage to the occipito-temporal region that also have both visual and haptic agnosia (Feinberg, Rothi, & Heilman, 1986; Morin, Rivrain, Eustache, Lambert, & Courtheoux, 1984; Ohtake et al., 2001), suggesting that LOtv may not only be *involved* in bimodal object shape processing, but may be *necessary* for object shape processing.

Other neuroimaging studies suggest that there are other cortical areas in addition to LOtv that are involved in haptic macrogeometry perception of objects. Positron emission tomography (PET) and fMRI studies have shown the parieto-occipital cortex (POC) to be sensitive to orientation discrimination (Sathian, Zangaladze, Hoffman, & Grafton, 1997; Sergent, Ohta, & MacDonald, 1992). A follow-up study (Zangaladze, Epstein, Grafton, & Sathian, 1999) using transcranial magnetic stimulation (TMS) demonstrated that TMS application at the site where POC is located impaired haptic macrogeometric discrimination of grating orientation, but did not impair haptic microgeometric discrimination of grating texture.

Besides the involvement of POC in haptic macrogeometry perception, the anterior part of the intraparietal sulcus (aIPS; shown in Figure 6.1) is often found to be involved in haptic object processing.

Patients with lesions in aIPS exhibit an inability to recognize haptic objects, supporting the involvement of aIPS in haptic object recognition (Binkofski, Kunesch, Classen, Seitz, & Freund, 2001). The inability of these patients to recognize haptic objects, however, may be because they cannot execute appropriate finger movements to explore objects. However, fMRI studies in healthy individuals have shown that aIPS (as well as sometimes POC) is sensitive to orientation discrimination with gratings (Kitada et al., 2006; Van Boven, Ingeholm, Beauchamp, Bikle, & Ungerleider, 2005; Zhang et al., 2005). In addition to these studies that showed macrogeometry selectivity in aIPS using simple orientation or raised letters, some other fMRI studies (Grefkes, Weiss, Zilles, & Fink, 2002; Kim & James, 2010; Miquee et al., 2008; Stilla & Sathian, 2008) used more complex objects and also showed shape selectivity in IPS. Taken together, POC, IPS, and LOtv represent higher levels of the hierarchical haptic object processing system and are specifically involved in shape processing.

Neural Pathways of Microgeometric Properties: Texture

Microgeometric properties, such as texture, roughness, and hardness, are also used for haptic object recognition. Microgeometric properties are very salient for haptic perception, and the haptic system processes information about microgeometric properties of objects, especially roughness, more effectively than information about macrogeometric properties (Klatzky, Lederman, & Reed, 1987).

Microgeometric surface features of objects are processed as early as the peripheral afferent neurons such as SA1 and the Pacinian afferents (Hollins & Bensmaia, 2007; Hollins, Bensmaia, & Washburn, 2001; Johnson, 2001), which project to SI. Evidence for the selective involvement of SI in haptic texture processing comes from both lesion and single-unit recording studies in nonhuman primates. Lesions in Area 1 impair texture discrimination, while lesions in Area 3b impair both texture and shape discrimination (Randolph & Semmes, 1974). Stimulation of the digits with two-dimensional textured surfaces produces significant responses in neurons in Areas 3b and 1 (Darian-Smith, Sugitani, Heywood, Karita, & Goodwin, 1982). Similarly, Iwamura (1998) suggested that Area 3b is responsible for processing fine features of objects such as texture and roughness that can be perceived at the level of fingertips, while Area 2 is responsible for processing global features of objects such as size and shape that can be perceived at the level of relatively large finger or hand areas. In addition to the primate lesion and neurophysiological studies, a study using TMS in human subjects showed that roughness judgments are disrupted by TMS over SI and interdot distance ratings are disrupted by TMS over medial occipital cortex (MOC; Merabet et al., 2004).

There is also evidence for the involvement of cortical regions beyond SI in haptic texture processing. A few decades ago, a cortical ablation study in nonhuman primates (Garcha & Ettlinger, 1978) showed evidence for texture selectivity in SII, demonstrating that removal of SII produced deficits in texture discrimination. Their finding was supported later by Sinclair and Burton's study (1993) that found texture-sensitive cells in monkey SII using single-unit recording. The involvement of SII in haptic texture perception has been shown in the human brain as well. Clinical case studies of patients with tactile agnosia (Bohlhalter, Fretz, & Weder, 2002; Caselli, 1991) and at least one fMRI study (Reed, Shoham, & Halgren, 2004) have proposed that human SII is involved in haptic object recognition. These studies used real objects as stimuli, which were not systematically controlled for differences in macrogeometric and microgeometric properties; therefore, they do not provide direct evidence for the role of SII in haptic microgeometry processing. However, other neuroimaging studies (Kitada et al., 2006; Roland, O'Sullivan, & Kawashima, 1998; Servos, Lederman, Wilson, & Gati, 2001; Stilla & Sathian, 2008; Stoesz et al., 2003) have directly compared processing of macrogeometric and microgeometric properties of objects. Most of these studies showed that SII was involved in processing microgeometric properties more than macrogeometric properties. Therefore, despite some inconsistencies in results across studies, the evidence generally suggests that SII plays a greater role in processing microgeometric properties than macrogeometric properties.

Some researchers have found tactile/haptic texture-selective regions in other cortical areas in human brain besides SI and SII. An fMRI study of vibrotactile stimulation on the fingertips produced activation in brain areas SI and SII, but also in pINS (McGlone et al., 2002). Another study by Kitada and colleagues (2006) found that a roughness discrimination task produced activation in SII and the insula. In Stilla and Sathian's (2008) fMRI study, haptic texture perception was directly contrasted with haptic shape perception; results indicated that texture produced greater activation than shape in SII and pINS as well as the MOC.

Taken together, the literature reviewed in this section suggests that microgeometric properties are processed in a hierarchical pathway that is at least partially distinct from the hierarchical pathway that processes macrogeometric properties. The texture-selective pathway involves SI, SII, pINS, and possibly areas of the early visual cortex.

CONVERGING PATHWAYS OF HAPTIC AND VISUAL OBJECT PROCESSING

Over the last half century, many studies have provided strong evidence that the primate visual system is organized hierarchically. Anatomically and functionally distinct brain regions process visual information at different stages of the system (Felleman & Van Essen, 1991; Lennie, 1998; Lerner, Hendler, Ben-Bashat, Harel, & Malach, 2001). Along with the evidence for a hierarchical organization, vision researchers have also developed considerable evidence for dual-pathway theories of visual processing within the hierarchical organization. One of the most influential dual-pathway theories considers a ventral cortical pathway for perception or identification and a dorsal cortical pathway for visually guided action or spatial vision (Goodale & Milner, 1992; Ungerleider & Mishkin, 1982). Evidence cited in the previous sections suggests that the somatosensory system, like vision, is also organized hierarchically. Perhaps not surprisingly, researchers have recently begun to develop dual-pathway theories of haptic object processing (Dijkerman & de Haan, 2007; James, Kim, & Fisher, 2007; Reed, Klatzky, & Halgren, 2005). Of particular interest is the suggestion that the two hypothesized pathways for haptic object processing may converge with the analogous pathways for visual object processing. The next section of the chapter focuses on evidence for this hypothesized convergence and examines the interaction with the distinct haptic shape and texture pathways described earlier.

Visuo-Haptic Convergence in Shape Processing

Vision and touch are the two human sensory modalities best adapted for processing macrogeometric shape properties of objects, and there has been behavioral evidence for crossmodal transfer between vision and touch in object shape perception. Gibson (1963) documented that normal healthy people could distinguish tangible objects across senses, suggesting a crossmodal transfer of global shape between vision and touch. In a relatively recent study, Norman, Norman, Clayton, Lianekhammy, and Zielke (2004) also reported that participants were able to transfer shape information across visual and haptic modalities during three-dimensional (3D) shape-matching tasks. Not only adults, but also young infants showed visual-haptic crossmodal transfer abilities for object shape processing (Rose, Gottfried, & Bridger, 1983; Streri & Gentaz, 2004), suggesting that visuo-haptic convergence of shape information develops early. Given the behavioural evidence, information about object shape appears to be shared and integrated across visual and haptic modalities.

For behavioral multisensory transfer or integration to occur, information from vision and touch must converge in the brain. Many studies have suggested that the neural substrates for vision and touch overlap at several cortical sites. Sathian and Zangaladze (1997) investigated crossmodal interactions between vision and touch using PET and demonstrated that tactile discrimination of grating orientation activated a region in the extrastriate visual cortex. In the same study, by showing that TMS application over a similar region disrupted participants' performance in the tactile discrimination task, they suggested that this extrastriate visual cortex is not only involved in, but also necessary for, tactile orientation processing. Notably, the involvement of the visual cortex was found only during tactile discrimination of orientation, but not during spatial frequency, suggesting that the extrastriate visual cortical region involved in tactile perception they found was sensitive to macrogeometric properties of objects, but not microgeometric properties.

The finding that visual and haptic shape processing shared a common neural substrate in the extrastriate cortex was supported by other neuroimaging studies. Amedi and his colleagues (2001, 2002) compared brain activation with visual 3D objects and textures and also with haptic 3D objects and textures. They found object selectivity in a subregion of LOC (LOtv) for both vision and haptics. Furthermore, they tested whether or not LOtv specifically processed visuo-haptic bimodal shape information, as opposed to being an "association" area in which bimodal activation was essentially an epiphenomenon mediated by nonsensory feedback from amodal processes. They found that any possible confounding factors, such as naming or visual imagery, played only a minor role in producing bimodal activation in LOtv (Amedi et al., 2001). LOtv was found to be sensitive to graspable objects that contain geometrical shape, and this region was only sensitive to visual and haptic objects, not to auditory objects that rarely contained shape information of objects, suggesting that LOtv activation is correlated with processing geometrical shape of objects (Amedi et al., 2002).

In another fMRI study, James and his colleagues (2002) examined neural facilitative effects of previous exposure to stimuli on the perception of subsequent stimuli to test interactions between vision and touch in the human brain, notably with novel 3D objects with no names associated with the objects to prevent semantic systems from mediating any priming effects. In addition, all the objects were made from the same material so that they could be identified only by their shapes not by their textures. Participants studied the objects either visually or haptically and then were tested visually in fMRI sessions. They found that both visually and haptically primed objects enhanced the brain activation in MOC and LOC compared with nonprimed objects. Their results suggest that the visual and haptic systems share a common substrate for object shape recognition in the extrastriate visual cortex and show that the visuo-haptic crossmodal priming effect occurs both behaviorally and neurally. These findings of overlapping neural substrates for visual and haptic object processing are supported by many follow-up neuroimaging studies (e.g., Kim & James, 2010; Stilla & Sathian, 2008; Tal & Amedi, 2009).

Neural convergence between vision and touch is also supported by the case study of patient D.F. (James et al., 2005) which was described in an earlier section. D.F. was diagnosed with visual agnosia, which was caused by bilateral lesions in her lateral occipital cortex at the same coordinates as LOtv. When D.F. was tested visually and haptically, it was found that her performance on haptic object recognition tasks was similar to her ability with visual recognition. Importantly, the objects used for the haptic and visual tasks were the same and could only be discriminated based on their macrogeometric properties. The findings with D.F. suggest not only that LOtv is involved in haptic object recognition, but that recruitment of LOtv is necessary for successful and efficient visual and haptic shape recognition.

IPS is another brain area where visuo-haptic convergence is commonly observed. James, Culham, Humphrey, Milner, and Goodale (2003) suggested that aIPS was involved in processing visual shape information, particularly for visually guided reaching and grasping movements, and an earlier PET study showed that IPS was activated during visual discrimination of grating orientation (Vandenberghe et al., 1996), which is important for the visual control of hand movement (Murata, Gallese, Luppino, Kaseda, & Sakata, 2000). Along with these results in the visual domain, another PET study showed that tactile discrimination of shape activated aIPS (Bodegard et al., 2001) and a later fMRI study also found that this area was involved in tactile orientation discrimination (Zhang et al., 2005). Other groups of researchers examined haptic shape selectivity in the human brain and found that aIPS was sensitive to grating orientation (Kitada et al., 2006; Van Boven et al., 2005). Besides the evidence for the involvement of IPS found independently with visual and haptic object shape processing, other neuroimaging studies suggest that aIPS is a bimodal sensory region that receives inputs from both vision and touch (Grefkes et al., 2002; Kim & James, 2010; Tal & Amedi, 2009; Zhang, Weisser, Stilla, Prather, & Sathian, 2004). These studies suggest that shape information from vision and haptics converges in IPS, with most studies specifically reporting aIPS. Interestingly, IPS is considered to be not only a part of the somatosensory or visual system but also a part of the motor system (Binkofski et al., 1999), suggesting that aIPS in the dorsal pathway integrates bimodal sensory information from the somatosensory/visual systems with information from the motor system, perhaps for the execution of visually guided actions (Culham & Valyear, 2006; Gardner et al., 2007; Tunik, Rice, Hamilton, & Grafton, 2007).

Visuo-Haptic Convergence in Texture Processing

Similar to shape processing, there has been behavioral evidence for crossmodal transfer of texture processing between vision and touch in adults (Guest & Spence, 2003) and young children (Picard, 2007). Compared to the studies of shape processing, however, there have been fewer studies of visuo-haptic convergence for texture processing. Given the relatively few studies, it is notable that Stilla and Sathian (2008) showed that microgeometric tasks such as texture discrimination recruited putative visual brain areas. Using fMRI, they compared brain activation with texture and shape across vision and touch. The results showed that haptic texture evoked bilateral activation in SII, pINS, and MOC, an early visual processing area. Although it is only a single study, their results suggest that visual-haptic convergence of texture information may occur in the early stages of hierarchical processing. To support this hypothesis, they examined effective connectivity of modality-specific areas during haptic perception with right hand exploration (Deshpande, Hu, Stilla, & Sathian, 2008). They found that somatosensory inputs progressed from the left postcentral sulcus (PoCS; shown in Figure 6.1) and right pINS into visual cortical areas, both the texture-selective right MOC and the shape-selective right LOC. Thus, there is a growing body of evidence that suggests the existence of visuo-haptic sites of neural convergence for texture that are distinct from those for shape.

There are other brain regions that are thought to be convergence sites for vision and touch. Bruce, Desimone, and Gross (1981) showed that macaque STS was sensitive to somesthetic stimulation as well as visual and auditory stimulation. In a more recent fMRI study, Beauchamp, Yasar, Frye, and Ro (2008) demonstrated that posterior STS in humans responds to vibrotactile stimulation as well as visual and auditory stimulation, concluding that human STS is important for integrating information from multiple senses, including the sense of touch. Still, the results did not distinguish between different properties of objects, and it is not clear whether or not STS is specialized for the visuo-haptic processing of macrogeometric, microgeometric, or both types of properties in object perception.

CONCLUSIONS

In this chapter, we reviewed the hierarchically organized neural pathways of haptic object processing in human and nonhuman primate brains and compared the neural pathways of haptic object processing with those of visual object processing. Recent findings suggest convergences of neural pathways for haptic and visual object processing of both macrogeometric and microgeometric properties of objects. We briefly discussed a tentative dual-stream system of haptic object processing in the ventral and dorsal pathways.

Study of the neural mechanisms of haptic object perception and visuo-haptic multisensory integration is an emerging field in cognitive neuroscience. Study has been largely confined, however, to the adult brain, with relatively few electrophysiological or fMRI studies conducted in the developing brain. There are technical challenges associated with conducting neuroimaging studies of haptic object processing in adults, and these challenges would only be exacerbated when studying children. It would, however, be interesting and worthwhile to put forth the effort to investigate the neural substrates of visuo-haptic object processing across different age groups, and in particular the development of visual imagery and modality-specific dominance. Examining how the neural system of visuo-haptic object processing changes over the course of development and how individual experience with age can influence the development of this system would increase our understanding of the general mechanisms of the interaction between vision and haptics and object processing.

REFERENCES

Amedi, A., Jacobson, G., Hendler, T., Malach, R., & Zohary, E. (2002). Convergence of visual and tactile shape processing in the human lateral occipital complex. *Cerebral Cortex, 12*, 1202–1212.

Amedi, A., Malach, R., Hendler, T., Peled, S., & Zohary, E. (2001). Visuo-haptic object-related activation in the ventral visual pathway. *Nature Neuroscience, 4*, 324–330.

Beauchamp, M. S., Yasar, N. E., Frye, R. E., & Ro, T. (2008). Touch, sound and vision in human superior temporal sulcus. *Neuroimage, 41*, 1011–1020.

Binkofski, F., Buccino, G., Stephan, K. M., Rizzolatti, G., Seitz, R. J., & Freund, H. J. (1999). A parieto-premotor network for object manipulation: Evidence from neuroimaging. *Experimental Brain Research, 128*, 210–213.

Binkofski, F., Kunesch, E., Classen, J., Seitz, R. J., & Freund, H. J. (2001). Tactile apraxia: Unimodal apractic disorder of tactile object exploration associated with parietal lobe lesions. *Brain, 124*(Pt 1), 132–144.

Bodegard, A., Geyer, S., Grefkes, C., Zilles, K., & Roland, P. E. (2001). Hierarchical processing of tactile shape in the human brain. *Neuron, 31*, 317–328.

Bohlhalter, S., Fretz, C., & Weder, B. (2002). Hierarchical versus parallel processing in tactile object recognition: A behavioural-neuroanatomical study of aperceptive tactile agnosia. *Brain, 125*, 2537–2548.

Bruce, C., Desimone, R., & Gross, C. G. (1981). Visual properties of neurons in a polysensory area in superior temporal sulcus of the macaque. *Journal of Neurophysiology, 46*, 369–384.

Burton, H., Fabri, M., & Alloway, K. (1995). Cortical areas within the lateral sulcus connected to cutaneous representations in areas 3b and 1: A revised interpretation of the second somatosensory area in macaque monkeys. *Journal of Comparative Neurology, 355*, 539–562.

Caselli, R. J. (1991). Rediscovering tactile agnosia. *Mayo Clinic Proceedings, 66*, 129–142.

Culham, J. C., & Valyear, K. F. (2006). Human parietal cortex in action. *Current Opinion in Neurobiology, 16*, 205–212.

Darian-Smith, I., Sugitani, M., Heywood, J., Karita, K., & Goodwin, A. (1982). Touching textured surfaces: Cells in somatosensory cortex respond both to finger movement and to surface features. *Science, 218*, 906–909.

Deshpande, G., Hu, X., Stilla, R., & Sathian, K. (2008). Effective connectivity during haptic perception: A study using Granger causality analysis of functional magnetic resonance imaging data. *Neuroimage, 40*, 1807–1814.

DiCarlo, J. J., Johnson, K. O., & Hsiao, S. S. (1998). Structure of receptive fields in area 3b of primary somatosensory cortex in the alert monkey. *The Journal of Neuroscience, 18*, 2626–2645.

Dijkerman, H. C., & de Haan, E. H. (2007). Somatosensory processes subserving perception and action. *Behavioral and Brain Sciences, 30*, 189–201; discussion 201–239.

Disbrow, E., Roberts, T., & Krubitzer, L. (2000). Somatotopic organization of cortical fields in the lateral sulcus of Homo sapiens: Evidence for SII and PV. *Journal of Comparative Neurology, 418*, 1–21.

Disbrow, E., Roberts, T., Poeppel, D., & Krubitzer, L. (2001). Evidence for interhemispheric processing of inputs from the hands in human S2 and PV. *J Neurophysiology, 85*, 2236–2244.

Duffy, F. H., & Burchfiel, J. L. (1971). Somatosensory system: Organizational hierarchy from single units in monkey area 5. *Science, 172*, 273–275.

Eickhoff, S. B., Amunts, K., Mohlberg, H., & Zilles, K. (2006). The human parietal operculum. II. Stereotaxic maps and correlation with functional imaging results. *Cereb Cortex, 16*, 268–279.

Eickhoff, S. B., Schleicher, A., Zilles, K., & Amunts, K. (2006). The human parietal operculum. I. Cytoarchitectonic mapping of subdivisions. *Cerebral Cortex, 16*, 254–267.

Feinberg, T. E., Rothi, L. J., & Heilman, K. M. (1986). Multimodal agnosia after unilateral left hemisphere lesion. *Neurology, 36,* 864–867.

Felleman, D. J., & Van Essen, D. C. (1991). Distributed hierarchical processing in the primate cerebral cortex. *Cerebral Cortex, 1,* 1–47.

Frackowiak, R. S. J., Ashburner, J. T., Penny, W. D., Zeki, S., Friston, K. J., Frith, C. D.,...Price, C. J. (2004). *Human Brain Function.* New York, NY: Elsevier Academic Press.

Friedman, D. P., Jones, E. G., & Burton, H. (1980). Representation pattern in the second somatic sensory area of the monkey cerebral cortex. *Journal of Comparative Neurology, 192,* 21–41.

Garcha, H. S., & Ettlinger, G. (1978). The effects of unilateral or bilateral removals of the second somatosensory cortex (area SII): A profound tactile disorder in monkeys. *Cortex, 14,* 319–326.

Gardner, E. P., Babu, K. S., Reitzen, S. D., Ghosh, S., Brown, A. S., Chen, J.,...Ro, J. Y. (2007). Neurophysiology of prehension. I. Posterior parietal cortex and object-oriented hand behaviors. *Journal of Neurophysiology, 97,* 387–406.

Gibson, J. J. (1963). The useful dimensions of sensitivity. *American Psychologist, 18,* 1–15.

Goodale, M. A., & Milner, A. D. (1992). Separate visual pathways for perception and action. *Trends in Neuroscience, 15,* 20–25.

Grefkes, C., Weiss, P. H., Zilles, K., & Fink, G. R. (2002). Crossmodal processing of object features in human anterior intraparietal cortex: An fMRI study implies equivalencies between humans and monkeys. *Neuron, 35,* 173–184.

Guest, S., & Spence, C. (2003). Tactile dominance in speeded discrimination of textures. *Experimental Brain Research, 150,* 201–207.

Hollins, M., & Bensmaia, S. J. (2007). The coding of roughness. *Canadian Journal of Experimental Psychology, 61,* 184–195.

Hollins, M., Bensmaia, S. J., & Washburn, S. (2001). Vibrotactile adaptation impairs discrimination of fine, but not coarse, textures. *Somatosensory and Motor Research, 18,* 253–262.

Hsiao, S. S., Johnson, K. O., & Twombly, I. A. (1993). Roughness coding in the somatosensory system. *Acta Psychologica, 84,* 53–67.

Hyvärinen, J., & Poranen, A. (1978). Receptive field integration and submodality convergence in the hand area of the post-central gyrus of the alert monkey. *The Journal of Physiology, 283,* 539–556.

Iwamura, Y. (1998). Hierarchical somatosensory processing. *Current Opinion in Neurobiology, 8,* 522–528.

Iwamura, Y. (2003). Somatosensory association cortices. *International Congress Series, 1250,* 3–14.

Iwamura, Y., & Tanaka, M. (1978). Postcentral neurons in hand region of area 2: Their possible role in the form discrimination of tactile objects. *Brain Research, 150,* 662–666.

James, T. W., Culham, J., Humphrey, G. K., Milner, A. D., & Goodale, M. A. (2003). Ventral occipital lesions impair object recognition but not object-directed grasping: An fMRI study. *Brain, 126*(Pt 11), 2463–2475.

James, T. W., Humphrey, G. K., Gati, J. S., Servos, P., Menon, R. S., & Goodale, M. A. (2002). Haptic study of three-dimensional objects activates extrastriate visual areas. *Neuropsychologia, 40,* 1706–1714.

James, T. W., James, K. H., Humphrey, G. K., & Goodale, M. A. (2005). Do visual and tactile object representations share the same neural substrate? In M. A. Heller & S. Ballesteros (Eds.), *Touch and blindness: Psychology and neuroscience* (pp. 139–155). Mahwah, NJ: Lawrence Erlbaum.
James, T. W., Kim, S., & Fisher, J. S. (2007). The neural basis of haptic object processing. *Canadian Journal of Experimental Psychology, 61,* 219–229.
Johnson, K. O. (2001). The roles and functions of cutaneous mechanoreceptors. *Current Opinion in Neurobiology, 11,* 455–461.
Johnson, K. O., & Hsiao, S. S. (1992). Neural mechanisms of tactual form and texture perception. *Annual Review of Neuroscience, 15,* 227–250.
Kim, S., & James, T. W. (2010). Enhanced effectiveness in visuo-haptic object-selective brain regions with increasing stimulus salience. *Human Brain Mapping, 31,* 678–693.
Kitada, R., Kito, T., Saito, D. N., Kochiyama, T., Matsumura, M., Sadato, N.,...Lederman, S. J. (2006). Multisensory activation of the intraparietal area when classifying grating orientation: A functional magnetic resonance imaging study. *The Journal of Neuroscience, 26,* 7491–7501.
Klatzky, R. L., Lederman, S. J., & Reed, C. L. (1987). There's more to touch than meets the eye: The salience of object attributes for haptics with and without vision. *Journal of Experimental Psychology: General, 116,* 356–369.
Kopietz, R., Sakar, V., Albrecht, J., Kleemann, A. M., Schopf, V., Yousry, I., ...Wiesmann, M. (2009). Activation of primary and secondary somatosensory regions following tactile stimulation of the face. *Klinische Neuroradiologie, 19,* 135–144.
Krubitzer, L., Huffman, K. J., Disbrow, E., & Recanzone, G. (2004). Organization of area 3a in macaque monkeys: Contributions to the cortical phenotype. *Journal of Comparative Neurology, 471,* 97–111.
Lennie, P. (1998). Single units and visual cortical organization. *Perception, 27,* 889–935.
Lerner, Y., Hendler, T., Ben-Bashat, D., Harel, M., & Malach, R. (2001). A hierarchical axis of object processing stages in the human visual cortex. *Cerebral Cortex, 11,* 287–297.
Maldjian, J. A., Gottschalk, A., Patel, R. S., Pincus, D., Detre, J. A., & Alsop, D. C. (1999). Mapping of secondary somatosensory cortex activation induced by vibrational stimulation: An fMRI study. *Brain Research, 824,* 291–295.
McGlone, F., Kelly, E. F., Trulsson, M., Francis, S. T., Westling, G., & Bowtell, R. (2002). Functional neuroimaging studies of human somatosensory cortex. *Behavioural Brain Research, 135,* 147–158.
Merabet, L., Thut, G., Murray, B., Andrews, J., Hsiao, S., & Pascual-Leone, A. (2004). Feeling by sight or seeing by touch? *Neuron, 42,* 173–179.
Miquee, A., Xerri, C., Rainville, C., Anton, J. L., Nazarian, B., Roth, M., & Zennou-Azogui, Y. (2008). Neuronal substrates of haptic shape encoding and matching: A functional magnetic resonance imaging study. *Neuroscience, 152,* 29–39.
Morin, P., Rivrain, Y., Eustache, F., Lambert, J., & Courtheoux, P. (1984). Visual and tactile agnosia. *Revue Neurologique (Paris), 140,* 271–277.
Murata, A., Gallese, V., Luppino, G., Kaseda, M., & Sakata, H. (2000). Selectivity for the shape, size, and orientation of objects for grasping in neurons of monkey parietal area AIP. *Journal of Neurophysiology, 83,* 2580–2601.

Murray, E. A., & Mishkin, M. (1984). Relative contributions of SII and area 5 to tactile discrimination in monkeys. *Behavioural Brain Research, 11*, 67–83.

Norman, J. F., Norman, H. F., Clayton, A. M., Lianekhammy, J., & Zielke, G. (2004). The visual and haptic perception of natural object shape. *Perception and Psychophysics, 66*, 342–351.

Ohtake, H., Fujii, T., Yamadori, A., Fujimori, M., Hayakawa, Y., & Suzuki, K. (2001). The influence of misnaming on object recognition: A case of multimodal agnosia. *Cortex, 37*, 175–186.

Picard, D. (2007). Tactual, visual, and cross-modal transfer of texture in 5- and 8-year-old children. *Perception, 36*, 722–736.

Pietrini, P., Furey, M. L., Ricciardi, E., Gobbini, M. I., Wu, W. H., Cohen, L., ... Haxby, J. V. (2004). Beyond sensory images: Object-based representation in the human ventral pathway. *Proceedings of the National Academy of Sciences of the United States of America, 101*, 5658–5663.

Randolph, M., & Semmes, J. (1974). Behavioral consequences of selective subtotal ablations in the postcentral gyrus of Macaca mulatta. *Brain Research, 70*, 55–70.

Reed, C. L., Klatzky, R. L., & Halgren, E. (2005). What vs. where in touch: An fMRI study. *Neuroimage, 25*, 718–726.

Reed, C. L., Shoham, S., & Halgren, E. (2004). Neural substrates of tactile object recognition: An fMRI study. *Human Brain Mapping, 21*, 236–246.

Roland, P. E., O'Sullivan, B., & Kawashima, R. (1998). Shape and roughness activate different somatosensory areas in the human brain. *Proceedings of the National Academy of Sciences of the United States of America, 95*, 3295–3300.

Rose, S. A., Gottfried, A. W., & Bridger, W. H. (1983). Infants cross-modal transfer from solid objects to their graphic representations. *Child Development, 54*, 686–694.

Ruben, J., Schwiemann, J., Deuchert, M., Meyer, R., Krause, T., Curio, G., ... Villringer, A. (2001). Somatotopic organization of human secondary somatosensory cortex. *Cerebral Cortex, 11*, 463–473.

Sathian, K., Zangaladze, A., Hoffman, J. M., & Grafton, S. T. (1997). Feeling with the mind's eye. *Neuroreport, 8*, 3877–3881.

Sergent, J., Ohta, S., & MacDonald, B. (1992). Functional neuroanatomy of face and object processing. A positron emission tomography study. *Brain, 115(Pt 1)*, 15–36.

Servos, P., Lederman, S., Wilson, D., & Gati, J. (2001). fMRI-derived cortical maps for haptic shape, texture, and hardness. *Cognitive Brain Research, 12*, 307–313.

Sinclair, R. J., & Burton, H. (1993). Neuronal activity in the second somatosensory cortex of monkeys (Macaca mulatta) during active touch of gratings. *Journal of Neurophysiology, 70*, 331–350.

Stilla, R., & Sathian, K. (2008). Selective visuo-haptic processing of shape and texture. *Human Brain Mapping, 29*, 1123–1138.

Stoesz, M. R., Zhang, M., Weisser, V. D., Prather, S. C., Mao, H., & Sathian, K. (2003). Neural networks active during tactile form perception: Common and differential activity during macrospatial and microspatial tasks. *International Journal of Psychophsiology, 50*, 41–49.

Streri, A., & Gentaz, E. (2004). Cross-modal recognition of shape from hand to eyes and handedness in human newborns. *Neuropsychologia, 42*, 1365–1369.

Tal, N., & Amedi, A. (2009). Multisensory visual-tactile object related network in humans: Insights gained using a novel crossmodal adaptation approach. *Experimental Brain Research, 198*, 165–182.

Tunik, E., Rice, N. J., Hamilton, A., & Grafton, S. T. (2007). Beyond grasping: Representation of action in human anterior intraparietal sulcus. *Neuroimage, 36*(Suppl. 2), T77–86.
Ungerleider, L. G., & Mishkin, M. (1982). Two cortical visual systems. In D. J. Ingle, M. A. Goodale, & R. J. Mansfield (Eds.), *The analysis of visual behavior* (pp. 549–586). Cambridge, MA: MIT Press.
Van Boven, R. W., Ingeholm, J. E., Beauchamp, M. S., Bikle, P. C., & Ungerleider, L. G. (2005). Tactile form and location processing in the human brain. *Proceedings of the National Academy of Sciences of the United States of America, 102,* 12601–12605.
Vandenberghe, R., Dupont, P., De Bruyn, B., Bormans, G., Michiels, J., Mortelmans, L., & Orban, G. A. (1996). The influence of stimulus location on the brain activation pattern in detection and orientation discrimination. A PET study of visual attention. *Brain, 119*(Pt 4), 1263–1276.
Woolsey, C. N. (1943). "Second" somatic receiving areas in the cerebral cortex of cat, dog and monkey. *Federation Proceedings, 2,* 55–56.
Zangaladze, A., Epstein, C. M., Grafton, S. T., & Sathian, K. (1999). Involvement of visual cortex in tactile discrimination of orientation. *Nature, 401,* 587–590.
Zhang, M., Mariola, E., Stilla, R., Stoesz, M., Mao, H., Hu, X., & Sathian, K. (2005). Tactile discrimination of grating orientation: fMRI activation patterns. *Hum Brain Mapping, 25,* 370–377.
Zhang, M., Weisser, V. D., Stilla, R., Prather, S. C., & Sathian, K. (2004). Multisensory cortical processing of object shape and its relation to mental imagery. *Cognitive, Affective and Behavioral Neuroscience, 4,* 251–259.

7

The Organization and Function of Somatosensory Cortex

SLIMAN J. BENSMAIA AND JEFFREY M. YAU

When we interact with an object, much information about the object is conveyed through signals from the hand. Information about the shape of the object, its texture, its compliance, and its thermal properties is carried in the pattern of activity evoked in a variety of receptors embedded in the skin, in the joints, and in the muscles. This information allows us to recognize objects based on tactile exploration alone, when, for instance, our visual system is not available, as is the case in the dark or when the object is occluded by another. One of the hallmarks of tactile object recognition is that it involves movement between the skin and the object. Because scanning is such an important part of tactile object recognition, information about the motion of the sensory sheet relative to the object is important to extract information about its spatial properties. Probably the most important sensory role the hand plays is in guiding the rapid and accurate manipulation of objects. For instance, information about the orientation of a pen relative to the first three digits of the hand helps guide the delicate motor behavior, that is, writing.

While tactile perception begins with the activation of receptors embedded in the skin, the extraction of meaningful features from this pattern of activation across the sensory sheet requires that these signals be processed in the brain. Different aspects of the peripheral response convey information about different aspects of the stimulus. For instance, information about stimulus motion is conveyed by different signals than is information about stimulus form or surface texture, despite the fact that these signals stem from overlapping populations of mechanoreceptors. Neurons in the brain must therefore perform different computations, depending on whether they are part of a pathway for processing form, motion, texture, or temperature. In this chapter, we investigate how different aspects of a haptically explored stimulus are represented and processed in the brain.

SPATIAL FORM

When you reach into your pocket to fish out your keys or when you pick up your morning cup of coffee, you rely on your sense of touch to guide your actions. Haptic form perception refers to the appreciation of the spatial features of an object through direct contact with the skin and plays an important role in facilitating our dexterous manipulation of objects. When we manipulate an object, we acquire information about its shape, for instance, about the presence and orientation of corners and edges, how these are arranged with respect to each other, etc. Because of the importance of acquiring information about objects haptically, we have developed strategic and highly stereotyped hand motions for object exploration and manipulation (Lederman & Klatzky, 1987; Thakur, Bastian, & Hsiao, 2008). Although the visual system is better at conveying information about object geometry than is the somatosensory system (Lederman, Klatzky, Chataway, & Summers, 1990; Magee & Kennedy, 1980), the ability to discriminate and identify spatial patterns using vision and touch have been shown to be comparable under certain experimental conditions (Loomis, Klatzky, & Lederman, 1991; Phillips, Johnson, & Browne, 1983). The most celebrated instance of haptic form perception is probably the human ability to read Braille. Skilled Braille readers can read Braille at rates of 70–90 words per minute and many read at higher rates (Nolan & Kederis, 1969). This remarkable sensibility is not restricted to highly trained Braille readers, as untrained individuals can very capably identify haptically explored embossed letters (Loomis, 1982; Vega-Bermudez, Johnson, & Hsiao, 1991). A primary goal of somatosensory research has been to elucidate the mechanisms that mediate our ability to perceive form through haptic exploration.

The Somatosensory Periphery

The first stage in somatosensory form processing consists of converting a pattern of deformation of the skin into a pattern of activation in a population of receptors in the skin, a process known as mechanotransduction. The representation of spatial patterns applied to the skin in mechanoreceptive afferents, which carry the signals from the skin to the brain, has been extensively studied and is well characterized (Johnson, 2001). The high spatial resolution of signals stemming from slowly adapting type I (SAI) and rapidly adapting (RA) afferents make these mechanoreceptive afferent fibers well suited to convey information about the spatial configuration of the stimulus impinging upon the skin. Populations of these afferents convey to the brain an isomorphic representation of the stimulus, that is, the spatial pattern of activation in mechanoreceptive afferents matches the spatial configuration of the stimulus. This spatial isomorphism has been demonstrated using a wide range of spatial patterns, including Braille characters (Johnson & Lamb, 1981), Roman alphabet letters (Phillips, Johnson, & Hsiao, 1988), straight and curved two-dimensional (2D) bars (Wheat & Goodwin, 2001), and surface curvature (Khalsa, Friedman, Srinivasan, & LaMotte, 1998; LaMotte, Friedman, Lu, Khalsa, & Srinivasan, 1998). The point-by-point correspondence between the stimulus and its neural representation results from the simple structure of the receptive fields (RFs) of SA1 and RA afferents. Indeed, individual SA1 or RA afferents respond to stimulation of very restricted region of the skin and provide information about deformations of the skin at that location alone. Information about the shape of an object is carried in the response of a population of afferents.

Signals from mechanoreceptive afferents propagate centrally through the dorsal column and principal trigeminal nuclei, in the midbrain, to the ventral posterior thalamic nuclei and into primary somatosensory cortex (SI). The RFs of subcortical and thalamic neurons resemble those of peripheral afferents, suggesting that signals from the skin arrive at the brain relatively unprocessed (Gynther, Vickery, & Rowe, 1995; Sahai et al., 2006). Thus, the representation of form is isomorphic until it reaches SI. A major focus of research in sensory neuroscience has been to elucidate how distributed, isomorphic representations of objects are processed in the brain to form compact and stable neural representations that can be used to interact with the objects and stored in memory.

The Somatosensory Cortex

In primates, SI is located in the postcentral gyrus and comprises four distinct, densely interconnected areas (moving toward the back of the brain from the central sulcus): Brodmann Areas 3a, 3b, 1, and 2 (Kaas, Nelson, Sur, Lin, & Merzenich, 1979; Kaas et al., 1981; Figure 7.1). These

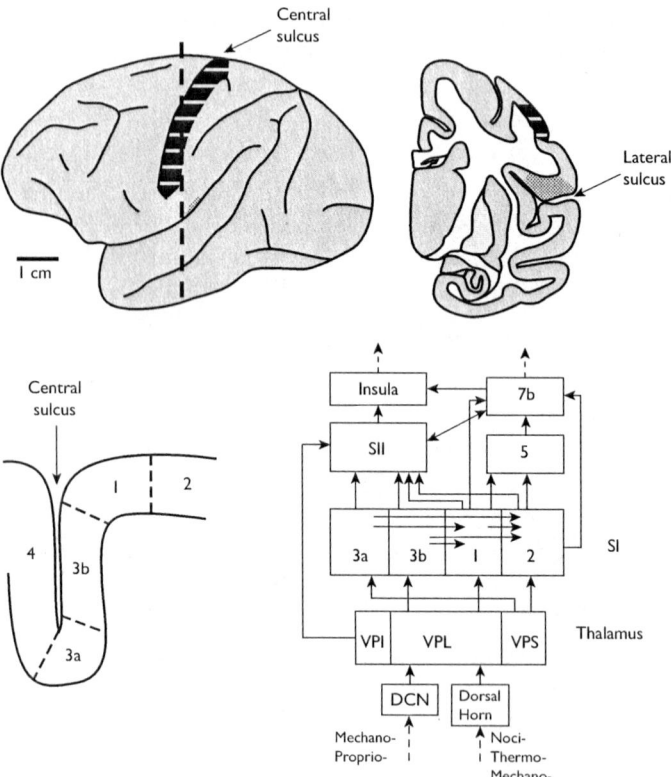

FIGURE 7.1 Diagrams showing the positions of the primary (horizontal lines) and secondary (textured patch) somatosensory cortices in the brain. The top left panel shows a view of the brain as seen from the left, and the top right panel shows a slice of the brain as seen from the front. Bottom left panel shows the four areas that form SI, namely Brodmann Areas 3a, 3b, 1, and 2. Area 4 is the primary motor cortex. The diagram in the bottom right shows the flow of information in the somatosensory system.

areas contain separate somatotopic representations of the body form, that is, each area contains a complete map of the body in which neighboring neurons respond to stimulation of adjacent and overlapping regions on the skin. Each anatomical area in SI receives input from the thalamus, albeit with different strengths and from different parts of the thalamus: Areas 3b and 1 respond to stimulation of the skin, whereas Area 3a responds to changes in limb position or body posture. Neurons in Area 2 respond to both stimulation of the skin and movement of the joints. Most, if not all, somatosensory information funnels through Areas 3a and 3b, which receive the densest thalamocortical projections. Thus, when Area 3b is surgically removed, neurons in Area 1 become unresponsive (Garraghty, Florence, & Kaas, 1990) and sensitivity to stimulation of the skin is abolished (Randolph & Semmes, 1974). Because Areas 3a and 3b form an earlier processing stage than Areas 1 and 2, they are often considered to be the SI proper (Kaas, 1983); in this view, Areas 1 and 2 are intermediate levels of cortical processing between SI proper and the secondary somatosensory cortex (SII).

Signals from SI are elaborated along two cortical pathways, the first passing through posterior parietal cortex by way of Areas 5 and 7. This pathway is thought to be involved in the planning of motor actions (Mountcastle, Lynch, Georgopoulos, Sakata, & Acuna, 1975). The other pathway projects to SII, located in the superior bank of the lateral sulcus (Sylvian fissure; Figure 7.1). SII receives its own input from thalamic nuclei, as well as extensive corticocortical projections from each SI region. SII is further along the somatosensory processing hierarchy than is SI as evidenced by the fact that responses of neurons in SII are abolished when SI is removed or inactivated (Pons, Garraghty, Friedman, & Mishkin, 1987; Pons, Garraghty, & Mishkin, 1992). There are functionally distinct regions in SII: a central region, in which neurons respond primarily to deformation of the skin, flanked by two cortical fields containing neurons that exhibit mixed proprioceptive (joint) and cutaneous responses (Fitzgerald, Lane, Thakur, & Hsiao, 2004). SII sends projections to insular cortex, which, in turn, sends distributed projections to frontal and temporal lobe regions (Augustine, 1996). This second pathway—comprising SII and insular cortex—may be analogous to the ventral processing stream described for the visual system (Ungerleider, Mishkin, Ingle, Goodale, & Mansfield, 1982). In both vision and touch, the ventral processing stream is involved in object perception and these ascending pathways can be regarded as successive stages of an image-processing chain (Bankman, Johnson, & Hsiao, 1990; Johnson, 1980).

RFs in SI

Each neuron in Area 3b, like peripheral neurons, responds to stimulation of very restricted regions of skin, its so-called RF. RFs tend to be smallest on the fingertips and the lips and larger in other skin regions. Specifically, RFs increase gradually as one proceeds from the fingertips, to the palm, to the lower arm, etc. (Sur, Merzenich, & Kaas, 1980). On average, RFs of Area 3b neurons are ~30 mm^2 on the fingertips, whereas they can cover tens of square centimeters on the back where RFs are largest. The size of RFs in Area 3b is related to the acuity with which spatial patterns are perceived; accordingly, we can make out finer details of objects when these are explored with our fingers than when they are explored with our backs (Weinstein & Kenshalo, 1968). More cortical volume is dedicated to highly acute areas, such as the lips and fingertips, than to areas with lower spatial resolution (e.g., the back), as reflected in famous renderings of the somatosensory homunculus (Figure 7.2).

Typically, the activity of neurons in Area 3b will increase above their baseline activity when one region of skin is activated (the excitatory region) and will decrease below this baseline when another region of skin is activated (the inhibitory region; DiCarlo, Johnson, & Hsiao, 1998). The spatial configuration of these RF subregions confers to the neuron different stimulus preferences (DiCarlo & Johnson, 2000). For instance, if the RF of a neuron comprises an elongated excitatory region, flanked by two elongated inhibitory regions, then the neuron will respond to an extended stimulus (e.g., a bar) that impinges upon the excitatory region but not the inhibitory regions (Bensmaia, Denchev, Dammann, Craig, & Hsiao, 2008; Figure 7.3).

The size of the RFs tends to increase as one proceeds upstream along the somatosensory pathway. For instance, neurons in SII respond to stimulation of entire limbs or, in some cases, the entire body (Robinson & Burton, 1980; Whitsel, Petrucelli, & Werner, 1969). The complexity of RFs also increases at successive stages of processing. While the RF of a neuron in Area 3b can easily be mapped by indenting different regions

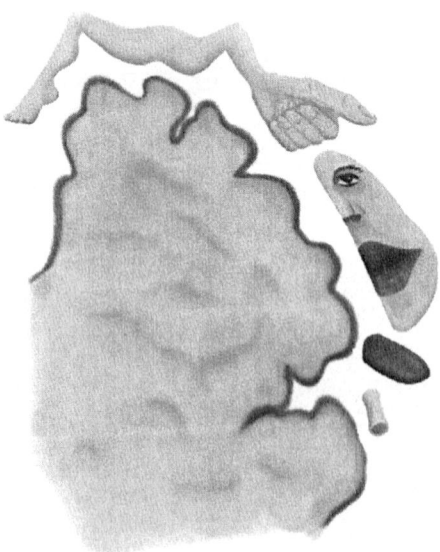

FIGURE 7.2 The somatosensory homunculus. The homunculus, meaning "little man," is a representation of the body surface in cortex. Two key features are observed in the homunculus. First, the somatosensory cortex is organized somatotopically; adjacent neurons respond to adjacent (often overlapping) skin regions. Second, more brain volume is dedicated to certain body parts (e.g., the lips) than others (e.g., the back). Illustration courtesy of Matthew Best and Allison Wu.

CHAPTER 7 FUNCTIONS OF SOMATOSENSORY CORTEX 167

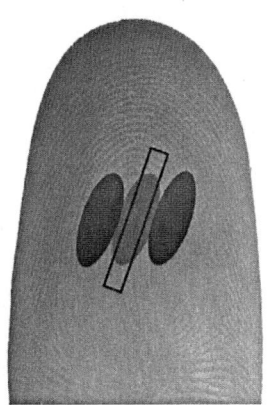

FIGURE 7.3 RF structure of a hypothetical neuron in Area 3b laid over a human fingertip. An excitatory region (red) is typically flanked by one or more inhibitory regions (blue). Because of the spatial configuration of this neuron's RF, it will respond most strongly to an elongated bar presented in its excitatory subregion, at the center of the fingerpad. To the extent that the bar extends into the inhibitory subregions, the neuron's response will decrease.

of skin and determining whether its response increases or decreases, neurons upstream from Area 3b require more complex patterns to become excited (Bensmaia, Denchev, Dammann, Craig, & Hsiao, 2008; Sripati, Yoshioka, Denchev, Hsiao, & Johnson, 2006). For instance, some neurons in Area 1 do not respond to stimuli indented into the skin but rather require that stimuli be scanned in a particular direction to produce a response (see below).

Representation of Spatial Form in SI

In the first stage of visual processing, stimuli are represented as a set of contours, each at a specific location and orientation. Specifically, individual neurons in primary visual cortex (V1) respond when contours at a specific orientation are present within a specific region of the visual field, namely their RF (Hubel & Wiesel, 1968). This representational transformation has been shown to minimize the number of neurons necessary to produce a useful representation of form (Olshausen & Field, 1996; Vinje & Gallant, 2000). Analogously to their counterparts in V1, many neurons in SI are sensitive to the orientation of bars pressed into the skin (Hyvarinen & Poranen, 1978; Pubols & LeRoy, 1977; Warren, Hamalainen, & Gardner, 1986). These orientation-sensitive neurons in SI are similar to those found in V1 in that they respond most strongly when a bar impinging upon their RF is at a given orientation, and their response decreases as the orientation of the bar diverges from this "preferred" orientation (Figure 7.4). More than half of the neurons in Areas 3b and 1 are orientation selective (Bensmaia, Denchev, Dammann, Craig, & Hsiao, 2008). The orientation

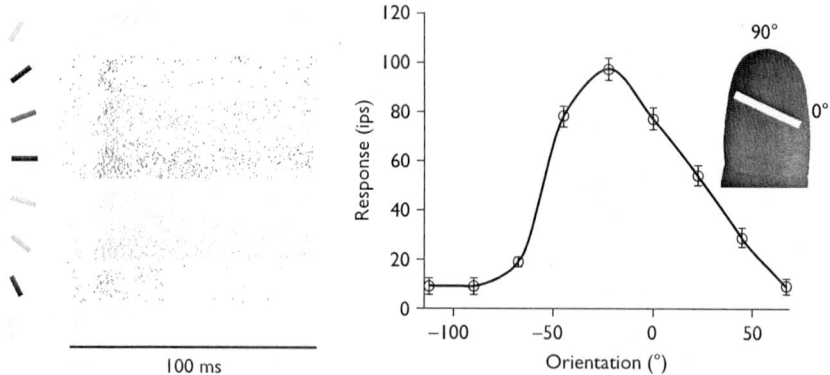

FIGURE 7.4 Left: Raster plot showing the responses of a neuron to 90 repeated presentations of bars at eight different orientations. The neuron responds most strongly to a bar oriented approximately transversally relative to the long axis of the finger. Right: Orientation-tuning curve showing the neuron's response as a function of the bar's orientation. The neuronal response peaks at about −22.5° (the inset to the right denotes the coordinate system).

selectivity of SI neurons is preserved across a variety of conditions and so provides robust information about the shape of an object in contact with the skin. Because both visual and tactile objects comprise continuous edges, it is no surprise that the two systems have evolved similar representational schemes.

As mentioned earlier, different populations of afferents convey different types of information about the stimulus. To what extent do SA1 and RA signals contribute to our ability to perceive stimulus orientation, and by extension spatial form? SA1 and RA afferents exhibit very stereotyped responses to indentations of the skin: SA1 fibers produce a response that is sustained throughout the indentation, whereas RA afferents only respond at the onset and the offset of the indentation. Given these differences in the temporal profiles of afferent responses, examination of the time course at which the orientation signal develops in cortex can yield insight into the peripheral origin (SA1 or RA) of this signal. Pacinian corpuscle (PC) afferents are unlikely contributors to the orientation signal because they innervate the skin too sparsely. The temporal profile of SI responses to indentations ranges from purely RA-like, i.e., responding only at the onset and offset of the stimulus, to strongly SA1-like, responding throughout the stimulation interval. The wide range of cortical responses to indentations suggests that signals from SA1 and RA afferents converge onto individual SI neurons (Pei, Denchev, Hsiao, Craig, & Bensmaia, 2009). The temporal analysis of the orientation signal in SI revealed that neurons that produced sustained responses to indented bars tended to convey more information about stimulus orientation than did neurons that only produced transient responses (Bensmaia, Denchev, Dammann, Craig, & Hsiao, 2008). Thus, it is likely that signals from SA1 afferents contribute to orientation selectivity, and by extension to form perception. This conclusion is consistent with the finding that these afferents convey finer spatial information than do their RA counterparts (Phillips & Johnson, 1981a; Srinivasan & LaMotte, 1987). In fact, when RA afferents are desensitized, our ability to make out fine spatial details improves (Bensmaia, Craig, & Johnson, 2006).

Representation of Spatial Form Beyond SI

While it is well established that stimulus shape is represented in the responses of populations of orientation-tuned neurons in Areas 3b and 1, less is known about how this early representation of form is elaborated at higher processing stages. Neurons in Area 2 and SII have large RFs that cover multiple digits and, in the case of SII, are often bilateral (in other words, these neurons have RFs that cross the midline). When these areas are lesioned, the ability to perceive and remember haptically explored objects is impaired, which implicates them in tactile form processing (Carlson, 1981; Murray & Mishkin, 1984). Higher-order somatosensory neurons also exhibit orientation selectivity, but over larger areas of skin (Hyvarinen & Poranen, 1978). For example, some Area 2 neurons signal the orientation of an indented bar regardless of where it was presented on the monkey's hand. Position-invariant responses, a hallmark of higher-order form representations, require more complex neural processing than position-specific responses and are critical to producing stable percepts. The independence of orientation selectivity from contact position is even more prevalent in SII. RFs in SII span multiple digits (Fitzgerald, Lane, Thakur, & Hsiao, 2006a) and are often bilateral. Many SII neurons exhibit selective responses to oriented bars presented anywhere within their RFs, and the preferred orientation is often similar or identical across skin regions (Fitzgerald, Lane, Thakur, & Hsiao, 2006b). Neurons with bilateral RFs can display similar orientation selectivity across hands (Nakama et al., 2000).

Because RFs are dramatically larger at higher-order stages of processing, the nature of form representations in these neurons reflects stimulus features typically encountered at these larger scales. While at small scales contours are relatively straight, stimuli at larger scales often comprise contours that exhibit smooth or sharp changes in orientation.

Accordingly, the responses of neurons at intermediate stages of visual processing (e.g., Area V4) demonstrate selectivity for contour curvature (Pasupathy & Connor, 1999, 2001). Similarly, neurons in SII encode curvature along the plane parallel to the surface of the skin (Yau, Pasupathy, Fitzgerald, Hsiao, & Connor, 2009). Specifically, a subpopulation of SII neurons exhibit selective responses for curved contours pointing in a specific direction (Figure 7.5). Interestingly, these neurons do not discriminate between sharp and smooth changes in orientation, that is, they respond equally to angles and arcs. This finding likely reflects the spatial filtering of the skin (Phillips & Johnson, 1981b; Sripati, Bensmaia, & Johnson, 2006); indeed, the forces exerted on the surface of the skin are dispersed throughout the tissue before they activate receptors embedded in the skin. At the depth where receptors are located, some of the finer stimulus features present at the surface may thus be obscured (in vision, it is equivalent to wearing blurring lenses). Importantly, the curvature preference of many SII neurons is the same across multiple positions on the distal finger pad. Together, results from neurophysiological studies in Area 2 and SII suggest

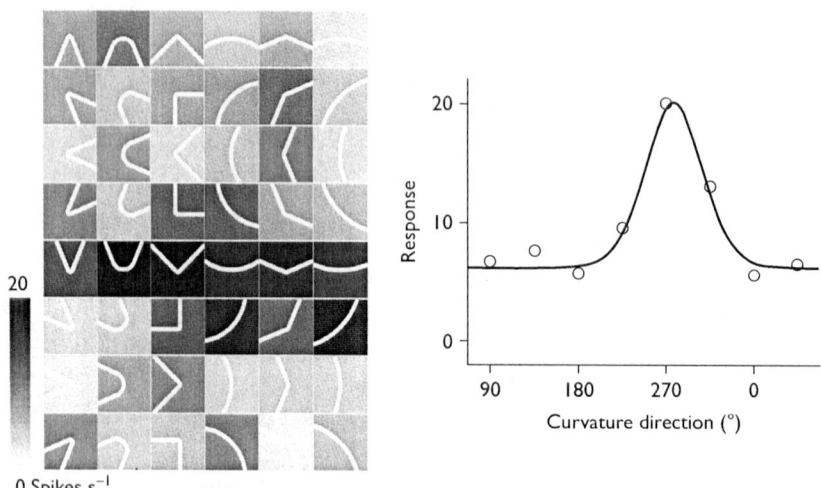

FIGURE 7.5 Left: Embossed curvature stimuli (shown here as white icons) were indented into the distal finger pad of a monkey. The background gray levels indicate the average responses of an example SII neuron to five presentations of each stimulus (see scale bar). Right: Tuning curve showing the neuron's response as a function of curvature direction (i.e., the direction in which angles and curves are typically described as pointing toward). This SII neuron responds selectively to downward-pointing stimuli and the tuning function shows a corresponding peak at 270° (coordinate system as in Fig 7.4).

that spatial form information is elaborated along a cortical hierarchy. The spatial features to which neurons are sensitive grow in complexity at intermediate levels of the somatosensory perceptual pathway, ultimately building toward sparse and invariant representations. Sparseness entails that few neurons are needed to fully represent an object or object feature, invariant means that these representations are robust across various stimulus conditions (e.g., neurons with position-invariant tuning will respond to the presence of a feature regardless of where it is located on the receptor sheet).

Acquiring the Representation of an Object in Three Dimensions

The somatosensory system faces a unique problem in form perception in that the receptor sheet (embedded in the skin) is deformable in a way that the retina, for example, is not. Consequently, to perceive a three-dimensional (3D) object through haptic exploration, it is necessary to integrate information about the stimulus impinging upon each digit (cutaneous information) and information about the relative locations of the digits in space (proprioceptive information). Area 2 and SII may be candidate areas for this integration to take place because both contain neurons that exhibit cutaneous and proprioceptive responses (i.e., they respond to both stimulation of the skin and movement of the joints). The haptic perception of 3D objects may also rely on brain structures outside the primary and secondary somatosensory areas. In human neuroimaging studies, regions in posterior parietal cortex and extrastriate visual cortex that are activated during haptic form recognition tasks have been identified (Amedi, Jacobson, Hendler, Malach, & Zohary, 2002; Amedi, Malach, Hendler, Peled, & Zohary, 2001; Lacey, Tal, Amedi, & Sathian, 2009; Peltier et al., 2007). The representation of haptic object information at the level of single neurons in these areas remains to be elucidated.

Another important question that remains to be addressed regards how tactile information is integrated over time. Because palpated objects may be considerably larger than our hands and because we have the highest spatial acuity at our fingertips, our manual interactions with an object involve actively repositioning the object in our grasp (or repositioning our hand with respect to the object) to acquire a complete view of it. Thus, haptic form perception relies on integrating limited spatial information over time. Future studies, then, must consider how this cutaneous and proprioceptive information is integrated over time to yield a global percept of the 3D shape of objects.

TEXTURE AND VIBRATION

When exploring a surface haptically, we have the ability to perceive a multitude of its textural properties. Though information about texture can be obtained both visually (Heller, 1989) and auditorily (Lederman, 1979), touch yields much finer and more complex textural information than do the other sensory modalities. When we run our fingers across a surface, we may perceive the surface as being rough, like sandpaper, or smooth, like glass; the surface may also vary along other sensory continua, such as hardness (e.g., stone) versus softness (e.g., felt) and stickiness (e.g., eraser rubber) versus slipperiness (e.g., soap). Also, whether a texture is thermally isolating (e.g., plastic) or thermally conductive (like metal) contributes to the textural percept (Bensmaia & Hollins, 2005; Hollins, Bensmaia, Karlof, & Young, 2000).

The size of and spacing between textural features that can contribute to the perceived texture range over several orders of magnitude, spanning hundreds of nanometers to millimeters. As is the case with spatial form processing, coarse textural features are initially represented in the spatial pattern of activity in populations of SA1 afferents at the somatosensory periphery. For example, the roughness of a surface is determined by differences in the activity it evokes in different SA1 afferents. If all SA1 afferents are equally active, then a surface is perceived as being smooth; to the extent that there are large differences in the activation of SA1 afferents innervating different parts of the finger, perceived roughness increases. For finer features (up to hundreds of micrometers), however, the distance between adjacent elements is shorter than that between adjacent mechanoreceptors in the skin. Thus, SA1 afferents do not provide information at a sufficiently high resolution to encode information about fine surface texture. However, we are still able to discriminate surfaces with different microgeometries. Over this range, the spatial properties of surface elements are conveyed through vibrations elicited in the skin during the haptic exploration of surfaces, which typically involves movement between surface and finger (Lederman & Klatzky, 1987). During scanning movements, small vibrations are produced in the skin, which are then transduced by cutaneous mechanoreceptors that are exquisitely sensitive to mechanical oscillations of the skin, namely PCs. In fact, fingerprint skin is thought to play a role in enhancing these texture-elicited vibrations (Scheibert, Leurent, Prevost, & Debregeas, 2009). Discrimination of fine textures is abolished in the absence of movement between skin and surface (Hollins & Risner, 2000) or when PC afferents are desensitized through extended suprathreshold vibratory stimulation at high frequencies (i.e., vibratory adaptation; Hollins, Bensmaia, & Washburn, 2001).

The properties of these texture-elicited vibrations have been shown to be strongly dependent on the surface microgeometry, and the percepts of surface texture are related to these vibrations (Bensmaia & Hollins, 2003, 2005). For example, the perceived roughness of a finely textured surface is determined by the energy of the vibrations it evokes in the skin. However, the perception of textures cannot be accounted for along the intensive dimension alone. For instance, the ridged surface of corduroy evokes periodic vibrations that are fundamental in determining the way corduroy is perceived. More generally, each textured surface elicits vibrations with specific temporal and intensive characteristics and we rely largely on these vibrations to identify textures and, by extension, objects. To understand how texture is processed in the brain, then, it is also necessary to understand how vibrations are processed.

Representation of Texture in Somatosensory Cortex

While ablation of Area 3b results in an almost complete inability to perform any tactile discrimination, lesions in Area 1 result in specific deficits in texture discrimination (Randolph & Semmes, 1974; Semmes & Turner, 1977). This area thus seems to be part of a pathway specialized for texture processing. Furthermore, many neurons in SI signal changes in surface texture (Jiang, Tremblay, & Chapman, 1997; Sinclair & Burton, 1991). Johnson and colleagues have advanced the hypothesis that a subpopulation of SI neurons implement the necessary computation to extract roughness (Yoshioka, Gibb, Dorsch, Hsiao, & Johnson, 2001), but this hypothesis remains to be tested.

In most, if not all, studies of texture processing, stimuli—embossed dot patterns or gratings—comprised coarse surface features. Such features have been shown to be encoded in the spatial pattern of activity in populations of mechanoreceptive afferents, particularly of SA1 fibers (Darian-Smith, Davidson, & Johnson, 1980; Darian-Smith & Oke, 1980). As mentioned earlier, however, a wide range of distinguishable textures comprise features that are too small and close together to be encoded this way; these textures are perceived on the basis of vibrations they produce in the skin during haptic exploration.

Human observers can discriminate the amplitude and frequency of vibrations applied to their skin. At the somatosensory periphery, the neural codes that mediate these discriminative abilities have been established in paired psychophysical and neurophysiological studies. The perceived intensity of a stimulus has been shown to be determined by the strength of the response it elicits in populations of cutaneous mechanoreceptive afferents—SA1, PC, and RA—weighted by fiber type (Muniak, Ray, Hsiao, Dammann, & Bensmaia, 2007). The strength of the response of a subpopulation of neurons in somatosensory cortex increases with increases in stimulus intensity (LaMotte & Mountcastle, 1975), and so the perceived intensity of a stimulus is thought to be encoded in the strength of the response it evokes in the brain.

The tactile perception of vibratory frequency is thought to rely on temporal patterning in the afferent response. Indeed, when stimulated with sinusoidal stimuli, afferents produce a burst of action potentials on each stimulus cycle that is confined to a restricted portion of the cycle (Figure 7.6). At low stimulus intensities, this phase locking or entrainment breaks down. The ability of human observers to discriminate the frequency of vibratory stimuli also breaks down at low stimulus intensities and this transition into atonality coincides with the point at which afferent responses stop entraining (Talbot, Darian-Smith, Kornhuber, & Mountcastle, 1968). This concurrence is interpreted as evidence that the tactile perception of vibratory frequency relies on this patterning. Stimulus frequency may be represented similarly in SI, namely in the temporal patterning of the neuronal response (temporal code, see Mountcastle, Talbot, Sakata, & Hyvarinen, 1969). Alternatively, neurons in SI may encode stimulus frequency in the strength of their response (rate

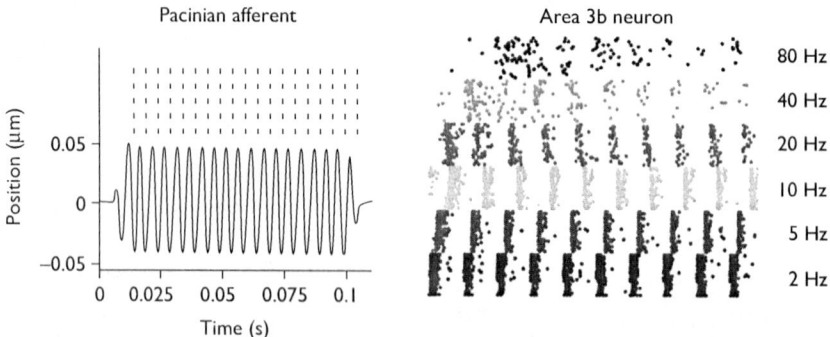

FIGURE 7.6 Left: Temporally patterned (entrained) response of a PC afferent (rasters) to five repeated presentations of a sinusoidal vibration at 200 Hz (bottom trace). Right: Responses of a neuron in Area 3b to vibratory stimuli ranging in frequency from 2 to 80 Hz. Cortical neurons exhibit entrained responses to vibratory stimuli. However, entrainment weakens and disappears at high stimulus frequencies.

code, see Salinas, Hernandez, Zainos, & Romo, 2000): The response of some neurons increases and that of others decreases as the stimulus frequency increases. Importantly, many studies of frequency coding have used stimuli in the so-called flutter range (between 10 and 50 Hz). Information about vibratory stimuli in the flutter range and that about stimuli at higher frequencies (above 100 Hz) may be elaborated along distinct processing streams (Talbot, Darian-Smith, Kornhuber, & Mountcastle, 1968; Tommerdahl et al., 2005). Although humans can perceive and discriminate stimuli at frequencies above 100 Hz, the neural code for frequency within this range remains to be conclusively elucidated. Indeed, phase locking of neurons in SI breaks down for frequencies above ~80 Hz (Figure 7.6). A population of neurons in SII responds to high-frequency stimulation of the skin, and the responses of these neurons exhibit weak temporal patterning (Burton & Sinclair, 1991; Ferrington & Rowe, 1980). It is not clear that this temporal patterning is strong enough to convey information about stimulus frequency, however.

As mentioned earlier, the perception of texture and vibration are intimately linked. To understand how information about surface texture is processed in the brain, it will be necessary to elucidate how vibrations are processed, particularly high-frequency vibrations. Indeed, the vibrations elicited in the skin during the exploration of textured surfaces often comprise high-frequency components (Bensmaia & Hollins, 2005).

MOTION

As mentioned earlier, a hallmark of haptic exploration is that it involves motion between skin and object. The rate at which object features move across a given skin region and the sequence in which they impinge upon the skin depend on the spatial configuration of the features and the motion of the object with respect to the skin. Thus, information about motion must be taken into account when interpreting signals about object shape and texture emanating from the skin. Because performance in a tactile shape identification task is the same whether tactile shapes are actively scanned by the observer or passively scanned across his or her skin (Vega-Bermudez, Johnson, Fasman, & Hsiao, 1989), our ability to compensate for the motion of the object when exploring its shape seems to rely primarily on cutaneous cues rather than proprioceptive ones. There are two main components to the perception of motion: One is the perception of the direction in which a stimulus moves across the skin, and the other is the perception of the speed at which it moves.

While individual mechanoreceptive afferents convey little to no information about direction of motion (Wheat, Salo, & Goodwin, 2009), a subpopulation of neurons in SI is sensitive to the direction in which stimuli are scanned across the skin (Costanzo & Gardner, 1980; Pei, Hsiao, Craig, & Bensmaia, 2010, 2011; Ruiz, Crespo, & Romo, 1995). Specifically, these neurons respond most strongly when a stimulus is scanned in a particular direction, and their response decreases as the scanning direction deviates from this "preferred" direction (Figure 7.7). At the earliest stage of cortical processing, namely in Area 3b, neurons exhibit direction-tuned responses to scanned bars. For instance, a neuron in this area might respond most strongly to a bar oriented perpendicular to the long axis of the finger and moving toward its tip while it will respond much more weakly to the same bar moving toward the palm. Neurons in Area 3b, however, exhibit only poor direction tuning when more spatially complex patterns, for instance gratings, are scanned across the skin (Pei et al., 2011). These neurons "cannot see the forest for the trees." In contrast, neurons in Area 1 exhibit strongly direction-tuned responses to complex moving stimuli such as gratings and embossed dot patterns, in addition to simple bars. This suggests that information about motion is elaborated as it ascends the somatosensory pathway from Area 3b to Area 1.

The motion signal in Area 1 can account for our ability to distinguish direction of motion (Pei et al., 2010). For instance, when two gratings, moving in different directions, are superimposed to form a plaid, the direction of the resulting stimulus, as measured in human subjects,

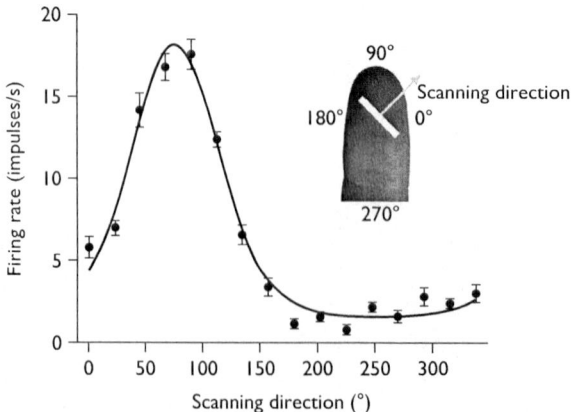

FIGURE 7.7 Direction-tuning curve for a neuron in Area 1. This neuron responded most strongly when a bar oriented perpendicular to the long axis of the finger was scanned toward the tip of the finger. Inset shows the coordinate system for the scanning directions.

can be predicted from the responses of neurons in Area 1. Certain combinations of gratings produce perceptual illusions in which the perceived direction of motion does not match the objective direction (Pei et al., in review). These illusions can be traced back to the responses of neurons in Area 1; in other words, these neurons signal the perceived rather than the veridical direction.

As discussed earlier, neurons in Area 1 convey more stable and robust information about direction of motion than do their counterparts in Area 3b. Interestingly, neurons in Area 2, a higher processing stage in the somatosensory hierarchy, are not as sensitive to motion direction as are their counterparts in Area 1. It thus seems that Area 1 plays a specialized role in processing tactile motion, although it has other roles as well (in form and texture perception). The elaboration of motion signals from Area 3b to Area 1 is thought to proceed as follows: Neurons in Area 3b encode the direction of motion of individual stimulus features, including edges and terminators (the intersections between two edges, or extremities of extended contours). Signals from these simple motion detectors then converge onto neurons in Area 1, where they are combined to convey information about the motion of the stimulus as a whole (Pei et al., in review). The perceived direction of the stimuli is then determined by the responses of this subpopulation of neurons in Area 1.

The representation of tactile speed in the brain has yet to be elucidated. However, the speed of a stimulus is strongly influenced by the rate at which stimulus features are scanned across a given region of skin. Thus, if two gratings are scanned across the skin at the same speed, the grating with the shorter period will be perceived as moving faster than the grating with the longer period (Depeault, Meftah el, & Chapman, 2009). Accordingly, the representation of tactile speed may rely in part on the processing of temporal frequency, described earlier.

Area 1 seems to be involved in the processing of motion, in addition to that of form and texture. The contiguity of form, texture, and motion representations in somatosensory cortex is not surprising given that motion is a hallmark of tactile exploration. Information about motion may indeed be necessary to resolve the spatial relationships between stimulus features during scanning (Ageranioti-Belanger & Chapman, 1992).

TEMPERATURE AND PAIN

Our ability to perceive temperature contributes yet another perceptual component to our multidimensional somatosensory experience.

Indeed, we are exquisitely sensitive to the thermal properties of objects. This sensitivity is useful for identifying and discriminating objects, but, more importantly, it plays an essential role in preventing tissue injury. Indeed, if an object is too hot or too cold, it may cause damage to the skin. Not surprisingly, our perception of temperature is intimately linked with our experience of pain (Green, 2004). Accordingly, temperature and pain processing involve many common neural structures. Temperature perception is further complicated by the fact that we not only perceive the thermal properties of contacted objects, but we also sense the thermal state of our corporeal selves. Coincidence of thermal and mechanoreceptive sensations or the lack thereof may be what distinguishes these two thermal perceptual processes (Craig, 2003a); that is, perceived temperature is assigned to an object along with other properties like shape and texture based on the temporal and spatial coincidence of mechanical and thermal signals.

The peripheral mechanisms underlying thermal transduction have been well characterized (Caterina, 2007). Briefly, families of membrane proteins have been identified that confer temperature selectivity to thermally sensitive neurons whose cell bodies reside in the dorsal horn of the spinal cord. These proteins, known as transient receptor potential (TRP) channels, signal temperature over specific ranges, as well as the presence of specific molecular compounds. For example, TRPV1 (also known as VR1) responds to a narrow range of temperatures, with thresholds centered around 42°C (Caterina et al., 1997), to low pH conditions, and to capsaicin, the active compound in hot peppers. Neurons located in the dorsal horn of the spinal cord exhibit a variety of responses to temperature. Some spinal-thalamic tract (STT) neurons respond exclusively to cold, cool, warm, or hot temperatures. Others display complex temperature and nociceptive responses (nociceptive responses denote responses to potentially damaging stimuli). Many STT neurons, known as wide-dynamic-range neurons, are sensitive to temperature and pain and also respond to mechanical stimulation. STT neurons can be generally grouped into two distinct populations (Craig, 2003b). Neurons in one group, located in Lamina I of the spinal cord, are highly selective and are believed to be involved in the discriminative aspects of temperature and pain processing. Neurons in the second group, located in Lamina V of the spinal cord, respond to the combination of thermal, nociceptive, and mechanical stimulation. These neurons are thought to mediate reflexive responses like the rapid withdrawal of a body part when it comes into contact with a potentially damaging stimulus (Lundberg, Malmgren, & Schomburg, 1987).

The characterization of temperature and pain representations in the brain has been limited by the fact that neurons exhibiting responses to temperature and pain are rarely encountered in neurophysiological recording experiments (Bushnell et al., 1999; Kenshalo, Iwata, Sholas, & Thomas, 2000). Temperature-sensitive neurons have been identified in the posterior portion of the ventral medial thalamic nucleus (VMpo) in human and nonhuman primates, and damage to this area produces deficits in the perception of temperature and pain (Davis et al., 1999; Dostrovsky, 2000; Lenz, Seike, Lin, et al., 1993). Moreover, the injection of small electrical currents through fine stimulating electrodes positioned in VMpo produces sensations of graded cold and pain in humans (Davis et al., 1999; Lenz, Seike, Richardson, et al., 1993).

In neuroimaging studies, SI, SII, the posterior insula, the prefrontal cortex, and the cerebellum have been implicated in the processing of innocuous temperature information (Casey, Minoshima, Morrow, & Koeppe, 1996; Craig, Chen, Bandy, & Reiman, 2000; Davis, Kwan, Crawley, & Mikulis, 1998). These cortical areas are also involved in the perception of stimuli that are potentially damaging, although the extended cortical networks activated by extreme temperatures and pain also include anterior insula and anterior cingulate cortex (Peyron, Laurent, & Garcia-Larrea, 2000). Insular cortex activations appear to reflect the subjective experience of temperature, rather than the actual temperature of the skin (Davis, Pope, Crawley, & Mikulis, 2004). Insular cortex activation also correlates with the perceived intensity of pain stimuli (Baliki, Geha, & Apkarian, 2009). These results imply a higher-order cognitive role for the insular cortex rather than a purely sensory one.

The current view is that thermal and painful experiences arise from neural activity across many neural populations in the peripheral and central nervous system. Neural coding of temperature and pain is distributed such that no single thalamic nucleus or cortical area appears to be essential for the perception of temperature or pain (Mountcastle, 2005). While the cortical regions involved in thermal and pain processing have been identified, future human and animal studies are needed to fully characterize this complex perceptual experience. A critical question that needs to be resolved regards the representation of temperature and pain at the single neuron level. The robust activations to thermal and pain stimulation observed in neuroimaging experiments need to be reconciled with the apparent dearth of cortical neurons showing selectivity to temperature and pain.

CONCLUSION

The somatosensory modality is a composite sense. Indeed, it is involved in processing a variety of different types of information relating to the state of the body and to stimuli impinging upon it. The different types of receptors embedded in the skin, muscle, and joints convey different information, which is then processed and interpreted in the brain. The visual and somatosensory systems share the common problem of inferring information about the shape and motion of a stimulus from a spatiotemporal pattern of activation over a 2D sensory sheet (the retina and the skin, respectively). As described earlier, the representation of form and motion are similar in the two systems. However, the somatosensory sensory sheet is deformable to a much greater extent than is its visual counterpart (the eyes can move somewhat relative to one another). Thus, signals emanating from the skin must be combined with signals about body state in order to be interpreted. How these two types of signals are combined remains to be elucidated. Given the overlapping functions of the two systems (both convey information about shape and motion, for instance), it is no wonder that information from the two systems is often combined in natural perception (Stein & Meredith, 2004). The somatosensory system also shares some common properties with the auditory system. Indeed, both systems are sensitive to environmental oscillations over an overlapping range of frequencies (Yau, Olenczak, Dammann, & Bensmaia, 2009). In fact, one brain area may be involved, under certain conditions, in processing vibrations, whether they are transduced in the skin or in the ear (Foxe et al., 2002; Fu et al., 2003). Again, tactile and auditory information is often combined in everyday sensory experience (Stein & Meredith, 2004). For instance, how a surface feels can be altered if the sounds that are made during the exploration of the surface are distorted (Jousmaki & Hari, 1998).

In addition to its role in guiding our identification and manipulation of objects, touch also plays an important affective role. Skin-to-skin contact is important in forming certain types of social bonds (Loken, Wessberg, Morrison, McGlone, & Olausson, 2009; McGlone, Vallbo, Olausson, Loken, & Wessberg, 2007), and pain comprises a very strong affective component (Craig, 2002, 2003a). The neural mechanisms underlying affective touch are not nearly as well understood as are their discriminative counterparts. The affective importance of touch is brought home by the words of Christopher Reeve, a famous quadriplegic: "To be able to feel the lightest touch really is a gift."

REFERENCES

Ageranioti-Belanger, S. A., & Chapman, C. E. (1992). Discharge properties of neurones in the hand area of primary somatosensory cortex in monkeys in relation

CHAPTER 7 FUNCTIONS OF SOMATOSENSORY CORTEX   181

to the performance of an active tactile discrimination task. II. Area 2 as compared to areas 3b and 1. *Experimental Brain Research, 91*(2), 207–228.

Amedi, A., Jacobson, G., Hendler, T., Malach, R., & Zohary, E. (2002). Convergence of visual and tactile shape processing in the human lateral occipital complex. *Cerebral Cortex, 12,* 1202–1212.

Amedi, A., Malach, R., Hendler, T., Peled, S., & Zohary, E. (2001). Visuo-haptic object-related activation in the ventral visual pathway. *Nature Neuroscience, 4,* 324–330.

Augustine, J. R. (1996). Circuitry and functional aspects of the insular lobe in primates including humans. *Brain Research Brain Research Reviews, 22,* 229–244.

Baliki, M. N., Geha, P. Y., & Apkarian, A. V. (2009). Parsing pain perception between nociceptive representation and magnitude estimation. *Journal of Neurophysiology, 101*(2), 875–887.

Bankman, I. N., Johnson, K. O., & Hsiao, S. S. (1990). Neural image transformation in the somatosensory system of the monkey: Comparison of neurophysiological observations with responses in a neural network model. *Cold Spring Harbor Symposia on Quantitative Biology, 55,* 611–620.

Bensmaia, S. J., Craig, J. C., & Johnson, K. O. (2006). Temporal factors in tactile spatial acuity: Evidence for RA interference in fine spatial processing. *Journal of Neurophysiology, 95,* 1783–1791.

Bensmaia, S. J., Denchev, P. V., Dammann, J. F., III, Craig, J. C., & Hsiao, S. S. (2008). The representation of stimulus orientation in the early stages of somatosensory processing. *Journal of Neuroscience, 28,* 776–786.

Bensmaia, S. J., & Hollins, M. (2003). The vibrations of texture. *Somatosensory and Motor Research, 20,* 33–43.

Bensmaia, S. J., & Hollins, M. (2005). Pacinian representations of fine surface texture. *Perception and Psychophysics, 67,* 842–854.

Burton, H., & Sinclair, R. J. (1991). Second somatosensory cortical area in macaque monkeys: 2. Neuronal responses to punctate vibrotactile stimulation of glabrous skin on the hand. *Brain Research, 538,* 127–135.

Bushnell, M. C., Duncan, G. H., Hofbauer, R. K., Ha, B., Chen, J. I., & Carrier, B. (1999). Pain perception: Is there a role for primary somatosensory cortex? *Proceedings of the National Academy of Sciences of the United States of America, 96,* 7705–7709.

Carlson, M. (1981). Characteristics of sensory deficits following lesions of Brodmann's areas 1 and 2 in the postcentral gyrus of Macaca mulatta. *Brain Research, 204,* 424–430.

Casey, K. L., Minoshima, S., Morrow, T. J., & Koeppe, R. A. (1996). Comparison of human cerebral activation pattern during cutaneous warmth, heat pain, and deep cold pain. *Journal of Neurophysiology, 76,* 571–581.

Caterina, M. J. (2007). Transient receptor potential ion channels as participants in thermosensation and thermoregulation. *American Journal of Physiology, Regulatory, Integrative and Comparative Physiology, 292*(1), R64–76.

Caterina, M. J., Schumacher, M. A., Tominaga, M., Rosen, T. A., Levine, J. D., & Julius, D. (1997). The capsaicin receptor: A heat-activated ion channel in the pain pathway. *Nature, 389*(6653), 816–824.

Costanzo, R. M., & Gardner, E. P. (1980). A quantitative analysis of responses of direction-sensitive neurons in somatosensory cortex of awake monkeys. *Journal of Neurophysiology, 43,* 1319–1341.

Craig, A. D. (2002). How do you feel? Interoception: The sense of the physiological condition of the body. *Nature Reviews Neuroscience, 3*, 655–666.

Craig, A. D. (2003a). A new view of pain as a homeostatic emotion. *Trends in Neurosciences, 26*, 303–307.

Craig, A. D. (2003b). Pain mechanisms: Labeled lines versus convergence in central processing. *Annual Review of Neuroscience, 26* 1–30.

Craig, A. D., Chen, K., Bandy, D., & Reiman, E. M. (2000). Thermosensory activation of insular cortex. *Nature Neuroscience, 3*, 184–190.

Darian-Smith, I., Davidson, I., & Johnson, K. O. (1980). Peripheral neural representation of spatial dimensions of a textured surface moving across the monkey's finger pad. *Journal of Physiology, 309*, 135–146.

Darian-Smith, I., & Oke, L. E. (1980). Peripheral neural representation of the spatial frequency of a grating moving across the monkey's finger pad. *Journal of Physiology, 309*, 117–133.

Davis, K. D., Kwan, C. L., Crawley, A. P., & Mikulis, D. J. (1998). Functional MRI study of thalamic and cortical activations evoked by cutaneous heat, cold, and tactile stimuli. *Journal of Neurophysiology, 80*, 1533–1546.

Davis, K. D., Lozano, R. M., Manduch, M., Tasker, R. R., Kiss, Z. H., & Dostrovsky, J. O. (1999). Thalamic relay site for cold perception in humans. *Journal of Neurophysiology, 81*, 1970–1973.

Davis, K. D., Pope, G. E., Crawley, A. P., & Mikulis, D. J. (2004). Perceptual illusion of "paradoxical heat" engages the insular cortex. *Journal of Neurophysiology, 92*(2), 1248–1251.

Depeault, A., Meftah el, M., & Chapman, C. E. (2009). Tactile perception of roughness: Raised-dot spacing, density and disposition. *Experimental Brain Research, 197*(3), 235–244.

DiCarlo, J. J., & Johnson, K. O. (2000). Spatial and temporal structure of receptive fields in primate somatosensory area 3b: Effects of stimulus scanning direction and orientation. *Journal of Neuroscience, 20*, 495–510.

DiCarlo, J. J., Johnson, K. O., & Hsiao, S. S. (1998). Structure of receptive fields in area 3b of primary somatosensory cortex in the alert monkey. *Journal of Neuroscience, 18*, 2626–2645.

Dostrovsky, J. O. (2000). Role of thalamus in pain. *Progress in Brain Research, 129*, 245–257.

Ferrington, D. G., & Rowe, M. J. (1980). Differential contributions to coding of cutaneous vibratory information by cortical somatosensory areas I and II. *Journal of Neurophysiology, 43*, 310–331.

Fitzgerald, P. J., Lane, J. W., Thakur, P. H., & Hsiao, S. S. (2004). Receptive field properties of the macaque second somatosensory cortex: Evidence for multiple functional representations. *Journal of Neuroscience, 24*(49), 11193–11204.

Fitzgerald, P. J., Lane, J. W., Thakur, P. H., & Hsiao, S. S. (2006a). Receptive field (RF) properties of the macaque second somatosensory cortex: RF size, shape, and somatotopic organization. *Journal of Neuroscience, 26*, 6485–6495.

Fitzgerald, P. J., Lane, J. W., Thakur, P. H., & Hsiao, S. S. (2006b). Receptive field properties of the macaque second somatosensory cortex: Representation of orientation on different finger pads. *Journal of Neuroscience, 26*, 6473–6484.

Foxe, J. J., Wylie, G. R., Martinez, A., Schroeder, C. E., Javitt, D. C., Guilfoyle, D.,...Murray MM. (2002). Auditory-somatosensory multisensory processing

in auditory association cortex: An fMRI study. *Journal of Neurophysiology, 88,* 540–543.
Fu, K. M., Johnston, T. A., Shah, A. S., Arnold, L., Smiley, J., Hackett, T. A.,... Schroeder CE. (2003). Auditory cortical neurons respond to somatosensory stimulation. *Journal of Neuroscience, 23,* 7510–7515.
Garraghty, P. E., Florence, S. L., & Kaas, J. H. (1990). Ablations of areas 3a and 3b of monkey somatosensory cortex abolish cutaneous responsivity in area 1. *Brain Research, 528,* 165–169.
Green, B. G. (2004). Temperature perception and nociception. *Journal of Neurobiology, 61,* 13–29.
Gynther, B. D., Vickery, R. M., & Rowe, M. J. (1995). Transmission characteristics for the 1:1 linkage between slowly adapting type II fibers and their cuneate target neurons in cat. *Experimental Brain Research, 105,* 67–75.
Heller, M. A. (1989). Texture perception in sighted and blind observers. *Perception and Psychophysics, 45,* 49–54.
Hollins, M., Bensmaia, S. J., Karlof, K., & Young, F. (2000). Individual differences in perceptual space for tactile textures: Evidence from multidimensional scaling. *Perception and Psychophysics, 62,* 1534–1544.
Hollins, M., Bensmaia, S. J., & Washburn, S. (2001). Vibrotactile adaptation impairs discrimination of fine, but not coarse, textures. *Somatosensory and Motor Research, 18,* 253–262.
Hollins, M., & Risner, S. R. (2000). Evidence for the duplex theory of tactile texture perception. *Perception and Psychophysics, 62,* 695–705.
Hubel, D. H., & Wiesel, T. N. (1968). Receptive fields and functional architecture of monkey striate cortex. *Journal of Physiology, 195,* 215–243.
Hyvarinen, J., & Poranen, A. (1978). Movement-sensitive and direction and orientation-selective cutaneous receptive fields in the hand area of the postcentral gyrus in monkeys. *Journal of Physiology, 283,* 523–537.
Jiang, W., Tremblay, F., & Chapman, C. E. (1997). Neuronal encoding of texture changes in the primary and the secondary somatosensory cortical areas of monkeys during passive texture discrimination. *Journal of Neurophysiology, 77,* 1656–1662.
Johnson, K. O. (1980) Sensory discrimination: Neural processes preceding discrimination decision. *Journal of Neurophysiology, 43,* 1793–1815.
Johnson, K. O. (2001). The roles and functions of cutaneous mechanoreceptors. *Current Opinion in Neurobiology, 11,* 455–461.
Johnson, K. O., & Lamb, G. D. (1981). Neural mechanisms of spatial tactile discrimination: Neural patterns evoked by Braille-like dot patterns in the monkey. *Journal of Physiology, 310,* 117–144.
Jousmaki, V., & Hari, R. (1998). Parchment-skin illusion: Sound-biased touch. *Current Biology, 8,* R190.
Kaas, J. H. (1983). What, if anything, is SI? Organization of first somatosensory area of cortex. *Physiological Reviews, 63,* 206–231.
Kaas, J. H., Nelson, R. J., Sur, M., Lin, C. S., & Merzenich, M. M. (1979). Multiple representations of the body within the primary somatosensory cortex of primates. *Science, 204,* 521–523.
Kaas, J. H., Nelson, R. J., Sur, M., Merzenich, M. M., (1981). Organization of somatosensory cortex in primates. In F. O. Schmitt, F. G. Worden, G, Adelman, &

Dennis, S. G. (eds.), *The organization of the cerebral cortex* (pp. 237–261). Cambridge, MA: MIT Press.

Kenshalo, D. R., Iwata, K., Sholas, M., & Thomas, D. A. (2000). Response properties and organization of nociceptive neurons in area 1 of monkey primary somatosensory cortex. *Journal of Neurophysiology, 84*, 719–729.

Khalsa, P. S., Friedman, R. M., Srinivasan, M. A., & LaMotte, R. H. (1998). Encoding of shape and orientation of objects indented into the monkey fingerpad by populations of slowly and rapidly adapting mechanoreceptors. *Journal of Neurophysiology, 79*, 3238–3251.

Lacey, S., Tal, N., Amedi, A., & Sathian, K. (2009). A putative model of multisensory object representation. *Brain Topography, 21*(3–4), 269–274.

LaMotte, R. H., Friedman, R. M., Lu, C., Khalsa, P. S., & Srinivasan, M. A. (1998). Raised object on a planar surface stroked across the fingerpad: Responses of cutaneous mechanoreceptors to shape and orientation. *Journal of Neurophysiology, 80*, 2446–2466.

LaMotte, R. H., & Mountcastle, V. B. (1975). Capacities of humans and monkeys to discriminate between vibratory stimuli of different frequency and amplitude: A correlation between neural events and psychophysical measurements. *Journal of Neurophysiology, 38*, 539–559.

Lederman, S. J. (1979). Auditory texture perception. *Perception, 8*, 93–103.

Lederman, S. J., & Klatzky, R. L. (1987). Hand movements: A window into haptic object recognition. *Cognitive Psychology, 19*, 342–368.

Lederman, S. J., Klatzky, R. L., Chataway, C., & Summers, D. C. (1990). Visual mediation and the haptic recognition of two-dimensional pictures of common objects. *Perception and Psychophysics, 47*, 54–64.

Lenz, F. A., Seike, M., Lin, Y. C., Baker, F. H., Rowland, L. H., Gracely, R. H., Richardson RT. (1993). Neurons in the area of human thalamic nucleus ventralis caudalis respond to painful heat stimuli. *Brain Research, 623*, 235–240.

Lenz, F. A., Seike, M., Richardson, R. T., Lin, Y. C., Baker, F. H., Khoja, I., ... Gracely R.H. (1993). Thermal and pain sensations evoked by microstimulation in the area of human ventrocaudal nucleus. *Journal of Neurophysiology, 70*, 200–212.

Loken, L. S., Wessberg, J., Morrison, I., McGlone, F., & Olausson, H. (2009). Coding of pleasant touch by unmyelinated afferents in humans. *Nature Neuroscience, 12*(5), 547–548.

Loomis, J. M. (1982). Analysis of tactile and visual confusion matrices. *Perception and Psychophysics, 31*, 41–52.

Loomis, J. M., Klatzky, R. L., & Lederman, S. J. (1991). Similarity of tactual and visual picture recognition with limited field of view. *Perception, 20*, 167–177.

Lundberg, A., Malmgren, K., & Schomburg, E. D. (1987). Reflex pathways from group II muscle afferents. 3. Secondary spindle afferents and the FRA: A new hypothesis. *Experimental Brain Research, 65*(2), 294–306.

Magee, L. E., & Kennedy, J. M. (1980). Exploring pictures tactually. *Nature, 283*, 287–288.

McGlone, F., Vallbo, A. B., Olausson, H., Loken, L., & Wessberg, J. (2007). Discriminative touch and emotional touch. *Canadian Journal of Experimental Psychology, 61*(3), 173–183.

Mountcastle, V. B. (2005). *The sensory hand: Neural mechanisms in somatic sensation* Cambridge, MA Harvard University Press.

Mountcastle, V. B., Lynch, J. C., Georgopoulos, A. P., Sakata, H., & Acuna, C. (1975). Posterior parietal association cortex of the monkey: Command functions for operations within extrapersonal space. *Journal of Neurophysiology, 38*, 871–908.

Mountcastle, V. B., Talbot, W. H., Sakata, H., & Hyvarinen, J. (1969). Cortical neuronal mechanisms in flutter-vibration studied in unanesthetized monkeys. Neuronal periodicity and frequency discrimination. *Journal of Neurophysiology, 32*(3), 452–484.

Muniak, M. A., Ray, S., Hsiao, S. S., Dammann, J. F., & Bensmaia, S. J. (2007). The neural coding of stimulus intensity: Linking the population response of mechanoreceptive afferents with psychophysical behavior. *Journal of Neuroscience, 27*, 11687–11699.

Murray, E. A., & Mishkin, M. (1984). Relative contributions of SII and area 5 to tactile discrimination in monkeys. *Behavioural Brain Research, 11*, 67–85.

Nakama, T., Lane, J. W., Fitzgerald, P. J., Sripati, A., Johnson, K. O., Yantis, S., Hsiao SS. (2000). Attentional modulation of bilateral neuronal responses in the secondary somatosensory cortex during an orientation discrimination task. *Society for Neuroscience Abstracts, 788, 8.*

Nolan, C. Y., & Kederis, C. J. (1969). *Perceptual factors in Braille word recognition*. New York, NY: American Foundation for the Blind.

Olshausen, B. A., & Field, D. J. (1996). Emergence of simple-cell receptive field properties by learning a sparse code for natural images. *Nature, 381*(6583), 607–609.

Pasupathy, A., & Connor, C. E. (1999). Responses to contour features in macaque area V4. *J Neurophysiol, 82*(5), 2490–2502.

Pasupathy, A., & Connor, C. E. (2001). Shape representation in area V4: Position-specific tuning for boundary conformation. *Journal of Neurophysiology, 86*(5), 2505–2519.

Pei, Y. C., Denchev, P. V., Hsiao, S. S., Craig, J. C., & Bensmaia, S. J. (2009). Convergence of submodality-specific input onto neurons in primary somatosensory cortex. *Journal of Neurophysiology, 102*(3), 1843–1853.

Pei, Y. C., Hsiao, S. S., Craig, J. C., & Bensmaia, S. J. (2010). Shape-invariant coding of motion direction in somatosensory cortex. *PLoS Biology, 8*(2), e1000305.

Pei, Y. C., Hsiao, S. S., Craig, J. C., & Bensmaia, S. J. (2011). Neural mechanisms of motion integration in somatosensory cortex. *Neuron, 69*(3), 536–547.

Peltier, S., Stilla, R., Mariola, E., Laconte, S., Hu, X., & Sathian, K. (2007). Activity and effective connectivity of parietal and occipital cortical regions during haptic shape perception. *Neuropsychologia, 45*, 476–283.

Peyron, R., Laurent, B., & Garcia-Larrea, L. (2000). Functional imaging of brain responses to pain. A review and meta-analysis. *Neurophysiologie Clinique, 30*, 263–288.

Phillips, J. R., & Johnson, K. O. (1981a). Tactile spatial resolution: II. Neural representation of bars, edges, and gratings in monkey primary afferents. *Journal of Neurophysiology, 46*, 1192–1203.

Phillips, J. R., & Johnson, K. O. (1981b). Tactile spatial resolution: III. A continuum mechanics model of skin predicting mechanoreceptor responses to bars, edges, and gratings. *Journal of Neurophysiology, 46*, 1204–1225.

Phillips, J. R., Johnson, K. O., & Browne, H. M. (1983). A comparison of visual and two modes of tactual letter resolution. *Perception and Psychophysics, 34*, 243–249.

Phillips, J. R., Johnson, K. O., & Hsiao, S. S. (1988). Spatial pattern representation and transformation in monkey somatosensory cortex. *Proceedings of the National Academy of Sciences of the United States of America, 85,* 1317–1321.

Pons, T. P., Garraghty, P. E., Friedman, D. P., & Mishkin, M. (1987). Physiological evidence for serial processing in somatosensory cortex. *Science, 237,* 417–420.

Pons, T. P., Garraghty, P. E., & Mishkin, M. (1992). Serial and parallel processing of tactual information in somatosensory cortex of rhesus monkeys. *Journal of Neurophysiology, 68,* 518–527.

Pubols, L. M., & LeRoy, R. F. (1977). Orientation detectors in the primary somatosensory neocortex of the raccoon. *Brain Research, 129,* 61–74.

Randolph, M., & Semmes, J. (1974). Behavioral consequences of selective ablations in the postcentral gyrus of Macaca mulatta. *Brain Research, 70,* 55–70.

Robinson, C. J., & Burton, H. (1980). Somatotopographic organization in the second somatosensory area of M. fascicularis. *Journal of Comparative Neurology, 192,* 43–67.

Ruiz, S., Crespo, P., & Romo, R. (1995). Representation of moving tactile stimuli in the somatic sensory cortex of awake monkeys. *Journal of Neurophysiology, 73,* 525–537.

Sahai, V., Mahns, D. A., Robinson, L., Perkins, N. M., Coleman, G. T., & Rowe, M. J. (2006). Processing of vibrotactile inputs from hairy skin by neurons of the dorsal column nuclei in the cat. *Journal of Neurophysiology, 95,* 1451–1464.

Salinas, E., Hernandez, A., Zainos, A., & Romo, R. (2000). Periodicity and firing rate as candidate neural codes for the frequency of vibrotactile stimuli. *Journal of Neuroscience, 20,* 5503–5515.

Scheibert, J., Leurent, S., Prevost, A., & Debregeas, G. (2009). The role of fingerprints in the coding of tactile information probed with a biomimetic sensor. *Science, 323*(5920), 1503–1506.

Semmes, J., & Turner, B. H. (1977). Effects of cortical lesions on somatosensory tasks. *Journal of Investigative Dermatology, 69,* 181–189.

Sinclair, R. J., & Burton, H. (1991). Neuronal activity in the primary somatosensory cortex in monkeys (*Macaca mulatta*) during active touch of textured surface gratings: Responses to groove width, applied force, and velocity of motion. *Journal of Neurophysiology, 66,* 153–169.

Srinivasan, M. A., & LaMotte, R. H. (1987). Tactile discrimination of shape: Responses of slowly and rapidly adapting mechanoreceptive afferents to a step indented into the monkey fingerpad. *Journal of Neuroscience, 7,* 1682–1697.

Sripati, A. P., Bensmaia, S. J., & Johnson, K. O. (2006). A continuum mechanical model of mechanoreceptive afferent responses to indented spatial patterns. *Journal of Neurophysiology, 95,* 3852–3864.

Sripati, A. P., Yoshioka, T., Denchev, P., Hsiao, S. S., & Johnson, K. O. (2006). Spatiotemporal receptive fields of peripheral afferents and cortical area 3b and 1 neurons in the primate somatosensory system. *Journal of Neuroscience, 26,* 2101–2114.

Stein, B. E., & Meredith, M. A. (2004). *The merging of the senses.* Cambridge, MA: MIT Press.

Sur, M., Merzenich, M. M., & Kaas, J. H. (1980). Magnification, receptive-field area, and hypercolumn size in areas 3b and 1 of somatosensory cortex in owl monkeys. *Journal of Neurophysiology, 44,* 295–311.

Talbot, W. H., Darian-Smith, I., Kornhuber, H. H., & Mountcastle, V. B. (1968). The sense of flutter-vibration: Comparison of the human capacity with response patterns of mechanoreceptive afferents from the monkey hand. *Journal of Neurophysiology, 31,* 301–334.

Thakur, P. H., Bastian, A. J., & Hsiao, S. S. (2008). Multidigit movement synergies of the human hand in an unconstrained haptic exploration task. *Journal of Neuroscience, 28,* 1271–1281.

Tommerdahl, M., Hester, K. D., Felix, E. R., Hollins, M., Favorov, O. V., Quibrera, P. M., et al. (2005). Human vibrotactile frequency discriminative capacity after adaptation to 25 Hz or 200 Hz stimulation. *Brain Research, 1057,* 1–9.

Ungerleider, L. G., Mishkin, M., Ingle, D. J., Goodale, M. A., & Mansfield, R. J. (1982). Two cortical visual systems. In *Analysis of Visual Behavior* (pp. 549–586). Cambridge, MA: M.I.T. Press.

Vega-Bermudez, F., Johnson, K. O., Fasman, K. H., & Hsiao, S. S. (1989). Active vs passive touch in a letter recognition task: Human performance and velocity effects. *Society for Neuroscience Abstracts, 313.*

Vega-Bermudez, F., Johnson, K. O., & Hsiao, S. S. (1991). Human tactile pattern recognition: Active versus passive touch, velocity effects, and patterns of confusion. *Journal of Neurophysiology, 65,* 531–546.

Vinje, W. E., & Gallant, J. L. (2000). Sparse coding and decorrelation in primary visual cortex during natural vision. *Science, 287,* 1273–1276.

Warren, S., Hamalainen, H. A., & Gardner, E. P. (1986). Coding of the spatial period of gratings rolled across the receptive fields of somatosensory cortical neurons in awake monkeys. *Journal of Neurophysiology, 56,* 623–639.

Weinstein, S., & Kenshalo, D. R. (1968). Intensive and extensive aspects of tactile sensitivity as a function of body part, sex and laterality. In *The Skin Senses* (pp. 195–222). Springfield, IL: C.C.Thomas.

Wheat, H. E., & Goodwin, A. W. (2001). Tactile discrimination of edge shape: Limits on spatial resolution imposed by parameters of the peripheral neural population. *Journal of Neuroscience, 21,* 7751–7763.

Wheat, H. E., Salo, L. M., & Goodwin, A. W. (2009). Cutaneous afferents from the monkeys fingers: Responses to tangential and normal forces. *Journal of Neurophysiology, 103,* 950–961.

Whitsel, B. L., Petrucelli, L. M., & Werner, G. (1969). Symmetry and connectivity in the map of the body surface in somatosensory area II of primates. *Journal of Neurophysiology, 32,* 170–183.

Yau, J. M., Olenczak, J. B., Dammann, J. F., & Bensmaia, S. J. (2009). Temporal frequency channels are linked across audition and touch. *Current Biology, 19,* 561–566.

Yau, J. M., Pasupathy, A., Fitzgerald, P. J., Hsiao, S. S., & Connor, C. E. (2009). Analogous intermediate shape coding in vision and touch. *Proceedings of the National Academy of Sciences of the United States of America, 106*(38), 16457–16462.

Yoshioka, T., Gibb, B., Dorsch, A. K., Hsiao, S. S., & Johnson, K. O. (2001). Neural coding mechanisms underlying perceived roughness of finely textured surfaces. *Journal of Neuroscience, 21,* 6905–6916.

8

Crossmodal Interactions in Tactile Perception

CHARLES SPENCE AND ANDREW J. BREMNER

Until recently, most textbooks on human perception considered each of the major senses (e.g., vision, hearing, touch, olfaction, and taste) in isolation, as if each represented an independent perceptual system. In many situations, however, our senses receive correlated information about the same external objects and events, and this information is typically combined by the brain to yield the rich multisensory percepts that fill our everyday lives (see Calvert, Spence, & Stein, 2004). Here, we explore how multisensory interactions impact on our perception of the objects/events in the environment as sensed through the tactile modality. We review the evidence both from the well-established literature on adults and also from the growing body of research investigating the multisensory aspects of tactile perception in infants and children.

Haptic perception (i.e., tactile perception that involves active as opposed to passive touch) allows us to gain information about objects and surfaces; information concerning both the substance (hardness, weight, temperature, texture, etc.) and structural properties (size, shape, and volume) of the objects with which we are interacting (see Lederman & Klatzky, 2009; and Spence & Gallace, 2008, for recent reviews). In the first part of this chapter, we examine how multisensory interactions shape haptic perception, reviewing the literature on auditory, olfactory, and visual contributions to tactile and haptic perception. In addition to providing information about the external environment through haptics, tactile stimuli that impinge on the body surface also play an important role in framing our representations of our own bodies and the disposition of our limbs with respect to ourselves and the external environment. Thus, we will also examine how multisensory interactions involving the tactile modality determine our perception of both the external environment and the relation of our bodies to the outside world. Finally, we discuss how recent findings from infants and young children can inform our growing understanding of how multisensory contributions to tactile perception develop.

MULTISENSORY TOUCH AND THE EXTERNAL ENVIRONMENT: HAPTICS

The majority of research into multisensory interactions in haptic perception has focused on the interaction of touch and vision. In particular, a great deal of effort has been devoted to understanding whether and why vision dominates over touch when people make judgments about multisensory objects. Before we enter into this debate, however, we will first describe the research that has examined crossmodal influences on haptic perception between two of the other major senses, namely, audition and olfaction. Although people often do not consider these senses when thinking about multisensory tactile (and haptic) perception, the available evidence shows that they can have a significant influence on what we feel.

Auditory Contributions to Tactile Perception

Researchers have demonstrated that manipulating the sounds that people hear when they touch a surface can have a dramatic effect on the perceived roughness of the surface (e.g., Guest, Catmur, Lloyd, & Spence, 2002; Jousmäki & Hari, 1998). What is more, people's perception of the pleasantness, powerfulness, and forcefulness of many different products has also been shown to be influenced by the sounds that they make when used (e.g., Spence & Zampini, 2007; Zampini, Guest, & Spence, 2003). For example, Jousmäki and Hari reported a particularly dramatic demonstration of the auditory modulation of tactile perception, known as the "parchment-skin" illusion. They showed that people's perception of the "feel" of the palmar skin of their own hands could be changed simply by changing the sounds that they heard (over headphones) when they rubbed them together in front of a microphone.

In a follow-up study reported by Guest et al. (2002), participants either heard the actual sound of their hands being rubbed together (which was picked up by a microphone and played back over headphones) or else the sound was manipulated to reduce the overall sound intensity level (by either 20 or 40 dB) or to amplify or attenuate just the high-frequency components of the sounds (i.e., those above 2 kHz) by 12 dB. The participants in this study had to make separate ratings concerning how rough and how moist their hands felt. Interestingly, the participants rated their hands as feeling significantly dryer when listening to the louder hand-rubbing sounds or when just the high-frequency components of the sounds were boosted. Changing the auditory feedback also had a small but significant effect on participants' ratings of the roughness of their hands. These results therefore highlight the significant role that auditory cues can play in influencing people's evaluation of the "feel" of a surface, even for a surface that may be as familiar to them as the skin of their own hands. The auditory modulation of tactile experience is not, however, restricted to the perception of our own skin/bodies: Guest et al. went on to show that people's perception of the texture (roughness) of sandpapers varying in roughness (or grit) value was also modified simply by varying the auditory feedback that they heard when touching them. In this case, the amplification of the high-frequency sounds appeared to result in an increased perception of sandpaper roughness, while the attenuation of these sounds made the touched surfaces feel smoother instead.

A growing body of applied research has now demonstrated that auditory cues also play an important role in people's perception of many everyday products (see Spence & Zampini, 2006, for a review). For example, Zampini et al. (2003) reported a study showing that people's perception of the pleasantness and powerfulness of an electric toothbrush was influenced by the particular sounds that it made when people brushed their front teeth with it. Similarly, Spence and Zampini (2007) have demonstrated that the perceived forcefulness and pleasantness of an aerosol spray can similarly be influenced by changing the particular spectral profile of the spraying sounds it makes when used. Results such as these, together with findings from a large number of other published studies, demonstrate just how important auditory cues are to our perception of many everyday objects, products, and surfaces (see Schifferstein & Spence, 2008).

Olfactory Contributions to Tactile Perception

To date, less research has been directed at investigating the nature of any crossmodal influence of olfaction on the sense of touch (see Demattè, Sanabria, Sugarman, & Spence, 2006; Laird, 1932, for exceptions). Laird, in a now classic study, described a house-to-house survey in which each of 250 housewives was presented with four pairs of silk stockings and then asked to judge the pair that had the highest quality. The housewives were allowed to look at, touch, and stretch the stockings. The stockings were actually identical except for the fact that one pair had a synthetic fragrance, another had a fruity fragrance, a third pair had a "sachet" scent, and the fourth pair had a slightly rancid smell. Half of the housewives in this study reported that they preferred the synthetic, narcissus-scented hosiery (24% preferred the fruity scent, 18% preferred the sachet scent, and the remainder preferred the rancid scent). Crucially, however, the majority of the housewives attributed their preferences not to the smell of the scented hosiery (which only six housewives noticed), but to the texture, durability, sheen, weight, or weave of the stockings instead (i.e., to their tactile and/or visual qualities).

More recently, Demattè et al. (2006) investigated whether or not the presence of an odor would modulate people's perception of the *softness* of fabric samples under rather more controlled laboratory conditions. The participants in Demattè et al.'s study sat in front of a rotating wheel on which a number of different swatches of fabric were hung (to allow for a naturalistic rubbing of the materials between the participant's thumb and forefinger). On each trial, the participants felt one of the swatches (the participants were not allowed to see the fabric samples) and rated its softness. While the participants were evaluating the feel of a particular fabric swatch, a lemon or an animal-like odor was occasionally delivered direct to the participant's nostrils. On each trial, the participants first had to classify any odor as either pleasant or unpleasant, or else respond that no odor had been presented. (Unsurprisingly, for the majority of participants, the lemon odor was judged as pleasant while the animal odor was judged as unpleasant.) Next, the participants had to indicate how soft the fabric felt between their fingers. The participants rated the fabrics as feeling significantly softer when presented at the same time as the pleasant lemon odor than when presented together with the "unpleasant" animal odor instead.

In a subsequent experiment, Demattè et al. (2006) went on to demonstrate that olfactory cues (in this case, the smell of lavender and/or "animal"—the smell of Greek goat according to one of the first author's PhD students) also influenced people's judgments of fabric softness when it was applied directly to the fabric swatches themselves (i.e., using a more ecologically valid experimental design). However, it is, at present, unclear whether the olfactory modulation of tactile perception highlighted by previous research is restricted to the perception of fabrics (i.e., to surfaces/materials that are commonly scented, as after washing), or whether instead such crossmodal influences can also modify people's perception of other surfaces (such as, e.g., sandpaper) that may not normally be associated with any particular fragrance. Nevertheless, the two studies reported in this section do demonstrate that olfactory cues can modulate tactile perception.

Visual Contributions to Tactile Perception

Traditionally, philosophers, when considering the relationship between the senses, believed that touch dominated over vision (and presumably the other senses too). Indeed, Bishop Berkeley (1709/1948) argued that touch "tutors" vision through development, by informing vision about the third dimension (see Rock & Harris, 1967). This view was based on the assumption that only tactile exploration could provide veridical information about the three-dimensional environment, whereas depth cues were lost on the two-dimensional retinal (i.e., visual) image. However, over the last 75 years or so, psychologists have conducted many studies demonstrating that vision frequently dominates over the sense of touch. For example, in one early study, Gibson (1943) reported that when people ran their fingers up and down a straight rod they perceived it as being curved if they simultaneously looked through lenses that made the rod look curved. As soon as the participants closed their eyes, however, the rod was reported as feeling straight again. Similar results were reported by Irvin Rock and his colleagues in a now-classic series of experiments in which the participants had to rate their impression of the size of a small object which they could either see (through a distorting lens), feel (under a cloth that hid their hand from view), or both see and feel at the same time (see Rock & Harris, 1967; Rock & Victor, 1964). The results showed that that people perceived squares to be rectangular if that was how they looked and that the size of an object was nearly entirely determined by what the participants saw. This kind of visual dominance over the perceived size and shape of haptically explored objects is so strong (and automatic) that it cannot easily be overridden by instruction. In fact, Rock and Harris (1967, p. 96) went so far as to state that "...vision completely dominates touch & even shapes it...."

Taken together, these and many other results published subsequently (see Spence & Gallace, 2008, for a review) show that vision typically dominates over the haptic perception of both the substance and structural properties of objects when the senses are put into intersensory conflict. Interestingly, those who are in some sense experts in using their hands (e.g., potters) have been shown to exhibit just as much visual dominance as naïve participants (see Spence & Gallace, 2008, for a review). Researchers have also demonstrated that visual dominance effects tend to be more pronounced when the stimuli presented in the two modalities originate (or at least are perceived to originate) from the same spatial location at more or less the same time (Gepshtein, Burge, Ernst, & Banks, 2005; Miller, 1972). However, Helbig and Ernst (2007a) have shown that people can still integrate visual and haptic information in a near-optimal manner when they come from different locations, just so long as the participants believe that what they are seeing and feeling refer to the same object (as, e.g., when one looks in a mirror in one location to see an object that is being haptically explored at a different location; see also Miller, 1972, on this issue).

Over the years, various different theories have been put forward to try to account for the apparent ubiquity of the visual dominance effects observed in the laboratory, including the "directed attention" hypothesis (Posner, Nissen, & Klein, 1976) and the "modality-appropriateness" hypothesis (Welch & Warren, 1980, 1986). According to the directed attention hypothesis, people tend to direct their attention more toward visual inputs to compensate for the poor alerting, or arousing, qualities of visual stimuli. This attentional bias results in (attended) visual inputs (i.e., those sensory impressions that people are concentrating on) being weighted more heavily than those from the other relatively "less attended" sensory modalities (e.g., such as touch; see Posner et al., 1976; Spence, Shore, & Klein, 2001). By contrast, according to the modality-appropriateness hypothesis, our brains tend to favor (i.e., to weight more highly) information from the sense that is most appropriate for the task at hand. The argument being that visual information frequently dominates because vision is the sense that normally provides the most accurate information concerning the judgment being made (at least for the kinds of perceptual judgments, regarding an object's size, shape, and position, that psychologists are fond of asking participants to make). Consistent with this latter view, researchers investigating the multisensory perception of surface texture have shown that both visual and tactile cues contribute to people's perception of the felt texture (or roughness) of a surface, with the extent to which one sense is preferred over another depending on the particular surface being evaluated (Guest & Spence, 2003a, 2003b; Spence & Gallace, 2008; see Lederman & Klatzky, 2004, for a review). Interestingly, touch has been shown to dominate when people have to evaluate very fine surface textures, but vision is dominant when judgments about rougher surfaces are required (Heller, 1989).

MODELING SENSORY DOMINANCE

Ernst and Banks (2002) brought some much-needed mathematical rigor to the field of sensory dominance research. They demonstrated that "maximum likelihood estimation" (MLE) can provide an excellent quantitative account of modality appropriateness. In their study, participants had to judge the height of a bar using visual and tactile/haptic cues (participants could see and also feel the "virtual" bar between the thumb and index finger of one hand). Ernst and Banks showed that adding noise to the visual signal (presented via computer) resulted in their participants increasingly relying on haptic information when making their judgments. Participants' judgments were updated on a trial-by-trial basis, depending on how much noise had been added to the visual signal, thus showing that visual dominance is not hardwired. According to the MLE account of sensory dominance, the human brain combines sensory inputs in a manner that is very close to that of a statistically optimal multisensory integrator. That is, the multisensory integration of disparate unisensory inputs maximally reduces the uncertainty of (or variance associated with) our multisensory estimates of external stimulus qualities (given that all sensory estimates are intrinsically noisy; note that the MLE approach assumes that the noise associated with each sense is independent and has a Gaussian distribution). Since Ernst and Banks' original paper was published, several research groups have successfully used MLE to model the sensory dominance observed in a number of other behavioral paradigms in both adults (see, e.g., Ernst, 2006; Helbig & Ernst, 2007b; Hillis, Ernst, Banks, & Landy, 2002; van Beers, Wolpert, & Haggard, 2002), children (Gori, Del Viva, Sandini, & Burr, 2008), and now monkeys (Morgan, DeAngelis, & Angelaki, 2008). MLE, then, provides an entirely bottom-up account of sensory dominance (see Ernst & Bülthoff, 2004).

In the majority of early studies of sensory dominance (including that of Ernst & Banks', 2002), only a single stimulus was presented in each sensory modality at any given time, and hence, there was essentially no binding problem to be solved (i.e., no problem associated with deciding which stimulus from each modality should be bound together). However, given that we typically operate in more complex multistimulus environments, the binding problem soon becomes much more apparent. This has led researchers in subsequent studies to move to a Bayesian decision theory account of sensory dominance, that is, to an account that incorporates both prior knowledge (so-called "Bayesian priors") and likelihood functions (e.g., Ernst & Bülthoff, 2004; Wozny, Beierholm, & Shams, 2008). By way of an example, one way in which researchers have suggested that prior knowledge can play a role in deciding what crossmodal stimuli to bind and integrate is by relying on the (prior) knowledge that multisensory stimuli typically arise from more or less the same spatial location (Gephstein et al., 2005; Helbig & Ernst, 2007a).

Given the excellent job that Bayesian decision theory has done in accounting for the empirical findings in the literature on sensory dominance, the question arises as to whether we need to retain any role for attention at all in multisensory integration (remember that in their influential review paper, Posner et al. (1976) argued that attention to the visual modality may have been responsible for visual dominance). Recently, Helbig and Ernst (2008) reported no effect of attentional manipulations (they used a dual-task manipulation to reduce the perceptual resources available in one sensory modality, vision) on the relative weightings of the unimodal inputs. (Of course, this is not to say that attentional manipulations will not influence people's responses under conditions of sensory conflict—see the discussion section of Helbig and Ernst' paper.) The latter results therefore support an "early," rather than "late," model of cue combination (i.e., whereby cue combination occurs prior to the influence of attention). However, as we shall see in the next section, it may be an oversimplification to suggest that many of the Bayesian priors Ernst and colleagues invoke are readily available. Take, for example, the prior of spatial colocation. Because the sensory surfaces of the body (the skin, the retina in the eyes, the tympanic membrane in the ear, etc.) move relative to one another when the body changes posture (e.g., when the eyes, hands, and head move—see Pöppel, 1973), it may be that such priors are only immediately available under a relatively limited set of circumstances. Future research will, then, need to address more thoroughly the ecological availability of Bayesian priors for multisensory integration.

The evidence that has been summarized thus far clearly demonstrates just how important the contributions of the other senses (in particular, vision, audition, and olfaction) can be to our haptic perception of objects, surfaces, and events. In the next section, we will move on to examine multisensory influences on tactile perception in a different representational context; namely, one in which touch is used to inform our perceptions of our own body and limbs and their disposition in space.

MULTISENSORY TOUCH AND THE INTERNAL WORLD: MULTISENSORY BODY REPRESENTATIONS

The ability to make sense of perceptual information about our own body and its relationship to the immediate (or "peripersonal") spatial environment (and the objects that fill it) is crucial for normal everyday functioning. Without a representation of the shape and extent of our body and the layout of our limbs in relation to ourselves and our environment we would be left helpless to interact with it in any meaningful way. The computational demands of forming functional body representations are quite complex, partly because our body parts often change their relative position. As we shall see later, this fact has important implications for how we integrate multisensory inputs about the body.

Visual Influences on the Perceived Location of Touch on the Body

The sense of touch provides unique information concerning our body and its relation to nearby objects. Typically, touch can only be stimulated by objects directly impinging on the body (the only exception being our distal perception of radiant heat sources, such as, e.g., the sun, and high-intensity, low-frequency sound sources). As such, touch informs us about the relationship between our body and the environment. Touch can also disambiguate which cues from our distal spatial senses (e.g., vision and audition) specify events that are located in our peripersonal environment, the environment that affords immediate action. The role of touch in representing the body and peripersonal space has now been confirmed by neuroscientific research findings in both human and nonhuman primates (see Graziano, Gross, Taylor, & Moore, 2004; Spence, Pavani, Maravita, & Holmes, 2004). However, behavioral and physiological studies also point toward the conclusion that it is the ways in which information from touch and proprioception are integrated with information from vision (and, on occasion, audition) that provides us with embodied representations of the environment and, in particular, peripersonal space (Rizzolatti, Fadiga, Fogassi, & Gallese, 1997). For instance, both single-unit recording studies on monkeys (Graziano et al., 2004) and fMRI of humans (Makin, Holmes, & Zohary, 2007) have uncovered robust evidence that neural circuits (particularly in ventral premotor cortex) responding to objects/events situated in peripersonal space are, to a large extent, multisensory. Likewise, the circuits underlying our representation of body posture and limb position (the "body schema") also rely on multisensory inputs (Maravita, Spence, & Driver, 2003).

Perhaps the most convincing behavioral data concerning multisensory influences on the perceived location of tactile stimuli comes from research using the crossmodal congruency task (see Spence, Pavani, & Driver, 2004). In the most commonly used variant of this

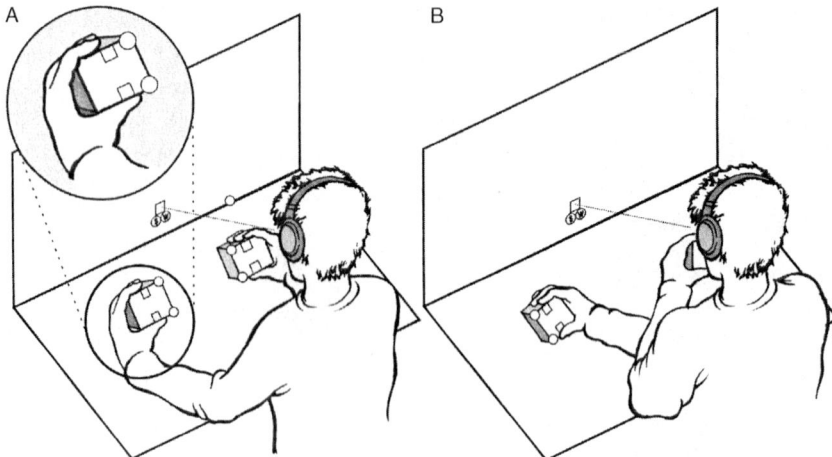

FIGURE 8.1 Schematic view of a participant adopting both (A) an uncrossed and (B) a crossed-hands posture while performing the crossmodal congruency task. Two vibrotactile stimulators (small rectangles) and two visual distractor lights (small circles) were embedded in each of the two foam cubes, held by the participants between their thumbs and index fingers. The participants made speeded elevation discrimination responses (by raising the toe or heel of their right foot), in response to vibrotactile targets presented either from the "top" by the index finger of either hand or from the "bottom" by either thumb, respectively. The largest crossmodal congruency effects are elicited by visual distractors placed closest to the location of the vibrotactile target (i.e., on the same foam cube), no matter whether the hands are held in an uncrossed or crossed posture. Reprinted with permission from "Multi-sensory interactions," by C. Spence, F. Pavani, A. Maravita, and N. P. Holmes, in *Haptic Rendering: Foundations, Algorithms, and Applications* (pp. 21–52) by M. C. Lin & M. A. Otaduy (Eds.), 2008, Wellesley, MA: AK Peters.

task, participants hold two foam blocks, one in either hand (see Figure 8.1A for a schematic illustration of the experimental setup). A vibrator and an LED are embedded at the top and bottom of each block. On each trial, a vibrotactile target and a visual distractor are presented randomly and independently from one of four possible stimulus locations. Vibrotactile targets (normally consisting of pulsed vibrations) are briefly presented to the index finger or thumb of either hand. Visual distractors consist of the pulsed illumination of one of the four LEDs. Participants make speeded elevation discrimination responses (i.e., "above," when the target is presented to the index finger; or "below," when the target is presented to the thumb) in response to the vibrotactile targets, while trying to ignore any visual distractors that happen to be presented at around the same time.

Although the visual distractors are just as likely to be presented from the same elevation as the vibrotactile target, as from a different elevation, participants are typically much worse (i.e., they are both slower and more error prone) at discriminating the elevation of the vibrotactile targets when the visual distractors are presented from an incongruent elevation (i.e., when the vibrotactile target is presented from the top and the visual distractor from the bottom, or vice versa) than when they are presented from the same (congruent) elevation (i.e., when both the target and vibrator are presented either from the top or from the bottom). The crossmodal congruency effect is calculated as the difference in performance between incongruent and congruent distractor trials for a particular pair of distractor LEDs (i.e., for the two LEDs on a particular cube as shown in Figure 8.1). By now, many studies have shown that visuotactile crossmodal congruency effects are largest when the target and distractor are presented from the *same* azimuthal location (i.e., when the distracting lights are situated by the hand receiving the vibrotactile target) and decline as the visual distractor and vibrotactile target hand are moved further and further away from each other (see Spence, Pavani, Maravita, & Holmes, 2008, for a review).

The magnitude of the crossmodal congruency effect has therefore been taken by many researchers to provide a behavioral index of which locations in visual and tactile space are considered to match. The assumption is that the crossmodal congruency effect should be maximal when the target and distractor are presented from more or less the same location (see also Zopf, Savage, & Williams, 2010). Interestingly, Poliakoff, Ashworth, Lowe, and Spence (2006) have gone on to show that the spatial modulation of the crossmodal congruency effect is substantially present in 65- to 72-year-olds, but is absent in 76- to 92-year-olds, suggesting that aging may compromise the spatial aspects of crossmodal selective attention.

Tracking the Location of Touch on the Body

The multisensory integration required to form such spatial representations with respect to the body is, though, by no means simple. A particular challenge, which we have already mentioned earlier, is the inconsistency in the spatial alignment of tactile stimuli with the other senses (most especially vision) due to on-going changes in limb position. When the posture of our hands changes, the relation of tactile locations to visual locations changes as well, and thus, to integrate tactile and visual space, a remapping between sensory frames of reference is required. Indeed, more generally, crossmodal integration faces a problem with accommodating postural change, as the integration of visual with auditory locations requires a neural mechanism that can take account of movements of the eyes within their orbits (e.g., Avillac, Denève, Olivier, Pouget, & Duhamel, 2005; Pöppel, 1973; Spence, McDonald, & Driver, 2004).

Spence, Pavani, Driver (2004) investigated the consequences of various basic postural manipulations on the crossmodal congruency effect. They showed, for instance, that the magnitude of the crossmodal congruency effect elicited by a particular pair of visual stimuli tends to decrease as the hand receiving the vibrotactile target is moved further away from them. However, the most frequently used manipulation for investigating our ability to remap body-centered locations across changes in postures is to cross participants' hands across the midline (Figure 8.1B). This manipulation changes the spatial correspondence of body sense information to distal locations such that hemispheric correspondence between tactile and visual stimuli is reversed. Under such conditions, Spence and his colleagues found that it is the visual distractors next to the current target hand position that elicit the largest crossmodal congruency effects; this despite the fact that the afferent signals from the vibrotactile targets presented to the crossed hand initially project predominantly to the opposite cerebral hemisphere with respect to the visual distractors. Results such as this suggest that when integrating tactile and visual stimuli, humans link these senses according to an external (rather than an anatomical frame of reference). To achieve this across changes in posture, we have to remap the relations between visual and tactile cues whenever our limbs move.

Such remapping processes may operate very early in neural processing. It has been reported that, if saccades are made immediately following a tactile stimulus applied to a hand crossed over the midline, a proportion of saccades are initially directed toward the visual hemispace where the tactile stimulus would normally be (Groh & Sparks, 1996b). However, if saccadic orienting responses to tactile stimuli are delayed by 600–1,000 ms, then they are directed correctly to the actual location of the stimulus in space, even when the tactile stimulus is in the visual hemifield opposite to that where the hand would normally be. Thus, it seems that an integrative mechanism, one that is sensitive to posture, is needed to make correct gaze-orienting responses to the hands when they are placed in atypical locations (see also Azañón & Soto-Faraco, 2008). Interestingly, it appears that adults are only conscious of such tactile sensations once they have been remapped (Azañón & Soto-Faraco, 2008; Kitazawa, 2002).

These processes of postural remapping have also been isolated physiologically. The same brain areas identified as sites of crossmodal integration (see above) have also been implicated in processes of postural remapping. Neurons that remap sensory correspondences across changes in posture have been reported in the monkey superior colliculus (auditory to visual: Jay & Sparks, 1984; visual to tactile: Groh & Sparks, 1996a, 1996b) and ventral premotor cortex (visual to tactile: Graziano & Gross, 1993; Graziano, Yap, & Gross, 1994). Ventral premotor cortex neurons represent the location of visual and tactile stimuli with respect to body-part-centered coordinates across changes in the position of the limbs (Graziano, Hu, & Gross, 1997). To respond to visual stimuli in body-part-centered coordinates, such neurons have to rely on up-to-date inputs concerning limb position provided by visual and proprioceptive cues (Lloyd, Shore, Calvert, & Spence, 2003). However, as we shall see in the next section, there is evidence that the brain does not, in all circumstances at least, take precise account of proprioceptive cues when locating tactile stimuli in space.

On the Capture of the Location of Tactile Stimuli on the Body by Visual Limbs

In the previous section on haptics, we discussed how vision can exert a dominant effect on the tactile identification and exploration of objects. Such processes of visual dominance also have an influence on our perception of tactile stimuli on the body (see also Kennett, Taylor-Clarke, & Haggard, 2001). According to the MLE account (Ernst & Banks, 2002), under certain circumstances, this is an adaptive process. The relatively greater weighting of the visually derived location of the limb over the proprioceptive location will normally lead to accurate localization of our limbs, due to the visual information having greater spatial reliability. That said, otherwise highly reliable visual information can be misleading and result in striking bodily illusions, such as the "rubber hand" and "mirror" illusions (Botvinick & Cohen, 1998; Ehrsson, Spence, & Passingham, 2004; Holmes, Crozier, & Spence, 2004; Moseley et al., 2008; see Makin, Holmes, & Ehrsson, 2008, for a review), in which the sight of a hand in one location leads people to mislocalize their limb.

Pavani et al. (2000) used the crossmodal congruency task to examine the relative contributions of visual and proprioceptive cues to the localization of tactile stimuli in peripersonal space. They modified Spence and colleagues' (Spence, Pavani, Driver, 2004) visual–tactile crossmodal congruency paradigm by introducing a pair of rubber hands. The participants in Pavani et al.'s study wore a pair of rubber washing-up gloves and held two foam cubes on each of which were mounted two vibrators. The participants could not see their own hands since they were hidden below an opaque screen (see Figure 8.2). The magnitude of the crossmodal congruency effect elicited by the visual distractors *increased* when a pair of rubber arms (actually a pair of stuffed rubber washing-up gloves) were placed in a plausible posture (on top of the occluding screen in front of the participants), apparently "holding" the visual distractors (see also Kanayama, Sato, & Ohira, 2009). In a subsequent experiment, Pavani et al. went on to show that the magnitude of the crossmodal congruency effect was unaffected by the presence of the rubber arms if they were placed in an implausible posture for the

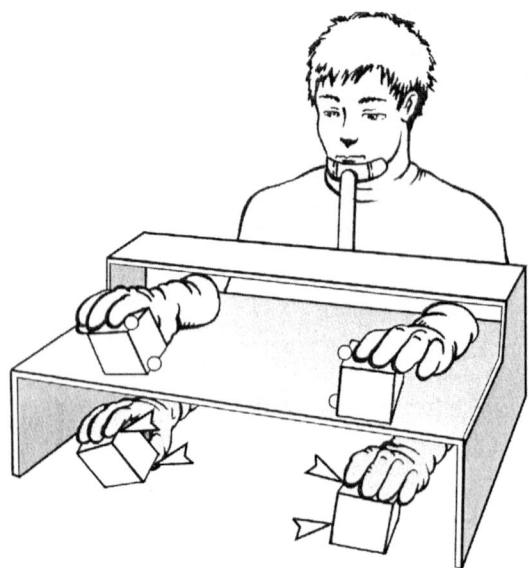

FIGURE 8.2 Schematic view of the experimental setup used in Pavani et al.'s (2000) "rubber hand" experiment, highlighting the location of the vibrotactile stimulators (indicated by the four arrows) on the foam cubes held by the participant below an occluding screen and the visual distractor lights (four open circles on the upper cubes) held by the rubber hands that, when present, were aligned with the participant's own hands. Note that in some conditions (not shown), the rubber arms were placed at 90° with respect to the participant's own arms (i.e., in a posture that the participant could not possibly adopt). Reprinted with permission from "Multi-sensory interactions," by C. Spence, F. Pavani, A. Maravita, and N. P. Holmes, in *Haptic Rendering: Foundations, Algorithms, and Applications* (pp. 21–52) by M. C. Lin & M. A. Otaduy (Eds.), 2008, Wellesley, MA: AK Peters.

participants (i.e., when placed at 90° with respect to the participant's own body).

Pavani et al. (2000) argued that the increased crossmodal congruency effects reported in the plausible rubber hands condition could be attributed to the "apparent" perception of the vibrotactile targets as being close to the distractor lights. In other words, they claimed that *tactile* stimuli were mislocalized toward the apparent visual location of the seen limb (really a stuffed rubber washing-up glove). In fact, the participants in Pavani et al.'s study only experienced the rubber hand illusion (as revealed by their responses to a questionnaire) in those blocks of trials in which the rubber hands were placed in a plausible posture for the participants to have adopted. What is more, the magnitude of this increase in the crossmodal congruency effect in the plausible rubber hands condition was also shown to correlate with subjective reports concerning the vividness of the rubber hand illusion, as indexed by participant's agreement with the statements: "I felt as if the rubber hands were my hands," and "It seemed as if I were feeling the vibration in the location where I saw the rubber hands."

The greater weighting of a visual frame of reference can also be observed in the absence of direct visual spatial cues to the location of the hand. When adults make temporal order judgments (TOJs) concerning tactile stimuli presented first on one hand and then on the other in quick succession, performance is much less accurate in the unusual crossed-hands posture than in the more typical uncrossed-hands posture (Schicke & Röder, 2006; Shore, Spry & Spence, 2002; Yamamoto & Kitazawa, 2001). Since these crossed-hands deficits do not occur in congenitally blind participants (Röder, Rösler, & Spence, 2004), the conclusion that follows is that representations of tactile stimuli rely on a visual frame of reference that relies on the typical layout of the body (see Eimer, 2004).

Thus, multisensory interactions with touch play an important role in framing our spatial representations of our bodies and the space just around them (peripersonal space). Visual stimuli close to the body and information (sometimes illusory) about the layout of the body bias our perceptions of the spatial location of tactile stimuli on the body surface. These multisensory influences on tactile perception play a very important role in enabling us to keeping track of where the body surfaces are when we move our limbs or change posture (e.g., when the arms cross over). Studies with human adults have demonstrated that we achieve these visual–tactile integrations in an effortless way, dynamically updating the way we integrate across sensory reference frames in response to changes in body and limb posture.

DEVELOPMENT OF MULTISENSORY INFLUENCES ON TOUCH

Developing Crossmodal Influences on Haptic Perception

The question of whether infants and young children are able to perceive spatial correspondences between tactile inputs and the other senses is one that has occupied philosophers and psychologists since the time of Locke (1690). The first empirical approaches attempted to discern whether children and, later, infants could recognize an object in one sensory modality which had previously been presented only in another (this is known as the "crossmodal transfer task"). Birch and Lefford (1963), the pioneers of this technique in children, observed that the accuracy of children's crossmodal matching of stimuli between vision and touch increased from the ages of 5 to 11 years of age. However, their conclusion that crossmodal integration of these senses undergoes extended development across childhood has since been heavily criticized. In particular, Bryant and his colleagues (Bryant, 1974; Bryant, Jones, Claxton, & Perkins, 1972; Hulme, Smart, Moran, & Raine, 1983) refuted Birch and Lefford's finding of age-related developments in crossmodal matching, by noting that they could be explained by corresponding developments in unimodal perceptual matching instead.

Bryant et al. (1972) went on to argue that, contrary to Birch and Lefford's (1963) account, the crossmodal integration of touch and vision is, in fact, present in early infancy and backed this up with evidence that 6- to 12-month-old infants are able to identify shapes visually which they had only previously experienced through touch. More recently, Streri and her colleagues confirmed that an ability to perceive commonalities between touch and vision is substantially present at birth, by demonstrating that newborn infants are capable of some visual–tactile crossmodal transfer of shape recognition (see Sann & Streri, 2007; Streri & Gentaz, 2003, 2004; see also Meltzoff & Borton, 1979). Thus, it now seems fairly well established that soon after birth, humans are able to register some kinds of visual–tactile spatial correspondences; exposure to visual stimuli influences newborns' later haptic recognition and vice versa. Importantly, however, it remains to be seen whether the senses interact in determining perceptual recognition. For instance, we do not know whether inputs from vision (or for that matter other senses) about an object influence infants' concurrent haptic perception as it is known to do in adults (see above). However, the observation that young infants' manual behavior varies significantly depending on the particular visual input they are receiving suggests that this is a strong possibility (see von Hofsten, 2004, for a review).

Despite these very early multisensory interactions in haptic perception, a number of recent articles have reported findings which, contrary to the claims of Bryant (e.g., Bryant, 1974), suggest that multisensory integration in haptic perception does indeed continue to develop beyond infancy and well into childhood. For instance, Picard (2007) reports a crossmodal transfer task in which children are asked to match fabric textures presented visually to one of a pair of later-presented tactile stimuli (this is known as a crossmodal delayed matching-to-sample task). Picard observed improvements in this task between 5 and 8 years, which occurred over and above any developments in intrasensory matching abilities. Gori et al. (2008), examining 5- to 10-year-old children's use of MLE in haptic–visual integration found similarly prolonged development. In their study, children were given two multisensory form discrimination tasks (in which participants had visual and haptic inputs concerning the stimuli). These researchers found that the young children's (in this case 5-year-olds') discrimination responses were dominated by one particular sensory modality depending on the task. Five-year-olds' judgments were dominated by haptics in a height discrimination task and by vision in an orientation discrimination task. Older children (8–10 years) and adults, by contrast, integrated optimally according to an MLE model in which the modalities were weighted relative to their task-specific reliabilities. But what developmental processes underlie age-related changes in ability in these tasks?

Gori et al. (2008) proposed that optimal multisensory integration might be delayed this long in development to provide a point of reference for crossmodal comparisons which are vital for recalibrating the senses as the body and limbs grow. Very recently, they have provided additional evidence for such a process of crossmodal calibration. In particular, Gori, Sandini Martolini, and Burr (2010) examined haptic size and orientation discrimination performance in congenitally blind children. Compared with sighted controls (who nevertheless had no vision of the stimuli), the blind children performed comparably at size discrimination, which is weighted toward haptics in typical development, but much worse at orientation discrimination which is typically weighted toward vision instead. Thus, it seems likely that vision is required to calibrate touch, specifically in those tasks at which touch in not particularly reliable (i.e., orientation discrimination). Picard's (2007) crossmodal transfer findings might also be explained by such a process of crossmodal calibration. Remember that Picard found prolonged development of an ability to match fabric textures between visual and tactile presentations. It is possible that touch, which is typically dominant for discriminating fine textures (see Heller, 1989; Spence &

Gallace, 2008), takes some time to calibrate the visual discrimination of texture. Returning then to Berkeley's (1709/1948) suggestion that *"touch educates vision,"* this evidence suggests that it is the most accurate sense that calibrates the other (touch/haptics for size, vision for orientation, and perhaps touch for texture).

The evidence that the senses calibrate each other is clear (Gori et al., 2010). But how convincing is Gori et al.'s (2008) argument that multisensory integration is delayed across childhood to allow calibration to occur? They argue that because the body and limbs continue to grow across childhood and adolescence, recalibration is constantly required, and so integration does not take place until the body has stopped growing substantially (see also King, 2004, for a similar argument in the ferret). It remains unclear, however, how such a process of delay in or inhibition of integration might come about, or indeed whether multisensory integration would adversely affect recalibration. Another possible explanation for this extended period of development of multisensory integration is that suboptimal integration in Gori et al.'s (2008) and Picard's (2007) tasks may instead be explained by working memory limitations which ameliorate gradually over childhood (e.g., Gallace & Spence, 2009, for a review).

Gori et al. (2008) examine the relationship between age and the ability to optimally integrate the senses by weighting the modalities in accordance with their relative precisions within any given situation or task. They show unequivocally that optimal multisensory integration in the context of the tasks they administered improved well into childhood; children's spatial judgments change from being dominated (or "captured") by just one sensory modality to a situation in which they are made with reference to an optimally integrated multisensory representation. However, it is critical to note that Gori et al.'s paradigm involved memory because of the fact that they use a successive (rather than a simultaneous) discrimination task. Picard's (2007) paradigm also involved a memory component, as the participants had to make delayed matching-to-sample judgments between vision and touch. As performance in both of these tasks is constrained by multisensory integration *and* memory, developments in either may be responsible for the age-related differences in performance that they report.

But which explanation is more plausible? Research with human infants indicates that multisensory integration in representations of the body (Bremner, Holmes, & Spence, 2008) and also the enhancement of orienting responses to bimodal relative to unimodal stimuli (a signature of multisensory integration; Neil, Chee-Ruiter, Scheier, Lewkowicz, & Shimojo, 2006) develops during the first year of life. Given that multisensory integration is available in early infancy and working memory undergoes prolonged development throughout childhood, we argue that working memory developments offer a plausible explanation of age-related changes in crossmodal integration in these tasks. Further research, in which memory demands are reduced, will be needed to determine whether optimal integration in multisensory perception really does continue to develop across childhood.

Developing Crossmodal Influences on the Tactile Sense of the Body

We have also only just begun to answer questions concerning whether infants can locate tactile sensations on their bodies. While recognizing and discriminating haptically explored objects, an ability which newborn infants possess (e.g., Sann & Streri, 2007), indicates that some kind of spatial representation of the skin surface is available, it is unclear from this research whether infants are able to form representations of the body as being separate from the external environment. Given young infants' skill with representing external spatial frames of reference (Bremner, Bryant, Mareschal, & Volein, 2007), it is quite plausible that haptic recognition and crossmodal transfer between touch and vision occur with respect to a frame of reference that is unrelated to intrinsic spatial coordinates, or a specific body representation (Bremner, Holmes, et al., 2008). To determine whether infants or children are able to encode tactile stimuli with respect to themselves, we need to consider their orienting responses.

Spatial orienting to tactile stimuli is observable in a range of neonatal reflexes. One example of a spatially specific orienting reflex is observable in newborn crossed extension (Fényes, Gergely, & Tóth, 1960; Zappella & Simopoulos, 1966). Thus, if a newborn infant is touched close to the inguinal canal at the top of the leg, they will flex and extend their other leg (Fényes et al., 1960). Neonatal grasping, another orienting response to tactile stimulation, is present even before birth, appearing as early as 11 weeks in utero (see Tan & Tan, 1999). Moreau, Helfgott, Weinstein, and Milner (1978) have also observed the habituation of neonatal head turning in response to tactile stimulation.

Bremner, Mareschal, Lloyd-Fox, and Spence (2008) recently traced the development of orienting to tactile stimuli in 6.5- and 10-month-old infants, by measuring their spontaneous manual and visual (crossmodal) orienting responses to tactile stimuli presented to the infants' hands when placed in both the uncrossed- and crossed-hands postures. Accurate visual orienting to tactile stimuli increased markedly in both occurrence and speed between these ages, suggesting that an ability to locate tactile stimuli within the visual field develops during the period between 6 and 10 months. Both age groups demonstrated accurate manual orienting responses to tactile stimuli in the uncrossed-hands posture. Interestingly, the 6.5-month-old infants demonstrated a bias to respond manually to the side of the body where the hand would typically rest (i.e., to the left of space for a vibration in the left hand), regardless of the posture (uncrossed or crossed) of the hands. This indicates a reliance on the typical location of the tactile stimulus in an external spatial reference system, suggesting that these younger infants are able to represent tactile locations beyond a simply anatomical frame of reference. Later, at 10 months of age, manual responses were made appropriately irrespective of the posture of the hands, suggesting that they become better at integrating information arriving from proprioception and vision when locating tactile stimuli on the body across changes in posture.

Research with blind participants suggests that the ability to locate tactile stimuli in an external frame of reference may to some extent be dependent upon early visual experience. Röder, Rösler, and Spence (2004) tested sighted, blindfolded sighted, late blind, and congenitally blind adults on a tactile TOJ task which requires participants to decide which hand receives a tactile stimulus first. In this task, poorer discrimination of tactile temporal order in the crossed-hands posture than in a typical uncrossed-hands posture is taken as an indication that participants code tactile stimuli according to an external (rather than an anatomical) frame of reference (Shore et al., 2002; Yamamoto & Kitazawa, 2001). Röder et al. found that congenitally blind participants showed a significant advantage over sighted and late blind participants in the crossed-hands posture. The fact that the late blind participants (one of whom had been blind for more than 40 years) showed similar crossed-hands impairments to those of the sighted participants suggests that early visual experience is necessary for the typical development of tactile spatial perception (Eimer, 2004).

It is interesting to speculate about when exactly visual experience is required for typical development of tactile spatial perception. Bremner, Mareschal, et al.'s (2008) finding that 6.5-month-old infants use an external frame of reference for locating tactile stimuli suggests that visual input might play a role in reshaping tactile spatial representations as early as the first year of life. However, using a tactile TOJ task, Pagel, Heed, and Röder (2009) have recently demonstrated that improvements in the ability to detect the temporal sequence of tactile stimuli presented across the hands in the uncrossed posture between 5 and 10 years of age were not matched by improvements in the crossed-hands posture. Pagel et al. thus argue that the development of use of an external frame of reference for locating tactile stimuli continues through early childhood. It is our view that developments in the perception of tactile location on the body are likely happening at both of these ages. Only further research will determine which period of development is the most crucial for developing a sense of the tactile body.

CONCLUSIONS

In conclusion, our awareness of the objects in the world around us is determined by a constant interplay between haptics, vision, and the other senses (e.g., audition, olfaction, etc.), and as such, multisensory integration (or cue combination) is now (rightly) considered the norm, rather than the exception in perception research. A large body of cognitive neuroscience research currently supports the view that our tactile/haptic perception of both the structural and surface properties of objects is profoundly influenced by what we see, when touching, interacting with, and/or evaluating them. What we smell and hear can also play a role. One outstanding question in this area that has yet to receive a satisfactory answer is whether there are any substantive individual differences (perhaps attributable to differences in practice or expertise) in the way in which people integrate haptic, visual, auditory, and/or olfactory information (see Spence, 2007, for a review). Are there, for example, individual differences in the extent to which vision dominates over tactile/haptic perception? Only further research will tell. Though see Saito, Okada, Honda, Yonekura, and Sadato (2007), for some interesting recent research in this area conducted on mah-jong players.

In 1690, John Locke wrote of a question posed to him by William Molyneux. Molyneux asked whether a blind man who had learned to distinguish objects through touch would then be able to recognize those objects if sight was restored to him. Despite Locke's assured answer that this was not possible without the man first learning the relationships between the senses, we now have quite a clear affirmative answer to Molyneux's query. Within days of birth, infants are able to encode information in one sense (e.g., touch) and recognize it in another (e.g., vision; e.g., Sann & Streri, 2007). Nonetheless, significant developments are evident in how infants and children integrate touch with vision to maximize the efficiency of their multisensory perceptual estimates and also how they represent touch stimuli with respect to their intrinsic spatial frame of reference—their body (Bremner,

TABLE 8.1 Developmental changes in multisensory influences on tactile perception across infancy and early childhood. Hypothetical developmental drivers of emerging perceptual abilities are indicated in the right-hand column

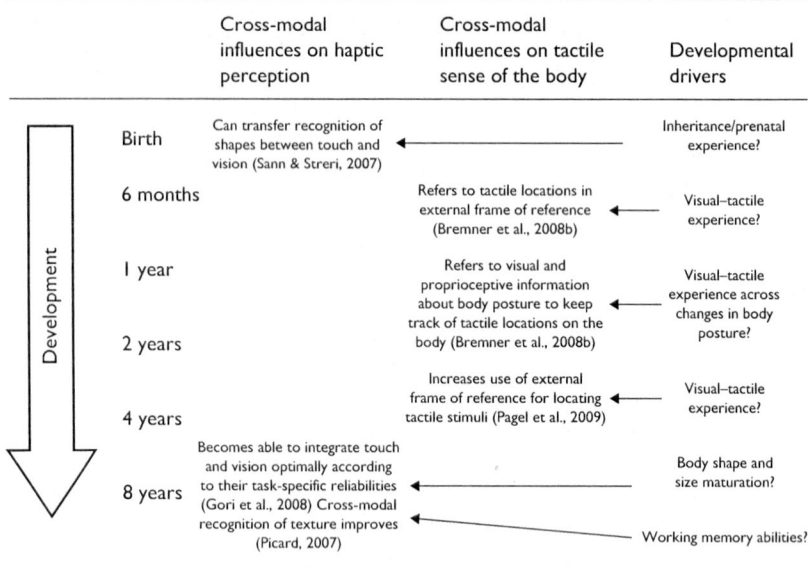

Mareschal, et al., 2008; Pagel et al., 2009, see Table 8.1). Future research will hopefully shed light on the causal processes of change which underlie developments in how we use touch in combination with our other senses (and we are not just talking about vision).

REFERENCES

Avillac, M., Denève, S., Olivier, E., Pouget, A., & Duhamel, J. R. (2005). Reference frames for representing visual and tactile locations in parietal cortex. *Nature Neuroscience*, 8, 941–949.

Azañón, E., & Soto-Faraco, S. (2008). Changing reference frames during the encoding of tactile events. *Current Biology*, 18, 1044–1049.

Berkeley, G. (1948). An essay toward a new theory of vision (originally published in 1709). In W. Dennis (Ed.), *Readings in the history of psychology* (pp. 69–80). East Norwalk, CT: Appleton-Century-Crofts.

Birch, H. G., & Lefford, A. (1963). Intersensory development in children. *Monographs of the Society for Research in Child Development*, 28, 1–37, 39–43, 45–48.

Botvinick, M., & Cohen, J. (1998). Rubber hands 'feel' touch that eyes see. *Nature*, 391, 756.

Bremner, A. J., Bryant, P. E., Mareschal, D., & Volein, Á. (2007). Recognition of complex object-centred spatial configurations in early infancy. *Visual Cognition, 15,* 896–926.
Bremner, A. J., Holmes, N. P., & Spence, C. (2008). Infants lost in (peripersonal) space? *Trends in Cognitive Sciences, 12,* 298–305.
Bremner, A. J., Mareschal, D., Lloyd-Fox, S., & Spence, C. (2008). Spatial localization of touch in the first year of life: Early influence of a visual code and the development of remapping across changes in limb position. *Journal of Experimental Psychology: General, 137,* 149–162.
Bryant, P. E., Jones, P., Claxton, V., & Perkins, G. H. (1972). Recognition of shapes across modalities by infants. *Nature, 240,* 303–304.
Calvert, G. A., Spence, C., & Stein, B. E. (Eds.). (2004). *The handbook of multisensory processes.* Cambridge, MA: MIT Press.
Demattè, M. L., Sanabria, D., Sugarman, R., & Spence, C. (2006). Cross-modal interactions between olfaction and touch. *Chemical Senses, 31,* 291–300.
Ehrsson, H. H., Spence, C., & Passingham, R. E. (2004). That's my hand! Activity in premotor cortex reflects feeling of ownership of a limb. *Science, 305,* 875–877.
Eimer, M. (2004). Multisensory integration: How visual experience shapes spatial perception. *Current Biology, 14,* R115–R117.
Ernst, M. O. (2006). A Bayesian view on multimodal cue integration. In G. Knoblich, I. M. Thornton, M. Grosjean, & M. Shiffrar (Eds.), *Human body perception from the inside out* (pp. 105–131). Oxford: Oxford University Press.
Ernst, M. O., & Banks, M. S. (2002). Humans integrate visual and haptic information in a statistically optimal fashion. *Nature, 415,* 429–433.
Ernst, M. O., & Bülthoff, H. H. (2004). Merging the senses into a robust percept. *Trends in Cognitive Sciences, 8,* 162–169.
Fényes, I., Gergely, C., & Tóth, S. (1960). Clinical and electromyographic studies of "spinal reflexes" in premature and full-term infants. *Journal of Neurology, Neurosurgery & Psychiatry, 23,* 63–68.
Gallace, A., & Spence, C. (2009). The cognitive limitations and neural correlates of tactile memory. *Psychological Bulletin, 135,* 380–406.
Gepshtein, S., Burge, J., Ernst, M. O., & Banks, M. S. (2005). The combination of vision and touch depends on spatial proximity *Journal of Vision, 5,* 1013–1023.
Gibson, J. J. (1943). Adaptation, after-effect and contrast in the perception of curved lines. *Journal of Experimental Psychology, 16,* 1–31.
Gori, M., Del Viva, M., Sandini, G., & Burr, D. C. (2008). Young children do not integrate visual and haptic information. *Current Biology, 18,* 694–698.
Gori, M., Sandini, G., Martinoli, C., & Burr, D. (2010). Poor haptic orientation discrimination in nonsighted children may reflect disruption of cross-sensory calibration. *Current Biology, 20,* 223–225.
Graziano, M. S. A., & Gross, C. G. (1993). A bimodal map of space: Somatosensory receptive fields in the macaque putamen with corresponding visual receptive fields. *Experimental Brain Research, 97,* 96–109.
Graziano, M. S. A., Gross, C. G., Taylor, C. S. R., & Moore, T. (2004). A system of multimodal areas in the primate brain. In C. Spence & J. Driver (Eds.), *Crossmodal space and crossmodal attention* (pp. 51–67). Oxford: Oxford University Press.
Graziano, M. S. A., Hu, X. T., & Gross, C. G. (1997). Visuospatial properties of ventral premotor cortex. *Journal of Neurophysiology, 77,* 2268–2292.

Graziano, M. S. A., Yap, G. S., & Gross, C. G. (1994). Coding of visual space by premotor neurons. *Science, 266*, 1054–1057.

Groh, J. M., & Sparks, D. L. (1996a). Saccades to somatosensory targets: 2. Motor convergence in primate superior colliculus. *Journal of Neurophysiology, 75*, 428–438.

Groh, J. M., & Sparks, D. L. (1996b). Saccades to somatosensory targets: 3. Eye-position dependent somatosensory activity in primate superior colliculus. *Journal of Neurophysiology, 75*, 439–453.

Guest, S., Catmur, C., Lloyd, D., & Spence, C. (2002). Audiotactile interactions in roughness perception. *Experimental Brain Research, 146*, 161–171.

Guest, S., & Spence, C. (2003a). Tactile dominance in speeded discrimination of pilled fabric samples. *Experimental Brain Research, 150*, 201–207.

Guest. S., & Spence, C. (2003b). What role does multisensory integration play in the visuotactile perception of texture? *International Journal of Psychophysiology, 50*, 63–80.

Helbig, H. B., & Ernst, M. O. (2007a). Knowledge about a common source can promote visual-haptic integration. *Perception, 36*, 1523–1533.

Helbig, H. B., & Ernst, M. O. (2007b). Optimal integration of shape information from vision and touch. *Experimental Brain Research, 179*, 595–606.

Helbig, H. B., & Ernst, M. O. (2008). Visual-haptic cue weighting is independent of modality-specific attention. *Journal of Vision, 8*(10):21, 1–16.

Heller, M. A. (1989). Texture perception in sighted and blind observers. *Perception & Psychophysics, 45*, 49–54.

Hillis, J. M., Ernst, M. O., Banks, M. S., & Landy, M. S. (2002). Combining sensory information: Mandatory fusion within, but not between, senses. *Science, 298*, 1627–1630.

Holmes, N., Crozier, G., & Spence, C. (2004). When mirrors lie: "Visual capture" of arm position impairs reaching performance. *Cognitive, Affective, & Behavioral Neuroscience, 4*, 193–200.

Hulme, C., Smart, A., Moran, G., & Raine, A. (1983). Visual, kinaesthetic and cross-modal development relationships to motor skill development. *Perception, 12*, 477–483.

Jay, M. F., & Sparks, D. L. (1984). Auditory receptive fields in primate superior colliculus shift with changes in eye position. *Nature, 309*, 345–347.

Jousmäki, V., & Hari, R. (1998). Parchment-skin illusion: Sound-biased touch. *Current Biology, 8*, 869–872.

Kanayama, N., Sato, A., & Ohira, H. (2009). The role of gamma band oscillations and synchrony on rubber hand illusion and crossmodal integration. *Brain and Cognition, 69*, 19–29.

Kennett, S., Taylor-Clarke, M., & Haggard, P. (2001). Noninformative vision improves the spatial resolution of touch in humans. *Current Biology, 11*, 1188–1191.

King, A. (2004). Development of multisensory spatial integration. In C. Spence & J. Driver (Eds.), *Crossmodal space and crossmodal attention* (pp. 1–24). Oxford: Oxford University Press.

Kitazawa, S. (2002). Where conscious sensation takes place. *Consciousness and Cognition, 11*, 475–477.

Laird, D. A. (1932). How the consumer estimates quality by subconscious sensory impressions: With special reference to the role of smell. *Journal of Applied Psychology, 16*, 241–246.

Lederman, S. J., & Klatzky, R. L. (2004). Multisensory texture perception. In G. A. Calvert, C. Spence, & B. E. Stein (Eds.), *The handbook of multisensory processes* (pp. 107–122). Cambridge, MA: MIT Press.
Lederman, S. J., & Klatzky, R. L. (2009). Haptic perception: A tutorial. *Attention, Perception, & Psychophysics, 71*, 1439–1459.
Lloyd, D. M., Shore, D. I., Spence, C., & Calvert, G. A. (2003). Multisensory representation of limb position in human premotor cortex. *Nature Neuroscience, 6*, 17–18.
Locke, J. (1690). *An essay concerning human understanding.* London: Edward Mory.
Makin, T. R., Holmes, N. P., & Ehrsson, H. H. (2008). On the other hand: Dummy hands and peripersonal space. *Behavioural Brain Research, 191*, 1–10.
Makin, T. R., Holmes, N. P., & Zohary, E. (2007). Is that my hand? Multisensory representation of peripersonal space in human intraparietal sulcus. *Journal of Neuroscience, 24*, 731–740.
Maravita, A., Spence, C., & Driver, J. (2003). Multisensory integration and the body schema: Close to hand and within reach. *Current Biology, 13*, R531–R539.
Meltzoff, A. N., & Borton, R. W. (1979). Intermodal matching by human neonates. *Nature, 282*, 403–404.
Miller, E. A. (1972). Interaction of vision and touch in conflict and nonconflict form perception tasks. *Journal of Experimental Psychology, 96*, 114–123.
Moreau, T., Helfgott, E., Weinstein, P., & Milner, P. (1978). Lateral differences in habituation of ipsilateral head-turning to repeated tactile stimulation in the human newborn. *Perceptual and Motor Skills, 46*, 427–436.
Morgan, M. L., DeAngelis, G. C., & Angelaki, D. E. (2008). Multisensory integration in macaque visual cortex depends on cue reliability. *Neuron, 59*, 662–673.
Moseley, G. L., Olthof, N., Venema, A., Don, S., Wijers, M., Gallace, A., & Spence, C. (2008). Psychologically induced cooling of a specific body part caused by the illusory ownership of an artificial counterpart. *Proceedings of the National Academy of Sciences USA, 105*, 13168–13172.
Neil, P. A., Chee-Ruiter, C., Scheier, C., Lewkowicz, D. J., & Shimojo, S. (2006). Development of multisensory spatial integration and perception in humans. *Developmental Science, 9*, 454–464.
Pagel, B., Heed, T., & Röder, B. (2009). Change of reference frame for tactile localization during child development. *Developmental Science, 12*, 929–937.
Pavani, F., Spence, C., & Driver, J. (2000). Visual capture of touch: Out-of-the-body experiences with rubber gloves. *Psychological Science, 11*, 353–359.
Picard, D. (2007). Tactual, visual, and cross-modal transfer of texture in 5- and 8-year-old children. *Perception, 36*, 722–736.
Poliakoff, E., Ashworth, S., Lowe, C., & Spence, C. (2006). Vision and touch in ageing: Crossmodal selective attention and visuotactile spatial interactions. *Neuropsychologia, 44*, 507–517.
Pöppel, E. (1973). Comments on "Visual system's view of acoustic space." *Nature, 243*, 231.
Posner, M. I., Nissen, M. J., & Klein, R. M. (1976). Visual dominance: An information-processing account of its origins and significance. *Psychological Review, 83*, 157–171.
Rizzolatti, G., Fadiga, L., Fogassi, L., & Gallese, V. (1997). The space around us. *Science, 277*, 190–191.
Rock, I., & Harris, C. S. (1967, 17 May). Vision and touch. *Scientific American, 216*, 96–104.

Rock, I., & Victor, J. (1964). Vision and touch: An experimentally created conflict between the two senses. *Science, 143,* 594–596.

Röder, B., Rösler, F., & Spence, C. (2004). Early vision impairs tactile perception in the blind. *Current Biology, 14,* 121–124.

Saito, D. N., Okada, T., Honda, M., Yonekura, Y., & Sadato, N. (2007). Practice makes perfect: The neural substrates of tactile discrimination by Mah-Jong experts include the primary visual cortex. *BMC Neuroscience, 7:79.*

Sann, C., & Streri, A. (2007). Perception of object shape and texture in human newborns: Evidence from cross-modal transfer tasks. *Developmental Science, 10,* 399–410.

Schicke, T., & Röder, B. (2006). Spatial remapping of touch: Confusion of perceived stimulus order across hand and foot. *Proceedings of the National Academy of Sciences USA, 103,* 11808–11813.

Schifferstein, H. N. J., & Spence, C. (2008). Multisensory product experience. In H. N. J. Schifferstein & P. Hekkert (Eds.), *Product experience* (pp. 133–161). Amsterdam, The Netherlands: Elsevier.

Shore, D. I., Spry, E., & Spence, C. (2002). Confusing the mind by crossing the hands. *Cognitive Brain Research, 14,* 153–163.

Spence, C. (2007). Making sense of touch: A multisensory approach to the perception of objects. In E. Pye (Ed.), *The power of touch: Handling objects in museums and heritage contexts* (pp. 45–61). Walnut Creek, CA: Left Coast Press.

Spence, C., & Gallace, A. (2007). Recent developments in the study of tactile attention. *Canadian Journal of Experimental Psychology, 61,* 196–207.

Spence, C., & Gallace, A. (2008). Making sense of touch. In H. Chatterjee (Ed.), *Touch in museums: Policy and practice in object handling* (pp. 21–40). Oxford, UK: Berg Publications.

Spence, C., McDonald, J., & Driver, J. (2004). Exogenous spatial cuing studies of human crossmodal attention and multisensory integration. In C. Spence & J. Driver (Eds.), *Crossmodal space and crossmodal attention* (pp. 277–320). Oxford, UK: Oxford University Press.

Spence, C., Pavani, F., & Driver, J. (2004). Spatial constraints on visual-tactile crossmodal distractor congruency effects. *Cognitive, Affective, & Behavioral Neuroscience, 4,* 148–169.

Spence, C., Pavani, F., Maravita, A., & Holmes, N. (2004). Multisensory contributions to the 3-D representation of visuotactile peripersonal space in humans: Evidence from the crossmodal congruency task. *Journal of Physiology (Paris), 98,* 171–189.

Spence, C., Pavani, F., Maravita, A., & Holmes, N. P. (2008). Multi-sensory interactions. In M. C. Lin & M. A. Otaduy (Eds.), *Haptic rendering: Foundations, algorithms, and applications* (pp. 21–52). Wellesley, MA: AK Peters.

Spence, C., Shore, D. I., & Klein, R. M. (2001). Multisensory prior entry. *Journal of Experimental Psychology: General, 130,* 799–832.

Spence, C., & Zampini, M. (2006). Auditory contributions to multisensory product perception. *Acta Acustica united with Acustica, 92,* 1009–1025.

Spence, C., & Zampini, M. (2007). Affective design: Modulating the pleasantness and forcefulness of aerosol sprays by manipulating aerosol spraying sounds. *CoDesign, 3* (Suppl. 1), 109–123.

Streri, A., & Gentaz, E. (2003). Cross-modal recognition of shape from hand to eyes and handedness in human newborns. *Somatosensory & Motor Research, 20,* 13–18.

Streri, A., & Gentaz, E. (2004). Cross-modal recognition of shape from hand to eyes and handedness in human newborns. *Neuropsychologia, 42,* 1365–1369.

Tan, U., & Tan, M. (1999). Incidences of asymmetries for the palmar grasp reflex in neonates and hand preference in adults. *Neuroreport, 10,* 3253–3256.

Van Beers, R. J., Wolpert, D. M., & Haggard, P. (2002). When feeling is more important than seeing in sensorimotor adaptation. *Current Biology, 12,* 834–837.

von Hofsten, C. (2004). An action perspective on motor development. *Trends in Cognitive Sciences, 8,* 266–272.

Welch, R. B., & Warren, D. H. (1980). Immediate perceptual response to intersensory discrepancy. *Psychological Bulletin, 3,* 638–667.

Welch, R. B., & Warren, D. H. (1986). Intersensory interactions. In K. R. Boff, L. Kaufman, & J. P. Thomas (Eds.), *Handbook of perception and performance: Vol. 1. Sensory processes and perception* (pp. 25–1–25–36). New York: Wiley.

Wozny, D. R., Beierholm, U. R., & Shams, L. (2008). Human trimodal perception follows optimal statistical inference. *Journal of Vision, 8,* 1–11.

Yamamoto, S., & Kitazawa, S. (2001). Reversal of subjective temporal order due to arm crossing. *Nature Neuroscience, 4,* 759–765.

Zampini, M., Guest, S., & Spence, C. (2003). The role of auditory cues in modulating the perception of electric toothbrushes. *Journal of Dental Research, 82,* 929–932.

Zappella, M., & Simopoulos, A. (1966). The crossed-extension reflex in the newborn. *Annales Paediatriae Fenniae, 12,* 30–33.

Zopf, R., Savage, G., & Williams, M. A. (2010). Crossmodal congruency measures of lateral distance effects on the rubber hand illusion. *Neuropsychologia, 48,* 713–725.

III

Measurement of Touch

9

Measurement of Tactile Response and Tactile Perception

CATANA BROWN, DIANE L. FILION, AND SANDRA J. WEISS

Response to touch is highly individualized. The same tactile input may be barely noticed by one, perceived as pleasurable by another, and noxious and intolerable to someone else. For example, a wool sweater feels cozy and warm to some and scratchy and itchy to others. The ubiquitous nature of touch means that people are constantly responding and adjusting to a somatosensory experience although this response is often outside of awareness. Therefore, most individuals are unlikely to characterize their own touch response because it is not part of the popular vernacular. Consequently, the measurement of touch response requires methods that can capture both the perceived and this frequently unrecognized tactile experience. The two most common and highly distinct methods of measuring response to touch are behavioral measures and physiological approaches. This chapter will review existing measures, describe their methods and psychometric properties, and consider future areas of development for improved measurement of response to touch.

BEHAVIORAL MEASURES OF TOUCH

Behavioral measures are made up of multiple items or coding categories that describe an individual's response to different types of tactile experience. Some behavioral measures of response to touch collect data using a survey or questionnaire method obtaining either a self or informant report of either an individual's attitudes toward being touched or behavioral reactions to touch. Other measures use observation of an individual's actual response to tactile stimuli that are administered by a researcher or clinician. Responses to these specific stimuli are then recorded using a structured coding system. These two types of behavioral measure can be further divided into (1) those that focus exclusively on touch and (2) global measures of sensory processing that include touch scales or tests.

Specific Touch Measures

Measures that focus specifically on response to touch are generally oriented toward assessing (1) receptivity to interpersonal touch, (2) tactile perception, and/or (3) tactile defensiveness in response to tactile stimuli. Receptivity to touch reflects an individual's appraisal of his/her own cognitive and emotional responses to being touched or touching others. Assessments of receptivity to touch are often used to understand how different responses to touch may influence health or psychosocial outcomes (Jones & Brow, 1996; Weiss & Wilson, 2006; Wilhelm, Kochar, Roth, & Gross, 2001). Tactile perception includes responses associated with discrimination of the location and intensity of tactile sensations as well as recognition of shape, texture, or form through touch. Measures of tactile perception are commonly used to identify tactile responses associated with neurological impairment or injury (Brown, Lewis, McCarthy, Doyle, & Hurvitz, 2010; Carey, Oke, & Matyas, 1997; Soler et al., 2010). Tactile defensiveness is an aversive reaction or hypersensitivity to tactile stimuli that most individuals would perceive as benign (Miller & Lane, 2000). Measures of tactile defensiveness are frequently used to assess children with disabilities such as attention-deficit hyperactivity disorder (ADHD; Broring, Rommelse, Sergeant, & Scherder, 2008), autism (Baranek, Boyd, Poe, David, & Watson, 2007), and developmental disabilities (Baranek & Berkson, 1994; Baranek et al., 2002) though they have also been used to characterize typically developing children (Goldsmith, Van Hulle, Arneson, Schreiber, & Gernsbacher, 2006). Table 9.1 provides a general overview of measures that include a component assessing behavioral response to touch.

Touch Inventory for Preschoolers. The Touch Inventory for Preschoolers (TIP; Royeen, 1987) includes 46 items of responses to daily life situations that indicate tactile defensiveness (e.g., do tags in shirts bother the child and does it bother the child if his/her hands are dirty?). A parent or teacher that knows the child well typically completes the measure based on behaviors observed over the last 2 weeks. The TIP uses a

TABLE 9.1 Structured measures of response to touch

Measure	Dimensions	Method	Age for Use
Physical Contact Assessment (Weiss et al., 2000)	Overall receptivity to touch Felt security with touch	Self-report questionnaire	Adolescents/adults
Social Touch Questionnaire (Wilhelm et al., 2001)	Attitudes toward touch	Self-report questionnaire	Adolescents/adults
Tactile Somatosensory Dysfunction Checklist (Ghanizadeh, 2008)	Hypersensitivity to touch Hyposensitivity to touch Tactile perception/discrimination	Parent questionnaire	Children
Tactile Vulnerability Assessment (Weiss & Wilson, 2006)	Physiologic reactivity Behavioral reactivity Tolerance for stimulating touch	Administration of touch protocol Behavioral coding Physiologic monitoring	Infants
TACTYPE (Deethardt & Hines, 1983)	Attitudes toward touch	Self-report questionnaire	Adolescents/adults
Touch Avoidance Measure (Andersen & Leibowitz, 1982)	Avoidance of Touch	Self-report questionnaire	Adolescents/adults
Touch Inventory for Preschoolers (Royeen, 1987)	Tactile defensiveness	Parent questionnaire	2–5 years of age
Touch Inventory for Elementary-School-Aged Children (Royeen & Fortune, 1990)	Tactile defensiveness	Parent questionnaire	6–12 years of age
Touch Test (Fromme et al., 1989)	Comfort with touch	Self-report questionnaire	Adolescents/adults

1- to 5-point scale from "never" to "always." A higher score indicates greater levels of tactile defensiveness. The measure appears to have good internal consistency; however, there has been minimal psychometric work to determine overall reliability and validity. Although no norms are available, the author suggests that a score of 104 or greater (one standard deviation above the mean in the pilot study sample) may indicate behaviors associated with tactile defensiveness.

In a study that used the TIP to classify children with ADHD as being either tactually defensive or not, children with tactile defensiveness had a stronger response to an electrical stimuli of the median nerve (measured using somatosensory evoked potentials) supporting the discriminant validity of the TIP (Parush, Sohmer, Steinberg, & Kaitz, 2007). This study also provides preliminary physiological support for the construct of tactile defensiveness.

Touch Inventory for Elementary-School-Aged Children. The Touch Inventory for Elementary-School-Aged Children (TIE) is a 26-item measure designed for use with children between ages 6 and 12 (Royeen & Fortune, 1990). The child acts as the respondent to questions such as "Does it bother you to have your hair combed by others?" The three responses of "no," "a little," or "a lot" are scored using a three-point scale from 1 to 3. A single total score is calculated by summing the points for each of the 26 items. This score reflects the child's degree of aversion in response to touch. The measure and normative data based on 415 children are available in Royeen and Fortune (1990). Royeen and Fortune indicate that the measure is appropriate for use with children who have significant communication or learning disabilities but should not be used with children who have physical disabilities, such as cerebral palsy, that may affect their tactile discrimination.

A study of test–retest reliability found moderate agreement when the TIE was administered twice, 1 week apart (Bennett & Peterson, 1995). The same study had mothers complete the TIE along with the child and found that the correlation between the two responses was weak, with mothers consistently scoring lower than the child. Parush, Doryon, and Katz (2006) also found a weak correlation between child and parent report and recommended that the child be considered as the preferred respondent. Another study found that the TIE was stable in assessing levels of tactile defensiveness in American and European cultures (Royeen & Mu, 2003). In a study of gender differences in ADHD, the TIE indicated higher levels of tactile defensiveness for females (Broring et al., 2008). Siblings without ADHD did not have higher levels of tactile defensiveness. This study provides some evidence for discriminant validity of the TIE.

Tactile Somatosensory Dysfunction Checklist. Ghanizadeh (2008) developed the Tactile Somatosensory Dysfunction Checklist specifically for a study examining sensory dysfunction in children with ADHD. This checklist assesses three components of the tactile response: (1) hypersensitivity to touch (tactile defensiveness), (2) hyposensitivity to touch, and (3) poor tactile perception and discrimination. The measure includes 16 items on the hypersensitivity subscale (e.g., doesn't like to be kissed by others, distressed when his/her face is washed), 8 items on the hyposensitivity subscale (e.g., may not be aware that his/her face or hands are dirty, enjoys messy play with things such as soil or glue), and 4 items on the poor tactile perception and discrimination subscale (e.g., has trouble doing fine motor tasks). Each item is rated on a four-point scale from 0 (never) to 3 (always).

Preliminary examination of the measure's psychometric properties has occurred. Psychiatrists and psychologists with content expertise examined the face validity of the measure and items were revised based on their feedback. Internal consistency for each of the subscales using Cronbach's alpha coefficients suggested reasonable reliability with values ranging from 0.75 to 0.78. The study also indicated that the measure distinguished children with comorbid ADHD and oppositional defiant disorder, as these children had greater hypersensitivity to touch. Unlike the study with the TIE (Broring et al., 2008), Ghanizadeh did not find gender differences in hypersensitivity (tactile defensiveness).

Touch Test. The purpose of this questionnaire is to measure an individual's degree of comfort with touch (Fromme et al., 1989). It has 12 items that ask for an evaluation of how comfortable the person is with a specific touch behavior on a five-point scale from very uncomfortable to very comfortable. For instance, items ask about comfort with kissing a loved one in a shopping mall or being touched on the hand, arm, or shoulder by a stranger. The measure yields a total score for overall comfort with touch. Predictive validity was established through comparing scores on the Touch Test with individual willingness to participate in situations involving touch. Authors reported a test–retest reliability of $r = 0.73$.

TACTYPE. Deethardt and Hines (1983) developed a brief questionnaire to assess general attitudes toward touch. Their measure has 15 items on a five-point scale from strongly agree to strongly disagree. Items examine preferences in situations such as wanting to be touched by a friend in times of distress or unhappiness and wanting to be touched by a loved one as a demonstration of her love. Factor analysis indicated that items fell into three dimensions: (1) touch involving members of the opposite sex with whom one was close or intimate, (2) touch involving an opposite sex acquaintance, and (3) touch involving a same-sex acquaintance. However, only reliability for the total measure has been established, with an alpha of 0.87.

Touch Avoidance Measure. The Touch Avoidance Measure (TAM; Andersen & Leibowitz, 1978) provides a total score for an individual's predisposition to avoid touch as well as two separate scores for same-sex (TAM1) and opposite-sex (TAM2) interactions. These two subscales were supported by factor analysis and have internal reliabilities of 0.82 and 0.88. The original alpha for internal consistency of the total scale was 0.81. There are 18 items in the measure, each on a five-point scale from strongly agree to strongly disagree. Examples of items are "I like it when members of the opposite sex touch me" and "I find it difficult to be touched by a member of my own sex."

Guerrero and Andersen (1991) supported the validity of this self-report measure by demonstrating its relationship to actual observations of touch. The measure has also been correlated with logs of touch behavior, but only for women (Jones & Brown, 1996). Jones and Brown found no relationship between tactile attitudes and tactile behavior for men. The TAM has also been shown to predict the degree of distance people maintain between themselves and others (Andersen & Sull, 1985) as well as their response to being touched in a lab experiment (Sorensen & Beatty, 1988). Studies indicate that scores on the Touch Test, TACTYPE, and TAM are significantly correlated with one another (Jones & Brown, 1996).

The Physical Contact Assessment. This self-report measure of response to touch provides a profile of an individual's receptivity to interpersonal touch and felt security with the touch they have experienced (Weiss, 2000). It has three scales which are each scored separately because of the different responses they measure. The first scale includes 10 items on four-point scales that assess general responses to touch, with higher scores indicating greater receptivity to touch. Examples of items include "I appreciate a hug when I need comforting" and "I don't like it when people touch me if they are not very close family or friends." The other scales each have six items that assess the person's responses to the touch they received in the family of origin (second section) and in their current relationships (third section). Higher scores in the second and third scales reflect greater feelings of emotional security regarding the touch they received as children or that they experience in their current lives.

Internal reliability of the three scales has ranged from 0.83 to 0.89 (Weiss & Goebel, 2003; Weiss & Wilson, 2006; Weiss, Wilson, Hertenstein, & Campos, 2000). Relationships among the scales have also been found: felt security regarding the touch received in one's family of origin is associated with general attitudes toward touch (Weiss & Goebel, 2003) and attitudes toward touch are associated with felt security in current tactile relationships (Weiss et al., 2000). Validity has been supported through findings that felt security regarding touch in both past and current relationships predicts the frequency and quality of the actual touch used by parents with their infants (Weiss & Goebel, 2003). In addition, mothers who reported themselves as less comfortable with being touched were significantly more likely to have neonates who were physiologically and behaviorally more hypersensitive and aversive to touch at birth (Weiss & Wilson, 2006). This latter finding supports discriminant validity and suggests a potential inherited transmission of aversion or reactivity to touch.

Social Touch Questionnaire. The Social Touch Questionnaire (STQ) was designed to measure a broad sample of affects and attitudes regarding social touch (Wilhelm, Kochar, Roth, & Gross, 2001). It includes 20 statements on five-point scales from "not at all characteristic" of the person's response to touch to "extremely characteristic or true." Sample items are "It annoys me when someone touches me unexpectedly" and "I would rather avoid shaking hands with strangers." The questionnaire has only been tested in a sample of women where its internal consistency was 0.89. The total scale score significantly discriminated between women who were socially anxious versus those who were not. However, scores on the scale did not predict women's physiological responses to having their wrist held for 2 minutes by a male researcher.

Global Sensory or Neuropsychological Measures That Include Touch Components

A number of measures have been developed to assess responses across a variety of sensory or neuropsychological modalities. Each measure has a component addressing response to touch. Like the specific measures of touch, these global measures require either self-report or other report regarding how one responds to sensory experiences or evaluate an individual's actual response to tactile stimuli that are presented in a standardized way (see Table 9.2).

TABLE 9.2 Global measures of sensory response with a touch subscale or component

Measure	Tactile Dimension(s)	Method	Age for Use
Sensory Integration and Praxis Tests (Ayres, 1989)	Tactile discrimination	Administration of tactile stimuli Observation of response	4- to 8-year old Children
Sensory Over-Responsivity Assessment (Schoen et al., 2008)	Sensitivity to tactile stimuli	Administration of tactile stimuli Observation of response	Children and adults
Sensory Over-Responsivity Inventory (Schoen et al., 2008)	Sensitivity to tactile stimuli	Self or other questionnaire	Children and adults
Sensory Processing Measure School (Miller-Kuhaneck et al., 2005) Home (Parham & Ecker, 2005)	Tactile processing difficulties	Teacher questionnaire Parent/caregiver questionnaire	Elementary school Children
Sensory Profile Infant/Toddler (Dunn, 2002) Children (Dunn, 1999) Adolescent/Adult (Brown & Dunn, 2002)	Low registration of touch Touch (sensation) seeking behavior Tactile sensitivity Avoidance of touch	Self or other questionnaire	Infants/toddlers Children Adolescents/adults
Test of Sensory Functions (DeGangi & Greenspan, 1989)	Reactivity to touch	Administration of tactile stimuli Observation of response	Infants/toddlers
Halstead-Reitan Neurological Test Battery (Reitan & Wolfson, 1993)	Tactile discrimination Tactile form recognition Tactile neglect	Administration of tactile stimuli Observation of response	Children and adults
Luria–Nebraska Neuropsychological Battery (Golden, Purisch, & Hammeke, 1980)	Tactile discrimination Tactile localization Tactile form recognition Tactile sensitivity	Administration of tactile stimuli Observation of response	Children and adults

Sensory Processing Measure. Designed for elementary school children, the Sensory Processing Measure assesses the impact of sensory processing difficulties in the school (Miller-Kuhaneck, Henry, & Glennon, 2005) and home environment (Parham & Ecker, 2005). The home environment scale was formerly known as the Evaluation of Sensory Processing (Johnson-Ecker & Parham, 2000). There are three separate forms: (1) home (72 items), (2) main classroom (62 items), and (3) school environments (e.g., music, bus, recess), with 10–15 items for each environment. The measure includes norm-referenced scores for five sensory areas: visual, auditory, proprioceptive, vestibular, and tactile functioning. Therefore, a separate tactile scale with corresponding norms allows for separate assessment of this particular sensory modality. These norm-referenced scores utilize a categorization system with three levels: (1) typical, (2) problems, and (3) definite dysfunction.

A study of the Sensory Processing Measure—Home (Johnson-Ecker & Parham, 2000) found that the measure distinguished children with and without sensory integrative dysfunction. Twenty four of the 62 items in the home form are touch related. Likewise, in a study of the school version, the measure discriminated between children with and without sensory issues and indicated adequate internal consistency, with values for Cronbach's alpha ranging from 0.70 to 0.99 (Miller-Kuhaneck, Henry, Glennon, & Mu, 2007).

Sensory Profile. The Sensory Profiles (SPs) include several versions that are intended for particular age groups. Each version measures multiple domains of sensory processing that were developed and interpreted using Dunn's Model of Sensory Processing (1997). The Infant/Toddler SP (I/TSP; Dunn, 2002) is designed for children from birth to the age of 3; the SP (Dunn, 1999) is designed for children of ages 3–10; and the Adolescent/Adult SP (A/ASP; Brown & Dunn, 2002) is appropriate for those aged 11 and older. The A/ASP is a self-report measure whereas the SP and I/TSP are completed by a parent or caretaker. Each measure is a survey with questions focused on sensory responses to everyday life activities.

Each SP includes a set of items specifically devoted to touch. There are 13 touch items on the adolescent/adult version, 24 items on the child version, and 15 items on the infant/toddler version. These subsections can provide useful information in assessing response to touch according to a theoretical model. Using Dunn's (1997) Model of Sensory Processing as a guide, the tactile component of the measure is interpreted according to four subscale or quadrant scores: low registration or hyposensitivity to touch, tactile sensation seeking, tactile sensitivity, and avoidance of touch. An important distinction exists for scoring the adolescent/adult versus the child versions. A high score on the A/ASP indicates more of a particular attribute (e.g., sensory sensitivity) while a low score in the SP or I/TSP indicates more of an attribute. Adults with high scores on the sensory-sensitive items would notice touch more readily than others; conversely, adults with high scores on low registration would be less likely to notice tactile stimuli than others. Adults with high scores in the avoidance quadrant would engage in intentional behaviors to prevent exposure to tactile stimuli perceived as noxious, while adults with high scores in sensation seeking would find opportunities to experience touch.

Several studies support the reliability and validity of the SPs; however, the psychometric properties of the touch items have not been analyzed separately. Therefore, the reliability and validity of the measure as a whole should be applied cautiously when considering the touch items alone. Using factor analytic methods, studies support the integrity of the four subscales of sensory sensitivity, sensation avoiding, low registration, and sensation seeking (Brown, Tollefson, Dunn, Cromwell, & Filion, 2001; Dunn & Brown, 1997). Another study used skin conductance to further support the construct validity of the subscales (Brown et al., 2001). Several studies have found that the SPs discriminate between people with and without disabilities including adults with schizophrenia and bipolar disorder (Brown, Cromwell, Filion, Dunn, & Tollefson, 2002); adults with obsessive compulsive disorder (Rieke & Anderson, 2009); children with ADHD (Yochman, Parush, & Ornoy, 2004); and toddlers (Ben-Sasson et al., 2008), children (Tomcheck & Dunn, 2007), and adults (Crane, Goddard, & Pring, 2009) with autism.

Sensory Over-Responsivity Scales. The Sensory Over-Responsivity Scale (SensOR; Schoen, Miller, & Green 2008) is a newer measure, with use currently recommended for research purposes only. The measure is designed for both children and adults. The SensOR specifically measures sensitivity to sensory stimuli and includes both a caregiver/self report (the SensOR Inventory) and an examiner-administered performance measure (the SensOR Assessment). The SensOR is organized by sensory domains: tactile, auditory, visual, proprioceptive, olfactory, gustatory, and vestibular.

The SensOR Inventory is similar to the caregiver and self reports of the SP in that the items address sensory responses to daily-life activities; however, all items focus on sensory over-responsivity. The measure is used as a self-report for individuals over the age of 16, and caregivers provide the responses for children 16 years and younger. There is a similar stem for multiple questions such as "these aspects of self care bother me" (Schoen et al., 2008, p. 396) with a list of sample activities such as wiping face or getting dressed. Items are scored as applicable or nonapplicable and then scored in terms of total number of over-responsive behaviors endorsed.

For the SensOR Assessment, the respondent is exposed to different sensory stimuli that have the potential to be perceived as aversive. There are 16 activities that involve sensory exposure. The tactile activities include removing a Band-Aid from the hands or wrists, finding a toy animal hidden in "special goo," and experiencing an air puff or feather on the face. Each exposure is scored on a four-point scale in terms of the intensity of the response in the behavioral categories of startle, elimination (e.g., rubbing the spot that was touched), dislike, and negative-stop (e.g., refusing to engage in the activity).

Pilot testing found the SensOR to discriminate typical children and adults from children and adults previously identified as "over-responsive" according to the SP (Schoen et al., 2008). In addition, the same study found strong internal consistency for the subscales and the total measure (coefficient alpha = 0.90 for the Tactile subscale of the SensOR Assessment and 0.81 for the Tactile subscale of the SensOR Inventory). A study using the SensOR Inventory found that children with ADHD and sensory over-responsivity were more likely to experience anxiety than children with ADHD without anxiety (Reynolds & Lane, 2009). These findings support the measure's predictive validity.

The Sensory Integration and Praxis Tests. This assessment provides information in four major areas: form and space, praxis, vestibular and proprioceptive processing, and tactile discrimination (Ayres, 1989). It was developed for use with children of ages 4–8 who had mild to moderate learning or motor difficulties. The Sensory Integration and Praxis Test (SIPT) has 17 tests, with 4 tests focused specifically on tactile discrimination. These include a test assessing identification of individual fingers via touch, localization of tactile stimuli applied to arms or hands, matching tasks between touching and vision, and interpretation of writing on the hand (graphesthesia). The SIPT was standardized with a sample of 2,000 children in the United States and Canada. Evidence of construct and criterion-related validity has been shown for the entire SIPT. Concurrent validity and good reliability (inter-rater and test–retest) are evident for the tactile discrimination tests, although test–retest reliability for localization of touch was lower than others (Ayres & Marr, 2002; Kinnealey, 1989). Research has also supported the ability of the tactile discrimination tests to predict developmental delay (Case-Smith, 1991).

The Test of Sensory Functions. This criterion-referenced test was designed to assess tactile, vestibular, and motor functions of infants during their first 2 years of life (DeGangi & Greenspan, 1989). Three subtests from the measure assess tactile functions: deep pressure, light touch, and visual–tactile integration. The test of reactivity to pressure involves rubbing five different areas of the child's body with firm pressure for 10 seconds, three times for each body area. The second subtest involves responses to five different textured objects that are placed on different parts of the child's body. The test of light touch uses an air puff from an ear syringe on the child's cheek. Children are rated by the examiner on a five-point scale, from negative affect (frown, fuss, cry) to positive affect (smile, giggle). The child receives a total score for degree of reactivity based upon all tests, with scores at the positive end suggesting normal sensory function. Consistent scores in the middle indicate hyposensitivity and scores at the negative end represent hypersensitivity and aversion. The total test has shown predictive validity with other measures of sensory threshold, concurrent validity with measures of sensory function and good test–retest reliability (Beard and Goodman, 1999; DeGangi & Greenspan, 1989; Williamson & Anzalone, 2001).

The Luria–Nebraska Neuropsychological Battery. The original measure was designed to assess individuals aged 15 and older with potential neurological impairment (Golden, Purisch, & Hammeke, 1980). There is a children's version as well to assess children 8 years of age or older (Golden, 1986). Both versions are based upon Luria's theory of higher cortical functioning and examine 11 primary clinical areas of neuropsychological functioning, including sensory processes as well as cognitive and brain function tests. The measure has a Tactile Functions Scale consisting of 21 tests that assess localization of touch, varied types of tactile discrimination, tactile sensitivity and extinction, and different types of tactile recognition. Factor analysis has supported the integrity of the tactile function scale (Golden, Sweet, et al., 1980). The overall battery has shown the ability to distinguish among individuals with brain injury, seizure, and other forms of neurological impairment (Purisch, 2001). The specific tests within the tactile function scale have been widely used, with varied adaptations in a variety of research and clinical measures (e.g., Essick et al., 2010; High, Gough, Wright, & Fitch, 1998; Lundborg & Rosen, 2004; Minshew & Hobson, 2008; Morch, Andersen, Quevedo, Arendt-Nielsen, & Coghill, 2010).

The Halstead–Reitan Neuropsychological Test Battery. Like the Luria–Nebraska Battery, this measure provides for a broad assessment of neuropsychological functions, including sensory–motor integration (Reitan & Wolfson, 1993). It has versions that are appropriate for ages 5 and older. Among its 10 tests is a "Tactual Performance Test" that examines three areas of tactile function. These include tactile form recognition, finger discrimination, and tactile neglect or suppression. This latter test involves light touch to different body areas that is randomly varied between single and double simultaneous stimulation. Neglect is involved when an individual reports only single stimulation when actually double stimulation occurs. The battery discriminates between normal individuals and those with a variety of neurological and psychiatric impairments, as well as distinguishing between focal and diffuse neurological problems and various cortical areas and etiologies (Reitan & Wolfson, 2002). Recent studies indicate that the battery for children of ages 5–8 had a 100% classification rate with no false positives while the version for older children correctly classified 87.5% (Vanderslice-Barr, Lynch, & McCaffrey, 2008). The adult battery had excellent sensitivity but its specificity was fair (Horowitz, Lynch, McCaffrey, & Fisher, 2008). Although the Luria battery has more extensive coverage of different types of tactile response, the Halstead–Reitan battery is purported to provide more detailed assessment of responses that involve higher tactile processes (Goldstein, Hersen, & Beers, 2004).

PHYSIOLOGICAL MEASURES

The previous section describes the use of behavioral measures to investigate how people feel about and/or respond to tactile stimulation. For some situations and groups of people, however, behavioral measures have significant limitations. For example, understanding how infants and children respond to being touched is an area of great interest, but limitations in communication skills make self-report measures impossible. Parent or teacher reports may be used, but such reports rely exclusively on observable reactions and cannot provide insight into the sensory processes that may produce those reactions. Self-report measures may also be of limited utility for investigating responses to touch in people with cognitive or emotional challenges and those who are severely ill. These circumstances may interfere with accurate perception of touch or their ability to communicate their tactile experience. Lastly, there are times when the use of behavioral measures may be challenging because of demand characteristics or social desirability effects. In cases like these, where behavioral measures may provide insufficient or inaccurate information about sensory experiences, the use of physiological measures may provide a valuable alternative.

All sensory experiences, if they are detected by the sense receptors, produce some level of change in our physiological state. When sensory stimuli are initially detected, the pattern of physiological response can be viewed as an orienting response, a defensive response, or a startle response (Graham & Clifton, 1966; Sokolov, 1963). Orienting responses occur when detected sensory stimuli are perceived as novel. Orienting responses are the most widely studied of the physiological responses to sensory stimulation. Defensive responses occur when detected sensory stimuli are perceived as aversive, painful, or potentially dangerous. Startle responses occur when sensory stimuli are unexpected, have an abrupt onset, and are intense but not at the level of being aversive or painful. Each of these categories of response is actually a constellation of physiological changes—autonomic, motoric, and neurochemical—that occur within a short time window following stimulus onset. Because these physiological changes occur with any change in sensory stimulation that is detected by the sensory receptors, it is technically the case that *any* of these physiological variables could be used to study response to touch. Realistically, however, only a subset of the physiological changes associated with orienting, defensive, and startle responding are sufficiently large that they are readily detectable using standard physiological recording equipment and by placing sensors on the surface of the skin. Other smaller and more subtle change may only be detectable by more intensive or invasive measures of neuronal or biochemical change. These physiologic responses to touch can shed light on aspects of an individual's disposition toward touch or tactile temperament, including (1) initial sensitivity or threshold for perceiving touch, (2) the degree of arousal or reactivity experienced as a result of touch, and (3) the individual's tolerance for sensations associated with touch (Weiss, 2005). To date, physiological responses to touch stimuli have received relatively little research attention compared to other sensory stimuli. Of the studies that exist, the most widely studied physiological responses have been electrodermal activity (EDA) and heart rate.

Electrodermal Activity

EDA is an index of sympathetic nervous system activation and is related to changes in the "sweatiness" of the palms and finger tips (see Dawson, Schell, & Filion, 2007, for a review). EDA is typically measured by placing two recording electrodes on the palm or finger tips of one hand, passing a low level voltage between the electrodes, and measuring the conductivity of the skin to the passage of that current. Conductivity increases as the amount of sweat in the sweat glands under the electrodes increases. Skin conductance level, or the baseline level of conductivity in the absence of stimulation, can be used to index tonic sympathetic nervous system arousal, and the skin conductance response (SCR) can be used to index the sympathetic nervous system's response to discrete stimuli. The SCR to mild or innocuous stimuli is viewed as a component of the orienting response and is believed to index the allocation of attention to a new or significant stimulus. Recording the SCR to repeated discrete stimuli can additionally provide an index of habituation or the adaptive decline in response to a stimulus as it becomes familiar. SCRs can be reliably elicited by stimuli in any sensory modality. However, the intimate relationship between touch and the skin, along with the established sensitivity of the SCR to tactile stimuli, has made it a popular measure in studies of touch.

For example, Miller and colleagues have carried out a number of studies using electrodermal measures to study responses to tactile stimulation in children with sensory processing disorders (Mangeot et al., 2001; McIntosh, Miller, Shyu, & Hagerman, 1999; Miller et al., 1999; Shoen, Miller, Brett-Green, & Nielsen, 2009). In each of these studies, EDA was measured in response to a sensory challenge that included tactile stimulation in the form of a light touch with a feather. Although responses to the tactile stimulus were averaged with responses to other sensory stimuli in many of these studies, it is clear that there is an SCR to the tactile stimulus. Shoen and colleagues found the SCR to the tactile stimulus to be higher for children with sensory modulation disorder than children with autism spectrum disorder, providing evidence that the size of the SCR can discriminate between children with varied types of sensory processing disorder.

In addition to studies showing that EDA is sensitive to sensory processing disorders in children, there are also studies demonstrating that EDA is sensitive to touch of adults (e.g., Vrana & Rollick, 1998; Wilhelm, Kochar, Roth, & Gross, 2001). In these studies, EDA and other physiological measures were recorded during a brief touch to the wrist. Skin conductance increased significantly during the touch encounter. Interestingly, Wilhelm et al. found that skin conductance was even higher during the period when participants anticipated the touch than during the actual touch experience. This indicates that the SCR is sensitive not only to the experience of touch but also to states of touch anticipation. Such findings have implications for understanding receptivity to being touched or preferences resulting from individual traits or previous experiences.

Heart Rate

Heart rate is influenced by both the sympathetic and the parasympathetic branches of the autonomic nervous system. In studies of touch, it is often measured by placing one electrode on the left ankle and one on each wrist. Other approaches involve placement of electrodes on the chest wall and limbs. Complex assessment of heart rate and rhythm can occur using a 12-lead electrocardiogram (ECG) in studies involving individuals with cardiovascular or other health problems. Each of these configurations provides measurement of the electrical signals that occur each time the heart beats. Both heart rate and heart rate variability can be determined using the ECG. By measuring the number of times the heart beats over a specific time window, an average heart rate for that window can be computed. Heart rate is used as a measure of sympathetic nervous system function. Heart rate variability is the range or spread of the heart rate during exposure to touch and is often used as a measure of parasympathetic functioning or vagal tone. The simplest measure of variability is the difference between the lowest and highest heart rates within each cardiac cycle, but there are more complex approaches that examine the standard deviation of normalized beat to beat intervals or the percent of interbeat intervals that differ from neighboring intervals. Respiratory sinus arrhythmia can also be used as a measure of vagal tone; it is the difference between the longest interbeat interval corresponding to expiration and the shortest interbeat interval corresponding to inspiration. Many software programs exist to record and analyze the various measures of heart rate and heart rate variability.

The use of heart rate to investigate responses to touch began with a series of studies showing that dogs showed reliable decreases in heart rate when touched by a human (Lynch & McCarthy, 1969). Extending that work, Drescher, Gantt, and Whitehead (1980) replicated this effect in humans. Interestingly, these investigators found that the heart rate decrease occurred only when the participant was being touched by a second person and that there was no change in heart rate in a self-touch condition. Drescher, Whitehead, Morrill-Corbin, and Cataldo (1985) replicated the finding of decreased heart rate in response to touch and ruled out that the decrease was simply a part of a more generalized arousal reduction or relaxation response because the decrease in heart rate observed was found not to correlate with a variety of other physiological indicators of arousal.

These findings were again supported in a study of hospitalized cardiovascular patients (Weiss, 1990). Patients were given a standardized protocol of touch that included structured periods of different tactile stimuli in the form of physical assessment procedures and massage. Their heart rate and blood pressure were monitored throughout the 16-minute protocol. Both blood pressure and heart rate decreased as a result of touch, providing support for concurrent validity of the heart rate measure. However, Weiss and Puntillo (2001) found that certain traits can play an important role in determining response to touch. In their study, hospitalized patients who indicated less tolerance for sensory stimulation on a self-report questionnaire and who had greater basal heart rate were significantly more likely to have increased heart rate as a result of touch provided during a standardized caregiving protocol. These individuals also experienced more life-threatening changes in the normal rhythms of their heart in response to being touched.

Further documenting the sensitivity of heart rate as a measure of touch, Nilsen and Vrana (1998) found that an expected touch by a familiar person produced the same pattern of heart rate decrease as shown by others. However, their results indicated that heart rate would increase when participants were touched in a threatening way or an ambiguous context. These various studies suggest that both individual and environmental factors clearly affect response to touch.

Another way in which heart rate has been used to measure the effects of touch is in studies on the effects of touch on stress or pain. In these studies, participants are randomly assigned to a touch or a control condition prior to a stressful event or painful medical procedure. Heart rate is then monitored during and following the event. Heart rate differences between the touch and control groups are analyzed to determine if participants in the touch condition show heart rate responses indicative of less stress or pain. This technique has been used to study the effects of maternal touch on infant pain during heel stick (e.g., Cong, Ludington-Hoe, McCain, & Fui, 2009; Feldman, Singer, & Zagoory, 2010) and to investigate the effects of handholding on anxiety responses in older adults undergoing cataract surgery (Moon & Cho, 2001). In addition, measures of vagal tone or heart rate variability have been employed to study effects of massage therapy and gentle touch by nurses on preterm infant vulnerability to stress and overall arousal (Field, Diego, Hernandez-Reif, Deeds, & Figuereido, 2006; Harrison, Williams, Leeper, Stern, & Wang, 2000).

Heart rate has also been used to study the effects of touch more indirectly, by investigating the effects of touch as a form of stress inoculation.

In this study, Grewen, Anderson, Girdler, and Light (2003) randomly assigned adult participants to one of two conditions: a control condition or a warm partner contact condition. Participants in the contact condition spent 10 minutes with their partner in a private space engaged in comfortable touching, a short romantic movie, and a 20-second hug. Participants in the control condition spent the same 10-minute period alone. Participants were then required to give a 3-minute speech and to watch a replay of the speech on video, both conditions known to elicit a cardiovascular stress response. Heart rate and blood pressure responses were recorded during the speech and replay periods. Results indicated that both heart rate and blood pressure responses were lower for participants who were engaged in touching and hugging before the stressor than responses shown by the control group.

Overall, the existing literature suggests that heart rate can provide a sensitive measure of a person's immediate response to touch and can also provide an indirect measure of more long-lasting effects of touch such as reduction of anxiety or pain.

Issues in Physiologic Measurement

Unlike questionnaires or observational coding systems that have more traditional psychometric data, somewhat different approaches are used to assure the validity and reliability of physiologic measures of touch response. Physiologic measures must be calibrated on an ongoing basis to assure accuracy of their readings, checked for their precision to assure that the same value is achieved under the same conditions each time it is recorded, and acquired using standardized procedures and conditions that are repeated across subjects to assure reliability. In addition, investigators must control for artifact that is easily produced by movement or extraneous, confounding conditions in the environment. Ideally, they should also perform a number of trials to assure reliability of each individual's response and assess the relationship of one physiologic measure to other physiologic or behavioral measures. Ultimately, the more objective nature of physiologic measures can help to eliminate response and tester bias that exists when behavioral measures alone are used.

Additional Approaches to Measurement

A number of other biological measures are being explored for their utility in studying response to touch. For instance, salivary cortisol has been used to determine effects of touch on the stress levels of both infants and adults (Lindgren et al., 2010; Neu, Laudenslager, & Robinson, 2009; White-Traut, Schwertz, McFarlin, & Kogan, 2009). Electroencephalograms are being used to understand recognition of tactile stimuli and neural responsiveness to tactile stimulation (Aviles, Munoz, Kleinbohl, Sebastian, & Jimenez, 2010; Hotting, Friedrich, & Roder, 2009; Scher et al., 2009). Similarly, different types of brain imaging (e.g., PET, fMRI, MEG) can provide important information on cortical responses to touch (Bjornsdotter, Loken, Olausson, Vallbo, & Wessberg, 2009; Nebel et al., 2010; Wuhle, Mertiens, Ruter, Ostwald, & Braun, 2010).

In addition to these individual approaches, simultaneous measurement of multiple response systems is on the rise. Studies of high-risk infants have used a combination of measures such as heart rate, blood pressure, respiratory rate, oxygen saturation, and behavior to develop a more comprehensive understanding of response to touch (Field et al., 2006; Harrison, Leeper, & Yoon, 1990; Harrison, Williams, Berbaum, Stern, & Leeper, 2000; Weiss, 1992). Simultaneous measurement of multiple response systems (e.g., heart rate, blood pressure, heart rhythm, pupil size, cortisol, respiration, EEG, SCR, electromyograms, anxiety, and nonverbal behavior) also has been used to assess response to touch in both healthy populations (Holt-Lunstad, Birmingham, & Light, 2008; Lindgren et al., 2010; Vrana & Rollock, 1998; Wilhelm et al., 2001) and critically ill adults (Keller, Hulsdunk, & Muller, 2007; Li, Miaskowski, Burkhardt, & Puntillo, 2009; Weiss, 1990). These various studies have shown the ability of diverse measures to assess response to touch and provide emerging evidence of concurrent validity across many physiologic and behavioral measures.

Weiss and Wilson (2006) developed the Tactile Vulnerability Assessment (TVA) as a method to integrate scores from various physiologic and behavioral measures of response to touch by high-risk infants. Their measures included heart rate, respiratory rate, oxygen saturation, changes in skin color, facial expression, activity level, and vocalization. As shown in Table 9.1, the TVA has subscales for physiologic reactivity, behavioral reactivity, and tolerance for specific qualities of touch in response to a standardized protocol of touching. Internal consistency of the measure's items was 0.85 and the relationship of each subscale to the overall tactile vulnerability score was significant. Inter-rater reliability ranged from 0.81 to 0.89. Concurrent validity was established via correlations with ratings of the infant's typical tactile responses as assessed by the infant's primary nurse ($r = 0.45$, $p < 0.001$). The investigators found that the severity of the infants' medical problems and complications, fetal drug exposure, and their mother's own self-reported discomfort with being touched were key predictors of the infants' physiologic hyperarousal and behavioral distress when touched.

CONCLUSIONS

Initial development of measures to assess tactile response focused primarily on survey and psychophysical approaches. More recently, physiologic and multimethod approaches have increased in use. There is no one method of measuring response to touch that is inherently better than another. The method of choice depends upon the specific response being studied, the nature of the subjects or participants, and the overall study design.

More attention is needed to preliminary development and adequate testing of measures that assess response to touch. Many measures have been developed as part of an ongoing study rather than fully tested and refined prior to use. Others have been designed for clinical use and then incorporated into research projects at a later time. Future research that provides information on the relationship among various methods will be essential in examining the convergent validity of different measures. There is also the need for more detailed assessment of touch subscales or item sets that are part of global sensory or neuropsychological measures. The psychometric data available on these subscales are frequently limited, with dependence on validity and reliability findings for the global measure.

The spectrum of measurement approaches for studying response to touch is growing at a rapid pace. This increase in measurement options raises exciting possibilities for better understanding human response to touch. It also challenges investigators to assure that the methods being used are conceptually appropriate and empirically sound.

REFERENCES

Andersen, P. A., & Leibowitz, K. (1978). The development and nature of the construct of touch avoidance. *Environmental Psychology and Nonverbal Behavior, 3,* 89–106.

Andersen, P. A., & Sull, K. K. (1985). Out of touch, out of reach: Tactile predisposition as predictors of interpersonal distance. *Western Journal of Speech Communication, 49,* 57–72.

Aviles, J., Munoz, F., Kleinbohl, D., Sebastian, M., & Jimenez, S. (2010). A new device to present textured stimuli to touch with simultaneous EEG recording. *Behavioral Research Methods, 42,* 547–555.

Ayres, A. J. (1989). *Sensory Integration and Praxis Tests Manual.* Los Angeles: Western Psychological Services.

Ayres, A. J., & Marr, D. (2002). Sensory Integration and Praxis Tests. In A. Bundy, S. Lane, & E. Murray (Eds.), *Sensory integration: Theory and practice* (pp. 453–476). Philadelphia, PA: F.A. Davis Company.

Baranek, G. T., & Berkson, G. (1994). Tactile defensiveness in children with developmental disabilities: Responsiveness and habituation. *Journal of Autism and Developmental Disorders, 32,* 397–422.

Baranek, G. T., Boyd, B. A., Poe, M. D., David, F. J., & Watson, L. R. (2007). Hyperresponsive sensory patterns in young children with autism, developmental delay and typical development. *American Journal of Mental Retardation, 112,* 233–245.

Baranek, G. T., Chin, Y. H., Greiss Hess, L. M., Yankee, J. G., Hatton, D. D., & Hooper, S. R. (2002). Sensory processing correlates of occupational performance in children with Fragile X syndrome. Preliminary findings. *American Journal of Occupational Therapy, 56,* 538–546.

Beard, J., & Goodman, I. (1999, April). *Air puff and other measures of emotional reactivity to touch in high risk infants at six months.* Paper presented at the Society for Research in Child Development, Morgantown, WV.

Bennett, J. W., & Peterson, C. Q. (1995). The Touch Inventory for Elementary School Aged Children: Test-retest reliability and mother child correlations. *American Journal of Occupational Therapy, 49,* 795–801.

Ben-Sasson, A., Cermak, S. A., Orsmond, G. I., Tager-Flusberg, H., Kadlec, M. B., & Carter, A. S. (2008). Sensory clusters of toddlers with autism spectrum disorders: Differences in affective symptoms. *Journal of Child Psychology and Psychiatry, 49,* 817–825.

Bjornsdotter, M., Loken, L., Olausson, H., Vallbo, A., & Wessberg, J. (2009). Somatotopic organization of gentle touch processing in the posterior insular cortex. *Journal of Neuroscience, 29,* 9314–9320.

Broring, T., Rommelse, N., Sergeant, J., & Scherder, E. (2008). Sex differences in tactile defensiveness in children with ADHD and their siblings. *Developmental Medicine and Child Neurology, 50,* 129–133.

Brown, C., Cromwell, R. L., Filion, D., Dunn, W., & Tollefson, N. (2002). Sensory processing in schizophrenia: Missing and avoiding information, *Schizophrenia Research, 55,* 187–195.

Brown, C., & Dunn, W. (2002). *Adolescent/Adult Sensory Profile.* San Antonio, TX: Psychological Corporation.

Brown, C., Tollefson, N., Dunn, W., Cromwell, R., & Filion, D. (2001). The Adult Sensory Profile: Measuring patterns of sensory processing. *American Journal of Occupational Therapy, 55,* 75–82.

Brown, S., Lewis, C., McCarthy, J., Doyle, S., & Hurvitz, E. (2010). The effects of internet-based home training on upper limb function in adults with cerebral palsy. *Neurorehabilitation and Neural Repair, 24,* 575–583.

Carey, L., Oke, L., & Matyas, T. (1997). Impaired touch discrimination after stroke: A quantitative test. *Neurorehabilitation and Neural Repair, 11,* 219–232.

Case-Smith, J. (1991). The effects of tactile defensiveness and tactile discrimination on in-hand manipulation. *American Journal of Occupational Therapy, 45,* 811–118.

Cong, X., Ludington-Hoe, S. M., McCain, G., & Fui, P. (2009). Kangaroo Care modifies preterm infant heart rate variability in response to heel stick pain: A pilot study. *Early Human Development, 85,* 561–567.

Crane, L., Goddard, L., & Pring, L. (2009). Sensory processing in adults with autism spectrum disorders. *Autism, 13,* 215–228.

Dawson, M. E., Schell, A. M., & Filion, D. L. (2007). The sudomotor system. In J. T. Cacioppo, L. G. Tassinary, & G. Bernsten (Eds.), *Principles of psychophysiology: Physical, social, and inferential elements* (3rd ed.; pp. 159–181). Cambridge, MA: Cambridge University Press.

Deethardt, J. F., & Hines, D. (1983). Tactile communication and personality differences. *Journal of Nonverbal Behavior, 8,* 143–156.

DeGangi, G., & Greenspan, S. (1989). *Test of Sensory Functions in Infants.* Los Angeles, CA: Western Psychological Services.

Drescher, V. M., Gantt, W. H., & Whitehead, W. E. (1980). Heart rate response to touch. *Psychosomatic Medicine, 42,* 559–565.

Drescher, V. M., Whitehead, W. E., Morrill-Corbin, E. D., & Cataldo, M. F. (1985). Physiological and subjective reactions to being touched. *Psychophysiology, 22,* 96–100.

Dunn, W. (1997). The impact of sensory processing abilities on the daily lives of young children and their families: A conceptual model. *Infants and Young Children, 9,* 23–35.

Dunn, W. (1999) *Sensory Profile.* San Antonio, TX: Psychological Corporation.

Dunn, W. (2002) *Infant/Toddler Sensory Profile.* San Antonio, TX: Psychological Corporation.

Dunn, W., & Brown, C. (1997). Factor analysis on the sensory profile from a national sample of children without disabilities. *American Journal of Occupational Therapy, 51,* 490–495.

Essick, G., McGlone, F., Dancer, C., Fabricant, D., Ragin, Y., Phillips, N.,...Guest, S. (2010). Quantitative assessment of pleasant touch. *Neuroscience and Biobehavioral Reviews, 34,* 192–203.

Feldman, R., Singer, M., & Zagoory, O. (2010). Touch attenuates infants' physiological reactivity to stress. *Developmental Science, 13,* 271–278.

Field, T., Diego, M., Hernandez-Reif, M., Deeds, O., & Figuereido, B. (2006). Moderate versus light pressure massage therapy leads to greater weight gain in preterm infants. *Infant Behavior and Development, 29,* 574–578.

Fromme, D. K., Jaynes, W., Taylor, D., Hanold, E., Daniell, J., Rountree, J., & Fromme, M. (1989). Nonverbal behavior and attitudes toward touch. *Journal of Nonverbal Behavior, 13,* 3–14.

Ghanizadeh, A. (2008). Tactile sensory dysfunction in children with ADHD. *Behavioural Neurology, 20,* 107–112.

Golden, C. J. (1986). *Luria–Nebraska Neuropsychological Battery—Children's Version.* Los Angeles, CA: Western Psychological Services.

Golden, C. J., Purisch, A., & Hammeke, T. (1980). *Luria–Nebraska Neuropsychological Battery.* Los Angeles, CA: Western Psychological Services.

Golden, C. J., Sweet, J., Hammeke, T., Purisch, A., Graber, B., & Osmon, D. (1980). Factor analysis of the Luria–Nebraska Neuropsychological Battery: Motor, rhythm and tactile scales. *International Journal of Neuroscience, 11,* 91–99.

Goldsmith, H. H., Van Hulle, C. A., Arneson, C. L., Schreiber, J. E., & Gernsbacher, M. A. (2006). A population-based twin study of parentally reported tactile and auditory defensiveness in young children. *Journal of Abnormal Child Psychology, 34,* 393–407.

Goldstein, G., Hersen, M., & Beers, S. (2004). *Comprehensive Handbook of Psychological Assessment: Intellectual and Neuropsychological Assessment.* Hoboken, NJ: John Wiley & Sons.

Graham, F. K., & Clifton, R. K. (1966). Heart rate change as a component of the orienting response. *Psychological Bulletin, 65,* 305–320.

Grewen, K. M., Anderson, B. J., Girdler, S. S., & Light, K. C. (2003). Warm partner contact is related to lower cardiovascular reactivity. *Behavioral Medicine, 29,* 123–130.

Guerrero, L., & Andersen, P. (1991). The waxing and waning of relational intimacy: Touch as a function of relational stage, gender and touch avoidance. *Journal of Social and Personal Relationships, 8,* 147–165.

Harrison, L. L., Leeper, J., & Yoon, M. (1990). Effects of early parent touch on preterm infants' arterial oxygen saturation and heart rate levels. *Journal of Advanced Nursing, 15,* 877–885.

Harrison, L. L., Williams, A., Berbaum, M., Stern, J., & Leeper, J. (2000). Physiologic and behavioral effects of gentle human touch on preterm infants. *Research in Nursing and Health, 23,* 435–446.

Harrison, L. L., Williams, A., Leeper, J., Stern, J., & Wang, L. (2000). Factors associated with vagal tone responses in preterm infants. *Western Journal of Nursing Research, 22,* 776–792.

High, J., Gough, A., Wright, C., & Fitch, A. (1998). Tactile discrimination in children: The tactile assessment kit. *International Journal of Therapy and Rehabilitation, 5,* 47–51.

Holt-Lunstad, J., Birmingham, W., & Light, K. (2008). Influence of a "warm touch" support enhancement intervention among married couples on ambulatory blood pressure, oxytocin, alpha amylase, and cortisol. *Psychosomatic Medicine, 70,* 976–985.

Horowitz, J., Lynch, J., McCaffrey, R., & Fisher, J. (2008). Screening for neuropsychological impairment using Reitan and Wolfson's preliminary neuropsychological test battery. *Archives of Clinical Neuropsychology, 23,* 393–398.

Hotting, K., Friedrich, C., & Roder, B. (2009). Neural correlates of cross-modally induced changes in tactile awareness. *Journal of Cognitive Neuroscience, 21,* 2445–2461.

Johnson-Ecker, C. L., & Parham, L. D. (2000). The Evaluation of Sensory Processing: A validity study using contrasting groups. *American Journal of Occupational Therapy, 54,* 494–503.

Jones, S., & Brown, B. (1996). Touch attitudes and behaviors, recollections of early childhood touch, and social self-confidence. *Journal of Nonverbal Behavior, 20,* 147–163.

Keller, I., Hulsdunk, A., & Muller, F. (2007). The influence of acoustic and tactile stimulation on vegetative parameters and EEG in persistent vegetative state. *Functional Neurology, 22*, 159–163.

Kinnealey, M. (1989). Tactile functions in learning-disabled and normal children: Reliability and validity considerations. *Occupational Therapy Journal of Research, 16*, 75–97.

Li, D., Miaskowski, C., Burkhardt., D., & Puntillo, K. (2009). Evaluations of physiologic reactivity and reflexive behaviors during noxious procedures in sedated critically ill patients. *Journal of Critical Care, 24*, 472–479.

Lindgren, L., Rundgren, S., Winso, O., Lehtipalo, S., Wiklund, U., Karlsson, M.,...Brulin, C. (2010). Physiological responses to touch massage in healthy volunteers. *Autonomic Neuroscience, 158*, 105–110.

Lundborg, G., & Rosen, B. (2004). The two-point discrimination test—Time for a reappraisal? *Journal of Hand Surgery, 29*, 418–422.

Lynch, J. J., & McCarthy, J. F. (1969). Social responding to dogs: Heart rate changes to a person. *Psychophysiology, 5*, 389–393.

Mangeot, S. D., Miller, L. J., McIntosh, D. N., McGrath-Clarke, M. A., Simon, J., Hagerman, R. J., & Goldson, E. (2001). Sensory modulation dysfunction in children with attention-deficit-hyperactivity disorder. *Developmental Medicine and Child Neurology, 43*, 399–406.

McIntosh, D. N., Miller, L. J., Shyu, V., & Hagerman, R. J. (1999). Sensory modulation disruption, electrodermal responses, and functional behaviors. *Developmental Medicine and Child Neurology, 41*, 608–615.

Miller, L. J., & Lane, S. J. (2000). Towards a consensus in terminology in sensory integration theory and practice. Part I: Taxonomy of neurophysiological processes. *Sensory Integration Special Interest Quarterly, 23*, 1–4.

Miller, L. J., McIntosh, D. N., McGrath, J., Shyu, V., Lampe, M., Taylor, A. K., ...Hagerman, R. J. (1999). Electrodermal response to sensory stimuli in individuals with Fragile X syndrome: A preliminary report. *American Journal of Medical Genetics, 83*, 268–279.

Miller-Kuhaneck, H., Henry, D. A., & Glennon, T. J. (2005). *Sensory Processing Measure–School*. Los Angeles, CA: Western Psychological Services.

Miller-Kuhaneck, H., Henry, D. A., Glennon, T. J., & Mu, K. (2007). Development of the Sensory Processing Measure–School: Initial studies of reliability and validity. *American Journal of Occupational Therapy, 61*, 170–175.

Minshew, N., & Hobson, J. (2008). Sensory sensitivities and performance on sensory perceptual tasks in high-functioning individuals with autism. *Journal of Autism and Developmental Disorders, 38*, 1485–1498.

Moon, J. S., & Cho, K. S. (2001). The effects of handholding on anxiety in cataract surgery patients under local anaesthesia. *Journal of Advanced Nursing, 35*, 407–415.

Morch, C., Andersen, O., Quevedo, A., Arendt-Nielsen, L., & Coghill, R. (2010). Exteroceptive aspects of nociception: Insights from graphesthesia and two-point discrimination. *Pain*, Epub ahead of print.

Nebel, M., Folger, S., Tommerdahl, M., Hollins, M., McGlone, F., & Essick, G. (2010). Temporamandibular disorder modifies cortical response to tactile stimulation. *Journal of Pain*, Epub ahead of print.

Neu, M., Laudenslager, M., & Robinson, J. (2009). Co-regulation in salivary cortisol during maternal holding of premature infants. *Biological Research in Nursing, 10*, 226–240.

Nilsen, W. J., & Vrana, S. R. (1998). Some touching situations: The relationship between gender and contextual variables in cardiovascular responses to human touch. *Annals of Behavioral Medicine, 20,* 270–276.

Parham, L. D., & Ecker, C. (2005). *Sensory Processing Measure–Home.* Los Angeles, CA: Western Psychological Services.

Parush, S., Doryon, Y. D., & Katz, N. (2006). A comparison of self-report and informant report of tactile defensiveness amongst children in Israel. *Occupational Therapy International, 3,* 274–283.

Parush, S., Sohmer, H., Steinberg, A., & Kaitz, M. (2007). Somatosensory function in boys with ADHD and tactile defensiveness. *Physiology and Behavior, 90,* 553–558.

Purisch, A. D. (2001). Misconceptions about the Luria–Nebraska Neuropsychological Battery. *NeuroRehabilitation, 16,* 275–280.

Reitan, R., & Wolfson, D. (1993). *The Halstead–Reitan Neuropsychological Test Battery: Theory and Clinical Interpretation.* South Tucson, AZ: Neuropsychology Press.

Reynolds, S., & Lane, S. J. (2009). Sensory overresponsivity and anxiety in children with ADHD. *American Journal of Occupational Therapy, 63,* 433–440.

Rieke, E. F., & Anderson, D. (2009). Adolescent/Adult Sensory Profile and obsessive compulsive disorder. *American Journal of Occupational Therapy, 63,* 138–145.

Royeen, C., & Mu, K. (2003). Stability of tactile defensiveness across cultures: European and American children's responses to the Touch Inventory for Elementary School Aged Children (TIE). *Occupational Therapy International, 10,* 165–174.

Royeen, C. B. (1987). TIP–Touch Inventory for Preschoolers. *Physical and Occupational Therapy in Pediatrics, 7,* 29–40.

Royeen, C. B., & Fortune, J. C. (1990). Touch Inventory for Elementary School Aged Children. *American Journal of Occupational Therapy, 44,* 155–159.

Scher, M., Ludington-Hoe, S., Kaffashi, F., Johnson, M., Holditch-Davis, D., & Loparo, K. (2009). Neurophysiologic assessment of brain maturation after an 8-week trial of skin-to-skin contact on preterm infants. *Clinical Neurophysiology, 120,* 1812–1818.

Schoen, S. A., Miller, L. J., Brett-Green, B. A., & Nielsen, D. M. (2009). Physiological and behavioral differences in sensory processing: A comparison of children with Autism Spectrum Disorder and Sensory Modulation Disorder. *Frontiers in Integrative Neurosciences, 3,* 1–11.

Schoen, S. A., Miller, L. J., & Green, K. E. (2008). Pilot study of the Sensory Over-Responsivity Scales: Assessment and inventory. *American Journal of Occupational Therapy, 62,* 393–406.

Sokolov, E. N. (1963). *Perception and the conditioned reflex.* Oxford, UK: Pergamon.

Soler, M., Kumru, H., Vidal, J., Pelayo, R., Tormos, J., Fregni, F., ... Pascual-Leone, A. (2010). Referred sensations and neuropathic pain following spinal cord injury. *Pain,* Epub ahead of print.

Sorensen, G., & Beatty, M. J. (1988). The interactive effects of touch avoidance on interpersonal evaluations. *Communication Research Reports, 5,* 84–90.

Tomcheck, S. D., & Dunn, W. (2007). Sensory processing in children with and without autism: A comparative study using the short sensory profile. *American Journal of Occupational Therapy, 61,* 190–200.

Vanderslice-Barr, J., Lynch, J., & McCaffrey, R. (2008). Screening for neuropsychological impairment in children using Reitan and Wolfson's preliminary neuropsychological test battery. *Archives of Clinical Neuropsychology, 23,* 243–249.

Vrana, S. R., & Rollick, D. (1998). Physiological response to a minimal social encounter: Effects of gender, ethnicity, and social context. *Psychophysiology, 35,* 462–469.

Weiss, S. (1990). Effects of differential touch on nervous system arousal of patients recovering from cardiac disease. *Heart and Lung, 19,* 474–480.

Weiss, S. (1992). Psychophysiologic and behavioral effects of tactile stimulation on infants with congenital heart disease. *Research in Nursing and Health, 15,* 93–101.

Weiss, S. (2000). The Physical Contact Assessment. Available from the Department of Community Health Systems, Box 0608, University of California, San Francisco, 94143.

Weiss, S. (2005). Haptic perception and the psychosocial functioning of premature, low birth weight children. *Infant Behavior and Development, 28,* 329–359.

Weiss, S., & Goebel, P. (2003). Parents' touch of their preterm infants and its relationship to their state of mind regarding touch. *Journal of Prenatal and Perinatal Psychology and Health, 17,* 185–202.

Weiss, S., & Puntillo, K. (2001). Predictors of psychophysiologic responses to caregiving. *International Journal of Nursing Practice, 7,* 177–187.

Weiss, S., & Wilson, P. (2006). Origins of tactile vulnerability in high risk infants. *Advances in Neonatal Care, 6,* 25–36.

Weiss, S., Wilson, P., Hertenstein, M., & Campos, R. (2000). The tactile context of a mother's caregiving: Implications for attachment of low birth weight infants. *Infant Behavior and Development, 23,* 91–111.

White-Traut, R., Schwertz, D., McFarlin, B., & Kogan, J. (2009). Salivary cortisol and behavioral state responses of healthy newborn infants to tactile-only and multisensory interventions. *Journal of Obstetric and Gynecological Nursing, 38,* 22–34.

Wilhelm, F. H., Kochar, A. S., Roth, W. T., & Gross, J. J. (2001). Social anxiety and response to touch: Incongruence between self-evaluative and physiological reactions. *Biological Psychology, 58,* 181–202.

Williamson, G., & Anzalone, M. (2001). *Sensory Integration and Self Regulation in Infants and Toddlers.* Washington, DC: National Center for Infants, Toddlers and Families.

Wuhle, A., Mertiens, L., Ruter, J., Ostwald, D., & Braun, C. (2010). Cortical processing of near-threshold tactile stimuli: An MEG study. *Psychophysiology, 47,* 523–534.

Yochman, A., Parush, S., & Ornoy, A. (2004). Responses of preschool children with and without ADHD to sensory events in daily life. *American Journal of Occupational Therapy, 58,* 294–302.

10

Measurement of Touch Behavior

SANDRA J. WEISS AND SANDRA K. NIEMANN

Although interest in the measurement of touch perception emerged in the early 1800s with the work of Ernst Weber (Weber, 1834/1978), efforts to measure touch behavior did not arise until the 1950s. At that time, there was growing recognition that nonverbal communication was a profound factor in human relationships. The development of specific methods to measure tactile behavior was catalyzed by Frank's (1957) seminal monograph on the role of touching in human interaction, combined with new conceptualizations regarding methods to measure proxemics and kinesics (Birdwhistell, 1952; Hall, 1959). Substantial progress has occurred in designing measures of touch behavior from that time until now. This chapter provides an overview of these methods, including measures focused solely on tactile behavior as well as measures that include a touch subscale or touch component within a broader assessment of interaction or behavior. Recommendations to advance the sound measurement of touch are offered.

STRUCTURED MEASURES OF TOUCH BEHAVIOR

Most structured measures of touch behavior involve detailed systems for identifying and differentiating characteristics of touch that are observed in dyadic interaction. These systems entail prior training for those who will record the touch either in real time or from videotaped records of the interaction. However, a few measures use self-report to identify the nature of the individual's own touch behavior or touch that they receive from others.[1] The largest group of structured measures focuses on touch used in parent–child interaction. A second set of measures addresses touch used by adults with their peers. One measure examines touch behavior of nurses in health care relationships. Lastly, a few have the potential to assess touch used by anyone. See Table 10.1 for an overview of these measures.

Measures of Parent–Child Touch

Measures described below that assess maternal-infant touch involve behavioral coding of videotaped interactions during a structured situation called the still-face procedure (Tronick, Als, Adamson, Wise, Brazelton, 1978). One of these measures focuses on infant touch and two focus on maternal touch. A fourth measure of parent–child touch is a retrospective questionnaire regarding the touch a person remembers receiving as a child.

Infant Touch Scale. The Infant Touch Scale (ITS) has two distinct components. The core component of the measure, called the ITS, examines the type and location of touch used by infants during mother–infant interaction (Moszkowski & Stack, 2007). Seven categories of touch type are examined, including (1) static touch, (2) rub/caress/wipe/stroke, (3) grasp/clutch/clasp, (4) finger/manipulate/scrumble/poke/prod, (5) mouth, (6) pat/tap, and (7) pull/push/lift. Locations of touch include five categories of infant self-touch (face/head/neck area, mouth, hand/arm, feet/leg, and trunk) as well as instances of touching the mother or other objects (e.g., chair, clothing). Investigators reported the kappa coefficients for inter-rater agreement in categorizing types of touch as 0.80 and 0.84 for agreement on location of infant touch (Moszkowski, Stack, & Chiarella, 2009a). Although no formal validity testing has been reported, findings of studies indicate predictive validity of the measure. For instance, infants used more self-touch during still-face episodes of the data collection when they would be predicted to experience greater distress, supporting the sensitivity of the measure to contextual changes. Investigators viewed the infant's increased self-touching as attempts to self-sooth (Moszkowski et al., 2009a).

---

[1] Some of the self-report measures in the previous chapter (Measurement of Tactile Response and Tactile Perception) have certain items regarding personal use of touch or experiences with touch. However, those items contribute primarily to a better understanding of the individual's general comfort with touch or attitudes toward touch.

TABLE 10.1 Structured measures of touch

Measure	Dimensions of Touch	Method	Population Using Touch
Face-to-Face Touch Coding System (Koester et al., 2000)	Type Location Intensity Duration	Behavioral Coding	Parents
Functions of Touch Scale (Jean & Stack, 2009)	Function	Behavioral Coding	Parents
Infant Touch Scale (Moszkowski & Stack, 2007)	Type Location	Behavioral Coding	Infants
Functions of Infant Touch Scale (Chiarella, 2006; Moszkowski et al., 2009a)	Function Location	Behavioral Coding	Infants
Live Tactile Interaction Body Chart (Andersen & Guerrero, 2005; Guerrero & Andersen, 1991)	Frequency Duration	Behavioral Coding	Any Population
Observation Schedule for Nurse–Patient Touch (Oliver & Redfern, 1991; Porter et al., 1986)	Type Location Intensity Duration Context	Behavioral Coding	Nurses
Recollections of Early Childhood Touch Scale (Jones & Brown, 1996)	Amount	Self Report Questionnaire	Parents
Tactile Interaction Index (Weiss, 1992, 2000)	Action Location Intensity Duration Frequency Type Pattern	Behavioral Coding	Any Population
Tie Signs Coding Sheet and Functions Measure (Afifi & Johnson, 1999; 2005)	Type Intensity Function	Behavioral Coding Self Report Questionnaire	Adults
Touch Log Record (Jones 2005; Jones & Yarbrough, 1985)	Type Location Meaning Context Response	Self Report Log	Adults

A second component of the ITS is called the **Functions of Infant Touch Scale** (FITS; Chiarella, 2006; Moszkowski et al., 2009a). Functional categories of touch in the FITS are based on the communicative context accompanying each type of touch in the ITS. For example, soothing-regulatory touch is identified as a function that includes touch such as self-stroking or mouthing with the finger in an attempt to calm the self. A dysregulated function is described as using any type of touch while also crying. There are two published versions of the FITS, one having 11 categories of function (Moszkowski et al., 2009a) and the other having 8 categories (Moszkowski et al., 2009b). The latter version appears to combine certain functions of infant touch, such as different forms of play. The 11-item version includes intense play, light play, passive play, quiet acceptance, soothing-regulatory, reactive-regulatory/attention-seeking, exploratory, regulatory exploratory, dysregulated, partial engaged, and disengaged. The observer can also code "no apparent function." Investigators reported the kappa coefficient for inter-rater agreement of the FITS to be 0.94 (Moszkowski et al., 2009a). Previous research support for the measure's predictive validity has been shown by findings that infants demonstrated more reactive and dysregulated functions of touch during laboratory-based procedures when they were separated from their mothers (Moszkowski et al., 2009b). Research has also shown that maternal sensitivity predicted more playful and less disengaged touch among infants; in contrast, maternal hostility predicted more disengaged infant touch (Moszkowski et al., 2009a). While coding of the ITS occurs without sound to minimize contextual biases, the FITS is coded with sound because its operational definitions take the full context of interaction into consideration. Infants on whom the measure has been tested are primarily Caucasion and range from 4 to 6 months of age.

Functions of Touch Scale. Jean and Stack (2009) developed this measure to assess the functions of touch used by mothers with their infants, specifically the length of time mothers spent using each of nine tactile functions. Data were based upon videotapes of mothers and infants during a still-face procedure in the home. The measure's potential relevance to other maternal-child situations has not been described. The functions examined were (1) passive accompaniment (static touch that occurs along with another communication modality—such as verbal—when touch is not the focus), (2) active accompaniment (e.g., lifting or grabbing the infant in conjunction with another communication modality when touch is not the focus), (3) nurturing touch, (4) playful touch (e.g., to make the infant smile or laugh), (5) attention-getting touch, (6) accidental touch, (7) utilitarian touch (accomplishing a task), (8) harsh or negative touch (e.g., controlling, intrusive), and (9) touch with no apparent function. Like the FITS described earlier, the co-occurring context of other behaviors was considered important in coding the functions of maternal touch. The measure has been tested with mothers of infants who were ~5½ months old. No formal validity testing was described. Mothers used more nurturing touch when infants were distressed, providing some support for this functional category. Percent of inter-rater agreement across categories was 87.5.

Face-to-Face Touch Coding System. This measure of maternal touch (Koester, Brooks, & Traci, 2000) was developed to examine type, location, intensity, and duration of touch used by deaf mothers and their infants. Touch was assessed during warm-up and recovery periods of the still-face procedure. Types include (1) passive (no movement), (2) active (any movement such as tapping or stroking), (3) a combination of active and passive touch involving use of both hands, and (4) moving of the infant's limbs or body. Four location areas are identified: head/face, torso, arms/hands, or feet/legs. Intensity of touch has two levels: gentle/mild or strong/vigorous. Although not a primary focus of the measure, durations of less than 1 second, 1–10 seconds, and more than 10 seconds were also coded. The measure has been tested with both hearing and deaf mothers of 3- and 6-month-old infants who were primarily Caucasian. There is evidence of discriminant validity based on differences in type, location, intensity, and duration of touch depending on hearing status of both mother and infant. Inter-rater reliability was 84.7% for type of touch, 97.8% for location, and 77% for intensity.

Recollections of Early Childhood Touch Scale. This measure was developed to assess characteristics of early childhood touch from parents (or other salient primary caregivers) through retrospective self-report (Jones & Brown, 1996). The items were adapted from an early scale of familial touch orientation developed by Gladney and Barker (1979). The Recollections of Early Childhood Touch Scale is a 10-item questionnaire in which both male and female parents/caretakers are rated separately. Items acquire information on the general use or amount of touch received from these individuals when the respondent was a child. Questions address areas such as being kissed or hugged when leaving for school, having their hand held by the caretaker in a public place, sitting in the caretaker's lap, and getting a back rub or soothing touch at bedtime. The items yield scores for the likelihood that an individual's caretakers used touch as a typical part of the parent–child interaction.

Testing of the measure with college students showed that it had adequate internal consistency reliability for sections regarding both male (0.85) and female (0.83) caretakers and that the scores for these two sections correlated significantly with one another. Predictive validity of the measure was supported by its relationship to the attitudes of students who completed the scale regarding their comfort with touching and being touched. Their actual use of touch as adults (measured by behavioral logs) was correlated only with the component of the questionnaire measuring the touch received as a child from their mother (or female caretaker).

Touch Between Health Professionals and Patients

The Observation Schedule for Nurse–Patient Touch. This measure was initially developed by Porter, Redfern, Wilson-Barnett, and Le May (1986) to assess the touch between staff nurses and patients in a hospital setting. The schedule identified (1) type of touch as expressive or instrumental, (2) who initiated the touch, (3) when it occurred during the course of the encounter (e.g., approach, separation), (4) patient and nurse position when the touch occurred (e.g., laying down, walking), (5) location of touch on a body map, (6) intensity of touch, (7) duration of the touch, and (8) the response of the person being touched (none, positive, or negative). An open-ended section was also included to describe the accompanying verbal communication. Kappas for interobserver reliability ranged between 0.31 for intensity and 0.72 for type of touch.

In a later revision of the schedule (Le May & Redfern, 1987; Oliver & Redfern, 1991), the intensity measure was eliminated because of its poor reliability in previous testing. Investigators also modified the open-ended section describing the verbal interaction, replacing it with boxes that are checked for specific types of accompanying verbal communication during the touch (i.e., silence, treatment-oriented discussion, social chatting; emotional/psychosocial care). The refined version included 4 options for type of touch, 13 locations of touch, and 9 specific options for response to the touch (e.g., reciprocal touch, smile, cry). Testing of this version was performed in a setting with elderly patients, during 5-minute periods of nurse–patient interaction (Oliver & Redfern, 1991). Although the measure was developed to assess touch initiated by either patient or nurse, only the nurses' touch of patients was measured in this study. The section on type of touch achieved a kappa coefficient of 0.65. Inter-rater agreement on area of

CHAPTER 10   MEASUREMENT OF TOUCH BEHAVIOR   251

the body touched was 0.79 and 0.95 for patient response to the touch. No psychometric data addressing validity of either the original measure or its revisions were reported.

Measures of Adult–Adult Touch

Two measures have been developed specifically for adult touching in public places. One of these entails an individual logging his/her own touch interactions while the other involves observation of dyads by a trained rater in conjunction with a self-report component.

Touch Log Record.   The Touch Log Record and Observation Form (Jones, 2005; Jones & Yarbrough, 1985) is a participant observation technique to measure touch between adult dyads in public places. Individuals are trained to record events in which they are actually involved over a specified period of time. In the initial long version, participants were asked to record all touch events they experienced over a 3-day period, completing a standard observation form immediately after each touch occurred. The form acquires data on who initiates the touch, its degree of mutuality, areas of the body touched, and type of touch. Areas of the body touched are marked on a body diagram initially developed by Jourard (1966). The types of touch are based upon a tactility scale developed by Hall (1963) and include options such as handshake, accidental brushing against the other person, and prolonged holding. Information on a variety of contextual factors such as place of meeting and nature of the relationship is also acquired. As part of the initial instrument, investigators asked participants to give a verbal label to the meaning of each touch event. On the basis of these data, they identified 12 "distinct and unambiguous" categories of meaning, such as showing support, appreciation, and affection. In the revised short form of the measure (Jones, 2005), eight categories of meaning are included for participants to select as descriptive of each touch event. It is not clear how these 8 categories were derived from the original 12. The revised short form asks for a written description of the body parts contacted rather than using the body diagram that was initially included. The categories for types of touch also differ from the original form and are more specific.

Testing of the original touch log showed a high percent of agreement for most parts of the log among coders who observed the filmed tactile interactions of others (Jones & Yarborough, 1985). Agreement regarding who initiated the touch, body parts contacted, degree of mutuality, and acceptance of the touch ranged from 94% to 100%. Agreement on specific types of touch was 69%. Initially, the intent of the measure was for use in coding one's own tactile behavior, and so this reliability assessment does not directly address reliability of an individual's coding of his/her own behavior. However, data on day-to-day stability of individuals' coding of their own touch was examined, with correlations ranging from 0.41 to 0.46 for total touches initiated and received (Jones, 2005). In a study of the relationship between attitudes toward touch and actual use of touch, no relationship was found between individuals' reported attitudes and the frequency of logged touch events on the original Touch Log Record (Jones & Brown, 1996). No testing has been reported for the revised, short version of the measure.

Tie Signs Coding Sheet and Functions Measure. The Tie Signs Coding Sheet, developed by Afifi and Johnson (1999), is based upon the initial work of Goffman (1971) and Morris (1971) who described "tie signs" as tactile displays or haptic behaviors that communicate intimacy with another person. They designed the measure to be used for naturalistic observation of adult dyadic touching in public settings. The behaviors in the Tie Signs Function and Coding Sheet are the 14 tie signs identified by Morris (1971) in his ethnographic studies, such as handshake, shoulder embrace, pat, kiss, and mock attack. The signs can be grouped into categories of moderately intimate (e.g., linking arms), intimate (e.g., hugging), and very intimate (e.g., leaning head against head). Overall agreement among trained coders for the various tie signs in the measure for a 15-minute period of observation in a cocktail bar was 95%. In a revised version (2005), the investigators have included a rating scale from 1 to 7 for the intensity of each tie sign. No testing was reported for this new scale.

Afifi and Johnson (1999, 2005) also developed a Tie Sign Functions Scale, a self-report questionnaire that measures seven functions of touch. These functions were taken from Patterson's typology of the purposes of nonverbal communication, including items such as affect management, expressing intimacy, or social control (Patterson, 1988). The scale has seven Likert-type items, one for each function or purpose. Individuals are asked to rate each function for its applicability to the 14 tie signs. Typically, they are approached after observation and coding of their touch with the Tie Signs Coding Sheet to acquire consent to use their observational data. They are then asked if they would be willing to complete the Tie Signs Function Scale. In this way, investigators can combine public observations with self-report. The function scale acquires information, for example, about the degree to which a person would use a shoulder embrace to influence or control a person (i.e., the social control function of touch). The content validity of the functions was established in two studies in which individuals were asked the reasons that they used certain tie signs and why they thought that others had touched them. These qualitative data supported inclusion of the seven categories of tie sign functions in the measure. No data on reliability of the tie signs function measure was reported.

Measures of Touch With the Potential for Use Across Populations

Two measures of touch have applicability for use with a variety of age groups and relationships. One of these involves identification of touch characteristics from videotapes of a dyad either during structured situations or during spontaneous interaction. In the other measure, observers record real-time touch that occurs between dyads.

The Tactile Interaction Index. The Tactile Interaction Index (TII; Weiss, 1992, 2000) identifies characteristics associated with five qualities of touch: intensity, location, action, duration, and frequency of touch. Scores for these initial qualities of touch are then combined to create a variety of other conceptually important scores for types of touch and patterns of touch. The intensity index allows for coding of touch as strong, moderate, or light based on the degree of pressure to the skin. Deep intensity was initially included as a fourth category but eliminated in a later version because of difficulty differentiating deep and strong intensity. The location index specifies 19 different areas of the body that can be touched, such as abdomen, hand, or neck. Depending on the age of the person being studied, these locations are based upon body diagrams for an infant, child, or adult. The action index identifies different gestures or movements that can be used in touching (e.g., grab, push, rub, squeeze, or contact without movement). Ongoing testing has refined the measure by increasing the original number of actions from 21 to 28. The duration index determines the overall length of time a person uses touch throughout an observation period and the frequency index is the actual number of touches that occur, using number of tactile actions as the basis for what constitutes a single touch. These dimensions are coded from DVDs or videotapes using either slow motion or real-time microanalysis.

From raw scores on these initial qualities, eight types of touch can be determined. These types may have relevance for specific research programs where their effects on development or health are being studied or certain cultural values are being examined. From the location index, scores for (1) touch of highly innervated body areas (densely packed with many nerve endings, such as the face, hands, or feet) and (2) extent of contact with various areas of another person's body are identified (i.e., the number of locations touched out of the total 19 possible). From the action index, types of touch that can be scored are (3) nurturing or comforting touch (e.g., kissing, stroking), (4) harsh or painful touch (e.g., slap, hit), (5) cutaneous touch, involving sensations only on the surface of the skin (e.g., contact without movement), (6) proprioceptive touch, where stimulation affects deeper tissue, muscles, and joints (e.g., rubbing), (7) vestibular touch, with sensations affecting body alignment or position (e.g., lifting), and (8) diverse or varied touch (i.e., the number of different actions that are used out of the 28 possible).

Lastly, four patterns of touch can be determined from initial scores for quality and type of touch. Stimulating touch is computed by summing scores for (a) touching of body areas that are highly innervated, (b) use of strong intensity, and (c) actions involving proprioceptive sensation. Complexity of touch is identified by summing scores for (a) extent of body locations touched and (b) diversity of the actions used in touching. The affective nature of touch is the percent of nurturing/comforting touch that is used versus actions of a harsh or painful nature. Lastly, the overall amount of touch is the product of initial scores for duration and frequency.

The measure has been used in a variety of videotaped situations, including infant feeding and teaching, structured play with children, health care procedures in the intensive care unit, and spontaneous interactions in the home or laboratory setting. It requires training and employs a coding manual and videotape exemplars of various qualities of touch. Initial psychometric data supported content, concurrent and construct validity as well as inter-observer and retest reliability; this testing was based on a diverse sample of adults who were touching their children, friends, or spouses/partners (Weiss, 1990, 1992). More recent psychometric data with parents and infants supports the continuing reliability of the five qualities of touch in the measure as well as the validity of the tactile types and patterns generated with the measure. For instance, maternal use of touch that is more stimulating to the infant's nervous system is associated with better visual and motor development for the infant. In addition, use of more nurturing touch by mothers differentiates infants who have more secure attachment from those who do not (Weiss & Goebel, 2003; Weiss, Wilson, Hertenstein, & Campos, 2000; Weiss, Wilson, & Morrison, 2004; Weiss, Wilson, St. Jonn-Seed, & Paul, 2001).

Live Tactile Interaction Body Chart. This instrument was developed to measure the frequency, location, and duration of real-time touching that occurs between adult dyads in public places (Guerrero & Andersen, 1991, 1994). A picture is used as the basis of coding, with 13 areas of the body shown on a body chart. The measure involves tallying locations of any touch that occurs during each 10-second interval. Two different individuals code the dyad's touch, with each individual tallying touch events for one member of the dyad being observed. Coding periods typically occur for 2-minute blocks of time. The number of 10-second periods during which touch occurs determines duration. The number of tallies in each body area of the chart provides data on location and frequency.

Inter-rater reliability for the total body chart ranges from 0.88 to 0.99. Agreement on each of the specific body areas ranges from 0.90 to complete agreement. Convergent, divergent, and predictive validity of the chart also have been supported (Andersen & Guerrero, 2005). For example, scores for individuals on their touch avoidance are negatively related to frequency of touch shown on the body chart in real-time situations (Guerrero & Andersen, 1991). In addition, significant differences in body chart scores have been found for various cultural groups and nationalities (McDaniel & Andersen, 1998). Although this measure was developed for use with adults, its dimensions and methods have relevance for any age group.

STRUCTURED MEASURES WITH A TOUCH SUBSCALE

A number of instruments have subscales focused on tactile behavior, although their overall purpose is to measure broader aspects of interaction. The major emphasis of measures which have touch subscales is to examine harsh or abusive parenting practices. In the section that follows, these measures are divided into subsections for those measuring current parenting practices and those reporting on past parenting. In addition, one measure was designed to assess conflict behavior between adult partners. Another measure evaluates affectionate communication; it has relevance for a variety of dyadic relationships. Table 10.2 provides an overview of these assessments.

TABLE 10.2 Measures with a touch subscale

Measure	Dimensions of Touch	Method	Population Using Touch
Affectionate Communication Index (Floyd & Morman, 1998)	Affectionate touch	Self Report Questionnaire	Adults
Alabama Parenting Questionnaire (Frick, 1991)	Corporal punishment	Self Report Questionnaire Phone Interviews With Parent and Child	Parents
Assessing Environments (Berger et al., 1988)	Physical punishment	Self Report Questionnaire	Parents
Childhood Experience of Care and Abuse Questionnaire (Smith et al., 2002)	Physical abuse Sexual abuse	Self Report Questionnaire	Parents
Childhood Trauma Questionnaire (Bernstein et al., 2003)	Physical abuse Sexual abuse	Self Report Questionnaire	Parents
Comprehensive Child Maltreatment Scale for Adults (Higgins & McCabe, 2001)	Physical abuse Sexual abuse	Self Report Questionnaire	Parents
Conflict Tactics Scale (Straus et al., 1996)	Physical assault	Self Report Questionnaire	Adults
Daily Discipline Interview (Webster-Stratton & Spitzer, 1991)	Physical punishment	Parent Phone Interview	Parents
Dyadic Parent-Child Interaction Coding System, 3rd ed. (Eyberg et al., 2004)	Negative touch Positive touch	Behavioral Coding	Parents Children
Early Trauma Inventory (Bremner et al., 2007)	Physical punishment Sexual abuse	Self Report Questionnaire	Parents
Parent–Child Conflict Tactics Scales (Straus et al., 1998)	Physical assault	Self Report Questionnaire	Parents

Harsh or Negative Current Parenting Practices

Alabama Parenting Questionnaire. The overall purpose of this measure is to assess parenting practices with children who have disruptive behavior problems (Frick, 1991). The instrument includes a parent questionnaire and telephone interviews. It has a subscale on corporal punishment that asks parents about spanking, slapping, and hitting their child when he/she does something wrong. The alpha coefficient for internal consistency of the subscale was 0.81 and stability of responses across interviews was also 0.81 for the subscale. Good convergent and predictive validity also have been reported for the subscale using both questionnaire and interview formats. However, the subscale has shown a positive correlation with a measure of social desirability. The measure has been used with families who have children between 6 and 16 years of age. Some of these families were referred to a mental health clinic for their children's disruptive behavior while others were controls from the community (Shelton, Frick, & Wootton, 1996).

Daily Discipline Interview. Disciplinary approaches used by parents are examined with this tool (Webster-Stratton & Spitzer, 1991). Data are collected through phone interviews that are conducted regarding child misbehavior in the past 24-hour period. The interview has a subscale on physical force that asks about behaviors such as spanking, slapping, hitting, kicking, dragging, restraining, and pushing the child. It has been used with mothers of children who are 3–7 years of age. The total interview has shown construct validity. Inter-rater reliability is 0.94. Test–retest reliability is 0.45 and the reliability coefficient for internal consistency is 0.62. The physical force subscale has shown predictive validity with child behavior problems and has been correlated with mother's verbal criticism of the child in a laboratory observation.

Dyadic Parent–Child Interaction Coding System. This measure identifies the quality of parent–child interactions and was developed initially for use with families whose children had conduct problems (Eyberg, Nelson, Duke, & Boggs, 2004; Robinson & Eyberg, 1981). It is currently in its third edition, having been revised and expanded over time. It contains 25 categories that can be coded from videotaped interactions between a parent and a child, including vocalizations, verbalizations, and physical behaviors of both members of the dyad. The section on physical behaviors focuses entirely on touch that occurs within the parent–child dyad. Touches that occur are coded as either positive or negative touch, with neutral touches rated as positive. Only intentional touches are measured; accidental touches are not included. The manual provides examples of negative and positive touch used by parent and child as well as decision rules for situations that may present dilemmas in coding. For example, a negative touch by a parent would involve dragging the child by the arm or shaking the child. A positive touch by a child might involve putting an arm around a parent or playfully poking the parent's nose.

The psychometric data for the overall measure indicate good interrater reliability (means of 0.91 for parent behavior and 0.92 for child behavior). Discriminate validity has consistently been shown in distinguishing families with conduct problems from those without these problems. In general, convergent validity is also evident for the measure (Eyberg et al., 2004). Psychometric data specific to the touch subscale was not available.

Parent–Child Conflict Tactics Scale. This parent questionnaire measures different dimensions of maltreatment of the child (Straus, Hamby, Finkelhor, Moore, & Runyan, 1998), including a physical assault scale. The physical assault scale has items that reflect minor assault (e.g., shaking, spanking with bare hand), severe assault (e.g., slapping face, hitting with fist), and very severe assault (e.g., choking, burning, beating). There are supplemental questions that can be used on sexual touch. This scale assesses parental behavior during the past year, with either parents or children as respondents. The measure has been tested with diverse children of all ages as well as with adult children who recall earlier behavior of their parents. It has shown construct and discriminant validity. The internal consistency reliability of the physical assault scale is 0.55.

Harsh or Negative Past Parenting Practices

Assessing Environments. This measure examines punitive childhood experiences as recalled by adolescents or adults (Berger, Knutson, Mehm, & Perkins, 1988). It has a physical punishment scale that includes items such as being spanked, hit with objects or the parent's hand, punched, kicked, or severely beaten. Content validity and discriminant validity are reported for the physical punishment scale, with the measure differentiating children who were reported to social services for physical injuries from abuse. Internal consistency coefficients for the scales range from 0.65 to 0.79, with test–retest reliability ranging from 0.61 to 0.89. The measure was tested with college students.

Childhood Experience of Care and Abuse Questionnaire. This self-report questionnaire screens for past childhood adversity among adults (Smith, Lam, Bifulco, & Checkley, 2002). It has a physical abuse subscale that starts with yes/no items about being hit, punched, kicked, or burnt by someone in the household, followed by questions about the nature of the event(s). There is also a sexual abuse subscale that uses a similar approach. The measure has shown concurrent validity with the previous interview form. Test–retest reliability for the physical abuse scale was 0.83, and it correctly identified 93.3% of the cases of severe abuse identified through clinician interview. The sexual abuse scale has shown similarly high levels of agreement. Testing occurred with adults who have affective disorders.

Childhood Trauma Questionnaire. This self-report, short version of the measure screens for history of maltreatment (Bernstein et al., 2003). It has a physical abuse subscale that assesses tactile behaviors such as being hit so hard that it left bruises or marks. Confirmatory factor analysis showed a good fit for the subscale items across diverse samples. The physical abuse scale has demonstrated criterion validity with interviews administered by clinicians and with ratings by therapists for incidence of sexual and physical abuse. Coefficients for internal consistency of the physical abuse subscale have ranged from 0.81 to 0.86. Test–retest reliability over 3–6 months is 0.80. The measure also has a sexual abuse subscale that has shown excellent reliability. The questionnaire has been tested with adults who have mental health problems as well as community controls.

Comprehensive Child Maltreatment Scales for Adults. This measure assesses five types of maltreatment, including physical and sexual abuse (Higgins & McCabe, 2001). It is used to acquire retrospective reports of childhood experience as well as reports from parents about the current maltreatment of their own 5- to 12-year-old children. Both versions have shown adequate test–retest reliability (0.92) and internal consistency for each of the subscales (0.66–0.88). The subscales were also significantly correlated with related subscales of the Child Abuse Trauma Scale. The measure was developed and tested mostly with women who were involved in community and health organizations.

Early Trauma Inventory. This self-report questionnaire assesses history of maltreatment before the age of 18 (Bremner, Bolus, & Mayer, 2007). The physical punishment subscale asks questions about being slapped, burned, punched or kicked, hit with an object, pushed, or shoved. There also is a subscale on sexual events involving touch. The measure has shown discriminant validity for patients with known trauma history. Both the physical abuse and sexual abuse subscales have been correlated with measures of post-traumatic stress severity. All subscales have good internal consistency. The physical abuse subscale has an alpha coefficient of 0.78 and 0.91 for the sexual abuse scale. Testing of the measure has occurred with both healthy adults and those with known trauma and psychiatric disorders.

Conflict Between Adult Partners

Revised Conflict Tactics Scale. This questionnaire measures psychological and physical attacks between partners and their use of reasoning and negotiation to deal with conflicts (Straus, Hamby, Boney-McCoy, & Sugarman, 1996). Questions are asked about behaviors of both the respondent and his/her dating, cohabiting, or marital partner. The subscale on physical assault is constituted entirely of items specific to touch behavior. There is also a subscale for sexual coercion, with a few touch-related items. Construct and discriminant validity have been demonstrated. Internal consistency for subscales ranges from 0.79 to 0.95, with the physical assault scale having an alpha of 0.86. Testing has taken place with a broad-based and diverse sample.

Affectionate Communication

Affectionate Communication Index. This index was originally developed from a grounded theory study that interviewed respondents about the ways in which they communicated affection with people considered to be close relationships (Floyd & Morman, 1998). From that study, items were generated for the Affectionate Communication Index. It has three subscales that measure verbal expressions of affection, nonverbal (tactile) expression of affection, and social support behaviors. Items in the nonverbal subscale assess behaviors such as hugging, holding hands, sitting close to another, and kissing on the cheek. Each item is rated on a 7-point scale from "never" to "almost always."

The measure has been tested with adult males who have described affection toward their fathers and sons, as well as with both genders to describe affection toward their mothers, fathers, siblings, romantic partners, and friends. The touch subscale has shown internal consistency of 0.74 to 0.87 in various studies (Floyd & Mikkelson, 2005). The investigators report evidence of construct validity based upon confirmatory factor analysis (Floyd & Morman, 2000). Evidence of convergent, discriminant, and predictive validity is also summarized across a number of studies (Floyd & Mikkelson, 2005). For instance, the non-verbal (tactile) subscale has been associated with degree of involvement, satisfaction, and closeness with others. It has also discriminated between father's expression of tactile affection for their biological, adopted, and step sons.

OTHER MEASURES OF TOUCH BEHAVIOR

In addition to the measures described earlier, a variety of observational coding procedures and other questionnaires provide useful information regarding touch. These coding procedures typically integrate selected aspects of other touch measures or may not undergo comprehensive validity and reliability testing. Even so, they often provide valuable data regarding touch that helps investigators address their specific research aims. Certain questionnaires exist which are not developed to directly measure touch but do incorporate touch items. Examples of both types of measures are briefly described in the next section.

Coding Procedures for Observation of Touch Behavior

Numerous coding procedures for touch behavior have been developed as part of individual studies in developmental, social, and health care research. Some of these procedures are entirely focused on touch while others are part of larger assessments of more general behavior. Tactile coding systems in the developmental field have examined touch in parenting behavior with infants (Feldman, Eidelman, Sirota, & Weller, 2002; Ferber, Feldman, & Makhoul, 2008; Gordon, Zagoory-Sharon, Leckman, & Feldman, 2010; Herrera, Reissland, & Shepherd, 2004; Hsu & Fogel, 2003; Kaitz, Zvi, Levy, Berger, & Eidelman, 1995; Main & Stadtman, 1981; Millot, Filiatre, & Montagner, 1988) as well as changes in infant touch behavior as a function of development (Toda & Fogel, 1993). Coding procedures have also been designed to study patterns of family tactile interaction (Oveis, Gruber, Keltner, Stamper, & Boyce, 2009), peer and self-touch in adolescents (Field, 1999), and touch between college students (Goldberg & Rosenthal, 1986; Hertenstein, Holmes, McCullough, & Keltner, 2009; Hertenstein, Keltner, App, Bulient, & Jaskolka, 2006). Other coding procedures characterize touch between adult friends and partners (Guerrero, 1997, 2005; Julien, 2005), touch during interactions of health professionals and their patients (Barnett, 1972; Caris-Verhallen, Kerkstra, & Bensing, 1999; Gorawara-Bhat, Cook, & Sachs, 2007; Harrigan, 1985; Routasalo & Lauri, 1996), and adult touching of acquaintances or strangers in a variety of different professional and public settings (Goldstein & Jeffords, 1981;

Hall, 1996; Knofler & Imhof, 2007; Major, Schmidlin, & Williams, 1990; Shuter, 1976). These coding procedures examine many of the characteristics of touch discussed under earlier measures such as type and function of touch as well as its location, duration, and frequency. They typically involve training of observers to perform the coding and reliability testing to assure intercoder agreement.

Questionnaires That Involve Touch Items

A number of questionnaires with selected touch items exist. For instance, the Parent Behavior Inventory (Lovejoy, Weis, O'Hare, & Rubin, 1999) includes items regarding rough handling, spanking, hugging, or kissing the child, and touching the child affectionately. These are incorporated into subscales of hostile/coercive parenting behavior or supportive/engaged behavior. Another assessment of parent discipline, the Coercive Discipline Scale, also includes items related to physical punishment (Fagot, 1992). Parents use this scale to make choices regarding interventions they would select to handle child misbehaviors shown in videotapes. In a study of interpersonal touch experiences, a few Likert-type items were created to elicit the recall of college students regarding how often they had been touched by parents and peers during preschool and at different points during school age years (Takeuchi et al., 2010). Through this approach, investigators attempted to assess the touch experienced by individuals at various times during their development. Lastly, questionnaires have been developed to examine children's exposure to sexual abuse or the responses of adults to scenarios regarding sexual consent. Examples of these measures include the Checklist of Sexual Abuse and Related Symptoms (Spaccarelli, 1995), the Child Sexual Behavior Inventory (Friedrich et al., 1992), the Sexual Consent Scale (Hickman & Muehlenhard, 1999), and the Same-Sex Sexual Consent Scale (Beres, Herold, & Maitland, 2004). Such measures include items specific to sexual touch.

IMPLICATIONS FOR FUTURE MEASUREMENT OF TOUCH BEHAVIOR

Strengths in the Measurement of Touch

There has been substantial progress over the last few decades in the development and testing of measures that examine touch behavior.

Significant growth can be seen in the developmental and psychiatric fields where a number of observational and questionnaire methods have been designed to assess parent–child touch in current and past relationships. Assessments of current touch behavior are most prominent in the parent–infant relationship where measures can contribute to knowledge about the effects of parent touch on psychosocial and physical development of infants. In addition, new retrospective measures of harsh or punitive touch offer many psychometrically sound assessments from which to choose. The rich array of measures that examine physical punishment and abuse will enable researchers to more effectively identify the impact of early adversity on varied aspects of health and psychosocial function.

There has also been a growing trend to use behavioral indicators to study touch behavior rather than relying on self-report. This methodological advance helps to reduce potential bias that can occur with reliance only on self-report, enabling a multimethod approach to knowledge development that integrates subjective and objective data. Behavioral measures also are improving our ability to look at detailed characteristics of touch in both parent–child and adult–adult interactions. Slow motion and/or repeated observation of digitally preserved interactions makes possible more reliable assessment of dimensions of touch that are particularly challenging to measure. These new methods also allow for examination of multiple characteristics of touch that occur during one interaction, such as type, location, duration, context, and function. Such systems, while being resource intensive, are essential for understanding the nuanced properties of touch that may be associated with a variety of developmental, neurobiological, and psychosocial outcomes. Creative methods are also being used to acquire touch data, including phone interviews, participant observation, and response to video-based scenarios and vignettes.

In addition to these more detailed assessments, brief measures are available. At times, feasibility and efficiency may be important criteria for selecting a measure. This wide repertoire of methods available for studying touch will improve the quality and scope of what is measured as well as increase the portability and acceptability of measurement across the varied settings and contexts where touch occurs.

Facets of Touch Measurement That Deserve More Attention

Although some measures of touch behavior have solid theoretical grounding, the presence of a conceptual foundation is often missing. This leaves the field vulnerable to a focus on characteristics or even dimensions of touch that may lack validity. Similarly, refinements or revisions of measures are often not informed by empirical evidence or theoretical advances that indicate needed changes in items or categories of the measure.

A number of investigators have incorporated dimensions related to the functions or purpose of touch into their measurement tools. While this is an important contribution to touch measurement, there is a critical need for measures that assess aspects of meaning beyond function. For example, attempts to identify the specific emotions communicated through touch are an excellent basis for tool development (e.g., Hertenstein et al., 2006, 2009). Efforts to differentiate and measure the emotional and cognitive dimensions of the tactile message are needed. In addition, it is improbable that the type of touch alone will determine its meaning. Instead, unique combinations of the action, intensity, duration, and location of a touch will most likely create specific meaning for a particular touch. Understanding the language of touch will also require measuring the process of the tactile encounter. How it progresses from initiation to termination, the role of both participants in that progression, and their accompanying responses to touch must be examined. Some of the measures described in this chapter provide excellent groundwork for studying these contextual factors.

Increased focus on measurement of positive or rewarding characteristics of touch is also needed. As noted earlier, extensive progress has occurred in development of measures that examine negative or punitive touch. In contrast, few measures attempt to define and assess detailed qualities of nurturing or comforting touch that may have important implications for resilience and optimal well-being. Similarly, tactile deprivation requires careful, operational definition. Adequate measurement of tactile deprivation or neglect will involve far more than the absence or infrequency of touch. For instance, minimal use of stimulating or complex patterns of touch could constitute certain forms of deprivation, regardless of the amount of overall touch that is used.

Few efforts have been made to identify the role of factors such as gender, age, culture, and health status in the validity of touch measurement. Dimensions of touch are often included in a measure without apparent consideration of these issues. Likewise, the context or structure for measuring touch behavior is often assumed to be appropriate across populations. What ethnic or cultural implications might exist when measuring touch behavior during the still-face procedure or in very public situations such as a cocktail bar? How might gender, age, or culture differentially influence touch responses in videotaped situations or self-report of disciplinary practices? Greater emphasis also may be needed in development of measures appropriate for non-normative or special populations, with attention to unique dimensions of touch or tailored procedures that consider disability or health status.

Touch measures that have applicability for specific age groups are limited. Although a number of measures focus on infancy and young adulthood, few measures assess unique aspects of touch behavior during the elementary school years, adolescence, middle age, and old age. Methods to assess the touch used by children and adolescents are rare. Yet the child's tactile behavior plays an important role in the parent–child relationship, including its effects on the parent's touch behavior. In addition, touch that occurs between children or adolescents may have unique characteristics that have not been identified.

Enhanced focus on psychometric testing is essential. For many measures, especially various coding procedures for touch behavior, interrater reliability is often the only testing that is performed. As noted previously, greater conceptual grounding of tactile measures through content and construct validity testing would definitely strengthen the field. With the growth in availability of touch measures, concurrent and convergent validity testing is now very feasible. Validity testing should be expected as part of instrument development. Stability of touch measures is also rarely examined. Only a few investigators have identified the stability of observers' ratings of the same touch behavior on two or more occasions. Fewer yet have assessed the stability of a measure's reported or observed touch behavior for an individual over time in different situations.

Finally, efforts to use common, standardized measures whenever possible would serve the research community in furthering its measurement goals. New coding systems are frequently developed for a single study when measures that examine these same categories of touch exist. Rather than using existing questionnaires, new ones are designed which include items from previous questionnaires. While this tailoring of measures can be valuable and/or necessary at times, it can also result in duplication and preclude opportunities for more comprehensive testing of a core set of measures. By using common, standardized measures, results of varied studies can be compared and integrated more easily. In addition, measures can be more widely tested across diverse populations and settings. Ultimately, this cohesive, coordinated approach may advance knowledge regarding touch behavior at a greater pace.

REFERENCES

Affifi, W. A., & Johnson, M. L. (1999). The use and interpretation of tie signs in a public setting: Relationships and sex differences. *Journal of Social and Personal Relationships, 16,* 9–38.

Affifi, W. A., & Johnson, M. L. (2005). The nature and functions of tie-signs. In V. Manusov (Ed.), *The sourcebook of nonverbal measures: Going beyond words* (pp. 189–198). Mahwah, NJ: Lawrence Erlbaum.

Andersen, P. A., & Guerrero, L. K. (2005). Measuring live tactile interaction: The body chart coding approach. In V. Manusov (Ed.), *The sourcebook of nonverbal measures: Going beyond words* (pp. 83–92). Mahwah, NJ: Lawrence Erlbaum.

Barnett, K. (1972). A survey of the current utilization of touch by health team personnel with hospitalized patients. *International Journal of Nursing Studies, 9,* 195–209.

Beres, M. A., Herold, E., & Maitland, S. B. (2004). Sexual consent behaviors in same-sex relationships. *Archives of Sexual Behavior, 23,* 475–486.

Berger, A. M., Knutson, J. F., Mehm, J. G., & Perkins, K. A. (1988). The self-report of punitive childhood experiences of young adults and adolescents. *Child Abuse & Neglect, 12,* 251–262.

Bernstein, D. P., Stein, J. A., Newcomb, M. D., Walker, E., Pogge, D., Ahluvalia, T.,...Zule, W. (2003). Development and validation of a brief screening version of the Childhood Trauma Questionnaire. *Child Abuse & Neglect, 27,* 169–190.

Birdwhistell, R. L. (1952). *Introduction to kinesics.* Louisville, KY: University of Louisville Press.

Bremner, J. D., Bolus, R., & Mayer, E. A. (2007). Psychometric properties of the Early Trauma Inventory—Self Report. *The Journal of Nervous and Mental Disease, 195,* 211–218.

Caris-Verhallen, W., Kerkstra, A., & Bensing, J. M., (1999). Non-verbal behavior in nurse-elderly patient communication. *Journal of Advanced Nursing, 29,* 808–818.

Chiarella, S. S. (2006). *Functions of Infant Touch Scale* [Unpublished manuscript]. Montreal, Quebec, Canada: Concordia University.

Eyberg, S. M., Nelson, M. M., Duke, M., & Boggs, S. R. (2004). *Manual for the Dyadic Parent-Child Interaction Coding System* (3rd ed.). http://www.PCIT.org

Fagot, B. L. (1992). Assessment of coercive parent discipline. *Behavioral Assessment, 14,* 387–406.

Feldman, R., Eidelman, A., Sirota, L., & Weller, A. (2002). Comparison of skin to skin (kangaroo) and traditional care: Parenting outcomes and preterm infant development. *Pediatrics, 110,* 16–26.

Ferber, S. G., Feldman, R., & Makhoul, R. I. (2008). The development of maternal touch across the first year of life. *Early Human Development, 84,* 363–370.

Field, T. (1999). American adolescents touch each other less and are more aggressive toward their peers as compared with French adolescents. *Adolescence, 34,* 753–758.

Floyd, K., & Mikkelson, A. C. (2005). The Affectionate Communication Index. In V. Manusov (Ed.), *The sourcebook of nonverbal measures: Going beyond words* (pp. 47–55). Mahwah, NJ: Lawrence Erlbaum.

Floyd, K., & Morman, M. T. (1998). The measurement of affectionate communication. *Communication Quarterly, 46,* 144–162.

Floyd, K., & Morman, M. T. (2000). Affection received from fathers as a predictor of men's affection with their own sons: Tests of the modeling and compensation hypotheses. *Communication Monographs, 67,* 347–361.

Frank, L. K. (1957). Tactile communication. *Genetic Psychology Monographs, 56,* 209–255.

Frick, P. J. (1991). *The Alabama Parenting Questionnaire.* Unpublished rating scale, University of Alabama at Tuscaloosa.

Friedrich, W., Grambsch, P., Damon, L., Hewitt, S., Koverola, C., Lang, R.,... Broughton, D. (1992). Child Sexual Behavior Inventory: Normative and clinical comparisons. *Psychological Assessments, 4,* 303–311.

Gladney, K., & Barker, L. (1979). The effects of tactile history on attitudes toward and frequency of touching behavior. *Sign Language Studies, 24,* 231–252.

Goffman, E. (1971). *Relations in public places.* New York, NY: Basic Books.

Goldberg, S., & Rosenthal, R. (1986). Self-touching behavior in the job interview: Antecedents and consequences. *Journal of Nonverbal Behavior, 10,* 65–76.

Goldstein, A. G., & Jeffords, J. (1981). Status and touching behavior. *Bulletin of the Psychonomic Society, 17,* 79–81.

Gorawara-Bhat, R., Cook, M. A., & Sachs, G. A. (2007). Nonverbal communication in doctor-elderly patient transactions (NDEPT): Development of a tool. *Patient Education and Counseling, 66,* 223–234.

Gordon, I., Zagoory-Sharon, O., Leckman, J. F., & Feldman, R. (2010). Prolactin, oxytocin, and the development of paternal behavior across the first six months of fatherhood. *Hormones and Behavior, 58,* 513–518.

Guerrero, L. K. (1997). Nonverbal involvement across interactions with same-sex friends, opposite-sex friends, and romantic partners: Consistency or change? *Journal of Social and Personal Relationships, 14,* 31–58.

Guerrero, L. K. (2005). Observer ratings of nonverbal involvement and immediacy. In V. Manusov (Ed.), *The sourcebook of nonverbal measures: Going beyond words* (pp. 221–235). Mahwah, NJ: Lawrence Erlbaum.

Guerrero, L. K., & Andersen, P. A. (1991). The waxing and waning of relational intimacy: Touch as a function of relational stage, gender and touch avoidance. *Journal of Social and Personal Relationships, 8,* 147–165.

Guerrero, L. K., & Andersen, P. A. (1994). Patterns of matching and initiation: Touch behavior and avoidance across romantic relationship stages. *Journal of Nonverbal Behavior, 18,* 137–153.

Hall, E. T. (1959). *The silent language.* Garden City, NY: Doubleday.

Hall, E. T. (1963). A system for the notation of proxemic behavior. *American Anthropologist, 65,* 1003–1026.

Hall, J. A. (1996). Touch, status, and gender at professional meetings. *Journal of Nonverbal Behavior, 20,* 23–44.

Harrigan, J. A. (1985). Self-touching as an indicator of underlying affect and language processes. *Social Science & Medicine, 20,* 1161–1168.

Herrera, E., Reissland, N., & Shepherd, J. (2004). Maternal touch and maternal child-directed speech: Effects of depressed mood in the postnatal period. *Journal of Affective Disorders, 81,* 29–33.

Hertenstein, M. J., Holmes, R., McCullough, M., & Keltner, D. (2009). The communication of emotion via touch. *Emotion, 9,* 566–573.

Hertenstein, M. J., Keltner, D., App, B., Bulient, B. A., & Jaskolka, A. R. (2006). Touch communicates distinct emotions. *Emotion, 6,* 528–533.

Hickman, S. E., & Muehlenhard, C. L. (1999). "By the semi-mystical appearance of a condom": How young women and men communicate sexual consent in heterosexual situations. *Journal of Sex Research, 36,* 258–272.

Higgins, D. L., & McCabe, M. P. (2001). The development of the Comprehensive Child Maltreatment Scale. *Journal of Family Studies, 7,* 7–28.

Hsu, H., & Fogel, A. (2003). Social regulatory effects of infant nondistress vocalization on maternal behavior. *Developmental Psychology, 39,* 976–991.

Jean, A. D. L., & Stack, D. M. (2009). Functions of maternal touch and infants' affect during face-to-face interactions: New directions for the still-face. *Infant Behavior & Development, 32,* 123–128.

Jones, S. E. (2005). The Touch Log Record: A behavioral communication measure. In V. Manusov (Ed.), *The sourcebook of nonverbal measures: Going beyond words* (pp. 67–81). Mahwah, NJ: Lawrence Erlbaum.

Jones, S. E., & Brown. B. C. (1996). Touch attitudes and behaviors, recollections of early childhood touch, and social self-confidence. *Journal of Nonverbal Behavior, 20,* 147–163.

Jones, S. E., & Yarbrough, A. E. (1985). A naturalistic study of the meanings of touch. *Communication Monographs, 52,* 19–56.

Jourard, S. M. (1966). An exploratory study of body-accessibility. *British Journal of Social and Clinical Psychology, 5,* 221–231.

Julien, D. (2005). A procedure to measure interactional synchrony in the context of satisfied and dissatisfied couples' communication. In V. Manusov (Ed.), *The sourcebook of nonverbal measures: Going beyond words* (pp. 199–208). Mahwah, NJ: Lawrence Erlbaum.

Kaitz, M., Zvi, H., Levy, M., Berger, A., & Eidelman, A. I. (1995). The uniqueness of mother-own-infant interactions. *Infant Behavior and Development, 18,* 247–252.

Knofler, T., & Imhof, M. (2007). Does sexual orientation have an impact on nonverbal behavior in interpersonal communication? *Journal of Nonverbal Behavior, 31,* 189–204.

Koester, L. S., Brooks, L., & Traci, M. A. (2000). Tactile contact by deaf and hearing mothers during face-to-face interactions with their infants. *Journal of Deaf Studies and Deaf Education, 5,* 127–139.

Le May, A. C., & Redfern, S. J. (1987). A study of nonverbal communication between nurses and elderly patients. In P. Fielding (Ed.), *Research in the nursing care of elderly people* (pp. 171–189). New York, NY: John Wiley and Sons.

Lovejoy, M. C., Weis, R., O'Hare, E., & Rubin, E. C. (1999). Development and initial validation of the Parent Behavior Inventory. *Psychological Assessment, 11,* 534–545.

Main, M., & Stadtman, J. (1981). Infant response to rejection of physical contact by the mother: Aggression, avoidance, and conflict. *Journal of the American Academy of Child Psychiatry, 20,* 292–307.

Major, B., Schmidlin, A. M., & Williams, L. (1990). Gender patterns in social touch: The impact of setting and age. *Journal of Personality and Social Psychology, 58,* 634–643.

McDaniel, E., & Andersen, P. A. (1998). Intercultural patterns of tactile communication: A field study. *Journal of Nonverbal Behavior, 22,* 59–76.

Millot, J. L., Filiatre, J. C., & Montagner, H. (1988). Maternal tactile behavior correlated with mother and newborn infant characteristics. *Early Human Development, 16,* 119–129.

Morris, D. (1971). *Intimate behavior.* New York, NY: Random House.

Moszkowski, R. J., & Stack, D. M. (2007). Infant touching behavior during mother-infant face-to-face interactions. *Infant and Child Development, 16,* 307–319.

Moszkowski, R. J., Stack, D. M., & Chiarella, S. S. (2009a). Infant touch with gaze and affective behaviors during mother-infant still-face interactions: Co-occurrence and functions of touch. *Infant Behavior and Development, 32,* 392–403.

Moszkowski, R. J., Stack, D. M., Girouard, N., Field, T., Hernandez-Reif, M., & Diego, M. (2009b). Touching behaviors of infants of depressed mothers during normal and perturbed interactions. *Infant Behavior and Development, 32,* 183–194.

Oliver, S., & Redfern, S. J. (1991). Interpersonal communication between nurses and elderly patients: Refinement of an observation schedule. *Journal of Advanced Nursing, 16,* 30–38.

Oveis, C., Gruber, J., Keltner, D., Stamper, J. L., & Boyce, W. T. (2009). Smile intensity and warm touch as thin slices of child and family affective style. *Emotion, 9,* 544–548.

Patterson, M. (1988). Functions of nonverbal behavior in close relationships. In S. W. Duck (Ed.), *Handbook of personal relationships: Theory, research and intervention.* Chichester, UK: John Wiley and Sons.

Porter, L., Redfern, S., Wilson-Barnett, J., & Le May, A. (1986). The development of an observation schedule for measuring nurse-patient touch, using an ergonomic approach. *International Journal of Nursing Studies, 23,* 11–20.

Robinson, E., & Eyberg, S. (1981). The dyadic parent-child interaction coding system: Standardization and validation. *Journal of Consulting and Clinical Psychology, 49,* 245–250.

Routasalo, P., & Lauri, S. (1996). Developing an instrument for the observation of touching. *Clinical Nurse Specialist, 10,* 293–299.

Shelton, K. K., Frick, P. J., & Wootton, J. (1996). Assessment of parenting practices in families of elementary school-age children. *Journal of Clinical Child Psychology, 25,* 317–329.

Shuter, R. (1976). Proxemics and tactility in Latin America. *Journal of Communication, 26,* 46–52.

Smith, N., Lam, D., Bifulco, A., & Checkley, S. (2002). Childhood Experience of Care and Abuse Questionnaire (CECAQ). *Social Psychiatry and Psychiatric Epidemiology, 37,* 572–579.

Spaccarelli, S. (1995). Measuring abuse, stress, and negative cognitive appraisals in child sexual abuse: Validity data on two new scales. *Journal of Abnormal Child Psychology, 23,* 703–726.

Straus, M. A., Hamby, S. L., Boney-McCoy, S., & Sugarman, D. B. (1996). The Revised Conflict Tactics Scales (CTS2): Development and preliminary psychometric data. *Journal of Family Issues, 17,* 283–316.

Straus, M. A., Hamby, S. L., Finkelhor, D., Moore, D. W., & Runyan, D. (1998). Identification of child maltreatment with the Parent-Child Conflict Tactics Scales: Development and psychometric data for a national sample of American parents. *Child Abuse & Neglect, 22,* 249–270.

Takeuchi, M. S., Miyaoka, H., Tomoda, A., Suzuki, M., Liu, Q., & Kitamura, T. (2010). The effect of interpersonal touch during childhood on adult attachment and depression: A neglected area of family and developmental psychology? *Journal of Child and Family Studies, 19,* 109–117.

Toda, S., & Fogel, A. (1993). Infant response to the still-face situation at 3 and 6 months. *Developmental Psychology, 29,* 532–538.

Tronick, E., Als, H., Adamson, L., Wise, S., & Brazelton, B. (1978). The infant's response to entrapment between contradictory messages in face-to-face interaction. *Journal of the American Academy of Child Psychiatry, 17,* 1–13.

Weber, E. H. (1978). *The sense of touch.* H. E. Ross, trans. New York, NY: Academic Press. (Original work [*De Tactu*] published in 1834).

Webster-Stratton, C., & Spitzer, A. (1991). Development, reliability, and validity of the daily telephone discipline interview. *Behavioral Assessment, 13,* 221–239.

Weiss, S. (1990). Parental touching: Correlates of body image in children. In K. Barnard and T. B. Brazelton (Eds.), *Touch: The foundation of experience* (pp. 425–460). New York, NY: International Universities Press.

Weiss, S. J. (1992). Measurement of the sensory qualities of tactile interaction. *Nursing Research, 41,* 82–86.

Weiss, S. J. (2000). *Tactile Interaction Index: Manual and Coding Guidelines.* Available from the Department of Community Health Systems, Box 0608, University of California, San Francisco, 94143–0608.

Weiss, S., & Goebel, P. (2003). Parents' touch of their preterm infants and its relationship to their state of mind regarding touch. *Journal of Prenatal and Perinatal Psychology and Health, 17,* 185–202.

Weiss, S., Wilson, P., Hertenstein, M., & Campos, R. (2000). The tactile context of a mother's caregiving: Implications for attachment of low birth weight infants. *Infant Behavior and Development, 23,* 91–111.

Weiss, S., Wilson, P., & Morrison, D. (2004). Maternal tactile stimulation and the neurodevelopment of low birth weight infants. *Infancy, 5,* 85–107.

Weiss, S., Wilson, P., St.Jonn-Seed, M., & Paul, S. (2001). Early tactile experience of low birth weight children: Links to later mental health and social adaptation. *Infant and Child Development, 10,* 93–115.

IV

Communication via Touch

11

Communicating Through Touch: Touching During Parent–Infant Interactions

DALE M. STACK AND AMELIE D. L. JEAN

Over the last decade, research in the area of touch has grown and this is also true for research on touching in the adult–child relationship. Significant progress has been made in animal models, uncovering the benefits of touch and massage for human infants and children, understanding the mechanisms and functions of touch, defining and extending the role(s) that touch plays, and discovering more about parental touch with children, at different ages, under different contexts, and in different cultures. Touch is also included and measured more in studies investigating the parent–child relationship, social interaction, and communication and even studied on its own. While still sparse, there are some investigations of infant and child touch, and touch between adults other than the parent with children, and the relationship of touching behaviors to other modalities, as well as direct and indirect relations of touch with other domains of development. The primary goal of this chapter is to provide a detailed overview of the empirical research regarding touch in the early adult–child relationship. Given the focus, the emphasis will be on touch as it occurs in a social context between the child and an adult, usually the caregiver. It is important to note that in most of the literature reviewed it is the mother who is the participant; there have been fewer studies conducted with fathers to date. However, we have drawn together the existing literature on touch in the father–child relationship in one section. The first objective of this chapter is to underscore the importance and functions of parental (largely maternal) touch in development, particularly social and emotional development, focusing on its role(s) during social interchange and communication. The goal is to provide evidence for the contributions of parental/adult touch to interactions and the developing relationship and to highlight the child's use of touch that has emerged in recent research. A second objective is to present a developmental picture by drawing together the research on touch in the adult–child relationship at different ages in early development, beginning with the fetus and continuing into the newborn, infant, and preschool periods. A third overarching objective is to compile some of the diverse lines of research on touch and physical contact and integrate these findings into an emerging body of literature underscoring the importance of touch and physical contact in the adult–child relationship. Emphasis is placed on the infancy period of the healthy, typically developing child's life.

IMPORTANCE OF TOUCH FOR HUMAN INFANTS

Touch is of central importance to human infants. The somesthetic system (kinesthetic and cutaneous processes) is the earliest sensory system to develop in the human embryo (Maurer & Maurer, 1988; Montagu, 1971), and the skin is the largest sensory system in the body. Consequently, it seems reasonable to expect that the somesthetic system plays a fundamental role in early development. Results from many studies have lead researchers to advocate that tactile stimulation is essential to psychological and physical health (e.g., Jones & Yarbrough, 1985; Montagu, 1986). Research in the last 10 years (e.g., Field, 2002; Rutter & English Romanian Adoptees Study Team, 1998) is indicative that in extreme forms limited touch affects children's growth and development, and there is an accumulating literature on massage that implicates touch in benefits for infant growth.

However, despite advances and the acknowledged importance of tactile stimulation, the specific contribution(s) of tactile stimulation to early development (e.g., first years of life) remains relatively undefined particularly with regard to socioemotional development. There is evidence to suggest that touch is involved in regulation (e.g., Brazelton, 1990; Montagu, 1986) and soothing (Birns, Blank, & Bridger, 1966; Korner & Thoman, 1972), control of arousal (behavioral state, i.e., maintaining alertness, reducing drowsiness, etc.), modulating the overall level of stimulation (Koester, Papousek, & Papousek, 1989), and inducing changes in behavioral state (e.g., Barrera & Maurer, 1981; Muir & Field, 1979), as well as communication and exploration (Stack, 2010).

CAREGIVER TOUCH DURING PARENT–INFANT INTERACTIONS

Although social relationships are necessary and important for all human beings, they are a particularly focal ingredient in children's growth and well-being (e.g., Shipman & Zeman, 2001; Sroufe, Duggal, Weinfield, & Carlson, 2000). The mother–child relationship is integral to this process; it is the first relationship to develop for the infant and it is the foundation for future relationships. It is also a primary means to communicate, teach, and learn. In addition, the patterns of coregulation established in the context of social relations are critical for growth within the developing relationship and for children's engagement in later interactions (e.g., Bowlby, 1969; Fogel, 1993; Vygotsky, 1978). Consequently, in the following sections, we outline touching behaviors in the fetal, newborn, infancy, and preschool life stages, largely taking place during parent–child interactions.

Fetal Response to Tactile Stimulation and Physical Contact Between Parent and Newborn

The socialization of newborns and their parents, that first relationship, begins early, even in the womb. Along with the early developmental timing of the somesthetic system, massage and tactile stimulation have been shown to have positive effects and are successful in facilitating fetal activity (Diego, Field, & Hernandez-Reif, 2004). It is known that fetuses respond to vibroacoustic stimulation (e.g., Kisilevsky, Fearon, & Muir, 1998; Lecanuet, Granier-Deferre, & Busnel, 1989). However, because the fetus is housed in a liquid environment, there is no way to independently stimulate the fetal tactile and auditory systems; auditory and tactile stimuli are generated by a vibrating body which then reaches the fetus as pressure disturbances that come in successive waves (Kisilevsky, Stack, & Muir, 1991). Thus, "vibroacoustic" stimulation refers to both auditory and tactile stimulation in fetal research and is considered multimodal stimulation (Fearon, Hains, Muir, & Kisilevsky, 2002). Both movement and cardiac responses have been shown to vibroacoustic stimulation, beginning as early as 26 and 28 weeks postconceptional age, respectively (Kisilevsky, Muir, & Low, 1992). Increased movement and heart rate acceleration (Kisilevsky & Muir, 1991; Pomerleau-Malcuit & Clifton, 1973) to tactile and vibrotactile stimuli have also been shown in full-term newborns.

Physical contact between parent(s) and their newborn, immediately following the birth as well as several months later, has also received some research attention. Beyond its survival value, contact and affection between mother and infant are likely to serve the infant's developing social and emotional needs. For example, Carlsson et al. (1978) found that extended body contact between mother and newborn immediately after delivery was related to an increase in what the authors refer to as affective components of maternal nursing behavior observed 2–4 days later; increased contact behaviors (e.g., rubbing, rocking, touching, and holding) were shown during nursing and there were fewer noncontact behaviors. Similarly, de Chateau (1976) found that mothers given 10–15 minutes of extra contact experience during the first postpartum hour showed more holding, encompassing, looking "en face," and less cleaning behaviors at 36 hours than mothers providing only routine care. At the 3-month follow-up observation, more smiling and less crying were shown by infants with extra contact.

Extending the associations of physical contact to the first year of life, Bystrova and colleagues (2009) demonstrated that early skin-to-skin contact was related to maternal sensitivity, infants' self-regulation, and dyadic mutuality when infants were 1 year of age. Beyond maternal contact and its long-term effects, Fransson, Karlsson, and Nilsson (2005) established the importance of physical contact for temperature regulation in newborns.

Whether there are commonalities in how mothers touch their newborns has also been examined to some degree (e.g., Carlsson et al., 1978; de Chateau, 1976); however, there is mixed evidence as to whether there is an argument favoring an invariant pattern of maternal tactile behavior (e.g., Trevathan, 1981; Tulman, 1985). Furthermore, Kaitz and colleagues (Kaitz, Lapidot, Bronner, & Eidelman, 1992; Kaitz, Meirov, Landman, & Eidelman, 1993) showed that mothers could recognize their own baby 5–79 hours after delivery by stroking the dorsal surface of their infant's hand, and this was without the added benefit of visual, auditory, and olfactory cues. Their findings suggest that mothers are uniquely sensitive to their newborns through the tactile sense and that they learn the special tactile characteristics of their infant during the course of routine contact and interaction.

Maternal Touch During Mother–Infant Interactions

Interactions between mothers and children are essential for studying the underpinnings of social relationships and are a primary context within which to study touching. However, investigations of the role of touch in early social interactions have had a rather short history. Mothers (and fathers) commonly employ touch during face-to-face interactions and play, along with their vocal and facial expressions. During face-to-face exchanges, the infant and adult (primarily the mother) are seated at eye level to each other during a series of brief interaction periods. Caregivers interact spontaneously, using their facial, vocal, and tactile expressions, while infants respond to and even initiate interactions. Face-to-face interactions have been one of the primary means used to study the infant's social communication (Kaye & Fogel, 1980), emotional expressions and responses to stressful episodes (Field, Vega-Lahr, Scafidi, & Goldstein, 1986), and the development of social expectations (Cohn & Tronick, 1983). However, typically, researchers have analyzed maternal and infant facial and vocal behavior, but not touch. This, despite the fact that incidental reports reveal that maternal touch occurs during 33–61% of brief interaction periods (e.g., Field, 1984; Kaye & Fogel, 1980; Symons & Moran, 1987), and infant touch occurs 85% of the time (Moszkowski & Stack, 2007).

Within mother–infant interactions, touch has been shown to convey security and tenderness, aid in the reduction of infants' stress and distress (Jean & Stack, 2009; Stack & Muir, 1990), and promote emotional regulation in infants (Hertenstein & Campos, 2001; Weiss, Wilson, Hertenstein, & Campos, 2000) and has been demonstrated to be effective in regulating infants' behavior, affect, and attention (Moszkowski & Stack, 2007; Peláez-Nogueras, Gewirtz, et al., 1996; Stack & Muir, 1990, 1992). In addition to its potential benefit for infants' socioemotional development, there is evidence to suggest a clear preference by infants for interactions which include tactile stimulation from their caregivers and that touch is a powerful reinforcer (Brossard & Decarie, 1968; Peláez-Nogueras, Gewirtz, et al.). Parent–infant games that include considerable touching and physical contact (such as *pat-a-cake, tickle games, I'm gonna get you games*) have also been demonstrated to elicit positive responses from infants (Fogel, Hsu, Shapiro, Nelson-Goens, & Secrist, 2006; Wolff, 1963). For example, Dickson, Walker, and Fogel (1997) found that it was physical play that included tactile stimulation that elicited the most play smiles (45% of the time) during parent–infant interactions.

While there is diverse methodology to address infants' preference for touch (directly or indirectly) as illustrated earlier, much of the work assessing the role and influence of maternal touch during interactions has been conducted using a modification of the face-to-face procedure, the still-face (SF) paradigm (Tronick, Als, Adamson, Wise, & Brazelton, 1978). In a typical SF procedure, the mother–infant interaction is divided into three brief periods (90–120 seconds). In period 1, mothers interact normally, using facial expressions, voice, and touch (Normal); in period 2, they assume a neutral, nonresponsive SF and provide neither vocal nor tactile stimulation (SF); and in period, 3 they resume normal interaction. During the SF, compared to Normal periods, infants typically decrease gazing and smiling at mothers (e.g., Gusella, Muir, & Tronick, 1988), increase neutral to negative affect, and increase vocalizing (Ellsworth, Muir, & Hains, 1993; Stack & Muir, 1990). This dramatic effect has been replicated numerous times and in various ways (see Adamson & Frick, 2003 for an overview and history).

In those studies that have measured touch, there are particular role(s) that the SF has played in revealing important effects. For example, Gusella et al. (1988) found that 3-month-olds exhibited the SF effect only when maternal touching was part of the prior Normal periods and their attention declined over time without the tactile stimulation. Koester, Brooks, and Traci (2000) demonstrated that mothers of 6-month-old infants touched their infants more in the Normal period following the SF than in the period prior to the SF. The authors speculated that the increased touching might be reflecting mothers' attempts at nurturing and comforting their infants following a stressful period. These findings highlight infants' sensitivity to maternal cues and suggest the regulatory and communicative nature of touch.

Studies examining infants' responsiveness to their mothers' touch and their sensitivity to touch when other forms of stimulation are absent provide important insight into why mothers use touch during the first 6 months of life. By comparing a standard SF with one where mothers could touch during the SF period (SF with touch), Stack and Muir (1990) showed that by adding touch infants were not distressed, they showed increased smiling, and they maintained the high levels of gaze that are typical in Normal interactions. This new role for touch in moderating the SF effect has been replicated a number of times (e.g., Peláez-Nogueras, Field, Hossain, & Pickens, 1996; Stack & LePage, 1996; Stack & Muir, 1992). Stack and Muir (1992) also demonstrated that it was the tactile and not the visual stimulation from the adults' hands that was responsible for the effects. In addition, infants' sensitivity to changes in their mothers' touch during the SF has been shown by providing mothers with different verbal instructions. For example, mothers can use touch to elicit specific behaviors from their infants (e.g., maximize their infants' smiling; Stack & LePage, 1996; shift infants' attention to their mothers' hands; Stack & Muir, 1992). Moreover, Stack and Arnold (1998) found that infants are sensitive to changes in maternal touch and hand gestures and that, when instructed, mothers appear successful in eliciting specific behaviors from their infants using only nonverbal channels of communication. For example, maternal touch and hand gestures attracted infants' attention to their mothers' faces even when the face was still and expressionless, and infants in the experimental group smiled more relative to the control group when mothers were instructed to engage their infants in a playful interaction.

Exploring infants' understanding of tactile behavior further, LePage and Stack (1997) investigated infants' abilities to perceive a tactile contingency (or the lack of contingency) during social interactions. Infants in the contingent condition were reinforced for gazing at the experimenter's neutral face with standardized tactile stimulation (SF interaction with touch as the reinforcer), while infants in the noncontingent condition received the same tactile stimulation as their matched counterparts regardless of their behaviors. All infants in the contingent condition learned the contingency reflected in their gaze behavior. Results from these studies underscore infants' responsiveness and sensitivity to maternal touch and highlight the prevalence of touch during interactions.

Maternal Patterns of Touch During Social Interactions

While the importance of the aforementioned studies is not in question, the functions and adaptability of touch were largely inferred based on evidence taken from infant behavior, rather than direct measures of caregiver touch. Even in those studies where touch has been directly assessed, the measures have largely been the duration of all touching (e.g., Gusella et al., 1988) or intensity levels (e.g., Stack & Muir, 1990). All touch may not be used or interpreted similarly; different types of touch and the way touch is applied may have different meanings (Hertenstein, 2002; Stack, 2001; Tronick, 1995). Consistent with this contention, several coding systems have been developed to examine different properties of touch in mothers (e.g., Feldman, Weller, Sirota, & Eidelman, 2002; Stack, 2001; Weiss, 1992) and in infants (e.g., Herrera, Reissland, & Shepherd, 2004; Moszkowski & Stack, 2007).

Results from a number of studies have demonstrated that mothers use different types of touch during mother–infant social exchanges (e.g., Ferber, Feldman, & Makhoul, 2008; Harrison & Woods, 1991; Polan & Ward, 1994). Stack, LePage, Hains, and Muir (1996; as cited in Jean, Stack, & Fogel, 2009) developed the Caregiver–Infant Touch Scale to measure types of touch and associated quantitative characteristics (e.g., intensity, speed) in social contexts such as mother–infant play and to examine changes across age. Following a period of natural face-to-face interaction, mothers and their 5½-month-old infants participated in three SF with touch periods: (1) normal touch, (2) touch to maximize infant smiling, and (3) touch restricted to one area of the body. The more tactilely active profile was revealed during the period where smiling was maximized: mothers used more active types of touch (lifting, tickling), more surface area, and greater intensity and speed. In contrast, when mothers were asked to touch their babies in only one area, there was increased stroking and less shaking and touching was also less intense and executed more slowly. It is clear that mothers' profiles of touching changed as a function of instruction, suggesting that what was being communicated through the touch was different.

Using their Tactile Interaction Index, Weiss, Wilson, St. John Seed, and Paul (2001) coded for 28 different gestures or touching behavior during their study of 3-month-old low birth weight infants. Findings indicated that about half of mothers' touch was nurturing followed by complex/diverse patterns of touching. In a study with failure to thrive infants (Polan & Ward, 1994), mothers were found to provide less touch stimulation to their infants, with a decrease in matter-of-fact touch during feeding and an increase in unintentional touch (a touch believed to be an indicator of mother–child proximity) during play, as compared to their normal-growing infant counterparts. As well, they used less proprioceptive stimulation (a touch hypothesized to promote growth in infants) during the play period. In a similar study, Feldman, Keren, Gross-Rozval, and Tyano (2004) documented that mothers of infants with feeding disorders used less affectionate, proprioceptive, and unintentional touch compared to control mothers. Combined, these results suggest that the types of touch in some at-risk groups are less than optimal.

In infants of depressed mothers, it has been shown that positive touch stimulation enhances positive affect and attention (Peláez-Nogueras, Field, et al., 1996), and positive touch also enhances maternal sensitivity (Ferber et al., 2005) and reduces depressed mood and anxiety levels in depressed mothers (Feijó et al., 2006). In their study of parenting stress, depression and anxiety and its relationship to behavior, Fergus, Schmidt, and Pickens (1998) found that mothers who reported more symptoms of depression touched their infants more relative to nondepressed mothers; however, the pattern of interaction was more intrusive and overstimulatory. Similarly, Cohn and Tronick (1989) described depressed mothers as using more poking and jabbing with their infants; these touching behaviors were associated with negative affect and gaze aversion on the part of infants. Depressed mothers were also found to use more negative touches such as tickling, poking, tugging, and pulling while interacting with their 3-month-old infants. Finally, Herrera et al. (2004) reported that depressed mothers restrained their infants more by lifting them, and Stepakoff (1999) found that they showed more object-mediated and less affectionate touch.

Combined, results underscore the importance of maternal types of touch and converge to suggest that the quality of touch might be more important than its mere presence or absence.

Functions of Maternal Touch During Interactions

In attempts to investigate the unique role for touch during mother–infant interactions, the verbal instructions given to mothers have been varied; with variations in instructions, mothers changed their touch and these changes in touch produced observable changes in infant behavior (e.g., Arnold, 2002; Stack et al., 1996). While these studies are clearly essential in demonstrating that different types of touch can serve various functions, a direct assessment of the functions of touch is imperative to understand the communicative properties of touch.

To investigate the different functions that maternal touch serves, several coding schemes have been developed (e.g., Ferber et al., 2008; Jean & Stack, 2009; Landau, Shusel, Eshel, & Ben-Aaron, 2003). As pointed out by several researchers, to understand the communicative properties of touch and its roles within face-to-face interactions, its evaluation should not be made in isolation; rather, it should take into account the nonverbal and verbal behavior that accompanies each function of touch and the context in which each function occurs (Hertenstein, 2002; Jones & Yarbrough, 1985; Muir, 2002; Stack, 2001). Hence, Jean and Stack (2009) developed the Functions of Touch Scale, a systematic observational measure used to assess the functions of maternal touch while taking into consideration other modalities of verbal and nonverbal communication such as mothers' verbalizations and infants' emotional displays and attention. Across periods of the SF, mothers were found to use mostly playful function of touch, active and passive accompaniment (i.e., touches that serve as an accompaniment to another modality of communication), followed by nurturing and attention-getting function of touch. In addition, they found that the attention-getting function of touch increased in the first Normal period of the SF while the nurturing function of touch increased in the Reunion Normal period.

Findings from these studies suggest that while interacting with their infants, mothers' touching serves various functions, implying that simple touch duration is not a sufficient index to characterize adult behavior. Qualitative and quantitative variations in touching are important to measure and describe. What is also underscored is that mothers use different types of touching for different functions.

Longitudinal Studies of Maternal Touch

The bulk of the studies presented thus far have had cross-sectional designs. Longitudinal designs, particularly prospective longitudinal studies, allow researchers to follow groups of infants and children over time to identify whether certain factors in children's lives (e.g., parent's touching behavior, child's behavior to the same tactile stimulation, parent–child relationships) are modified or change with age (Widom,

Raphael, & DuMont, 2004). Pertaining to parental touching with children, longitudinal studies are important in revealing age-related changes. For example, during a face-to-face interaction, Field, Vega-Lahr, Goldstein, and Scafidi (1987a) found that the overall amount of touching and moving of infant's limbs was found to decrease with age. Harrison and Woods (1991) found that both mothers and fathers touched their younger premature infants less (>28 weeks) than older infants (<28 weeks). In addition, the quality of tactile stimulation varied with infant's gestational age; younger infants received lighter and shorter durations of touching while older premature infants received more active touching. These results indicate that parents were sensitive to the development of their infants and adjusted their tactile stimulation accordingly.

Most of the available studies that have examined age-related changes have examined changes in the *durations* of touching. There are a few studies that have investigated age-related changes in the *types* of touch. Ferber and colleagues (2008) examined the development of maternal touch during natural caregiving and mother–child play using nine different types of touch that were aggregated into the three global touch categories of affectionate, stimulating, and instrumental. While affectionate and stimulating touch decreased during the second half year of life, dyadic reciprocity increased. Similarly, Crnic, Ragozin, Greenberg, Robinson, and Basham (1983) showed that mothers of full-term and preterm infants decreased the amount of affectionate touch provided to their infants at 4, 8, and 12 months of age. In a study examining maternal touch across age (1, 3, and 5 months), Jean, Stack, and Fogel (2009) demonstrated that mothers changed their touching as a function of age: although touching was consistently high, maternal touch decreased from 1 to 3 months. More static touch was used at 5 compared to 3 months, and more stroking was used at 1 and 5 months of age.

Taken together, these studies illustrate the beginnings of how maternal touch evolves across infant age and context. However, these findings underscore just some of the changes that are manifested in touching as the infant grows older, and this is just a beginning. More longitudinal research is warranted to continue this line of research.

Touch in the Father–Child Relationship

Up to this point in the chapter, the focus has largely been with mother–infant touching. Yet while sparse, there is an accumulating literature on fathers (e.g., Allen & Daly, 2002) and a small body of research that specifically examines touching during the father–child relationship. For example, using the SF paradigm with mothers and fathers with their infants at 3 and 6 months, Forbes, Cohn, Allen, and Lewinsohn (2004) demonstrated that during the Normal period mothers showed more positive affect and fathers used more physical play; however, parents did not use physical play more with boys than with girls. Jean, Moszkowski, Girouard, and Stack (2005) included systematic measurement of touch in their SF study and found that while there were some differences in the types, combinations, and locations of touch between mothers and fathers, there were no differences in the overall duration and frequency of touch used. Furthermore, mothers and fathers were as sensitive and responsive to their infants' needs. Examining dual-career parents during face-to-face interactions with their 8-month-olds, Field, Vega-Lahr, Goldstein, and Scafidi (1987b) demonstrated that in addition to smiling and vocalizing more, mothers touched their infants more than fathers, resulting in greater infant smiling and motor activity. Similar effects have been shown in a triadic interaction context, taking place in the home environment (Zaslow, Pedersen, Suwalsky, Cain, & Fivel, 1985).

Finally, there have been a few studies that have examined fathers' touching behavior with their preterm infants. For example, Harrison and Woods (1991) found that fathers provided less touching behavior than mothers and grandmothers. Levy-Shiff, Sharir, and Mogilner (1989) found that mothers engaged in more touching, talking, and caregiving, while fathers engaged in more play and stimulating behaviors. However, at the time of discharge, differences between parents diminished except for caregiving. Goebel (2002) found while fathers' overall amount of touching with their 3-month-olds varied widely, the locations touched most frequently were shoulders, back, torso, and face, and the most frequent types of touch were patting, lifting, and passive contact. Given the scarcity of studies that have examined fathers' touching, more research is essential, particularly pertaining to fathers' use and styles of touching during interactions and the implications that different amounts, styles, or patterns might have on specific domains such as emotion regulation and for later development.

INFANT TOUCH DURING INTERACTIONS

Infant Patterns of Touching During Social Interactions

While research on maternal and paternal touching is still sparse (albeit growing), even less research has been conducted on infant touch. Yet infants use touch to explore their environments and themselves, self-comfort, regulate, and communicate. Beyond exploration of their physical environments, infants use touch in social contexts to learn about themselves and others. However, few studies have included measurements of infants' tactile or manual behaviors during early social exchanges between mothers and their infants (Murray & Trevarthen, 1985; Toda & Fogel, 1993). Results from a few studies have shown that self-touch is a mode of self-regulation (Landau et al., 2003; Toda & Fogel); however, given the paucity of studies and the lack of specificity, little is known about the types of touch infants use and how they use touch to fulfill different functions and under what conditions.

A systematic examination of the qualitative and quantitative components of infant touching (types, locations, and duration of touch) was carried out by Moszkowski and Stack (2007). Using a SF procedure with full-term 5½-month-olds, they demonstrated that during the SF period when mothers were unavailable, infants touched themselves more and used more active, reactive, and soothing touching behaviors (e.g., stroke, finger, pat, pull). In contrast, during the Normal periods when mothers were available for interaction, they touched their mothers and used more passive touch (static touch). This study was an important first step in developing a methodology for measuring infant touch and in delineating the regulatory, exploratory, and communicative roles for infant touch.

Moszkowski and Stack extended their infant touch research to a population of depressed and nondepressed mothers of 4-month-olds (Moszkowski, Stack, Girouard, Field, Hernandez-Reif, & Diego, 2009). They examined infants' touching behaviors during periods of maternal emotional unavailability (SF) and physical unavailability [separation procedure; when mothers were physically absent for a brief period (Field et al., 1986)]. Results indicated that when mothers were unavailable, infants exhibited more patting and pulling, and during both the SF and separation periods, infants of depressed mothers used more reactive types of touch (such as grabbing and pulling). Similarly, results from Hentel, Beebe, and Jaffe's (2000) investigation of depressed mothers and their 4-month-old infants suggest that infants of depressed mothers exhibited more self-comforting regulatory behaviors, including self-touch. Furthermore, Herrera et al. (2004) found that infants of depressed mothers touched their mothers and toys less and touched themselves more, suggesting that they might use self-touch as a way to compensate for their mothers' lack of nurturing touch.

Functions of Infant Touch During Interactions

In the few existing studies on infant touch, the functions of touch were only indirectly examined. Moszkowski, Stack, and Chiarella (2009) established new ground by more directly measuring the functions of infant touch and demonstrating that these functions of touch and the way that the functions were organized with gaze and affect varied depending on the interaction period. For example, infants demonstrated more regulatory and exploratory touch during the SF period: passive touch co-occurred with gaze at mothers during the Normal periods, while soothing and reactive touch co-occurred with gaze away from mothers during the SF period.

Taken together, findings from research on the patterns of mother and infant touch reveal that touch is clearly an integral part of mother–infant interactions: both mothers and infants use different touching behaviors depending on context and age; there are specific functions that maternal and infant touch serve during interactions; these vary across interaction periods, birth status, and age; and infant touch is organized with other behaviors during interactions.

THE JOINT EXAMINATION OF MOTHER AND INFANT TOUCH

Despite the fact that studies examining maternal and infant touch have increased over the recent years, few studies have attempted to simultaneously measure infants' and mothers' tactile behavior. Just as with gaze, affect, and other more distal means of communication, mothers *and* infants use these modalities to communicate. In addition, they may both be using touch at the same time. Examining these joint behaviors and how types of touching are associated is one way to better understand the communicative functions of touch during interactions. Moszkowski, Jean, and Stack (2005a) investigated the touching behavior of 5½-month-old infants and their mothers during a SF period. Mothers engaged in playful forms of touch, while infants used active types of touch. Moreover, both mothers and infants used passive forms of touching when the other partner was not touching. Similarly, while comparing the frequency and function of touch during child–mother and child–metapelet exchanges, mothers and children were found to touch each other more frequently and to exhibit more responsiveness to each other's touches (Landau et al., 2003).

The joint examination of mother and infant touch has also been conducted within at-risk populations (e.g., Beebe et al., 2008; Feldman et al., 2004; Herrera et al., 2004). In their study on feeding disorder (FD) infants, Feldman et al. (2004) found that in response to their mother's touch, FD infants used less affectionate and more negative touches and responded with more withdrawal and rejection than control infants. In return, mothers of FD infants responded to infant-initiated touches with more rejection responses. The authors speculate that both mothers and FD infants might be uncomfortable with reciprocal intimacy. Finally, in an examination of self- and interactive regulation of mothers with depressive symptoms and their 4-month-old infants, mothers exhibiting higher depressive symptoms (Beebe et al., 2008) touched their infants less frequently, displayed more intrusive touch, and did not coordinate their touching behavior with infants' touch patterns relative to controls. In contrast, infants of depressed mothers displayed high touch coordination with their mothers' touches; that is, they touched themselves less when mothers became more intrusive and less affectionate. These behaviors might be detrimental to infants' abilities to adequately self-regulate using touch when needed. Together, these findings reveal the utility of examining simultaneous touching between mothers and infants and how the type and location (self, other) of touch lend insight into communication and the developing relationship.

TOUCH AND AFFECT

Touch and Infants' Smiling

While the examination of simultaneous touch is an important direction, to better understand the communicative properties of touch, it is essential to directly examine the relationship between touch and infants' affect. Hertenstein (2002) and Stack (2001, 2004) contend that examining how mothers' touch modulates infants' affect and how in return infants' affect influences mothers' tactile behavior is central to elucidating how mothers and infants use touch to communicate, as well as the role of touch in behavioral regulation (Stack, 2001). At the same time, it highlights mothers' sensitivity toward their infants' emotional displays. As previously stated, the mere presence of touch is effective in generating positive affect in infants yet only a few studies have investigated how specific tactile behaviors influence infants' affect. For example, in a comparison of the reinforcing nature of three types of tactile stimulation on infants' smiling, Peláez-Nogueras, Field, et al. (1996) demonstrated that stroking, as compared to tickling or poking, increased infants' smiling, attention, and vocalizing. In addition, Perez and Gewirtz (2004) in their study assessing three types of tactile stimulation at two different levels of tactile pressure found that infants preferred intense stroking the most and intense poking the least. Moszkowski, Jean, and Stack (2005b) investigated the co-occurrence between infant/maternal touch and infant smiling during a SF procedure. Infants spent the most time smiling when being actively stimulated by their mothers or themselves (when mothers were not available), thus implying that touch is a positive affective experience for infants. Consistent with these findings, Jean, Moszkowski, Girouard, and Stack (2008) demonstrated that while interacting with their 6-month-old infants, playful function of touch predicted infants' smiling, while nurturing function of touch predicted infants' fretting.

Results from these studies examining touch and affect and emotional displays, during and following touch, provide additional insight into the communicative and interactive nature of touching.

Touch and Emotion Regulation

Studies that examine touching and its role in emotion regulation add to the growing body of literature that links touch and affect and emotional displays. In their examination of infant affective and behavioral states across a series of conditions, Brown and Tronick (in preparation, cited in Tronick, 1995) found that the lowest levels of infant fussing and crying were displayed in the touch-only condition. Consistent with Stack and colleagues' findings (e.g., Stack & Arnold, 1998; Stack & LePage, 1996; Stack & Muir, 1990, 1992), touching had calming effects on the infants, reflected in their decreased fretting, and seemed to permit an openness to the stimulation, reflected in high levels of attention and continued smiling. On the basis of these findings and others, Tronick (1989, 1995) suggests that touch is a component of the mutual regulatory process of the caregiver–infant dyad. With a few exceptions (e.g., Hertenstein & Campos, 2001; Jean & Stack, 2009), studies in the infant social interaction literature have not been specifically designed to explore these relationships directly and systematically.

In their study with 5½-month-old full-term and very low birth weight preterm infants, Millman, Jean, and Stack (2009) examined maternal touching and infants' self-regulating abilities during a SF procedure. Mothers used more nurturing and playful touch following the SF rather than prior to the SF period. Moreover, for the full-term group, mothers increased their nurturing touching when their infants exhibited distress during the SF. Finally, the quality of maternal touch was related to infants' self-regulating abilities. For example, increased playful touch was associated with increased bidirectional exchanges while attention-getting touch was associated with increased gaze aversion and decreased bidirectional exchanges. These findings suggest that mothers and infants are attuned to each other's behavior and that functions of maternal touch and infants' self-regulatory behaviors are related.

Similarly, Jean and Stack (2009), using the typical SF procedure, demonstrated that maternal behavior immediately following the SF period and infant fretting during the Reunion period predicted the amount of maternal nurturing touch provided to infants during the Reunion period. Moreno, Posada, and Goldyn (2006) directly examined the regulatory functions of touch by linking the quality of parent–infant touch and the regulatory effects on the infant. While contrary to hypotheses, results indicated that there was more symmetrical coregulation when touch was prohibited, and affectionate touch was inversely related to infant activity level while stimulating touch was directly related to infant activity level. The regulatory effects of touch have also been shown with regard to infants' irritability level and their stress responses during innoculations (Calkins, Hungerford, & Dedmon, 2004; Jahromi, Puttham, & Stifter, 2004).

In an attempt to examine the effects of touch on infants' emotion, Hertenstein and Campos (2001) varied the tactile stimulation provided to infants while they sat on their mothers' laps and were presented with objects. Specific qualities of touch (i.e., tension increase condition, where the mother was instructed to tighten her grip around her infant's torso with her fingers for a brief period) reliably elicited negative expression from infants; however, they were not successful with the touch quality that was expected to elicit positive expressions.

Taken together, results from these studies add to the literature on touch during parent–child interactions, highlight the relation between touching and affect and emotion regulation, and underscore the importance of measuring touch.

TOUCH IN THE PRESCHOOL PERIOD

Thus far, the focus of the chapter has largely been on the importance of touch for infants, beginning with the fetus and newborn and emphasizing the research between caregivers and infants. However, while there is a growing literature on the importance of touch with infants, its role in mother–infant and infant–peer interactions with older infants (older than 1 year of age) has not received much attention. As the numbers of children attending daycare increases, investigating tactile behaviors between infants and their peers and infants and their daycare providers is warranted to better understand the importance of touch in the socioemotional development of children.

Of the available studies to date, most have examined the role of physical contact in daycare settings. For example, Fleck and Chavajay (2009) sought to investigate the quality of physical contact between preschoolers and kindergartners. Preschoolers were found to engage in more purposeful and incidental touches than kindergartners and they affectionately touched other preschoolers and their teachers more frequently. During free-play, Cigales, Field, Hossain, Peláez-Nogueras, and Gewirtz (1996) examined the touching behavior of preschoolers aged between 3 and 64 months. Although the duration of touching did not change across age, the types of touch children utilized while playing did. Younger infants received more positive touch while preschoolers received more negative touching behavior, and toddlers used more affective and communicative touches than younger infants. While teachers touched infants more than toddlers and preschoolers, they provided similar amounts of task-oriented, affective, communicative, and playful functions of touch regardless of child age.

While the positive *impact* of touch within a daycare setting was demonstrated earlier, Wheldall, Bevan, and Shortall (1986) demonstrated the positive *reinforcing* nature of touch for 5- to 6-year-olds in a classroom setting. When teachers were asked to incorporate touch while praising children for appropriate social or academic behaviors and to withhold touch in any other situations, children's on-task behaviors increased and their disruptive behaviors decreased. Similarly, Field et al. (1994) examined mutual touching between children and their daycare teachers. Since the frequency of touching was found to be low over 1 month, teachers were asked to increase its frequency for another month. Following this increase, teachers touched preschoolers more frequently. In addition, older children used more positive touch with each other compared to infants who received positive tactile behavior from their teachers. Observations of tactile behavior conducted during the reunion period with parents at the end of the day showed that parents provided more positive touch to their younger infants and that there were relationships between teachers' caregiving practices and parent–child holding; for example, children who reported liking to be touched by their teachers were touched more during the reunion period by their parents and received more positive touching from their teachers. Field and colleagues suggest that children receiving more touching at home might seek and elicit these tactile behaviors in others.

Although rare, results from studies examining peer and educator touching illustrate the importance of examining different interpersonal contexts and extend our knowledge of touching to the spheres of peer and educational environments.

CONCLUSIONS

In our quest to reveal and understand touching behaviors in early development, many questions and critical issues remain (e.g., Stack, in press). However, it is clear that there is abundant converging evidence to support the importance of touch and highlight its diversity and flexibility. Touch is an adaptable modality, a modality that while often used alone also accompanies other modalities and channels of communication. It is used frequently in the first years of human life by mothers, fathers, and infants, and it serves a multitude of purposes. It is an important means for parents and infants to maintain a connection with each other and with the environment and the self. Both partners have been shown to modify their behavior, adjust, and compensate for the context, and patterns of touching may be different, illustrating the utility, value, and communicability of the tactile system.

Despite the fact that studies on touch have grown, and this is also true for touching during interactions in early development, they are still relatively scarce. It is imperative that more research be conducted and in a number of important areas. More studies with full-term healthy infants are warranted. While research with at-risk infants is certainly beneficial, touch may be serving different needs in these populations and is likely used differently or in different types and amounts, depending on the nature of the population. Addressing the continuum of what we might call "normative" touching or typical patterns of touch across age in healthy infants with their parents is essential if we are to understand the contributions of touch in early development. In addition, how touching is integrated with the other communication channels that are available would benefit from continued investigation. Although understanding each component's discrete and independent roles is important, the context within which touching occurs is important, and the context within which much of early development occurs is social and multimodal. Context shapes meaning (Jones & Yarbrough, 1985) and is considered by some to be the "mortar" of caregiver–infant communication (Hertenstein, 2002). What accompanies a touch behavior is important to impart meaning and the same behavior may have different meanings depending on the context. Directions to address the roles of context and understanding meaning during interactions include studies manipulating context, integrating both microscopic and global measures, using naturalistic and experimental paradigms, and emphasizing the nature of mutual or coactive influences. Furthermore, studies of different cultures provide a means to study interactions and assess cultural similarities and differences as well as the potential universality of meaning in some touch.

Technology has advanced and goes beyond video-recorded interactions to software that permits coding of multiple behaviors, the merging and integration of behaviors that are time synchronized, integration with physiological measurement (e.g., heart rate), and has the capacity to analyze the data in various ways (e.g., co-occurrence and sequential analysis). This enables, among other things, emphasis of mutual or coactive influences from both parent and infants. Increased emphasis on coding and integrating touch and gesture in studies and coding systems is warranted to better understand their roles in communication. While software to integrate measures has undoubtedly improved, more development in this domain would serve as a catalyst for better and more integrative studies, including linking touch with emotion and affective behaviors and physiological indices.

While we have made progress in measuring types and more recently functions of touch, much remains to be done to demonstrate more fully the communicative nature and other roles that touch serves. Moreover, research efforts need to be directed to some of the more quantitative components of touch: behavioral coding systems are limited in the ways that they can measure quantitative components of touching such as intensity and speed. In addition, clustering touch with other behaviors to formulate constellations of behavior, styles, or expressions of communicative meaning and then subsequently validating these in independent studies would advance our understanding of touch, as well as its relation to emotion and communication, its measurement, and its potential mechanisms.

More research on touching at different ages and under varied contexts (e.g., peer play, educational or daycare contexts) is warranted, as well as expansion beyond mothers to fathers, siblings, peers, and other significant figures. While the field has started to move beyond maternal touch to include infant and caregiver touch, longitudinal studies on touching behavior (both caregiver and infant) over time are still rare and have remained largely in the descriptive realm and in the short term. As the age range is extended, the types and functions of touch can be examined, and investigations of how changes in touching might be associated with other developmental domains and relationship dimensions can take place. Further, research needs to move toward addressing the functions in different and more sophisticated ways and the mechanisms through which touch works, and these over the longer term.

The long-term implications of touching (or the absence of it) are notably lacking, outside of the literature on massage and some work with premature infants. In addition, models that conceptualize the functions and meaning of touch across periods of development are practically nonexistent. Consequently, studies designed to address specific tenets of a theoretically driven model or particular components of socioemotional development do not exist. The use of different paradigms and procedures would also be advantageous, and innovations in measurement are critical. For example, studies that tie touch and emotion and attention together and examine the regulatory roles for touch are warranted. Furthermore, individual differences in touch have not been explored in any depth. Finally, exploring the mechanisms that underlie the effects of touch is essential.

The future holds much promise, offering a rich foundation from which to develop new and innovative questions and build empirically and theoretically driven studies. While there are many unresolved questions and challenges that remain to be pursued, research is at a point where cutting-edge issues are surfacing, studies are accumulating, and findings are converging. We are on the cusp of discovering more about the way touch works, specifically its influence and mechanisms, and social interactions continue to be pivotal in launching research of this nature.

ACKNOWLEDGMENTS

This chapter was written with the support of the Social Sciences and Humanities Research Council (SSHRC) of Canada and Fonds Québécois de la Recherche sur la Société et la Culture (FQRSC). The authors express their gratitude to Irene Mantis for help with literature searches and preparation of the final version of the chapter. Some of the ideas and content of this chapter originated from Stack, D. M. (2010), Touch and physical contact during infancy: Discovering the richness of the forgotten sense. In J. Gavin Bremner & T. D. Wachs (Eds.), *Blackwell handbook of infancy research* (2nd ed., Vol. 1). *Basic processes*. Oxford, England: Blackwell. The publishers of this handbook are gratefully acknowledged.

REFERENCES

Adamson, L. B., & Frick, J. E. (2003). The Still Face: A history of a shared experimental paradigm. *Infancy, 4,* 451–473.

Allen, S., & Daley, K. (2002). The effects of father involvement: A summary of the research evidence. *Newsletter of the Father Involvement Initiative, 1,* 1–11.

Arnold, S. (2002). Maternal tactile-gestural stimulation and infants' nonverbal behaviors during early mother-infant face-to-face interactions: Contextual, age and birth status effects. *Dissertation Abstracts International: Section B: Sciences and Engineering, 63(10-B),* 4962.

Barrera, M. E., & Maurer, D. (1981). The perception of facial expressions by the three-month-old. *Child Development, 52,* 203–206.

Beebe, B., Jaffe, J., Buck, K., Chen, H., Cohen, P., Feldstein, S., & Andrews, H. (2008). Six-week postpartum maternal depressive symptoms and 4-month mother-infant self- and interactive contingency. *Infant Mental Health Journal, 29,* 442–471.

Birns, B., Blank, M., & Bridger, W. H. (1966). The effectiveness of various soothing techniques on human neonates. *Psychosomatic Medicine, 28,* 316–322.

Bowlby, J. (1969). *Attachment and loss.* Vol.1. New York, NY: Basic Books.

Brazelton, T. B. (1990). Touch as a touchstone: Summary of the round table. In K. E. Barnard & T. B. Brazelton (Eds.), *Touch: The foundation of experience.* Madison, CT: International Universities Press, Inc.

Brossard, L. M., & Decarie, T. (1968). Comparative reinforcing effect of eight stimulations on the smiling response of infants. *Journal of Child Psychology and Psychiatry, 9,* 51–59.

Bystrova, K., Ivanova, V., Edhborg, M., Matthiesen, A.S., Ransjö-Arvidson, A. B., Mukhamedrakhimov, R.,...Widström, A. M. (2009). Early contact versus separation: Effects on mother-infant interaction one year later. *Birth, 36,* 97–109.

Calkins, S. D., Hungerford, A., & Dedmon, S. E. (2004). Mothers' interactions with temperamentally frustrated infants. *Infant Mental Health Journal, 25,* 219–239.

Carlsson, S. G., Fagerberg, H., Horneman, G., Hwang, C. P., Larsson, K., Rodholm, M.,...Gundewall C. (1978). Effects of amount of contact between mother and child on the mother's nursing behavior. *Developmental Psychobiology, 11,* 143–150.

Cigales, M., Field, T., Hossain, Z., Peláez-Nogueras, M., & Gewirtz, J. (1996). Touch among children at nursery school. *Early Child Development and Care, 126,* 101–110.

Cohn, J. F., & Tronick, E. Z. (1983). Three-month-old infants' reaction to simulated maternal depression. *Child Development, 54,* 185–193.

Cohn, J. F., & Tronick, E. Z. (1989). Specificity of infants' response to mothers' affective behavior. *Journal of the American Academy of Child and Adolescent Psychiatry, 28,* 242–248.

de Chateau, P. (1976). The influence of early contact on maternal and infant behavior on primiparae. *Birth and the Family Journal, 3,* 149–155

Crnic, K., Ragozin, A. S., Greenberg, M. T., Robinson, N. M., & Basham, R. B. (1983). Social interaction and developmental competence of preterm and full-term infants during the first year of life. *Child Development, 54,* 1199–1210.

Dickson, K. L., Walker, H., & Fogel, A. (1997). The relationship between smile type and play type during parent-infant play. *Developmental Psychology, 33,* 925–933.

Diego, M., Field, T., & Hernandez-Reif, M. (2004). Fetal responses to foot and hand massage of pregnant women. In Field, T. (Ed), *Touch and massage in early child development* (pp. 49–81). U.S.A: Johnson & Johnson Pediatric Institute.

Ellsworth, C. P., Muir, D. W., & Hains, S. M. H. (1993). Social competence and person-object differentiation: An analysis of the still-face effect. *Developmental Psychology, 29,* 63–73.

Fearon, I., Hains, S. M. J., Muir, D. W., & Kisilevsky, B. S. (2002). Development of tactile responses in human preterm and full-term infants form 30 to 40 weeks postconceptional age. *Infancy, 31,* 31–51.

Feijó, L., Hernandez-Reif, M., Field, T., Burns, W., Valley-Gray, S., & Simco, E. (2006). Mothers' depressed mood and anxiety levels are reduced after massaging their preterm infants. *Infant Behavior & Development, 29,* 476–480.

Feldman, R., Keren, M., Gross-Rozval, O., & Tyano, S. (2004). Mother-Child touch patterns in infants feeding disorders: Relation to maternal, child, and environmental factors. *Journal of the American Academy of Child and Adolescent Psychiatry, 43*, 1089–1097.

Feldman, R., Weller, A., Sirota, L., & Eidelman, A. I. (2002) Skin-to-skin contact (Kangaroo Care) promotes self-regulation in premature infants: Sleep-wake cyclicity, arousal modulation, and sustained exploration. *Developmental Psychology, 38*, 194–207.

Ferber, S. G., Feldman, R., Kohelet, D., Kuint, J., Dollberg, S., Arbel, E., & Weller, A. (2005). Massage therapy facilitates mother–infant interaction in premature infants. *Infant Behavior and Development, 28*, 74–81.

Ferber, S. G., Feldman, R., & Makhoul, I. R. (2008). The development of maternal touch across the first year of life. *Early Human Development, 84*, 363–370.

Fergus, E. L., Schmidt, J., & Pickens, J. (1998, April). *Touch during mother–infant interactions: The effects of parenting stress, depression and anxiety.* Poster session presented at the biennial meeting of the International Society of Infant Studies, Atlanta, GA.

Field, T. M. (1984). Early interactions between infants and their postpartum depressed mothers. *Infant Behavior and Development, 7*, 517–522.

Field, T. M. (2002). Infants' need for touch. *Human Development, 45*, 100–103.

Field, T. M., Harding, J., Soliday, B., Lasko, D., Gonzalez, N., & Valdeon, C. (1994). Touching in infant, toddler, and preschool nurseries. *Early Child Development and Care, 98*, 118–120.

Field, T. M., Vega-Lahr, N., Goldstein, S., & Scafidi, F. (1987a). Face-to-face interaction behavior across early infancy. *Infant Behavior and Development, 10*, 111–116.

Field, T. M., Vega-Lahr, N., Goldstein, S., & Scafidi, F. (1987b). Interaction behavior of infants and their dual-career parents. *Infant Behavior and Development, 10*, 371–377.

Field, T. M., Vega-Lahr, N., Scafidi, F., & Goldstein, S. (1986). Effects of maternal unavailability on mother–infant interactions. *Infant Behavior and Development, 9*, 473–478.

Fleck, B., & Chavajay, P. (2009). Physical interactions involving preschoolers and kindergartners in a childcare center. *Early Childhood Research Quarterly, 24*, 46–54.

Fogel, A. (1993). *Developing Through Relationships: Origins of Communication, Self, and Culture.* Chicago, IL: The University of Chicago Press.

Fogel, A., Hsu, H. C., Shapiro, A. F., Nelson-Goens, C. G., & Secrist, C. (2006). Effects of normal and perturbed social play on the duration and amplitude of different types of infant smiles. *Developmental Psychology, 42*, 459–473.

Forbes, E. E., Cohn, J. F., Allen, N. B., & Lewinsohn, P. M. (2004). Infant affect during parent-infant interaction at 3 and 6 months: Differences between mothers and fathers and influence of parent history of depression. *Infancy, 5*, 61–84.

Fransson, A.-L., Karlsson, H., & Nilsson, K. (2005). Temperature variation in newborn babies: Importance of physical contact with the mother Archives of Disease in Childhood. *Fetal and Neonatal Edition, 90*, F500–F504.

Goebel, P. W. (2002). Fathers' touch in low birthweight infants. *Dissertation Abstracts International: Section B: Sciences and Engineering, 62(8-B)*, 3553.

Gusella, J. L., Muir, D. W., & Tronick, E. Z. (1988). The effect of manipulating maternal behavior during an interaction of 3- and 6-month olds' affect and attention. *Child Development, 59*, 1111–1124.

Harrison, L. L., & Woods, S. (1991). Early parental touch and preterm infants. *Journal of Obstetric, Gynecologic, and Neonatal Nursing, 20,* 299–306.

Hentel, A., Beebe, B., & Jaffe, J. (2000, July). *Maternal depression at 6 weeks is associated with infant self-comfort at 4 months.* Poster presented at the International Conference on Infant Studies, Brighton, England.

Herrera, E., Reissland, N., & Shepherd, J. (2004). Maternal touch and maternal child-directed speech: Effects of depressed mood in the postnatal period. *Journal of Affective Disorders, 81,* 29–39.

Hertenstein, M. J. (2002). Touch: Its communicative functions in infancy. *Human Development, 45,* 70–94.

Hertenstein, M. J., & Campos, J. J. (2001). Emotion regulation via maternal touch. *Infancy, 2,* 549–566.

Jahromi, L. B., Putnam, S. P., & Stifter, C. A. (2004). Maternal regulation of infant reactivity from 2 to 6 months. *Developmental Psychology, 40,* 477–487.

Jean, A. D. L., Moszkowski, R., Girouard, N., & Stack, D. M. (2008, March). *The functions of maternal touch during a face-to-face still-face procedure: Influences of maternal regulatory behaviors during the transition periods.* Poster presented at the Biennial International Conference on Infant Studies, Vancouver, British Columbia.

Jean, A. D. L., Moszkowski, R., Girouard, N., & Stack, D. M. (2005, April). *The quality of mother-infant and father-infant face-to-face interactions: Parental touching behavior across interaction contexts.* Poster presented at the Biennial Meeting of the Society for Research in Child Development, Atlanta, GA.

Jean, A. D. L., & Stack, D. M. (2009). Functions of maternal touch and infants' affect during face-to-face interactions: New directions for the still-face. *Infant Behavior and Development, 32,* 123–128.

Jean, A. D. L., Stack, D. M., & Fogel, A. (2009). A longitudinal investigation of maternal touching across the first six months of life: Age and context effects. *Infant Behavior and Development, 32,* 344–349.

Jones, S. E., & Yarbrough, A. E. (1985). A naturalistic study of the meanings of touch. *Communication Monographs, 52,* 19–56.

Kaitz, M., Lapidot, P., Bronner, R., & Eidelman, A. I. (1992). Parturient women can recognize their infant by touch. *Developmental Psychology, 28,* 35–39.

Kaitz, M., Meirov, H., Landman, I., & Eidelman, A. I. (1993). Infant recognition by tactile cues. *Infant Behavior and Development, 16,* 333–341.

Kaye, K., & Fogel, A. (1980). The temporal structure of face-to-face communication between mothers and infants. *Developmental Psychology, 16,* 454–464.

Kisilevsky, B. S., Fearon, I., & Muir, D. W. (1998). Fetuses differentiate vibroacoustic stimuli. *Infant Behavior and Development, 21,* 25–46.

Kisilevsky, B. S., & Muir, D. W. (1991). Human fetal and subsequent newborn responses to sound and vibration. *Infant Behavior and Development, 14,* 1–26.

Kisilevsky, B. S., Muir, D. W., & Low, J. A. (1992). Maturation of human fetal responses to vibroacoustic stimulation. *Child Development, 63,* 1497–1508.

Kisilevsky, B. S., Stack, D. M., & Muir, D. W. (1991). Fetal and infant response to tactile stimulation. In M. Salomon Weiss & P. R. Zelazo (Eds.), *Newborn attention: Biological constraints and the influence of experience* (pp. 63–98). Norwood, NJ: Ablex Publishing Corporation.

Koester, L. S., Brooks, L., Traci, M. A. (2000). Tactile contact of deaf and hearing mothers during face-to-face interactions with their infants. *Journal of Deaf Studies and Deaf Education, 5,* 127–139.

Koester, L. S., Papousek, H., & Papousek, M. (1989). Patterns of rhythmic stimulation by mothers with three-month-olds: A cross-modal comparison. *International Journal of Behavioral Development, 12*, 143–154.

Korner, A. F., & Thoman, E. B. (1972). The relative efficacy of contact and vestibular-proprioceptive stimulation in soothing neonates. *Child Development, 43*, 443–453.

Landau, R., Shusel, R., Eshel, Y., & Ben-Aaron, M., (2003). Mother-child and metapelet-child touch behavior with three-year-old kibbutz children in two contexts. *Infant Mental Health Journal, 24*, 529–546.

Lecanuet, J. P., Granier-Deferre, C., & Busnel, M. C. (1989). Differential fetal auditory reactiveness as a function of stimulus characteristics and states. *Seminars in Perinatology, 13*, 421–429.

LePage, D. E., & Stack, D. M. (1997, April). *Four- and 7-month-old infants' abilities to detect tactile contingencies in a face-to-face context*. Poster session presented at the Biennial Meeting of the Society for Research in Child Development, Washington, DC.

Levy-Shiff, R., Sharir, H., & Mogilner, M. B. (1989). Mother- and father-preterm infant relationship in the hospital preterm nursery. *Child Development, 60*, 93–102.

Maurer, D., & Maurer, C. (1988). *The world of the newborn*. New York, NY: Basic Books.

Millman, T. P., Jean, A., & Stack, D. M. (2009, April). *Infants' self-regulating abilities and maternal touch: Examining the impact of birth status and reaction to the Sill-Face period*. Poster presented at the Biennial Meeting of the Society for Research in Child Development, Denver, CO.

Montagu, A. (1971). *Touching: The human significance of the skin*. New York, NY: Columbia University Press.

Montagu, A. (1986). *Touching: The human significance of the skin*. 3rd ed. New York, NY: Harper and Row Publishers.

Moreno, A. J., Posada, G. E., & Goldyn, D. T. (2006). Presence and quality of touch influence coregulation in mother-infant dyads. *Infancy, 9*, 1–20.

Moszkowski, R. J., Jean, A., & Stack, D. M. (2005a, April). *The co-occurrence of mother and infant touching during early social exchanges*. Poster presented at the biennial meeting of the Society for Research in Child Development, Atlanta, GA.

Moszkowski, R. J., Jean, A., & Stack, D. M. (2005b, June). *Infant smiling as a function of mother and infant tactile behaviours during early social exchanges*. Poster presented at the annual meeting of the Canadian Psychological Association, Montreal, Canada.

Moszkowski, R. J., & Stack, D. M. (2007). Infant touching behavior during mother-infant face-to-face interactions. *Infant and Child Development, 16*, 307–319.

Moszkowski, R. J., Stack, D. M., & Chiarella, S. (2009). Infant touch with gaze and affective behaviors during mother-infant still-face interactions: Co-occurrence and functions of touch. *Infant Behavior and Development, 32*, 392–403.

Moszkowski, R. J., Stack, D. M., Girouard, N., Field, T. M., Hernandez-Reif, M., & Diego, M. (2009). Touching behaviors of infants of depressed mothers during normal and perturbed interactions. *Infant Behavior and Development, 32*, 183–194.

Muir, D. W. (2002). Adult communications with infants through touch: The forgotten sense. *Human Development, 45*, 95–99.

Muir, D., & Field, J. (1979). Newborn infants orient to sounds. *Child Development, 50*, 431–436.

Murray, L., & Trevarthen, C. (1985). Emotional regulation of interactions between two-month-olds and their mothers. In T. M. Field, & N. A. Fox (Eds.), *Social perception in infants* (pp. 177–197). Norwoods, NJ: Ablex Publishing.

Peláez-Nogueras, M., Field, T. M., Hossain, Z., & Pickens, J. (1996). Depressed mothers' touching increases infants' positive affect and attention in still-face interactions. *Child Development, 67*, 1780–1792.

Peláez-Nogueras, M., Gewirtz, J. L., Field, T., Cigales, M., Malphurs, J., Clasky, S., Sanchez, A. (1996). Infants' preference for touch stimulation in face-to-face interactions. *Journal of Applied Developmental Psychology, 17*, 199–213.

Perez, H., & Gewirtz, J. L. (2004). Maternal touch effects on infant behavior. In Field, T. (Ed), *Touch and massage in early child development* (pp. 39–48). U.S.A: Johnson and Johnson Pediatrics Institute.

Polan, H. J., & Ward, M. J. (1994). Role of the mother's touch in failure to thrive: A preliminary investigation. *Journal of the American Child and Adolescent Psychiatry, 33*, 1098–1105.

Pomerleau-Malcuit, A., & Clifton, R. K. (1973). Neonatal heart-rate response to tactile, auditory, and vestibular stimulation in different states. *Child Development, 44*, 485–496.

Rutter, M., & English and Romanian Adoptees (ERA) Study Team. (1998). Developmental catch-up, and deficit, following adoption after severe early privation. *Journal of Child Psychology and Psychiatry, 39*, 465–476.

Shipman, K. L., & Zeman, J. (2001). Socialization of children's emotion regulation in mother–child dyads: A developmental psychopathology perspective. *Development and Psychopathology, 13*, 317–336.

Sroufe, A., Duggal, S., Weinfield, N., & Carlson, E. (2000). In A. J. Sameroff, M. Lewis, & M. Suzanne (Eds.), *Handbook of developmental psychopathology* (2nd ed., pp. 75–91). Dordrecht, Netherlands: Kluwer Academic Publishers.

Stack, D. M. (2001). The salience of touch and physical contact during infancy: Unraveling some of the mysteries of the somesthetic sense. In G. Bremner & A. Fogel (Eds.), *Blackwell handbook of infant development* (pp. 351–378). Oxford, UK: Blackwell Publishing Ltd.

Stack, D. M. (2004). Touching during mother-infant interactions. In Field, T. (Ed), *Touch and massage in early child development* (pp. 49–81). U.S.A: Johnson and Johnson Pediatrics Institute.

Stack, D. M. (2010). Touch and physical contact during infancy: Discovering the richness of the forgotten sense. In J. Gavin Bremner & T. D. Wachs (Eds.), *Blackwell handbook of infancy research* (2nd ed., Vol 1). *Basic Processes*. England: Blackwell.

Stack, D. M., & Arnold, S. L. (1998). Changes in mothers' touch and hand gestures influence infant behavior during face-to-face interchanges. *Infant Behavior and Development, 21*, 451–468.

Stack, D. M., & LePage, D. E. (1996). Infants' sensitivity to manipulations of maternal touch during face-to-face interactions. *Social Development, 5*, 41–55.

Stack, D. M., LePage, D. E., Hains, S. M., & Muir, D. W. (1996). Qualitative changes in maternal touch as a function of instructional condition during face-to-face social interactions. *Infant Behavior and Development, 19*, 761.

Stack, D. M., & Muir, D. W. (1990). Tactile stimulation as a component of social interchange: New interpretations for the still-face effect. *British Journal of Developmental Psychology, 8*, 131–145.

Stack, D. M., & Muir, D. W. (1992). Adult tactile stimulation during face-to-face interactions modulates 5-month-olds' affect and attention. *Child Development, 63*, 1509–1525.

Stepakoff, S. A. (1999). Mother-infant tactile communication at four months: Effects of infant gender, maternal ethnicity, and maternal depression [Unpublished doctoral dissertation]. New York: St. John's University.

Symons, D. K., & Moran, G. (1987). The behavioral dynamics of mutual responsiveness in early face-to-face mother-infant interactions. *Child Development, 58*, 1488–1495.

Toda, S., & Fogel, A. (1993). Infant response to the still-face situation at 3 and 6 months. *Developmental Psychology, 29*, 532–538.

Trevathan, W. R. (1981). Maternal touch at 1st contact with the newborn infant. *Developmental Psychobiology, 14*, 549–558.

Tronick, E. Z. (1989). Emotions and emotional communication in infants. *American Psychologist, 44*, 112–119.

Tronick, E. Z. (1995). Touch in mother-infant interaction. In T. M. Field (Ed.), *Touch in early development* (pp. 53–65). Mahwah, NJ: Lawrence Erlbaum Associates, Inc.

Tronick, E. Z., Als, H., Adamson, L., Wise, S., & Brazelton, T. B. (1978). The infant's response to entrapment between contradictory messages in face-to-face interactions. *Journal of the American Academy of Child Psychiatry, 17*, 1–13.

Tulman, L. J. (1985). Mother's and unrelated persons' initial handling of newborn infants. *Nursing Research, 34*, 205–210.

Vygotsky, L. (1978). Interaction between learning and development. *Mind in society* (pp. 79–91). Cambridge, MA: Harvard University Press.

Weiss, S. J. (1992). Measurement of the sensory qualities in tactile interaction. *Nursing Research, 41*, 82–86.

Weiss, S. J., Wilson, P., Hertenstein, M., & Campos, R. (2000). The tactile context of a mother's caregiving: Implications for attachment of low birth weight infants. *Infant Behaviour and Development, 23*, 91–111.

Weiss, S. J., Wilson, P., St. John Seed, M., & Paul, S. M. (2001). Early tactile experience of low birth weight children: Links to later mental health and social adaptation. *Infant and Child Development, 10*, 93–115.

Widom, C. S., Raphael, K. G., & DuMont, K. A. (2004). The case for prospective longitudinal studies in child maltreatment research: Commentary on Dube, Williamson, Thompson, Felitti, and Anda (2004). *Child Abuse & Neglect, 28*, 715–722.

Wheldall, K., Bevan, K., Shortall, K. (1986). A touch of reinforcement: The effects of contingent teacher touch on the classroom behaviour of young children. *Educational Review, 38*, 207–216.

Wolff, P. H. (1963). Observations on the early development of smiling. In B. M. Foss (Ed.), *Determinants of infant behavior II*. London, England: Methuen & Co. Ltd.

Zaslow, M. J., Pederson, F. A., Suwalsky, J. T. D., Cain, R. L., & Fivel, M. (1985). The early resumption of employment by mothers: Implications for parent-infant interaction. *Journal of Applied Developmental Psychology, 6*, 1–16.

12

The Communicative Functions of Touch in Adulthood

MATTHEW J. HERTENSTEIN

Thanks to Darwinian natural selection, our skin and hands evolved to the finely tuned tactile communication system we know today (Jablonski, 2006; Keltner, 2009). Evolutionary biologists posit that we evolved the relatively hairless bodies we have due to thermoregulation. That is, our ancestors on the hot savannah evolved hairless bodies to more quickly dissipate the heat of their bodies. Moreover, hairless bodies may have resulted in reduced drinking water requirements, an adaptation that makes eminent sense on the savannah (Wheeler, 1992). In the evolutionarily adaptive spirit, we gained exquisite control over our hands as we became bipedal and began to construct and use tools (Young, 2003). Of course, now, our hands are central to the tactile communication system.

This chapter is not about the evolutionary origins of touch, but rather the communicative functions served by touch in adulthood, many of which have evolutionary origins. A significant body of research is mounting which shows that touch plays a critical role in communication not only in infancy (e.g., Field, 2001; Weiss & Campos, 1999), but throughout our adult lives (e.g., Hertenstein, Verkamp, Kerestes, & Holmes, 2006). This chapter delineates many of the major functions served by touch as they relate to social phenomena primarily and cognition secondarily. The chapter draws upon and updates previous reviews the author has written on the communicative functions served by touch (Hertenstein, 2002, in press; Hertenstein, Butts, & Hile, 2007; Hertenstein, Verkamp, et al., 2006).

Like all reviews, difficult decisions must be made regarding the best way to parse the literature. The goal of this chapter is not to review all the functions served by touch, but rather the core communicative functions on which investigators have focused. Thus, the review does not focus on those domains in which little work has been conducted or those domains in which investigators made little or no attempt to understand the unique contributions of the tactile modality as it pertains to a given communicative function (e.g., studies focusing on the effects of stimulus deprivation, including touch, on infants; Spitz, 1946). In addition, I do not discuss some of the functions of touch either because they are covered in other chapters (e.g., communication of power, see Chapter 13) or because they are beyond the scope of this chapter (e.g., touch in therapeutic settings and self-touch). Whether readers find the current review comprehensive or even representative will depend on their theoretical orientation(s) as well as where they draw the line in the sand on the aforementioned exclusion criteria.

In this chapter, I first discuss conceptual issues related to touch and communication. Second, I discuss methodological approaches researchers have adopted to study touch. Third, I discuss some important communication functions served by touch, including intimacy, emotions, the perception of touch, and compliance. Finally, I discuss individual differences in touch, how touch intersects with other modalities, and suggestions for future research in the field.

DEFINITIONAL AND CONCEPTUAL ISSUES

I focus on two broad phenomena in this chapter: touch and communication. Here, *touch* can refer to two dissociable phenomena (Hertenstein, 2002; Hertenstein, Verkamp, et al., 2006). The first refers to the action of an object on the skin, whereas the second refers to the registration of information by the sensory system. The pressure exerted on the skin would encompass the former sense of the word, whereas feeling ticklish would be an example of the second of the latter sense of the word (i.e., sensory registration). The sensory registration of touch usually involves both cutaneous receptors (mechanoreceptors and thermoreceptors) which register tactile stimuli, as well as kinesthetic receptors which sense movement of the body (Loomis & Lederman, 1986).

The relations between touch and communication differ depending on the facet of touch to which one refers. For example, a person may touch two people identically, but one person may perceive the touch positively and the other negatively. To help clarify this state of affairs, the words *touch*, *tactile stimulus*, and *tactile pattern* are used in this chapter to connote the action of touch on the skin, whereas the words *perception* or *feeling* are used to connote the sensory registration of touch.

In addition to *touch*, conceptual clarity is important when discussing *communication* (Hertenstein, 2002; Hertenstein, Verkamp, et al.,

2006). We draw from the nonverbal communication, ethological, and functionalist literatures that emphasize the behavioral and cognitive consequences of communication, rather than the information transfer between two conspecifics. Thus, tactile communication occurs when there are systematic changes in another's thoughts, feelings, perceptions, or behavior as a function of another's touch in relation to the context in which it occurs (Barrett & Nelson-Goens, 1997; Hertenstein, 2002). Note that this definition does not require information transfer to occur between people for communication to transpire. For example, a person may touch another on the shoulder and the target may experience warmth when, in fact, the person administering the touch is experiencing a negative emotional state. Nonetheless, communication has taken place because the target's thoughts were influenced by the tactile stimulus.

Three important points must be discussed briefly regarding communication and touch (Hertenstein, 2002; Hertenstein, Verkamp, et al., 2006). First, the communication need not be intentionally displayed (i.e., deliberate) and be goal directed for true communication to transpire (e.g., Watzlawick, Beavin, & Jackson, 1967); communication via touch may be accidental and not goal directed (e.g., Hinde, 1997). Second, any discussion of tactile communication must take seriously two fundamental principles: equifinality and equipotentiality. The principle of equifinality refers to the idea that the same communicative outcome can be achieved via a number of different means (e.g., anger may be communicated via a slap or a push). The principle of equipotentiality refers to the idea that the same type of touch can be assigned very different meanings or consequences (e.g., an arm around one's shoulders may be interpreted as loving or a display of dominance). Third, communication does not take place in isolation, but is always embedded in a context. Thus, one must remain mindful that all communication is surrounded by a local context and larger historical, social, and economic contexts (Bronfenbrenner & Morris, 1998). Moreover, other modalities typically covary with touch during communication, and so researchers must remain mindful when focusing only on touch. Finally, all communication is bidirectional; there is a constant and dynamic interplay between communicators (Fogel, 2000); one cannot touch, after all, without being touched (Montagu, 1986).

APPROACHES TO THE STUDY OF TOUCH

Researchers have adopted three general approaches to study tactile communication in adulthood, each with their own advantages and drawbacks: self-report, observational, and experimental methods (Hertenstein, Verkamp, et al., 2006; Thayer, 1986).

The self-report method provides an efficient and cost-effective means to investigate touch that transpires both in public and in private. In some studies, participants are asked to recall their tactile experiences (e.g., Jourard, 1966), whereas in others participants are asked to record their touch experiences just after they occur (e.g., Jones & Yarbrough, 1985; Willis & Rinck, 1983). Obviously, participants' abilities to accurately recall their tactile experiences present a methodological challenge of the former method.

In a seminal study, typical of the latter self-report method, Jones and Yarbrough (1985) asked students to notate their tactile experiences immediately following each time they touched were touched by someone else. From these data, the researchers derived several distinct meanings of touch, including support, appreciation, inclusion, sexual interest, affection, playful touch, compliance, and attention getting.

Researchers have also employed observational methods to study tactile communication (e.g., Hall, 1996; Jones, 1972; Willis & Dodds, 1998; Willis, Rinck, & Dean, 1978). Hall conducted an exemplary study using the observational method in which she unobtrusively recorded instances of interpersonal touch (quality, location, function, and duration) and participants' gender, age, and status (student vs. member, prestige of one's institution and department) at three professional academic conferences. Although status did not mediate touch initiation, status did mediate the quality of touch used. Specifically, lower-status individuals initiated more formalized touch such as handshakes, whereas high-status individuals were more likely to initiate discrete touches to the arm and shoulders that were sometimes affectionate.

Observational methods have both strengths and weaknesses (Hertenstein, Verkamp, et al., 2006). Recordings of naturally occurring touch can be accurately recorded with well-trained and reliable coders. Such coders are less likely to be biased, unlike methodologies which require subjects to report their own tactile interactions. With well-trained, reliable, and unobtrusive coders, recordings of touch can be accurate and participant bias is reduced because the coder is not also the participant like self-report methods. Moreover, observational studies can take place in the "real world" such that the ecological validity of such studies are greater than experimental studies. Nevertheless, there are some disadvantages. First, there is no control over the variables of interest so that inferences of causation are constrained. Second, touch is not a frequent and spontaneous behavior in many contexts; thus, observing natural tactile interactions can be very time consuming and resource intensive. Finally, touch that transpires in personal contexts, such as the home, is difficult, if not impossible, to observe. Observational methods are best suited for public tactile interactions.

Experimental studies of touch have the distinct advantage of allowing researchers to infer causation about the effects of touch on a wide variety of phenomena. However, there are some significant drawbacks to this research approach. Perhaps the most serious drawback is that other nonverbal behaviors may systematically change with manipulated tactile displays which may confound accurate causal inference. For example, a group of researchers instructed confederates to maintain constant nonverbal behavior while they either touched or did not touch participants on the elbow or forearm (Lewis, Derlega, Shankar, Cochard, & Finkel, 1997). The intention was to manipulate only tactile behavior. However, when coding the confederates' nonverbal behaviors, the experimenters found that confederates who touched systematically displayed fewer expressive hand gestures and more nervous gestures. Thus, any inference about the touch manipulation was confounded with other nonverbal behaviors (Hertenstein, Verkamp, et al., 2006).

I have described three predominant approaches to the study of touch. With this in mind, I now discuss some of the major domains in which touch plays a fundamental role in adult life.

INTIMACY

In a comprehensive review of the literature, researchers found that relational communication is characterized by at least 12 conceptually distinct themes (Burgoon & Hale, 1984). One of these themes—intimacy—was considered to be primary because it consistently appeared in almost all the literatures evaluated. Touch constitutes one of the primary means of communicating and fostering intimacy, especially touch leading to sexual intimacy (Hertenstein, Verkamp, et al., 2006). As Thayer (1986) wrote over two decades ago, "Touch is a signal in the communication process that, above all other communication channels, most directly and immediately escalates the balance of intimacy" (p. 8). Many researchers hold that touch is a fundamental immediacy behavior (e.g., Mehrabian, 1971; Patterson, Reidhead, Gooch, & Stopka, 1984) and plays a primary role in theories of intimacy (Argyle & Dean, 1965; Cappella & Greene, 1982; Patterson, 1976).

Several studies demonstrate the ubiquity of touch in the communication of intimacy (Jones & Yarbrough, 1985; Jourard, 1966; Willis & Rinck, 1983). College participants recorded their tactile interactions with others using a personal log method in one study (Willis & Rinck, 1983). The majority of tactile interactions took place in private settings and most of these touches were of a personal nature. The researchers also classified sexual touches such as a hand to a thigh or other sexually oriented part of the body. Though the sample size was less than desired, the data revealed that a majority of the women and just over one-third of the men reported at least one of these touches in the study (Hertenstein, Verkamp, et al., 2006).

Jones and Yarbrough (1985) identified three touch categories using the log method that nearly always fostered intimate experience: touches expressing sexual intent and attraction, touches expressing positive affection and general positive regard toward the other, and touches communicating togetherness usually involving lower body parts touching such as the knees. All these types of touch occurred most often in close cross-sex relationships.

Heterosexual romantic couples typically engage in a specific sequence of touch behaviors to communicate intimacy (Morris, 1971). In order, they include hand-to-hand contact, arm-to-shoulder contact, arm-to-waist contact, mouth-to-mouth contact, hand-to-head contact, hand-to-body contact, mouth-to-breast contact, hand-to-genitals contact, and, finally, genitals-to-genitals contact. Of course, this sequence is not strictly invariant for couples as much heterogeneity exists between couples. Moreover, some of these steps are skipped because of canonical forms of touch such as handshakes, kisses, or dancing (Hertenstein, Verkamp, et al., 2006).

A number of researchers have found that the quantity of touch between couples is minimal in the initial stage of relationships, waxes thereafter reaching the quantitative apex during the intermediate stages of relationships (usually when monogamously dating or engaged), and wanes after the first year of marriage (Emmers & Dindia, 1995; Guerrero & Andersen, 1991; McDaniel & Andersen, 1998; Willis & Briggs, 1992). In one study, researchers recorded participants' tactile interactions, and then a female experimenter approached the participants and asked them to describe their relationship (Willis & Briggs). Couples who had been married longer than 1 year touched each other significantly less than couples who had been married less than 1 year or who were engaged or dating. This study and others (Guerrero & Andersen; McDaniel & Andersen) indicate that high quantities of tactile interaction are present early in intimate relationships and men tend to initiate touch more often than women early in relationships.

The quantity and quality of touch between couples reflects the intimacy and happiness of their relationships (Beier & Sternberg, 1977; Heslin & Boss, 1980). Beier and Sternberg videotaped recently married couples while interviewing them about their adjustment to marriage and coded self-touching and other touching. Couples who reported the greatest amount of marital happiness touched each other more and themselves less, as compared with couples reporting low marital happiness. In another study, researchers unobtrusively observed travelers at an airport for the type of tactile involvement that occurred between them and someone waiting for them at a terminal. The data revealed that the more intimate the couples reported being, the more intimate touch they used (Heslin and Boss). Of course, these studies are correlational, and so other variables may be playing an important role in the mediation of touch and intimacy (Hertenstein, Verkamp, et al., 2006).

What do outside observers infer about the intimacy level of couples based on their tactile interactions? A number of researchers have been interested in this question (Burgoon, 1991; Burgoon, Buller, Hale, & DeTurck, 1984; Floyd & Voloudakis, 1999; Pisano, Wall, & Foster, 1986). Typically, researchers show participants a photo or a videotaped interaction and ask participants to rate how intimate the tactile interaction was or how intimate the relationship is on the basis of the touches observed in the interaction. For example, Floyd (1999) presented a video-recorded interaction of two actors embracing each other and manipulated the duration and form of the embraces. Both the form and duration of the embraces influenced participants' perceptions of intimacy. Similarly, Burgoon showed photos to participants and varied the type of tactile interactions between the models. Handholding and face touching expressed the most intimacy compared with other types of touch.

Although we know that touch communicates and fosters intimacy, there are some significant challenges to the study of this topic (Hertenstein, Verkamp, et al., 2006). Perhaps the most daunting challenge is that most touch that communicates intimacy takes place privately, making it difficult for researchers who want to study such interactions using methods other than self-report. Another task for researchers is to study how touch operates in gay or lesbian couples. This is a population that has received very little empirical attention. Finally, measuring encoders' attitudes and perceptions of tactile displays of intimacy would be important. Typically, the recipients of touch are asked about their experiences, but asking encoders may yield some significant insights into the communication of intimacy via touch.

COMMUNICATION OF EMOTIONS BETWEEN HUMANS

The word *emotion* is derived from the Latin "to move out," suggesting that one facet of emotions is bodily movement and action (Hertenstein, 2002). This notion sits well with contemporary theories of emotion

(Frijda, 2006; Niedenthal, 2007; Niedenthal & Maringer, 2009). Frijda, for example, holds that tendencies to act in relation to others are fundamental to the concept of emotion. Thus, movement of the body against others' bodies, as well as physiological indicators skin temperature, perspiration, and respiratory patterns, can all contribute to the communication of emotion. Despite the apparent importance of touch in the study of affect, its role in the communication of emotion has received preciously little attention compared to the face and voice (Hertenstein, 2002). Indeed, one finds almost no mention of touch in reference works in the field of emotion (Davidson, Scherer, & Goldsmith, 2003; Lewis, Haviland-Jones, & Barrett, 2008). Nevertheless, there has been some work done on the communication of emotion via tactile stimulation, particularly the hedonic value of touch.

Hedonics

The hedonics—the positive and negative emotional perception—of touch has been of longstanding interest to researchers (e.g., Nguyen, Heslin, & Nguyen, 1976, 1975). The skin contains receptors that directly generate hedonic values, either because there are portions of the skin that are erogenous or because there are nerve endings that are nociceptive, thereby generating positive and negative affect, respectively (Hertenstein, 2002). The perceived hedonic quality of touch is moderated not only by the type of touch, but by other contextual variables such as gender, relationship status, and overall context. Nguyen, Heslin, and Nguyen designed a series of studies to investigate the hedonic meaning people ascribe to touch (Heslin, Nguyen, & Nguyen, 1983; Nguyen et al., 1976; Nguyen et al., 1975). Nguyen et al. (1975) asked college-age participants to identify what it meant for them to be touched by a close person of the opposite sex (excluding family) on 11 different areas of the body. Subjects identified the meaning they attributed to each touch by scales that represented degrees of pleasantness, sexual desire, playfulness, friendship or fellowship, and warmth or love. The more that men perceived touch as sexual, the more they perceived it as pleasant, warm, and playful, whereas the more that women perceived touch as sexual, the less they perceived it as warm, loving, playful, or friendly. In a follow-up study including married and unmarried participants, Nguyen et al. (1976) found that married women perceived sexual touch as warm and as pleasant as unmarried men, but unmarried women did not. Also, although all men found sexual touch to be pleasant, warm, and playful, the correlation was stronger for unmarried men than for married men. The researchers found that type and location of touch impacted the meaning that participants attributed to them (Nguyen et al., 1976; Nguyen et al., 1975). Stroking was associated with warmth, love, and sexual desire, whereas squeezing and patting were associated with playful and friendly touches. Playfulness was associated with touch on the leg, whereas sexual desire was associated with touch on the genital area (Hertenstein, Verkamp, et al., 2006).

In a follow-up study conducted by the same research team, participants were asked to consider touch from strangers and people of the same sex (Heslin et al., 1983). Participants rated touch from opposite-sex friends, for both men and women, as less of an invasion of privacy and more pleasant than touch from same-sex friends or same-sex strangers. These differences were most dramatic for touches that were perceived as sexual. However, there was a significant gender difference. Women perceived touch from opposite-sex strangers to be unpleasant and an invasion of privacy, whereas men did not. Men perceived touch of all kinds from an opposite-sex stranger to be as pleasant as from a close female friend. Both men and women rated sexual touches from opposite-sex friends to be the most pleasant. Women's second highest rating was for stroking nonsexual touches by a close male friend, whereas men's second highest rating was for stroking sexual touches by a female stranger (Hertenstein, Verkamp, et al., 2006).

Three implications can be drawn from this line of research (Heslin & Alper, 1983; Heslin et al., 1983). First, to be perceived positively, the intimacy of touch must be congruent with the intimacy of the relationship, at least for women. Thus, sexual touch is perceived positively when it is presented by an intimate other. Second, men and women weigh the familiarity of the person touching them with different importance; men tend not to mind being touched by female strangers, but women dislike touch from opposite-sex strangers. Finally, same-sex touch, especially sexual touch and touch from strangers, is often perceived as unpleasant. Researchers have consistently shown that disdain for same-sex touch is greater for men compared with women (Hewitt & Feltham, 1982; Willis & Rawdon, 1994).

Another important component in the study of the hedonics of touch is the role that cognition plays. McCabe and her colleagues recently addressed this issue in a study examining how one's cognitive frame influenced the perception of touch (McCabe, Rolls, Bilderbeck, & McGlone, 2008). In the study, a female experimenter applied body lotion to the ventral surface of the left forearm. The cream was applied in a standardized fashion for all subjects such that the experimenter applied the cream with one finger smoothly and slowly for 8 seconds. Concurrent with the administration of the cream, the word label "Rich moisturizing cream" or "Basic cream" was presented on a projection screen, only visible to the subject (i.e., the experimenter was naïve to the experimental condition). After a 2-second delay, the subject rated the pleasantness of the tactile stimulus on a Likert scale. These conditions were presented to the same subject along with several other experimental conditions. The researchers found that the label of the cream shown on the screen significantly influenced the pleasantness of the tactile stimulus. Specifically, when "Rich moisturizing cream" was displayed, subjects rated the pleasantness of the touch significantly higher than when shown "Basic cream." Thus, the cognitive context in which touch occurs can influence the hedonic intensity of touch.

A final area in which the impact of touch can be observed is in the realm of security, a state related to positive hedonics. Levav and Argo (2010) conducted a series of studies in which participants were touched by an experimenter on the shoulder. The participants were then assessed on how financially risky they would be both with hypothetical and real payoffs, as well as their feelings of security. When subjects were touched by a female (but not a male), they took greater financial risks compared to untouched participants. Importantly, the data indicated that such results were attributable, in part, to touch providing a sense of security to the subjects.

Distinct Emotions

Two general claims have been offered regarding the role of touch in emotional communication. First, some researchers have held that touch communicates the hedonic quality of emotion (i.e., positivity or negativity) and have conducted their research in this tradition (e.g., Hertenstein & Campos, 2001; Jones & Yarbrough, 1985). Second, touch has been thought to intensify already existing emotions (Hertenstein, Holmes, McCullough, & Keltner, 2009; Hertenstein, Keltner, App, Bulleit, & Jaskolka, 2006). For example, abruptly grabbing one's shoulder would intensify the communication of anger with a simultaneous display of anger on the face.

Despite these two claims, there is theoretical justification to believe touch communicates more than the valence or intensity of emotion (Hertenstein, Keltner, et al., 2006). One feature of the "basic" emotions is multimodal specification; that is, emotions such as fear, disgust, surprise, anger, joy, and sadness are communicated by the face, voice, and even posture (Ekman, 1999; Scherer, 1986; Wallbott, 1998). Phenomena such as distance, speed, and direction that are multimodally specified in sight and sound are also specified by touch (Stern, 1985). Given this, some have hypothesized that touch may communicate distinct emotions like the face and voice between humans (e.g., Tronick, 1995).

To test this hypothesis, Hertenstein and his colleagues have conducted a series of studies examining the potential of touch to communicate distinct emotions (Hertenstein et al., 2009; Hertenstein, Keltner, et al., 2006). In the first, two unacquainted participants came to the lab at the same time and sat on opposite sides of a table. Participants were never allowed to see or hear each other before or during the test session and an opaque cloth barrier separated the dyad. At the beginning of each of the 12 trials, one participant (i.e., the decoder) was instructed to place his/her arm through an aperture in the cloth barrier so as to display an arm and hand to the other participant (i.e., the encoder). The experimenter instructed the encoder to communicate 12 different emotions, one per trial, in serial order to the decoder. After each trial, the decoder chose which emotion he/she thought the encoder communicated. There was also a *none of these terms are correct* option to help reduce artificial inflation of accuracy rates (Frank & Stennett, 2001).

The results of the study provided convincing evidence that touch does, in fact, communicate distinct emotions, even in a very constrained and controlled context. Anger, fear, disgust, love, gratitude, and sympathy were communicated well above chance levels (defined as 25%), whereas happiness, sadness, surprise, embarrassment, envy, and pride were not communicated accurately (see Figure 12.1—arm-only). To replicate and extend these findings, Hertenstein et al. (2006)

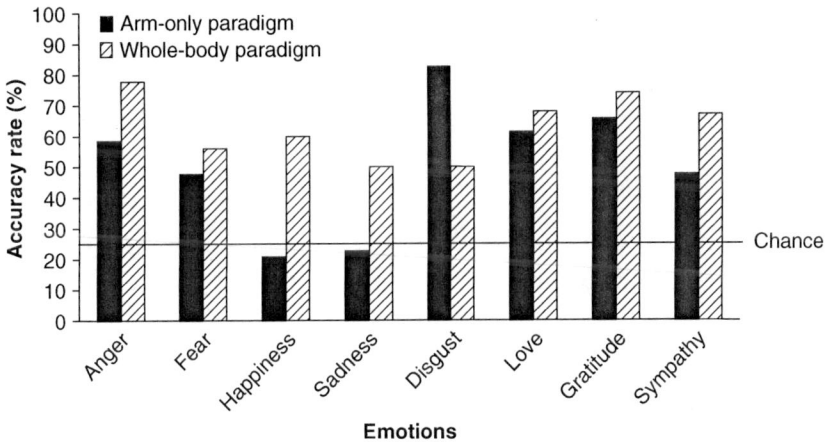

FIGURE 12.1 Percentage of decoding accuracy for each emotion.

employed the same experimental paradigm, though this time with four fewer emotions, in Spain. The same pattern of results were replicated with participants in Spain, a culture that is thought to highly value touch compared to some other Western cultures (Andersen, 1999; Hertenstein, Keltner, et al., 2006). In addition to the decoding findings, extensive behavioral coding of the U.S. sample identified specific tactile behaviors associated with each of the emotions. For example, sympathy was associated with stroking and patting, anger was associated with hitting and squeezing, disgust was associated with a pushing motion, and fear was associated with trembling.

Hertenstein and his colleagues conducted another study examining the communication of emotion; the researchers were guided by three motivations (Hertenstein et al., 2009). First, the study was designed to have greater ecological validity than the previous studies. In Hertenstein, Keltner, et al.'s (2006) previous studies, participants were allowed to touch only on the bottom half of the arm—a constrained context. In the follow-up study, encoders were allowed to touch the other member anywhere on the body that was appropriate. This more closely approximates how people rely on touch to communicate in more naturalistic settings. Second, Hertenstein et al. sought to investigate whether touch on the whole body could communicate more distinct emotions than known heretofore. Given the whole-body paradigm, touch could vary by location and encoders were allowed to apply a larger variety of touch qualities. Given the greater complexity of tactile signals permitted in the current paradigm, we predicted that touch on the whole body may communicate more emotions than previously discovered. Finally, we sought to identify the particular tactile types and location used to communicate each emotion.

In this study, the designated encoder entered the lab to find the decoder blindfolded. The decoder could not see the encoder, nor were the participants allowed to talk or make any sounds. Eight emotions words were displayed serially to the encoder and he/she was instructed to touch the decoder to communicate each of the emotions. Like the first set of studies, the decoder was asked to choose the emotion that was communicated.

Not only were the same emotions communicated as those in previous studies (Hertenstein, Keltner, et al., 2006), but two additional emotions were reliably communicated: happiness and sadness (see Figure 12.1—whole body). Moreover, specific tactile behaviors were associated with each of the emotions. Anger, for example, was associated with nuzzling and hugging; love was associated with hugging and stroking; and sympathy was associated with hugging and rubbing.

The studies reported earlier demonstrate that touch communicates at least four negatively valenced emotions—anger, fear, sadness, and disgust—and four positive or prosocial emotions—happiness, gratitude, sympathy, and love (Lazarus, 1991). Thus, there is considerable evidence to suggest that the tactile modality is just as differentiated, if not more so, as the face and voice when considering the communication of distinct emotions (see Bailenson, Yee, Brave, Merget, & Koslow (2007) for a study showing how handshakes communicate distinct emotions). This is particularly evident when considering positive emotions. Darwin (1872) foreshadowed this to some degree in *The Expression of the Emotions in Man and Animals* when he indicated that love did not differentiate itself in the face from other positive emotions. Instead, when discussing the emotion of love, he wrote "A strong desire to touch the beloved person is commonly felt; and love is expressed by this means more plainly than by any other." (p. 215).

The above studies demonstrate that touch is capable of communicating distinct emotions from one person to another. However, can observers decode distinct emotions from observations of other individuals communicating emotion via touch? To address this question, we presented a sample of observers with video clips of the tactile communications from the previous arm-only paradigm (Hertenstein, Keltner, et al., 2006). Each clip presented a view of the decoder's arm on which the encoder provided tactile stimulation to communicate an emotion. Like the behavioral studies of touch, of interest was how accurate observers could decode which emotion was being communicated between the dyads via touch. We found that anger, fear, happiness, disgust, love, and sympathy were communicated at above chance levels. These data lend additional support that touch communicates distinct emotions not only behaviorally, but by mere observation.

Although not related to communication between humans—the primary focus of this chapter—Clynes (1977) has investigated how humans can depress a pressure-sensitive button to associate states such as hatred, anger, reverence, and joy. Clynes claims that subjects universally depress the button in the same manner for a number of states. Clynes and Nettheim (1982) wanted to see if subjects could recognize states via fixed choice methods after practicing the specific motor pattern taught to them. On the whole, subjects accurately detected the states via button pressing. Unfortunately, some researchers have failed to replicate aspects of this line of work (Nettelbeck et al., 1989; Trussoni, O'Malley, & Barton, 1988), and the validity and theoretical underpinnings of the device used to collect the data have been questioned (Scherer & Zetner, 2001). Other researchers have investigated how emotions are communicated via other haptic devices as well (e.g., Salminen et al., 2008; Smith & MacLean, 2007).

LIKING

From the literature previously reviewed, we know that touch is perceived pleasantly under some circumstances and is an invasion of privacy in others. We also know that touch communicates distinct emotions. However, does touch increase or decrease liking of touchers? Researchers have designed a number of studies to address this question.

In a seminal study, a confederate library clerk momentarily touched men and women participants while handing back change (Fisher, Rytting, & Heslin, 1976). Participants who were touched reported greater positive affective states and liked the library clerk more than did participants who were not touched. This effect was not influenced by the sex of the toucher or whether or not the participants realized they were being touched. However, there was nearly a significant Touch × Sex of Participant interaction; women primarily carried the touch main effect, whereas men's ratings of the clerk were more variable.

Although the sex of the confederate did not affect participants' evaluations in the aforementioned study, others have shown evidence of an effect. In one study, women and men confederates greeted participants arriving for a study in one of three ways: (a) a polite nod with no touch, (b) a simple handshake, or (c) a handshake with a gentle squeeze on the right upper arm (Silverthorne, Micklewright, O'Donnell, & Gibson, 1976). Overall, the greater the amount of touch the confederate used, the more that the participants liked the confederate. However, there were some gender differences. The more touch that was involved in the initial contact when a male touched a female, the more the woman perceived the man as an acceptable marriage partner. In contrast, the more touch that was involved in the initial contact when a woman touched a man, the less the man perceived the woman as an acceptable marriage partner (Hertenstein, Verkamp, et al., 2006).

Another study indicated that males respond less positively to touch than do women (Whitcher & Fisher, 1979). A confederate female nurse either touched (on the hand and arm) or did not touch patients who were awaiting elective surgery. Men who were touched reported experiencing more anxiety leading up to their surgery and had higher blood pressure (both systolic and diastolic) following surgery than did men who were not touched. Women who were touched, compared with those who were not, perceived the nurse as more interested in them, were less anxious about their impeding surgery, and had lower blood pressure following surgery. Again, women responded significantly more positively to touch than did men (Hertenstein, Verkamp, et al., 2006).

The studies discussed thus far indicate that when touched by strangers (in a nonsexual manner), women like touchers more, whereas men's reactions to being touched are negative or neutral, particularly if they are touched by women (Fisher et al., 1976; Major, 1981; Silverthorne et al., 1976; Sussman & Rosenfeld, 1978; Whitcher & Fisher, 1979). However, not all researchers have found that men react negatively or neutrally to touch (Burgoon, Walther, & Baesler, 1992; Hornik, 1992; Jourard & Friedman, 1970; Silverthorne, Noreen, Hunt, & Rota, 1972). Jourard and Friedman, for example, found that both men and women reported more positive evaluations of a male interviewer after being touched by him. Overall, it appears that there are no clear overall and consistent gender effects when discussing the impact of touch on liking (Hertenstein, Verkamp, et al., 2006).

The literature on liking and bonding in humans has been linked to nonhuman primate evolution, in general, and grooming specifically (Dunbar, 2010). Dunbar has persuasively argued that grooming in nonhuman primates plays a foundational role in the positive consequences of touch in human communication. Moreover, Dunbar argues that the role of touch in social bonding and liking has a significant role to play in individuals' lifetime reproductive fitness.

COMPLIANCE

A large body of literature shows that tactile stimulation increases the compliance of the recipient in a number of important domains (Brockner, Pressman, Cabitt, & Moran, 1982; Crusco & Wetzel, 1984; Foehl & Goldman, 1983; Goldman & Fordyce, 1983; Goldman, Kiyohara, & Pfannensteil, 1985; Guéguen, 2002a, 2002b, 2002c, 2004; Guéguen & Fischer-Lokou, 2002, 2003; Guéguen, Jacob, & Boulbry, 2007; Hornik, 1991; Hornik & Ellis, 1988; Joule & Gueguen, 2007; Kaufman & Mahoney, 1999; Kleinke, 1977; Nannberg & Hansen, 1994; Patterson, Powell, & Lenihan, 1986; Paulsell & Goldman, 1984; Powell, Meil, Patterson, & Chouinard, 1994; Stephen & Zweigenhaft, 1986; Willis & Hamm, 1980). In a seminal study, Kleinke found that 51% of participants were more willing to return a lost dime in a phone booth to a confederate who touched them compared to only 29% of participants who were not touched (although, for a critique, see Hertenstein, Verkamp, et al., 2006).

The effects of touch on compliance go beyond returning money; people will *give* more money if touched (Hertenstein, Verkamp, et al., 2006). In one study, waitresses touched restaurant customers while returning their change (Crusco & Wetzel, 1984). Customers were randomly assigned to one of three conditions: (a) those who were touched by the waitress twice on the palm, (b) those who were touched on the shoulder, and (c) those who were not touched. The two touch conditions increased the amount of tips and these results were not influenced by gender, weather, day of the week, or the number of dining parties. A recent study, again conducted in a restaurant, showed that patrons who were touched by waiters while suggesting the chef's special were significantly more likely to accept the waiter's suggestion compared to a control condition in which patrons were not touched while hearing the suggestions (Guéguen et al., 2007).

Other researchers have investigated how touch increases compliance in other domains (Hertenstein, Verkamp, et al., 2006). In a study that has important health implications, Guéguen and Vion (2009) investigated how touch from medical practitioners influences patients' compliance in taking prescribed medicine. The researchers instructed male and female medical practitioners to either touch or not touch patients on the forearm as they informed the patients that it was important that they take their medication for pharyngitis. Patients who were touched complied with the medical practitioners' requests to a greater degree than those who were not touched; touched patients more faithfully consumed their medicine as instructed.

Willis and Hamm (1980) conducted two studies. In the first, a confederate asked participants to sign a petition for a local issue of concern, and in the second, participants were asked to fill out a questionnaire. In both studies, half of the participants were touched on the upper arm, whereas the other half were not touched, holding constant other nonverbal cues. In the first study, 81% of the touched participants signed the petition compared with 55% of the participants in the control group. Likewise, 70% of the touched participants in the second study completed the questionnaire, whereas only 40% of the participants who were not touched did so.

The foot-in-the-door effect in which a small request is asked of people in preparation for a more substantial request has also been investigated in relation to touch (Goldman et al., 1985; Patterson et al., 1986). In one study, participants were invited to a laboratory to fill out several questionnaires (Patterson et al., 1986). After completing the measures, they asked participants to stay longer and score some of the measures that were filled out previously by other participants. Half of the participants were touched on the shoulder during the request and the others were not. The former group spent significantly more time scoring inventories compared to the latter group.

A very different paradigm has been used to study the influence of touch. Kurzban (2001) invited small groups of participants to the lab to play what is known as a public goods game in which players are given tokens that can later be redeemed for money. The players are instructed that their tokens may be deposited into either a personal account or a public account. Ten rounds were played in which they were given this choice. At the end of the game, each player retains the tokens in the personal account, and the tokens in the public account are divided among the players. In a typical public goods game, players start the game by depositing some tokens into the public account. However, there is typically a gradual shift over the rounds for players to deposit fewer and fewer tokens into the public account.

How would touch affect giving to the public account? In one condition in the experiment, Kurzban (2001) instructed participants to give a brief touch to each other before each round. Kurzban found that touch significantly increased rates of giving in the game compared to a baseline condition in which subjects did not touch. However, the effect was driven primarily by male subjects. Related research suggests that giving behavior may be mediated by oxytocin release following tactile stimulation (Morhenn, Park, Piper, & Zak, 2008).

Gender effects are pervasive in studies of compliance, but they are unsystematic and thus militate against simplistic generalizations and conclusions (Brockner et al., 1982; Hornik & Ellis, 1988; Patterson et al., 1986; Paulsell & Goldman, 1984; Powell et al., 1994; Stephen & Zweigenhaft, 1986). Some studies, for example, indicate that the targets of touch help more when female confederates touch them (e.g., Hornik & Ellis; Paulsell & Goldman), whereas other studies indicate that targets help more when a confederate of the opposite sex touches them (e.g., Brockner et al.). However, it should be noted that several studies do not show gender effects (Crusco & Wetzel, 1984; Guéguen, 2002b; Guéguen & Fischer-Lokou, 2002, 2003; Nannberg & Hansen, 1994; Smith, Gier, & Willis, 1982; Willis & Hamm, 1980). Thus, gender effects may be evident with some compliance outcomes, but not with others. More systematic investigation is warranted to better understand gender's role in mediating compliance (Hertenstein, Verkamp, et al., 2006).

One recent study investigated the effects of homophobia on compliance. Dolinski (2010) carried out a series of experiments in which male and female confederates approached subjects in a railway station in Poland and asked them to deposit a letter into a mailbox for them. Half of the subjects received a light touch and the other half did not. The researcher found that touch increased compliance in all gender combinations except one: when male confederates touched male subjects. The researchers replicated this finding using a different paradigm in which subjects were asked by confederates to purchase a street product (again, half were touched). A final study showed that the more male subjects reported being homophobic as indexed in a self-report measure, the less compliant they were when men touched them. This study underscores that homophobia may influence observed gender differences in compliance.

Only a few studies have investigated the actual mechanism(s) that mediates the link between touch and compliance (Hertenstein, Verkamp, et al., 2006). The facilitating role of touch on compliance has most often been explained by the positive evaluation that a target can have after being touched by a person (Rose, 1990). An alternative suggestion has been offered in which one's history of tactile stimulation has been associated with mitigating stress arousal (Reite, 1990). Such an association, it is thought, results in the positive evaluation of the toucher resulting in compliance. Finally, relatively recent neuroscientific evidence offers another intriguing possibility (Gallace & Spence, 2010). The receptors in the skin that detect pleasant tactile stimulation may be neurally linked to stored information in the brain that has been positively associated with touch. Thus, this common neural system may mediate compliance. All the above possible mechanisms would benefit from programs of research that systematically test them.

INDIVIDUAL DIFFERENCES IN TOUCH

Individual differences are often neglected in the study of tactile communication. For example, we have little idea of what makes some people more likely to conform when touched by others compared to those who conform little. Or, why are some people more accurate at decoding distinct emotions than others? Researchers have tended to neglect these individual differences and focus on main effects or gender.

One construct serves as an exception to the neglect of individual differences: touch avoidance (Andersen & Leibowitz, 1978). Andersen, Andersen, and Lustig (1987) define touch avoidance as "...a trait or individual difference measure of a person's attitude toward touch.

The touch avoidance construct is not a direct index of how much a person actually touches or avoids being touched. Instead it is an index of a person's affect toward touch." (p. 90). Within the construct of touch avoidance, people high in touch avoidance are thought to experience negative affect when touching and being touched by others, whereas those low in avoidance tend to experience more positive affect when touched and being touched by others (Andersen et al., 1987). Touch avoidance is indexed by the touch avoidance measure (TAM) designed by Andersen and Leibowitz (1978). This instrument measures attitudes regarding avoidance for both same-sex touch and opposite-sex touch.

Several studies support the validity of the construct touch avoidance. Andersen and Sull (1985), for example, found that touch-avoidant people, in general, were more likely to maintain greater interpersonal distance in social interactions. This effect was particularly strong for males; a 0.57 correlation between scores on the TAM and males' interpersonal distance was evident in one study. That is, touch-avoidant males maintained less proximity to females compared to those low in touch avoidance. In addition, people who are touch avoidant also respond more negatively when touched by others, whereas people who report less touch avoidance experience less negative affect when touched (Sorensen & Beatty, 1988). Finally, others have found that touch avoidance is related to how much people actually touch each other, at least in dyadic relationships that are not long term (Guerrero & Andersen, 1994).

A number of correlates have been identified in touch avoidance. The most consistent correlates identified include the following:

1. Sex and gender: Males are more likely than females to be more same-sex touch avoidant, whereas females are more likely to be opposite-sex touch avoidant (Andersen, 2005). Moreover, men demonstrating more traditionally masculine characteristics (i.e., low in androgyny) tend to demonstrate greater same-sex touch avoidance.
2. Age: Opposite-sex touch avoidance increases with age, whereas same-sex touch avoidance does not (Andersen & Leibowitz, 1978). The research design of studies examining the impact of age have not been able to determine if this effect is maturational or a result of cohort effects (Andersen, 2005).
3. Self-esteem: People with high self-esteem, compared to those with low self-esteem, are less touch avoidant with the opposite sex (Andersen et al., 1987).
4. Culture: There are wide cultural differences in touch avoidance. These are discussed in Andersen's chapter (this volume).

Outside the touch avoidance construct, Dorros, Hanzal, and Segrin (2008) recently conducted a study examining the relationship between the big five personality constructs and participants' self-reported perceptions of touch. Dorris et al. identified two personality traits that correlated with perceptions of touch. People high in agreeableness, compared to those low in agreeableness, perceive intimate and nonintimate touch more positively. Moreover, openness to experience significantly predicted participants' positive perceptions of nonintimate touch. In sum, researchers have begun to understand how individual differences play a role in tactile communication, but many questions remain unanswered.

INTERSECTIONS BETWEEN TOUCH AND OTHER MODALITIES OF COMMUNICATION

Heretofore, the tactile modality has been considered independent from other modalities, including audition and vision. This approach was intended to draw attention to the independent role that touch plays in communication. However, we do not communicate using only one modality; there is a larger gestalt that must be taken into account. Although the communicative consequences of combining signal components from different modalities are poorly understood in general, it may be heuristic to consider how touch interacts with other modalities. To do so, I draw upon a theoretical framework of multimodal communication proposed by Partan and Marler (1999; see Figure 12.2).

The theoretical framework posits that the modalities used in communication may be redundant or nonredundant. Partan and Marler (1999) hold that redundancy (i.e., the modalities communicate the identical message) increases the probability that the message will be transmitted in the presence of environmental noise; in other words, the signal-to-noise ratio increases. While redundant messages transmit only one message, nonredundant ones (i.e., each of the modalities communicates a different message) are considered important because they can transmit more than one message concurrently.

According to Partan and Marler's (1999) framework, several outcomes are possible when modalities are combined during communication. Figure 12.2 represents the potential outcomes. When the modalities communicate redundant information, two outcomes are possible: (1) there is equivalence such that the message is the same strength as it would have been with only one modality; (2) the message

CHAPTER 12   FUNCTIONS OF TOUCH IN ADULTHOOD

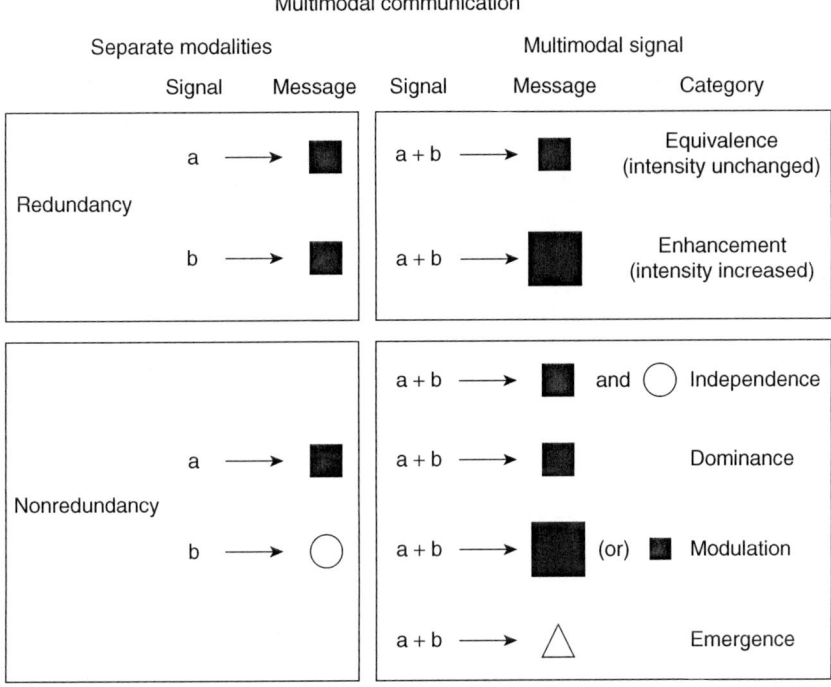

FIGURE 12.2   Interaction between modalities of communication. Adapted with permission from "Communication goes multimodal," by S. Partan and P. Marler, 1999, *Science, 283,* 1272–1273. Copyright 1999 by AAAS.

is strengthened when the two modalities are used simultaneously. When the modalities communicate nonredundant messages, four outcomes are possible: (1) the messages are independent; thus, two separate messages are communicated; (2) one of the messages is dominant over the other; thus, it supersedes the other; (3) one modality suppresses the message of the other; (4) the combination can produce a new message.

Partan and Marler's (1999) conceptual framework allows us to examine the possible relations between touch and the other modalities of communication. The degree to which Partan and Marler's framework maps onto reality, however, remains an empirical question. Their model seems to assume that all messages are of a discrete categorical nature, when in fact it is likely that the human utilizes gradient information related to temporal and spatial contours to understand the meaning of multimodal stimulation. Nevertheless, Partan and Marler's framework helps us conceptualize the possible relations between the tactile modality and other modalities.

FUTURE DIRECTIONS

This review has focused on some of the central functions served by touch in adulthood. Despite the fact that researchers have made great strides to understand the functions served by touch, several questions deserve empirical attention. For example, a persuasive evolutionary account of tactile communication in adulthood does not exist. If the field of touch will progress, an evolutionary analysis of the functions served by touch is needed.

In addition, researchers would be well served to extend the samples in their studies in two ways (Hertenstein, Verkamp, et al., 2006). First, given that gender continues to be an important variable in the study of touch, it seems appropriate to include people with varying sexual orientations. Second, the age of participants in most studies is restricted. Expanding the age range of studies to include the entire lifespan would help us better understand the developmental complexities that exist in tactile communication.

The field of touch would be well served to go beyond the positive functions served by touch, as well as recognize individual differences. The bias among touch researchers to study the positive consequences of touch is somewhat ironic given the positive psychology movement over the last decade. Better understanding how touch, or lack thereof, impacts human functioning and communication would be appropriate. Likewise, focusing on individual differences in tactile communication would be important as described earlier.

It is interesting that our language often systematizes major aspects of our lives in the form of idiomatic expressions (Hertenstein, 2002); Lakoff and Johnson (1980) have referred to these as "metaphors we live by." Perhaps it is no accident that numerous idioms exist referring to touch as communicatory. We speak of "rubbing" people the wrong way, and "stroking" them the right way. We speak of people who have "a happy touch," "a magic touch," "a human touch," "a soft touch," or "a delicate touch." We also say that we are "touched" by another person (Montagu, 1986). Undoubtedly, the "metaphors we live by" implicate touch as an important and invaluable modality of communication.

ACKNOWLEDGMENTS

This chapter was supported by the faculty development program at DePauw University. Significant portions of the chapter were excerpted and adapted from Hertenstein, Verkamp, Kerestes, and Holmes (2006) and Hertenstein (2002).

REFERENCES

Andersen, J. F., Andersen, P. A., & Lustig, M. W. (1987). Opposite-sex touch avoidance: A national replication and extension. *Journal of Nonverbal Behavior, 11,* 89–109.

Andersen, P. A. (1999). *Nonverbal communication: Forms and function.* Mountain View, CA: Mayfield Publishing.

Andersen, P. A. (2005). The touch avoidance measure. In V. Manusov (Ed.), *The sourcebook of nonverbal measures* (pp. 57–65). Mahwah, NJ: Erlbaum.

Andersen, P. A., & Leibowitz, K. (1978). The development and nature of the construct touch avoidance. *Environmental Psychology and Nonverbal Behavior, 3,* 89–106.

Andersen, P. A., & Sull, K. K. (1985). Out of touch, out of reach: Tactile predispositions as predictors of interpersonal distance. *Western Journal of Speech Communication, 49,* 57–72.

Argyle, M., & Dean, J. (1965). Eye-contact, distance, and affiliation. *Sociometry, 28,* 289–304.

Bailenson, J. N., Yee, N., Brave, S., Merget, D., & Koslow, D. (2007). Virtual interpersonal touch: Expressing and recognizing emotions through haptic devices. *Human-Computer Interaction, 22,* 325–353.

Barrett, K. C., & Nelson-Goens, G. C. (1997). Emotion communication and the development of the social emotions. In K. C. Barrett (Ed.), *The communication of emotion: Current research from diverse perspectives* (pp. 69–88). San Fransisco, CA: Jossey-Bass.

Beier, E. G., & Sternberg, D. P. (1977). Marital communication. *Journal of Communication, 27,* 92–97.

Brockner, J., Pressman, B., Cabitt, J., & Moran, P. (1982). Nonverbal intimacy, sex, and compliance: A field study. *Journal of Nonverbal Behavior, 6,* 253–258.

Bronfenbrenner, U., & Morris, P. A. (1998). The ecology of developmental processes. In R. M. Lerner (Ed.), *Handbook of child psychology: Theoretical models of human development.* (Vol. 1, pp. 993–1028). New York, NY: Wiley.

Burgoon, J. K. (1991). *Relational message interpretations of touch, conversational distance, and posture.* Netherlands: Kluwer Academic Publishers.

Burgoon, J. K., Buller, D. B., Hale, J. L., & DeTurck, M. A. (1984). Relational messages associated with nonverbal behaviors. *Human Communication Research, 10,* 351–378.

Burgoon, J. K., & Hale, J. L. (1984). The fundamental topoi of relational communication. *Communication Monographs, 51,* 193–214.

Burgoon, J. K., Walther, J. B., & Baesler, E. J. (1992). Interpretations, evaluations, and consequences of interpersonal touch. *Human Communication Research, 19,* 237–263.

Cappella, J. N., & Greene, J. O. (1982). A discrepancy-arousal explanation of mutual influence in expressive behavior for adult and infant-adult interaction. *Communication Monographs, 49,* 89–114.

Clynes, M. (1977). *Sentics: The touch of emotion*. New York, NY: Anchor/Doubleday.

Clynes, M., & Nettheim, N. (1982). The living quality of music: Neurobiologic patterns of communicating feeling. In M. Clynes (Ed.), *Music, mind and brain: The neuropsychology of music* (pp. 47–82). New York, NY: Plenum Press.

Crusco, A. H., & Wetzel, C. G. (1984). The Midas touch: The effects of interpersonal touch on restaurant tipping. *Personality & Social Psychology Bulletin, 10*, 512–517.

Darwin, C. (1872). *The expression of the emotions in man and animals*. London, England: John Murray.

Davidson, R. J., Scherer, K. R., & Goldsmith, H. H. (Eds.). (2003). *Handbook of affective sciences*. London, England: Oxford University Press.

Dolinski, D. (2010). Touch, compliance, and homophobia. *Journal of Nonverbal Behavior, 34*, 179–192.

Dorros, S., Hanzal, A., & Segrin, C. (2008). The Big Five personality traits and perceptions of touch to intimate and nonintimate body regions. *Journal of Research in Personality, 42*, 1067–1073.

Dunbar, R. I. M. (2010). The social role of touch in humans and primates: Behavioural function and neurobiological mechanisms. *Neuroscience and Biobehavioral Reviews, 34*, 260–268.

Ekman, P. (1999). Facial expressions. In T. Dalgleish & M. J. Power (Eds.), *Handbook of cognition and emotion* (pp. 301–320). New York, NY: Wiley.

Emmers, T. M., & Dindia, K. (1995). The effect of relational stage and intimacy on touch: An extension of Guerrero and Andersen. *Personal Relationships, 2*, 225–236.

Field, T. (2001). *Touch*. Cambridge, MA: MIT.

Fisher, J. D., Rytting, M., & Heslin, R. (1976). Hands touching hands: Affective and evaluative effects of an interpersonal touch. *Sociometry, 39*, 416–421.

Floyd, K. (1999). *All touches are not created equal: Effects of form and duration on observers' interpretations of an embrace*. Netherlands: Kluwer Academic Publishers.

Floyd, K., & Voloudakis, M. (1999). Affectionate behavior in adult platonic friendships: Interpreting and evaluating expectancy violations. *Human Communication Research, 25*, 341–369.

Foehl, J. C., & Goldman, M. (1983). Increasing altruistic behavior by using compliance techniques. *Journal of Social Psychology, 119*, 21–29.

Fogel, A. (2000). Developmental pathways in close relationships. *Child Development, 71*(5), 1150–1151.

Frank, M. G., & Stennett, J. (2001). The forced-choice paradigm and the perception of facial expressions of emotion. *Journal of Personality & Social Psychology, 80*, 75–85.

Frijda, N. (2006). *The laws of emotion*. Mahwah, NJ: Erlbaum.

Gallace, A., & Spence, C. (2010). The science of interpersonal touch: An overview. *Neuroscience and Biobehavioral Reviews, 34*, 246–259.

Goldman, M., & Fordyce, J. (1983). Prosocial behavior as affected by eye contact, touch, and voice expression. *Journal of Social Psychology, 121*, 125–129.

Goldman, M., Kiyohara, O., & Pfannensteil, D. A. (1985). Interpersonal touch, social labeling, and the foot-in-the-door effect. *Journal of Social Psychology, 125*, 143–147.

Guéguen, N. (2002a). Kind of touch, gender, and compliance with a request. *Studia Psychologica, 44*, 167–172.

Guéguen, N. (2002b). Status, apparel and touch: Their joint effects on compliance to a request. *North American Journal of Psychology, 4*, 279–286.
Guéguen, N. (2002c). Touch, awareness of touch, and compliance with a request. *Perceptual & Motor Skills, 95*, 355–360.
Guéguen, N. (2004). Nonverbal encouragement of participation in a course: The effect of touching. *Social Psychology of Education, 7*, 89–98.
Guéguen, N., & Fischer-Lokou, J. (2002). An evaluation of touch on a large request: A field setting. *Psychological Reports, 90*, 267–269.
Guéguen, N., & Fischer-Lokou, J. (2003). Tactile contact and spontaneous help: An evaluation in a natural setting. *Journal of Social Psychology, 143*, 785–787.
Guéguen, N., Jacob, C., & Boulbry, G. (2007). The effect of touch on compliance with a restaurant's employee suggestion. *International Journal of Hospitality Management, 26*, 1019–1023.
Guéguen, N., & Vion, M. (2009). The effect of a practitioner's touch on a patient's medication compliance. *Psychology, Health, & Medicine, 14*, 689–694.
Guerrero, L. K., & Andersen, P. A. (1991). The waxing and waning of relational intimacy: Touch as a function of relational stage, gender and touch avoidance. *Journal of Social & Personal Relationships, 8*, 147–165.
Guerrero, L. K., & Andersen, P. A. (1994). Patterns of matching and initiation: Touch behavior and avoidance across romantic relationship stages. *Journal of Nonverbal Behavior, 18*, 137–153.
Hall, J. A. (1996). Touch, status, and gender at professional meetings. *Journal of Nonverbal Behavior, 20*, 23–44.
Hertenstein, M. J. (2002). Touch: Its communicative functions in infancy. *Human Development, 45*, 70–94.
Hertenstein, M. J. (in press). Tactile stimulation. In S. Goldstein & J. Naglieri (Eds.), *Encyclopedia of child behavior and development*. New York, NY: Springer-Verlag.
Hertenstein, M. J., Butts, A., & Hile, S. (2007). The communication of anger: Beyond the face. In E. I. Clausen (Ed.), *Psychology of anger* (pp. 7–11). New York, NY: Nova.
Hertenstein, M. J., & Campos, J. J. (2001). Emotion regulation via maternal touch. *Infancy, 2*, 549–566.
Hertenstein, M. J., Holmes, R., McCullough, M., & Keltner, D. (2009). The communication of emotion via touch. *Emotion, 9*, 566–573.
Hertenstein, M. J., Keltner, D., App, B., Bulleit, B., & Jaskolka, A. (2006). Touch communicates distinct emotions. *Emotion, 6*, 528–533.
Hertenstein, M. J., Verkamp, J. M., Kerestes, A. M., & Holmes, R. M. (2006). The communicative functions of touch in humans, nonhuman primates, and rats: A review and synthesis of the empirical research. *Genetic, Social, and General Psychology Monographs, 132*, 5–94.
Heslin, R., & Alper, T. (1983). Touch: A bonding gesture. In J. M. Wiemann & R. P. Harrison (Eds.), *Nonverbal interaction* (pp. 47–75). Beverly Hills, CA: Sage Publications.
Heslin, R., & Boss, D. (1980). Nonverbal intimacy in airport arrival and departure. *Personality & Social Psychology Bulletin, 6*, 248–252.
Heslin, R., Nguyen, T. D., & Nguyen, M. L. (1983). Meaning of touch: The case of touch from a stranger or same sex person. *Journal of Nonverbal Behavior, 7*, 147–157.

Hewitt, J., & Feltham, D. (1982). Differential reaction to touch by men and women. *Perceptual & Motor Skills, 55*, 1291–1294.

Hinde, R. A. (1997). *Relationships: A dialectical perspective.* Hove, UK: Psychology Press.

Hornik, J. (1991). Shopping time and purchasing behavior as a result of in-store tactile stimulation. *Perceptual & Motor Skills, 73*, 969–970.

Hornik, J. (1992). Tactile stimulation and consumer response. *Journal of Consumer Research, 19*, 449–458.

Hornik, J., & Ellis, S. (1988). Strategies to secure compliance for a mall intercept interview. *Public Opinion Quarterly, 52*, 539–551.

Jablonski, N. G. (2006). *Skin: A natural history.* Berkeley, CA: University of California.

Jones, B. N. (1972). Categories of child-child interaction. *Ethological studies of child behaviour.* Oxford, England: Cambridge University Press.

Jones, S. E., & Yarbrough, A. E. (1985). A naturalistic study of the meanings of touch. *Communication Monographs, 52*, 19–56.

Joule, R., & Gueguen, N. (2007). Touch, compliance, and awareness of tactile contact. *Perceptual & Motor Skills, 104*, 581–588.

Jourard, S. M. (1966). An exploratory study of body-accessibility. *British Journal of Social & Clinical Psychology, 5*, 221–231.

Jourard, S. M., & Friedman, R. (1970). Experimenter-subject "distance" and self-disclosure. *Journal of Personality & Social Psychology, 15*, 278–282.

Kaufman, D., & Mahoney, J. M. (1999). The effect of waitresses' touch on alcohol consumption in dyads. *Journal of Social Psychology, 139*, 261–267.

Keltner, D. (2009). *Born to be good: The science of a meaningful life.* New York, NY: Norton.

Kleinke, C. L. (1977). Compliance to requests made by gazing and touching experimenters in field settings. *Journal of Experimental Social Psychology, 13*, 218–223.

Kurzban, R. (2001). The social Psychophysics of cooperation: Nonverbal communication in a public goods game. *Journal of Nonverbal Behavior, 25*, 241–259.

Lakoff, G., & Johnson, M. (1980). *Metaphors we live by.* Chicago, IL: University of Chicago Press.

Lazarus, R. (1991). *Emotion and adaptation.* New York, NY: Oxford University Press.

Levav, J., & Argo, J.J. (2010). Physical contact and financial risk taking. *Psychological Science, 21*, 804–810.

Lewis, M., Haviland-Jones, J., & Barrett, L. F. (Eds.). (2008). *Handbook of emotions* (3rd ed.). New York, NY: Guildford.

Lewis, R. J., Derlega, V. J., Shankar, A., Cochard, E., & Finkel, L. (1997). Nonverbal correlates of confederates' touch: Confounds in touch research. *Journal of Social Behavior & Personality, 12*, 821–830.

Loomis, J., & Lederman, S. (1986). Tactual perception. In K. Boff, L. Kaufman, & J. Thomas (Eds.), *Handbook of human perception and performance* (pp. 1–41). New York, NY: Wiley.

Major, B. (1981). Gender patterns in touching behavior. In C. Mayo & N. M. Henley (Eds.), *Gender and nonverbal behavior* (pp. 15–37). New York, NY: Springer-Verlag.

McCabe, C., Rolls, E. T., Bilderbeck, A., & McGlone, F. (2008). Cognitive influences on the affective representation of touch and the sight of touch in the human brain. *Social Cognitive and Affective Neuroscience, 3*, 97–108.
McDaniel, E., & Andersen, P. A. (1998). International patterns of interpersonal tactile communication: A field study. *Journal of Nonverbal Behavior, 22*, 59–75.
Mehrabian, A. (1971). *Silent messages.* Belmont, CA: Wadsworth Publishing Co.
Montagu, A. (1986). *Touching: The human significance of the skin* (3rd ed.). New York, NY: Harper & Row.
Morhenn, V. B., Park, J. W., Piper, E., Zak, P. J. (2008). Monetary sacrifice among strangers is mediated by endogenous oxytocin release after physical contact. *Evolution and Human Behavior, 29*, 375–383.
Morris, D. (1971). *Intimate behavior.* New York, NY: Random House.
Nannberg, J. C., & Hansen, C. H. (1994). Post-compliance touch: An incentive for task performance. *Journal of Social Psychology, 134*, 301–307.
Nettelbeck, T., Henderson, C., & Willson, R. J. (1989). Communicating emotion through sound: An evaluation of Clynes' theory of sentics. *Australian Journal of Psychology, 41*, 25–36
Nguyen, M. L., Heslin, R., & Nguyen, T. D. (1976). The meaning of touch: Sex and marital status differences. *Representative Research in Social Psychology, 7*, 13–18.
Nguyen, T. D., Heslin, R., & Nguyen, M. L. (1975). The meanings of touch: Sex differences. *Journal of Communication, 25*, 92–103.
Niedenthal, P. M. (2007). Embodying emotion. *Science, 316*, 1002–1005.
Niedenthal, P. M., & Maringer, M. (2009). Embodied emotion considered. *Emotion Review, 1*, 122–128.
Partan, S., & Marler, P. (1999). Communication goes multimodal. *Science, 283*, 1272–1273.
Patterson, M. L. (1976). An arousal model of interpersonal intimacy. *Psychological Review, 83*, 235–245.
Patterson, M. L., Powell, J. L., & Lenihan, M. G. (1986). Touch, compliance, and interpersonal affect. *Journal of Nonverbal Behavior, 10*, 41–50.
Patterson, M. L., Reidhead, S. M., Gooch, M. V., & Stopka, S. J. (1984). A content-classified bibliography of research on the immediacy behaviors: 1965 82. *Journal of Nonverbal Behavior, 8*, 360–393.
Paulsell, S., & Goldman, M. (1984). The effect of touching different body areas on prosocial behavior. *Journal of Social Psychology, 122*, 269–273.
Pisano, M. D., Wall, S. M., & Foster, A. (1986). Perceptions of nonreciprocal touch in romantic relationships. *Journal of Nonverbal Behavior, 10*, 29–40.
Powell, J. L., Meil, W., Patterson, M. L., & Chouinard, E. F. (1994). Effects of timing of touch on compliance to a request. *Journal of Social Behavior & Personality, 9*, 153–162.
Reite, M. (1990). Touch, attachment, and health: Is there a relationship? In K. E. Barnard & T. B. Brazelton (Eds.), *Touch: The foundation of experience: Full revised and expanded proceedings of Johnson & Johnson Pediatric Round Table X* (pp. 195–225): Madison, CT.
Rose, S. A. (1990). The sense of touch. In K. Bernard & T. B. Brazelton (Eds.), *Touch: The foundation of experience* (pp. 299–324). Madison, WI: International Universities Press.

Salminen K., Surakka, V., Lylykangas, J., Raisamo, J., Saarinen, R., Raisamo, R., ... Evreinov, G. (2008). Emotional and behavioral responses to haptic stimulation. *Proc. of Conference on Human Factors in Computing Systems,* 1555–1562.

Scherer, K. R. (1986). Vocal affect expression: A review and a model for future research. *Psychological Bulletin, 99,* 143–165.

Scherer, K. R., & Zentner, M. R. (2001). The emotional effects of music: Production rules. In P. N. Juslin & J. A. Sloboda (Eds.), *Music and emotion: Theory and research* (pp. 361–392). New York, NY: Oxford University Press.

Silverthorne, C., Micklewright, J., O'Donnell, M., & Gibson, R. (1976). Attribution of personal characteristics as a function of the degree of touch on initial contact and sex. *Sex Roles, 2,* 185–193.

Silverthorne, C., Noreen, C., Hunt, T., & Rota, L. (1972). The effects of tactile stimulation on visual experience. *Journal of Social Psychology, 88,* 153–154.

Smith, D. E., Gier, J. A., & Willis, F. N. (1982). Interpersonal touch and compliance with a marketing request. *Basic & Applied Social Psychology, 3,* 35–38.

Smith, J., & MacLean, K. (2007). Communicating emotion through a haptic link: Design space and methodology. *International Journal of Human-Computer Studies, 65,* 376–387.

Sorensen, G., & Beatty, M. J. (1988). The interactive effects of touch and touch avoidance on interpersonal perceptions. *Communication Research Reports, 5,* 84–90.

Spitz, R. A. (1946). Anaclitic depression: An inquiry into the genesis of psychiatric conditions in early childhood. *The Psychoanalytic Study of the Child, 2,* 313–342.

Stephen, R., & Zweigenhaft, R. L. (1986). The effect on tipping of a waitress touching male and female customers. *Journal of Social Psychology, 126,* 141–142.

Stern, D. N. (1985). *The interpersonal world of the infant.* New York, NY: Basic Books.

Sussman, N. M., & Rosenfeld, H. M. (1978). Touch, justification, and sex: Influences on the aversiveness of spatial violations. *Journal of Social Psychology, 106,* 215–225.

Thayer, S. (1986). History and strategies of research on social touch. *Journal of Nonverbal Behavior, 10*(1), 12–28.

Tronick, E. Z. (1995). Touch in mother-infant interaction. In T. M. Field (Ed.), *Touch in early development* (pp. 53–65). Mahwah, NJ: Erlbaum.

Trussoni, S., O'Malley, A., & Barton, A. (1988). Human emotion communication by touch: A modified replication of an experiment by Manfred Clynes. *Perceptual and Motor Skills, 66,* 419–424.

Wallbott, H. G. (1998). Bodily expression of emotion. *European Journal of Social Psychology, 28,* 879–896.

Watzlawick, P., Beavin, J. H., & Jackson, D. D. (1967). *Pragmatics of human communication: A study of interactional patterns, pathologies, and paradoxes.* New York, NY: W. W. Norton.

Weiss, S. J., & Campos, R. (1999). Touch. In C. A. Lindeman & M. McAthie (Eds.), *Fundamentals of contemporary nursing practice* (pp. 941–962). Philadelphia, PA: W. B. Saunders Company.

Wheeler, P. E. (1992). The influence of the loss of functional body hair on the water budgets of early hominids. *Journal of Human Evolution, 23,* 379–388.

Whitcher, S. J., & Fisher, J. D. (1979). Multidimensional reaction to therapeutic touch in a hospital setting. *Journal of Personality & Social Psychology, 37,* 87–96.

Willis, F. N., & Briggs, L. F. (1992). Relationship and touch in public settings. *Journal of Nonverbal Behavior, 16,* 55–63.

Willis, F. N., & Dodds, R. A. (1998). Age, relationship, and touch initiation. *Journal of Social Psychology, 138,* 115–123.

Willis, F. N., & Hamm, H. K. (1980). The use of interpersonal touch in securing compliance. *Journal of Nonverbal Behavior, 5,* 49–55.

Willis, F. N., & Rawdon, V. A. (1994). Gender and national differences in attitudes toward same-gender touch. *Perceptual & Motor Skills, 78,* 1027–1034.

Willis, F. N., & Rinck, C. M. (1983). A personal log method for investigating interpersonal touch. *Journal of Psychology, 113,* 119–122.

Willis, F. N., Rinck, C. M., & Dean, L. M. (1978). Interpersonal touch among adults in cafeteria lines. *Perceptual & Motor Skills, 47,* 1147–1152.

Young, R. W. (2003). Evolution of the human hand: The role of throwing and clubbing. *Journal of Anatomy, 202,* 165–174.

13

Gender and Status Patterns in Social Touch

JUDITH A. HALL

There are many reasons to link gender and status when thinking about human behavior, but the link has been especially close for psychologists interested in nonverbal communication, and touch in particular. To clarify what the reader may expect in this chapter, I use the term "gender" to designate the conventional categories of "men" and "women," not to designate gender-related psychological characteristics such as agency and communion. Because of the nature of the research literature, only heterosexual (or presumed heterosexual) men and women will be discussed. Only research on adolescents and adults will be discussed, and only touch that is not overtly aggressive will be considered unless indicated otherwise. Finally, because most of the research is done in the United States, this cultural setting will be assumed unless stated otherwise.

Ever since Nancy Henley's (1973, 1977) seminal statements on the topic of gender and touch, it is impossible to think of gender differences in nonverbal communication without also thinking of status, along with power, dominance, rank, and other definitions of the "vertical" dimension of social relations. For simplicity, I will treat these as roughly interchangeable, though of course they are not synonymous, a point often made in the literature (e.g., Ellyson & Dovidio, 1985; Hall, Coats, & Smith LeBeau, 2005).

Henley (1977) proposed that gender differences in nonverbal communication are rooted in social status, arguing that there are parallels between how men and women behave nonverbally and how people high and low in status, power, or dominance behave. This presumably reflects the role of status as the underlying cause of the gender differences. Important to this theory is the notion that nonverbal behavior can be a potent mechanism of social influence while remaining largely out of conscious awareness. Nonverbal behavior can therefore be a subtle means whereby men control others, including women, and whereby women signal their submissiveness to others, particularly men. Henley supplied a valuable framework within which to consider gender differences and one that has had a profound influence within this field of study.

Although Henley (1977) wrote about different kinds of nonverbal communication, her empirical studies focused on interpersonal touch (Henley, 1973; Henley & Harmon, 1985). A key notion was that men's higher status gives them touching privileges that result in an asymmetry such that men touch women more than vice versa. She also suggested that there are gender main effects for touch initiation and receipt, reflecting the "body politics" of nonverbal communication: men are freer to touch others and are therefore more likely to do so, while women are more likely to receive touch, which represents a kind of actual or symbolic victimization.

The goals of this chapter are to review the current state of research on gender and touch, and status and touch, and ways in which gender and status may come together regarding touch. Three ways of looking at gender differences will be considered—men's and women's attitudes and beliefs about touch, observed male and female touching behavior, and experimental studies asking how men and women respond to being touched. For status and touch, studies of beliefs, perceptions, and observed behavior will be discussed. I will draw on previous reviews (Hertenstein, Verkamp, Kerestes, & Holmes, 2006; Stier & Hall, 1984) in addition to describing other relevant studies.

In continuing the tradition of considering gender and status together I am not suggesting that these constructs necessarily must be linked, nor that status is the main framework within which we should consider gender and touch. The psychologies and life histories of men and women differ in many ways other than in terms of their relative social status. Indeed, as we shall see, the research does not yield an unequivocal basis for interpreting gender differences through the lens of status.

In fact, the origins of gender differences in nonverbal communication, including touch, remain obscure despite decades of interest among social psychologists. Potential explanations have been both biological (Andersen, 2006) and social, with the latter emphasizing not just status but also stereotypes, social expectations, roles and values, and personality (Hall, Carter, & Horgan, 2000; LaFrance, Hecht, & Levy Paluck, 2003; Noller, 1986). Though, conceivably, someone might argue that status is the causal antecedent of all other more proximal causes (stereotypes, expectancies, etc.), such an argument does not advance understanding because it renders the status hypothesis unfalsifiable except under very limited circumstances. Although descriptive research is abundant, empirical studies that relate nonverbal gender differences to possible explanatory factors are still much needed.

GENDER AND TOUCHING BEHAVIOR

Attitudes

Studies repeatedly find that women report more comfort with touch, especially same-gender touch, than men report (Andersen & Leibowitz, 1978; Fromme et al., 1989; Martin & Anderson, 1993; Roese, Olson, Borenstein, Martin, & Shores, 1992; Willis & Rawdon, 1994). Willis and Rawdon found this to be equally true in the United States, Malaysia, Spain, and Chile. Both men and women agree that male–male touch is less normal and appropriate than other kinds (Derlega, Catanzaro, & Lewis, 2001).

Men's greater discomfort with same-gender touch can be interpreted in several ways. One explanation sidesteps the question of how the gender difference originated and focuses instead on the self-perpetuating nature of a gender difference once it is entrenched in the culture and readily available for learning through processes of observation, modeling, and reinforcement. A cycle is easily created whereby the less one engages in the behavior, the more salient and potentially disturbing it becomes.

Another interpretation would be that men are in a perpetual (though often incipient) status contest with each other and that, because of this, men avoid touching each other to avoid an escalation of potentially dominance-claiming behaviors. Yet another interpretation focuses on the role of homophobia in regulating men's behavior with each other. Fear of being perceived (or perceiving oneself) as homosexual could easily be a factor in men's reluctance to touch each other.

Floyd (2000) showed participants photographs of same-gender couples embracing or not and described the couples as romantically involved or not. Respondents higher on homophobia rated the touching photographs described as romantic as less normal, especially when the embracers were both male. Roese et al. (1992) found that greater homophobia, especially among men, correlated negatively with their reported comfort with same-gender touching and in a second study found that both men and women who were observed to engage in less same-gender touching in a cafeteria reported having more homophobic attitudes when they later filled in a scale.

There are, of course, contexts in which women too would not be comfortable with physical contact, most notably when the touch is made by a man and is unwanted. Population surveys clearly show that both adolescent and adult females exceed their male counterparts in reporting instances of unwanted touch and that touch is closely tied to feeling sexually harassed (Uggen & Blackstone, 2004). Garlick (1994) asked college students to indicate appropriateness and comfort when imagining a hypothetical opposite-gender professor touching them in various ways. Women reported being less comfortable than men did for several kinds of touch (e.g., receiving a "playful" shoulder massage, being touched on the shoulder or arm while greeting), but not for being hugged while being congratulated. Apparently, the ritual nature of the latter touch removed any offensive overtones.

Struckman-Johnson and Struckman-Johnson (1993) asked participants to read vignettes describing various kinds of unexpected erotic touch by others of same and opposite gender. Women reported disliking male touch, while men were comfortable with female touch. A similar asymmetry occurs in other studies (Nguyen, Heslin, & Nguyen, 1976), though Hanzal, Segrin, and Dorros (2008) found an interesting reversal as a function of being married. In unmarried people, men had more positive attitudes toward opposite-sex intimate touch than women did, but this was reversed among married people, with further analysis showing that this was not due to marital status being confounded with age. This reversal bears an interesting relation to studies on male–female touch asymmetries reviewed in a later section.

Beliefs

Owing to the nonpublic nature of much interpersonal touching and the fact that touch is a low-frequency behavior in many situations, researchers have felt the need to supplement observational studies with people's reports of their own or others' touching behavior. Henley (1977) reported a study of undergraduates' beliefs about gender and the frequency of touch. Both males and females believed that females engaged in more same-gender touch than males did, and the females believed that male–female asymmetry in touch favored the males.

Willis and Rinck (1983) attempted to make participants' reports more objective by asking them to record touches in a personal log right after they happened. There was no overall gender difference in reported receipt of personal touch, but women were more likely to initiate personal (relative to impersonal) touch than men were. Jones

(1986) used a diary method and found that women reported touching men more than vice versa, especially for "control" touches. Overall, women reported touching others more than men did, and there was no difference between male–male and female–female touch.

Observational Studies

Stier and Hall (1984) performed a meta-analysis of observational studies of male and female touching. Here, we summarize those results and describe studies done since that review. Readers are referred to that review for an extended discussion of ambiguities in the literature. To illustrate one ambiguity regarding base rate information, the nature of a gender difference in touch and how one interprets it would be different if men and women have equal opportunity to touch others of same and opposite gender, as might be the case in a laboratory study, versus being in a more gender-segregated situation such as might exist in a school cafeteria or playground where people's chances of touching the opposite gender are much reduced.

Asymmetry between men and women. The seminal study addressing this question is Henley's (1973) observational study of intentional touches with the hand, in which young adult men were seen to touch young adult women significantly more than vice versa (23 male-to-female vs. 7 female-to-male). In that article, two other smaller samples representing different adult age groups did not show any difference. Henley interpreted the significant result to reflect the male prerogative to touch and control women through the subtle medium of touch.

Seven other studies on adolescents and adults that reported comparable analyses were reviewed by Stier and Hall (1984). Two of these had significant results, one showing a male asymmetry (232 male-to-female vs. 170 female-to-male; Major & Williams, 1980, reported in Major, 1981) and one showing a female asymmetry (38 female-to-male vs. 20 male-to-female; Willis, Rinck, & Dean, 1978). The remaining five studies were mixed in direction and far from significant. Using meta-analytic methods, Stier and Hall calculated the combined probability of the set of 10 studies to be $p = .22$ (nonsignificantly favoring men in direction), suggesting that, overall, there was no meaningful asymmetry.

Observations made in public places often yield little additional information about the people observed and contextual factors, making interpretations difficult. But Stier and Hall (1984) noted an important feature distinguishing the two studies that showed significant male asymmetry (Henley; Major and Williams): they were the only studies that counted only intentional touches with the hand.

Subsequent studies have clarified understanding of touch asymmetry. Hall and Veccia (1990), observing touching in public, found men and women to touch each other equally often (120 each), but also discovered both age and type of touch to be moderators of the difference. The asymmetry favored men for touches with the hand and for the "arm around" gesture, but favored women for arm-in-arm touch. Also, the asymmetry favored men in younger dyads but favored women in older dyads, such that in the over-40 group women touched men in a full 79% of the opposite-gender intentional touches.

Hall (1996) observed opposite-gender touches at academic conferences and found nonsignificant asymmetry, but with the direction showing more male-to-female than female-to-male touch overall (119 to 97) as well as with the hand (102 to 86). When examined as a function of the relative statuses of the individuals, there was no male–female asymmetry when there was a status disparity, but when the two individuals were of approximately equal status, the men did more of the touching than the women did (56 male-to-female vs. 38 female-to-male, $p < 0.06$). Hall (1996) suggested that this finding might fit with Expectation States Theory (Berger, Rosenholtz, & Zelditch, 1985), according to which gender serves as a "diffuse" status variable when there are not more clear-cut status indicators to guide behavior.

Remland, Jones, and Brinkman (1995) observed public touching and reported that asymmetry between the genders was not significant though it favored females slightly (11 to 7). DiBiase and Gunnoe (2004) observed touches in young opposite-gender couples in dance clubs in Rome, Prague, and Boston. For touches with the hand, the asymmetry (assessed with mean frequencies) favored men significantly but more so in Prague than in Boston; in Rome, the asymmetry favored women. For nonhand touches, the asymmetry favored women in all three cities, consistent with Hall and Veccia (1990), but this female advantage was only slight in Boston.

Later studies that examined relationship stage and touch asymmetry gave important clarification of the younger–older difference noted by Hall and Veccia (1990). Willis and Briggs (1992) observed opposite-gender couples in public places and then asked the couples about their relationship status. Relationship status was a significant moderator: among couples who were dating, engaged, or married less than 1 year, the asymmetry favored men (86 male-to-female vs. 60 female-to-male), but among couples married more than 1 year, women touched more (41 female-to-male vs. 32 male-to-female). Using the same methodology,

Guerrero and Andersen (1994) again found that among casual daters there was male asymmetry (22 male-to-female vs. 12 female-to-male) while among married couples there was female asymmetry (17 female-to-male vs. 8 male-to-female). Willis and Dodds (1998) used the same methodology and found again that relationship status moderated the touch asymmetry. Overall, women touched men more than vice versa (78 female-to-male vs. 50 male-to-female), but this difference was most pronounced in couples married more than 1 year (vs. courting or married less than 1 year). This series of studies is consistent with the age trends of Hall and Veccia (1990), Henley (1973), and DiBiase and Gunnoe (2004), who found male asymmetry in young adult samples.

Thus, accumulated research on the asymmetry question suggests that intentional touching in a public setting, particularly with the hand, is done more often by men in young and relationally uncommitted opposite-gender dyads. In more mature couples and relationships, the difference reverses itself and favors women, especially for nonhand touches, though in DiBiase and Gunnoe's (2004) study women used more nonhand touches even in young couples. Whether the asymmetry favoring women in more committed relationships reflects a reversal of the balance of power or the added safety and security of such a relationship cannot be said. Because men, in general, are more touch avoidant than women, it might simply reflect women's greater comfort with physical contact which is free to find expression under these circumstances. In less-developed relationships, women may feel inhibited about touching because it might be mistakenly interpreted as a sexual overture.

Whether the asymmetry findings, whichever way they go, reflect status and dominance is an unanswered question considering how little is known about the perceptions and intentions of the observed individuals, as noted by DiBiase and Gunnoe (2004). Men's touch with the hand, in younger or less-committed couples, might signify dominance in a direct way if it involves pulling, leading, or directing the other's movements. Or, it might be used more symbolically to signal possession. Obviously, too, in most cultures, women are considered sex objects more than men are, with the consequence that men probably find women's bodies to be a more magnetic object of touch than vice versa. It is also possible that the source of a male–female asymmetry lies not with the man but with the woman: to avoid risk of sexual assault or misunderstandings about their intentions, young women might not want to behave in too forward a way with male companions to whom they are not committed. Such hypothetical, and highly plausible, mechanisms, while clearly relevant to the psychology of pursuer and pursued and to the objectification of women in society, are not synonymous with the notion that men dominate women through touch. Therefore, finding that young men touch young women with the hand more than vice versa is not automatically indicative of either gender's dominance motives nor necessarily a sign than anyone has been dominated. Indeed, as we shall see later, wanting to touch another can be a testament to the *other's* high status rather than one's own.

A final asymmetry study is that of Grusky, Bonacich, and Peyrot (1984), who had families pose for a photograph. Fathers touched mothers in the photographs 11 times, while mothers never touched the fathers, a significant difference even with so small a sample. This finding, on couples married for an average of 16 years, contradicts the age and relationship duration findings described earlier. However, the request to pose for a family picture likely introduces demands into the situation that are quite different from those experienced in a spontaneous situation in which people are unaware of being observed. Possibly, in a posed family photograph, people conform to the cultural stereotype of the patriarch proudly displaying "his" family. Thus, though the status-related notions of possession and hierarchy are relevant in this case, the results might reflect more a stereotyped notion about how a family should pose for a photograph than the actual status and dominance dynamics of the couple.

Other gender comparisons. In Stier and Hall's (1984) review, women were observed to touch others more than men did. However, in a later study (Remland et al., 1995), men and women were seen equally often to touch another person, and this was also true in Hall and Friedman's (1999) study of employees in a company.

Stier and Hall (1984) found some support for Henley's (1977) prediction that women receive more touch than men. However, both this and the question of who initiates touch cannot be meaningfully discussed without consideration of same-gender touch: do men touch men at a different rate than women touch women? The self-report findings summarized earlier suggest that male–male touch might be particularly infrequent. On balance, the observational literature shows a preponderance of female–female over male–male touching (Kneidlinger, Maple, & Tross, 2001; Stier & Hall, 1984; Sugiyama, 1990), which is also consistent with Hall's (1984) meta-analysis, that showed that female dyads interact at closer distances than male dyads do.

Body parts and other qualitative differences. Authors have often noted gender differences for specific kinds of observed touch (Stier & Hall, 1984). I will not review all of these here, though as a general caveat it must be mentioned only nonaggressive touch is generally discussed.

A meta-analysis of aggressive touch found higher rates between men than between women, as well as, counter to stereotype, higher rates by women in opposite-gender relationships (Archer, 2000a,b).

Everyday experience suggests that shaking hands, at least in North American society, is more commonly initiated by men than women and that women are especially unlikely to shake hands with each other. Stier and Hall's (1984) meta-analysis found that male–male handshaking was more common than female–female handshaking. In a later study, Derlega, Lewis, Harrison, Winstead, and Costanza (1989) found that men engaged in less intimate touch with another man during a role-play of greetings than any other gender combination and that when men touched each other it was likely to be a handshake. Men's handshakes have also been found to be firmer than women's (e.g., Chaplin, Phillips, Brown, Clanton, & Stein, 2000).

It is commonly observed that men are more likely to engage in social touch with each other in the positively sanctioned domain of sport than in other public settings. Kneidlinger et al. (2001) compared male to female touching in gender-segregated softball and baseball games. Overall, women engaged in more touching than men, with significant differences for many distinct behaviors including hand slap, hand pile, and team hug. Men exceeded women on only two behaviors, butt slap and head shake. Similarly, female volleyball players touched each other more than male volleyball players did in the study of Sugiyama (1990). Thus, men in the same-gender sports setting are still more inhibited about touch than women are, though it is likely that the men are less inhibited than they would be in another setting.

GENDER AND REACTIONS TO BEING TOUCHED

Using experimental methodology, it is possible to gain direct insight into how men and women respond to being touched and therefore to go beyond people's self-reports. Quite a few experiments have been conducted in which confederates' touch is manipulated to see how it affects recipients (see Segrin, 1993, and Chapter 12, this volume, for reviews). These studies show that touch, usually operationalized as a confederate's brief touch to the hand, upper arm, or shoulder in a public setting, can be a potent source of social influence.

Much less clear is whether the psychological and behavioral responses of men and women differ when they are touched by confederates. A standard meta-analysis is not feasible because authors rarely report touch × recipient gender interactions in quantitative detail.

Nevertheless, a tally of studies that did and did not find significant touch × recipient gender interactions is instructive.

Table 13.1 lists nine studies that found women to respond more favorably than men to being touched. With only a couple of exceptions, the pattern in these studies was for touch to have a generally facilitative effect on whatever behavior served as the dependent variable, but more so for women than men. A set of studies conducted in Poland, not shown in the table, shows that compliance following touch was predictably high for all gender combinations except male–male, where the touch produced markedly low levels of compliance (Dolinski, in press). The author attributed this unusual result to the Polish culture which is said to be very homophobic.

Two additional studies (not shown in the table) found that men responded significantly *better* than women to being touched. Silverthorne, Micklewright, O'Donnell, and Gibson (1976) found this for liking of the toucher where the touch involved a handshake, and Guéguen (2002a) found this for compliance with a request where the touch was an attention-getting tap on the shoulder. These two studies are distinctive in that the touches were more impersonal than is typical in this literature, and indeed the handshaking gesture is actually male

TABLE 13.1 Experimental studies showing no significant gender difference in response to being touched

Study	Toucher	Toucher Gender	Outcome
Fisher, Rytting, & Heslin, 1976	Library clerk	3 F, 1 M	Evaluations, affect
Guéguen, 2002a	Passerby	4 F	Comply with request (give money for parking meter)
Guéguen & Jacob, 2006	Street vendor	2 F, 2 M	Taste, purchase product
Hornik, 1992	Store associate	3 F, 3 M	Shopping time[a]
Hornik, 1992	Server	4 F, 4 M	Tip, evaluations
Hornik, 1992	Store associate	4 F	Taste, purchase product
Stephen & Zweigenhaft, 1986	Server	1 F	Tip
Sussman & Rosenfeld, 1978	Experimenter	1 F, 1 M	Evaluations
Whitcher & Fisher, 1979	Nurse	>1 F	Evaluations, affect

[a] $p < 0.08$.

stereotypic. Whether men particularly like such touches or women particularly dislike them is a question for further study.

However, before concluding that the general trend shows women to have a more positive response to touch than men do, we must consider the large number of studies that found no significant interaction of touch with recipient gender (Table 13.2). It is unfortunate that hardly any of these studies reported enough information to allow effect sizes and directional trends to be calculated. However, many of these studies

TABLE 13.2 Experimental studies showing no significant gender difference in response to being touched

Study	Toucher	Toucher Gender	Outcome
Alagna, Whitcher, Fisher, & Wicas, 1979	Counselor	2 F, 2 M	Evaluations[a]
Bohm & Hendricks, 1997	Fellow shopper	1 F	Comply with request (move ahead in line)
Brockner, Pressman, Cabitt, & Moran, 1982	Passerby	2 F, 2 M	Comply with request (return dime), evaluations
Crusco & Wetzel, 1984	Server	3 F	Tip, evaluations
Goldman & Fordyce, 1983	Student researcher	1 M	Spontaneous help (pick up dropped items)
Guéguen, 2002b	Survey researcher	1 M	Comply with request (do questionnaire)
Guéguen, 2004	College instructor	1 M	Volunteer to go to blackboard
Guéguen & Jacob, 2004	Server	1 F	Tip
Guéguen & Fischer-Lokou, 2002	Passerby	1 F, 1 M	Comply with request (hold dog)
Guéguen & Fischer-Lokou, 2003	Passerby	1 M	Spontaneous help (pick up dropped items)
Guéguen, Jacob, & Boulbry, 2007	Server	2 F, 1 M	Comply with request (take server's menu suggestion)
Hornik, 1992	Store associate	3 F, 3 M	Evaluations, money spent
Hornik & Ellis, 1988	Student researcher	4 F, 4 M	Comply with request (do interview)

Continued

TABLE 13.2 Experimental studies showing no significant gender difference in response to being touched *Continued*

Study	Toucher	Toucher Gender	Outcome
Hubbard, Tsuji, Williams, & Seatriz, 2003	Server (restaurant)	1 F, 1 M	Tip
Hubbard et al., 2003	Server (bar)	1 F, 1 M	Tip[a]
Kaufman & Mahoney, 1999	Server	5 F	Alcohol consumed[b]
Kleinke, 1977	Fellow shoppers	8 F	Comply with request (lend a dime)
Lynn, Le, & Sherwyn, 1998	Server	1 M	Tip
Nannberg & Hansen, 1994	Survey researcher	1 F	Comply with request (extent of questionnaire completion)
Patterson, Powell, & Lenihan, 1986	Experimenter	2 F, 2 M	Comply with request (time spent helping experimenter)
Paulsell & Goldman, 1984	Survey researcher	1 F, 1 M	Spontaneous help (pick up dropped items)
Powell et al., 1994	Experimenter	7 F, 6 M	Evaluations, comply with request (help experimenter)[c]
Remland & Jones, 1994	Passerby	3 F	Comply with request (mail postcard)
Silverthorne, Noreen, Hunt, & Rota, 1972	Experimenter	1 F, 1 M	Evaluations
Smith, Gier, & Willis, 1982	Store associate	2 F, 2 M	Try, evaluate, purchase product
Steward & Lupfer, 1987	College instructor	2 F, 1 M	Evaluations, exam performance
Storrs & Kleinke, 1990	Interviewer	3 F, 3 M	Evaluations
Vaidis & Halimi-Falkowicz, 2008	Survey researcher	1 F	Comply with request (do survey)
Willis & Hamm, 1980	Survey researcher	4 F, 4 M	Comply with request (sign petition)
Willis & Hamm, 1980	Student researcher	4 F, 4 M	Comply with request (complete rating scale)

[a] Touch was more effective in opposite-gender dyads than same-gender dyads.
[b] No interaction with dyad type (MM, FF, MF); data were not analyzed for individual patrons.
[c] For compliance with request for help, touch had biggest impact in female–female dyads.

had large samples, meaning low statistical power may not account for the lack of gender interactions. It remains possible, of course, that there could be a consistent trend in the nonsignificant studies showing a more favorable female than male response. However, with so few details known, it is hard to reach any conclusion about the overall interaction effect and also about possible moderators (e.g., setting, toucher gender, nuances of touch, type of dependent variable). Inspection of Tables 13.1 and 13.2 suggests no methodological variables that clearly distinguish studies showing significant and nonsignificant interaction effects. Another unknown is the possibility of uncontrolled behaviors emitted by the (often few) confederates in touch experiments, which could obscure or produce touch × recipient gender interactions (see Lewis, Derlega, Shankar, Cochard, & Finkel, 1997, for a discussion of uncontrolled nonverbal behaviors in confederates).

STATUS AND TOUCH

Beliefs and Perceptions

In a meta-analysis of 19 studies that measured perceptions of status/dominance based on observed touch (e.g., perceivers' ratings based on photographs of people touching or not), nearly all of the studies showed that the initiation of touch produced perceptions of higher status (Hall et al., 2005). Sometimes, such studies show that, in the eyes of perceivers, touch both raises the status of the toucher and lowers the status of the recipient (Major & Heslin, 1982).

Carney, Hall, and Smith LeBeau (2005) asked participants to imagine hypothetical persons of high or low personality dominance, or high or low rank in an organization, and to rate how much each would engage in three kinds of touch. For invasive behavior (combination of standing too close, touching, and pointing) and touching the other's shoulder, back, or arm, participants rated the higher person as doing more, regardless of whether status/dominance was defined as personality dominance or rank in an organization. There was no believed status/dominance difference for "initiates shaking the other's hand."

Observational Studies

Both Henley (1973) and Major and Williams (1980, reported in Major, 1981) inferred the socioeconomic statuses (SESs) of people touching in public. It is hard to tell what was meant by SES in either study because the only example given (by Henley) was waitress–customer, which does not necessarily imply a difference in SES. In any case, both studies found more touching by the higher "SES" person than vice versa (significant in Henley, not significant in Major and Williams; combined $p = .02$ according to Stier & Hall, 1984).

Juni and Brannon (1981) used an experimental approach, manipulating status via how a potential recipient was dressed. They found a nonsignificant tendency for the lower-status person to be touched more than the higher-status person (25 higher-to-lower vs. 16 lower-to-higher). In a second experiment, status was manipulated by title of the potential recipient, and here there was no significant touching effect though in direction the higher status person was touched *more*, not less.

The possibility that people might touch high-status people more than they touch low-status people is actually consistent with everyday observation. We are all familiar with photographs of screaming fans reaching out to touch a famous rock star. The daughter of the revered Buddhist Panchen Lama is quoted as saying: "They told me that there were people lining the road for fifty miles. Thousands and thousands of people, all wanting to touch me" (Hilton, 2004). Even in more commonplace situations, people often find value in touching someone who is important in their eyes. They might say proudly, "I shook his hand!" In such a situation, the toucher feels that something of value has rubbed off, be it glory or fame or, as suggested by the perception studies reviewed earlier, some of the other person's high status. Touching can thus be motivated because of its potential to raise the status of an otherwise lower-status toucher.

The desire for lower-status people to touch higher-status people is suggested by Goldstein and Jeffords' (1981) study of intentional touch (excluding handshake) between male legislators in a state house of representatives while the legislature was in session. Status was determined objectively by using information on committee membership, committee standing, and past government service. The authors found that the lower in status initiated touch with the higher more than vice versa (84 vs. 62, $p = .07$). The authors noted that although the governor was touched by many, he did not initiate touch with anyone.

Hall (1996) adopted Goldstein and Jeffords' (1981) methodology to study the association of professional status to intentional touch at academic conferences. When two individuals were observed to engage in touch, observers unobtrusively recorded information about the touch and also about the individuals involved. By using archival information sources pertaining to the individuals and their institutions, a relative-status index was calculated which permitted an analysis of touching patterns between higher- and lower-status individuals. Over all kinds of touch, there was no status difference in touch. However, different kinds of touch showed different patterns. The lower-status person was significantly more likely to initiate handshake, whereas the higher-status person was nonsignificantly more likely to engage in affectionate and hand-to-shoulder and hand-to-arm touch. Comparisons between types of touch showed significant differences—for example, the difference in the relative-status index between formal touches (i.e., handshakes) and rated affectionate touch was significant. Thus, the lower-status person tended to touch in a polite, ritualized way while the higher-status person tended to touch in a relaxed and affectionate way suggestive of the touch license discussed by Henley (1977).

Hall and Friedman (1999) conducted a study of employees of a company, and rather than observe unobtrusively they paired dyads randomly and observed them during two structured interaction tasks. Rank within the company was determined objectively, based on administrative records. Higher- and lower-status individuals differed on a number of nonverbal behaviors, but not on touching. A factor analysis of measured variables showed that touching loaded with smiling, gazing, and rated warmth and expressiveness on a factor labeled "warm and direct." Touching did not load on the factor labeled "status," which included organizational rank, relaxed voice, and relaxed posture, further confirming that in this study touch did not connote or reflect status.

When these and other studies were combined in a meta-analysis of the touching behavior of people of known status (Hall et al., 2005), there was no overall status effect. However, as suggested by the Hall (1996) study, such an overall comparison can obscure differences according to the type of touch that is observed.

Touching on the part of winners and losers in sports competitions has been discussed as possibly reflecting status differences. Although victory or defeat in sports can be considered one kind of status, how to interpret any touching differences is unclear because the psychological processes are unknown. Winners might touch more because they feel endowed with the right to impose on others, but they might also touch more out of self-congratulation and exuberance, consistent with the "approach" tendencies documented for high-power holders in other situations (Keltner, Gruenfeld, & Anderson, 2003). They might, on the other hand, touch as a way of making it up to the loser—to show they are a good sport, show respect to the loser, or make the loser feel better by "reaching out" in a quite literal way. Losers, conversely, could suffer depressed mood that would reduce their motivation to touch the winner (or anyone else), or they might experience more generalized behavioral inhibition (Keltner et al.). Or, they might feel that the lower has no "right" to initiate touch (Henley, 1977). Thus, a touch difference between winners and losers might originate from a variety of different emotional, motivational, and cognitive processes.

Heckel (1993) counted intentional touches by winners and losers in tennis and racquetball games. Across both sports, winners touched losers more than vice versa ($p < .10$). In a similar analysis of college flag football games, touches were significantly more common from winners to losers than vice versa, with the majority of touches being handshakes (Heckel, Allen, & Blackmon, 1986). Here, unlike Hall (1996), handshaking was more frequently initiated by higher status individuals (i.e., winners) but this might be tied to specific traditions within the realm of sports.

In Anderton and Heckel's (1985) study of swimming races, observers counted all intentional touches but did not track who the recipient was, meaning that the asymmetry question could not be asked. Winners touched others far more than losers did, but they were also touched by others far more than losers were. This suggests the possibility that the touching was of the congratulatory kind and may further be due to more people surrounding the winners, creating a higher likelihood that any touch will occur.

Taken all together, the studies pertaining to status and touch reviewed in this chapter do not yield a simple or consistent picture. Sometimes higher-status people do more touching and sometimes the reverse is the case. Rarely in the literature were efforts made to separate the contributions of gender versus status. Sometimes the status-touch finding depends on what kind of touch it is, but even here studies are not consistent. One way to think about this inconsistency is to reflect on the motives of the individuals involved. I have already mentioned several variables that could be important, including the emotional state of the individuals and the nature of their goals in the situation. These goals (motives) could vary greatly and could be confounded with status. If the lower-status person is in a state of adoration vis-à-vis the other person, he might want to touch that person, but if the goal is to control the other person, greater touching might be done by the higher-status person. A low-status person might wish to elevate her relative status via touching a high-status person. A high-status person who is insecure about status or feels a need to display and enforce it might touch subordinates more, yet a high-status person who is secure might feel no need to engage in touch displays.

When investigating the relation of status to touch, as well as to other nonverbal behaviors, researchers need to be cognizant of potential confounders such as those just listed (Hall et al., 2005). When the psychological states (emotions, goals, motives, role construals) differ between high- and low-status individuals, it is these that may be determining their behavior rather than anything directly caused by their status. Confoundings between status and possible proximal (confounding) factors are hard to discern or control when naturalistic observation is done. In laboratory experiments, where status may be assigned, the situation is less ambiguous, but even here one must ask about the participants' states of mind. A high-status person who is motivated to be controlling might touch a very different amount from a high-status person who is motivated to be warm and supportive. Or, even if these two high-status people touch the same amount, it might be for different reasons and they might touch in different ways. Distinctions such as these, and many more, are likely to be operative in the situations in which touch is observed. If researchers are not able to measure the psychological processes and mechanisms involved, they should still discuss alternative explanations and interpretations.

BRINGING STATUS AND GENDER TOGETHER

Should gender and status be discussed together when we consider the subject of interpersonal touch? This review leads me to offer a very equivocal no, for the following reasons. First, the gender differences are complex and do not conform to a simple story about men's and women's status. As an example, the finding that male–female asymmetry in touch reverses itself as couple members are older and/or in more advanced relationships does not lend itself to a simplistic "women are weak" interpretation. On the other hand, one could argue that in young people, and in young relationships, men have a motive to dominate and that, in fact, women's relative status is weaker compared to more mature relationships where more equality may have been achieved. Whether this account is correct requires more data than we have at present. One could actually make the counterargument that younger people are more progressive (e.g., egalitarian) in their attitudes than older people, and therefore younger people might be more free from the stranglehold of a sexual politics of touch than older people would be. In this case, one would have to search for other explanations to account for the data.

Second, as implied by the preceding, other explanations besides status require consideration—for example, homophobia as an inhibitor of male–male touch. Furthermore, socialization histories that render women's interpersonal attitudes and nonverbal interaction style more open, warm, direct, and responsive than men's (Hall, 1984; Hall et al., 2000) could explain many of the gender differences without recourse to a status theory. As stated earlier, a theory that pronounces status inequality to be the root cause behind socialization differences would keep the status concept in the picture, but not in a way that is likely to be productive.

REFERENCES

Alagna, F. J., Whitcher, S. J., Fisher, J. D., & Wicas, E. A. (1979). Evaluative reaction to interpersonal touch in a counseling interview. *Journal of Counseling Psychology, 26*, 465–472.

Andersen, P. (2006). The evolution of biological sex differences in communication. In K. Dindia & D. J. Canary (Eds.), *Sex differences and similarities in communication* (pp. 117–135). Mahwah, NJ: Lawrence Erlbaum Associates.

Andersen, P. A., & Leibowitz, K. (1978). The development and nature of the construct touch avoidance. *Environmental Psychology and Nonverbal Behavior, 3*, 89–106.

Anderton, C. H., & Heckel, R. V. (1985). Touching behaviors of winners and losers in swimming races. *Perceptual and Motor Skills, 60*, 289–290.

Archer, J. (2000a). Sex differences in aggression between heterosexual partners: A meta-analytic review. *Psychological Bulletin, 126*, 651–680.

Archer, J. (2000b). Sex differences in physical aggression to partners: A reply to Frieze (2000), O'Leary (2000), and White, Smith, Koss, and Figueredo (2000). *Psychological Bulletin, 126*, 697–702.

Berger, J., Rosenholtz, S. J., & Zelditch, M., Jr. (1985). Status organizing processes. *Annual Review of Sociology, 6*, 479–508.

Bohm, J. K., & Hendricks, B. (1997). Effects of interpersonal touch, degree of justification, and sex of participant on compliance with a request. *Journal of Social Psychology, 137*, 460–469.

Brockner, J., Pressman, B., Cabitt, J., & Moran, P. (1982). Nonverbal intimacy, sex, and compliance: A field study. *Journal of Nonverbal Behavior, 6*, 253–258.

Carney, D. R., Hall, J. A., & LeBeau, L. S. (2005). Beliefs about the nonverbal expression of social power. *Journal of Nonverbal Behavior, 29*, 105–123.

Chaplin, W. F., Phillips, J. B., Brown, J. D., Clanton, N. R., & Stein, J. L. (2000). Handshaking, gender, personality, and first impressions. *Journal of Personality and Social Psychology, 79*, 110–117.

Crusco, A. H., & Wetzel, C. G. (1984). The Midas touch: The effects of interpersonal touch on restaurant tipping. *Personality and Social Psychology Bulletin, 10*, 512–517.

Derlega, V. J., Catanzaro, D., & Lewis, R. J. (2001). Perceptions about tactile intimacy in same-sex and opposite-sex pairs based on research participants' sexual orientation. *Psychology of Men and Masculinity, 2,* 124–132.

Derlega, V. J., Lewis, R. J., Harrison, S., Winstead, B. A., & Costanza, R. (1989). Gender differences in the initiation and attribution of tactile intimacy. *Journal of Nonverbal Behavior, 13,* 83–96.

DiBiase, R., & Gunnoe, J. (2004). Gender and culture differences in touching behavior. *Journal of Social Psychology, 144,* 49–62.

Dolinski, D. (2010). Touch, compliance, and homophobia. *Journal of Nonverbal Behavior, 34,* 179–192.

Ellyson, S. L., & Dovidio, J. F. (Eds.) (1985). *Power, dominance, and nonverbal behavior.* New York, NY: Springer-Verlag.

Fisher, J. D., Rytting, M., & Heslin, R. (1976). Hands touching hands: Affective and evaluative effects of an interpersonal touch. *Sociometry, 39,* 416–421.

Floyd, K. (2000). Affectionate same-sex touch: The influence of homophobia on observers' perceptions. *Journal of Social Psychology, 140,* 774–788.

Fromme, D. K., Jaynes, W. E., Taylor, D. K., Hanold, E. G., Daniell, J., Rountree, J. R., & Fromme, M. L. (1989). Nonverbal behavior and attitudes toward touch. *Journal of Nonverbal Behavior, 13,* 3–14.

Garlick, R. (1994). Male and female responses to ambiguous instructor behaviors. *Sex Roles, 30,* 135–158.

Goldman, M., & Fordyce, J. (1983). Prosocial behavior as affected by eye contact, touch, and voice expression. *Journal of Social Psychology, 121,* 125–129.

Goldstein, A. G., & Jeffords, J. (1981). Status and touching behavior. *Bulletin of the Psychonomic Society, 17,* 79–81.

Grusky, O., Bonacich, P., & Peyrot, M. (1984). Physical contact in the family. *Journal of Marriage and the Family, 46,* 715–723.

Guéguen, N. (2002a). Kind of touch, gender and compliance with a request. *Studia Psychologica, 44,* 167–172.

Guéguen, N. (2002b). Status, apparel and touch: Their joint effects on compliance to a request. *North American Journal of Psychology, 4,* 279–286.

Guéguen, N. (2004). Nonverbal encouragement of participation in a course: The effect of touching. *Social Psychology of Education, 7,* 89–98.

Guéguen, N., & Fischer-Lokou, J. (2002). An evaluation of touch on a large request: A field setting. *Psychological Reports, 90,* 267–269.

Guéguen, N., & Fischer-Lokou, J. (2003). Tactile contact and spontaneous help: An evaluation in a natural setting. *Journal of Social Psychology, 143,* 785–787.

Guéguen, N., & Jacob, C. (2004). The effect of touch on tipping: An evaluation in a French bar. *International Journal of Hospitality Management, 24,* 295–299.

Guéguen, N., & Jacob, C. (2006). The effect of tactile stimulation on the purchasing behaviour of consumers: An experimental study in a natural setting. *International Journal of Management, 23,* 24–33.

Guéguen, N., Jacob, C., & Boulbry, G. (2007). The effects of touch on compliance with a restaurant employee suggestion. *International Journal of Hospitality Management, 26,* 1019–1023.

Guerrero, L. K., & Andersen, P. A. (1994). Patterns of matching and invitation: Touch behavior and touch avoidance across romantic relationship stages. *Journal of Nonverbal Behavior, 18,* 137–153.

Hall, J. A. (1984). *Nonverbal sex differences: Communication accuracy and expressive style*. Baltimore, MD: The Johns Hopkins University Press.
Hall, J. A. (1996). Touch, status, and gender at professional meetings. *Journal of Nonverbal Behavior, 20*, 23–44.
Hall, J. A., Carter, J. D., & Horgan, T. G. (2000). Gender differences in the nonverbal communication of emotion. In A. H. Fischer (Ed.), *Gender and emotion: Social psychological perspectives* (pp. 97–117). Paris: Cambridge University Press.
Hall, J. A., Coats, E. J., & LeBeau, L. S. (2005). Nonverbal behavior and the vertical dimension of social relations: A meta-analysis. *Psychological Bulletin, 131*, 898–924.
Hall, J. A., & Friedman, G. B. (1999). Status, gender, and nonverbal behavior: A study of structured interactions between employees of a company. *Personality and Social Psychology Bulletin, 25*, 1082–1091.
Hall, J. A., & Veccia, E. M. (1990). More "touching" observations: New insights on men, women, and interpersonal touch. *Journal of Personality and Social Psychology, 59*, 1155–1162.
Hanzal, A., Segrin, C., & Dorros, S. M. (2008). The role of marital status and age on men's and women's reactions to touch from a relational partner. *Journal of Nonverbal Behavior, 32*, 21–35.
Heckel, R. V. (1993). Comparison of touching behaviors of winners and losers in racquetball and tennis. *Perceptual and Motor Skills, 77*, 1392–1394.
Heckel, R. V., Allen, S. A., & Blackmon, D. C. (1986). Tactile communication of winners in flag football. *Perceptual and Motor Skills, 63*, 553–554.
Henley, N. M. (1973). Status and sex: Some touching observations. *Bulletin of the Psychonomic Society, 2*, 91–93.
Henley, N. M. (1977). *Body politics: Power, sex, and nonverbal communication*. Englewood Cliffs, NJ: Prentice-Hall.
Henley, N. M., & Harmon, S. (1985). The nonverbal semantics of power and gender: A perceptual study. In S. L. Ellyson & J. F. Dovidio (Eds.), *Power, dominance, and nonverbal behavior* (pp. 151–164). New York, NY: Springer-Verlag.
Hertenstein, M. J., Verkamp, J. M., Kerestes, A. M., & Holmes, R. M. (2006). The communicative functions of touch in humans, nonhuman primates, and rats: A review and synthesis of the empirical research. *Genetic, Social, and General Psychology Monographs, 132*, 5–94.
Hilton, I. (2004, March 29). The Buddha's daughter. *The New Yorker*, 42–50.
Hornik, J. (1992). Tactile stimulation and consumer response. *Journal of Consumer Research, 19*, 449–458.
Hornik, J., & Ellis, S. (1988). Strategies to secure compliance for a mall intercept interview. *Public Opinion Quarterly, 52*, 539–551.
Hubbard, A. S. E., Tsuji, A. A., Williams, C., & Seatriz, V., Jr. (2003). Effects of touch on gratuities received in same-gender and cross-gender dyads. *Journal of Applied Social Psychology, 33*, 2427–2438.
Jones, S. E. (1986). Sex differences in touch communication. *Western Journal of Speech Communication, 50*, 227–241.
Juni, S., & Brannon, R. (1981). Interpersonal touching as a function of status and sex. *Journal of Social Psychology, 114*, 135–136.
Kaufman, D., & Mahoney, J. M. (1999). The effect of waitresses' touch on alcohol consumption in dyads. *Journal of Social Psychology, 139*, 261–267.
Keltner, D., Gruenfeld, D. H., & Anderson, C. (2003). Power, approach, and inhibition. *Psychological Review, 110*, 265–284.

Kleinke, C. L. (1977). Compliance to requests made by gazing and touching experimenters in field settings. *Journal of Experimental Social Psychology, 13,* 218–223.

Kneidinger, L. M., Maple, T. L., & Tross, S. A. (2001). Touching behavior in sport: Functional components, analysis of sex differences, and ethological considerations. *Journal of Nonverbal Behavior, 25,* 43–61.

LaFrance, M., Hecht, M. A., & Paluck, E. L. (2003). The contingent smile: A meta-analysis of gender differences in smiling. *Psychological Bulletin, 129,* 305–334.

Lewis, R. J., Derlega, V. J., Shankar, A., Cochard, E., & Finkel, L. (1997). Nonverbal correlates of confederates' touch: Confounds in touch research. *Journal of Social Behavior and Personality, 12,* 821–830.

Lynn, M., Le, J., & Sherwyn, D. S. (1998). Reach out and touch your customers. *Cornell Hotel and Restaurant Administration Quarterly, 39,* 60–65.

Major, B. (1981). Gender patterns in touching behavior. In C. Mayo & N. M. Henley (Eds.), *Gender and nonverbal behavior* (pp. 15–37). New York, NY: Springer-Verlag.

Major, B., & Heslin, R. (1982). Perceptions of cross-sex and same-sex nonreciprocal touch: It is better to give than to receive. *Journal of Nonverbal Behavior, 6,* 148–162.

Martin, M. M., & Anderson, C. M. (1993). Psychological and biological differences in touch avoidance. *Communication Research Reports, 10,* 141–147.

Nannberg, J. C., & Hansen, C. H. (1994). Post-compliance touch: An incentive for task performance. *Journal of Social Psychology, 134,* 301–307.

Nguyen, M. L., Heslin, R., & Nguyen, T. (1976). The meaning of touch: Sex and marital status differences. *Representative Research in Social Psychology, 7,* 13–18.

Noller, P. (1986). Sex differences in nonverbal communication: Advantage lost or supremacy regained? *Australian Journal of Psychology, 38,* 23–32.

Patterson, M. L., Powell, J. L., & Lenihan, M. G. (1986). Touch, compliance, and interpersonal affect. *Journal of Nonverbal Behavior, 10,* 41–50.

Paulsell, S., & Goldman, M. (1984). The effect of touching different body areas on prosocial behavior. *Journal of Social Psychology, 122,* 269–273.

Powell, J. L., Meil, W., Patterson, M. L., Chouinard, E. F., Collins, B., Kobus, T. J., ... Arnone, W. L. (1994). Effects of timing of touch on compliance to a request. *Journal of Social Behavior and Personality, 9,* 153–162.

Remland, M. S., & Jones, T. S. (1994). The influence of vocal intensity and touch on compliance gaining. *Journal of Social Psychology, 134,* 89–97.

Remland, M. S., Jones, T. S., & Brinkman, H. (1995). Interpersonal distance, body orientation, and touch: Effects of culture, gender, and age. *Journal of Social Psychology, 135,* 281–297.

Roese, N. J., Olson, J. M., Borenstein, M. N., Martin, A., & Shores, A. L. (1992). Same-sex touching behavior: The moderating role of homophobic attitudes. *Journal of Nonverbal Behavior, 16,* 249–259.

Segrin, C. (1993). The effects of nonverbal behavior on outcomes of compliance gaining attempts. *Communication Studies, 44,* 169–187.

Silverthorne, C., Noreen, C., Hunt, T., & Rota, L. (1972). The effects of tactile stimulation on visual experience. *Journal of Social Psychology 88,* 153–154.

Silverthorne, C., Micklewright, J., O'Donnell, M., & Gibson, R. (1976). Attribution of personal characteristics as a function of the degree of touch on initial contact and sex. *Sex Roles, 2,* 185–193.

Smith, D. E., Gier, J. A., & Willis, F. N. (1982). Interpersonal touch and compliance with a marketing request. *Basic and Applied Social Psychology, 3,* 35–38.

Stephen, R., & Zweigenhaft, R. L. (1986). The effect on tipping of a waitress touching male and female customers. *Journal of Social Psychology, 126,* 141–142.

Steward, A. L., & Lupfer, M. (1987). Touching as teaching: The effect of touch on students' perceptions and performance. *Journal of Applied Social Psychology, 17,* 800–809.

Stier, D. S., & Hall, J. A. (1984). Gender differences in touch: An empirical and theoretical review. *Journal of Personality and Social Psychology, 47,* 440–459.

Storrs, D., & Kleinke, C. L. (1990). Evaluation of high and equal status male and female touchers. *Journal of Nonverbal Behavior, 14,* 87–95.

Struckman-Johnson, C., & Struckman-Johnson, D. (1993). College men's and women's reactions to hypothetical sexual touch varied by initiator gender and coercion level. *Sex Roles, 29,* 371–385.

Sugiyama, Y. (1990). A sex difference in hand-to-hand touching behavior in volleyball games: A preliminary study. *Perceptual and Motor Skills, 71,* 1002.

Sussman, N. M., & Rosenfeld, H. M. (1978). Touch, justification, and sex: Influences on the aversiveness of spatial violations. *Journal of Social Psychology, 106,* 215–225.

Uggen, C., & Blackstone, A. (2004). Sexual harassment as a gendered expression of power. *American Sociological Review, 69,* 64–92.

Vaidis, D. C. F., & Halimi-Falkowicz, S. G. M. (2008). Increasing compliance with a request: Two touches are more effective than one. *Psychological Reports, 103,* 88–92.

Whitcher, S. J., & Fisher, J. D. (1979). Multidimensional reaction to therapeutic touch in a hospital setting. *Journal of Personality and Social Psychology, 37,* 87–96.

Willis, F. N., Jr., & Briggs, L. F. (1992). Relationship and touch in public settings. *Journal of Nonverbal Behavior, 16,* 55–63.

Willis, F. N., Jr., & Dodds, R. A. (1998). Age, relationship, and touch initiation. *Journal of Social Psychology, 138,* 115–123.

Willis, F. N., Jr., & Hamm, H. K. (1980). The use of interpersonal touch in securing compliance. *Journal of Nonverbal Behavior, 5,* 49–55.

Willis, F. N., Jr., & Rawdon, V. A. (1994). Gender and national differences in attitudes toward same-gender touch. *Perceptual and Motor Skills, 78,* 1027–1034.

Willis, F. N., & Rinck, C. M. (1983). A personal log method for investigating interpersonal touch. *Journal of Psychology, 113,* 119–122.

Willis, F. N., Rinck, C. M., & Dean, L. M. (1978). Interpersonal touch among adults in cafeteria lines. *Perceptual and Motor Skills, 47,* 1147–1152.

14

Tactile Traditions: Cultural Differences and Similarities in Haptic Communication

PETER A. ANDERSEN

Touch is arguably the most basic human sense. It constitutes the primary sense during fetal development, the most established sense during infancy (Montagu, 1978) and the most passionate and sexual sense during adulthood (Morris, 1971). Similarly, it is recognized that touch is essential to normal human development (Bowlby, 1969; Levine & Stanton, 1990; Montagu, 1978; Morris, 1971; Thayer, 1986) and indispensable to the maintenance of optimal physical and psychological heath (Burgoon, Guerrero, & Floyd, 2010; Field, 2001; Reite, 1990). It is at once the most sought and the most reviled, the source of the deepest sensual experiences (Andersen, 2008; Morris, 1971). All humans are tactile, but the degree, type, location, and nature of their tactile interactions vary considerably across culture. In this chapter, the numerous differences in tactile behavior among world cultures will be examined and the basis of these differences will be explored.

CROSS CULTURAL SIMILARITIES IN TOUCH

Imagine a visit to earth by interstellar social scientists from Alpha Centuri attempting to characterize this odd but intelligent species, the human being. Centurions would note that universal human tactile rituals include hugs, play, massage, sport, fighting, medical interventions, grooming, affectionate kissing, and sexual behavior, all of which involve substantial human tactile contact. This involvement is particularly true of adult–infant tactile interaction.

Touch With Human Infants

Centurions would unquestionably conclude that female human beings nourish their young through tactile contact, except for a few mothers in the most technologically advanced societies who believe that alternatives to breast milk are advantageous or more convenient. Even in countries like the United States about two-thirds of women breast feed (Healthy People, 2010). Happily, with encouragement from health communication campaigns, the number is increasing. Unfortunately, despite the increase in the developed world, breast feeding is decreasing in many parts of the world. In less-developed countries and throughout much of our own history, mothers nursed wearing little or no clothing, but most American mothers nurse their babies while fully dressed, reducing mother–infant tactile contact to contact with the nipple (Montagu, 1978). Nonetheless, even where breast feeding does not occur, or where it does not include skin-to-skin contact, Centurions would observe universally close tactile contact between human infants and their feeders and caregivers.

For the first year of life and beyond, humans throughout the world are not only fed, but carried, protected, taught, comforted, and loved through touch. Indeed, researchers suggest that severe tactile deprivation results in mental retardation, emotional problems, immunological problems, and even death (Andersen, 2008; Field, 2001; Montagu, 1978). Indeed studies show that adults touch infants around two-thirds of the time (Muir, 2002). Although culture and social class may dictate differing levels and kinds of tactile contact, touch is universally high between infants and their adult caregivers throughout the world.

Tactile Affection and Intimacy Among Adult Humans

Centurions would observe that a primary function of touch throughout the world is the expression of interpersonal closeness. From infants to seniors, touch creates feelings of comfort, warmth, affection, and relationship closeness (Andersen, 2008; Andersen & Guerrero, 1998; Floyd, 2006; Montagu, 1978). Touch is a central part of what constitutes human intimacy (Andersen, 2008; Andersen, Guerrero, & Jones, 2006; Prager, 1995), the construct of nonverbal immediacy (Andersen, 1985, 2008; Andersen, Hecht, Hoobler, & Smallwood, 2002; Andersen & Wang, 2006), and the concept of interpersonal affection (Floyd, 1997, 2000, 2006). Even in the most tactilely hesitant cultures, intimacy is expressed through touch in families, romantic dyads, and among close friends.

Indeed, there may be an underlying chemical basis for the positive feelings of interpersonal touch. Recent research shows that interpersonal touch releases oxytocin (Floyd, 2006; Floyd, Mikkleson, & Hesse, 2007; Morhenn, Park, Piper, & Zak, 2008), a chemical known to produce feelings of warmth, intimacy, and even love.

Touch and Human Sexuality

Though sexual interaction involves all human senses, the prototypic sexual sense is touch. Throughout the world, sexual interaction is ultimately a tactile activity whether for procreation, for recreation, or for relational enhancement (Guerrero, Andersen, & Afifi, 2007). Of course, cultures vary greatly in the rules surrounding sexual touch, including initiation and refusal, and rules regarding the appropriateness of who touches and who is touched. But to our interstellar observer, sexual touch would constitute a relatively ubiquitous human activity.

Humans overwhelmingly reproduce and share sexual intimacy through tactile contact, though a very small percentage of conceptions are via test-tube babies and surrogate moms. Most humans are sexually modest and wear clothing; even when they are naked they tend to be modest (Brown, 1991). Ostentatious public sexual displays occur in many cultures, but they tend to be noteworthy because they are unusual; sexual contact in humans typically occurs in private. Similarly, incest is a universal human taboo and is relatively rare in every culture (Brown, 1991). So while cultural variation in sexual touch certainly exists, humans are more similar than different in these activities.

Emotional Communication

As discussed earlier, touch has been shown across many studies to communicate positively valenced warmth, though it also has the capacity to communicate negatively valenced discomfort (Andersen, 2008; Hertenstein & Campos, 2001; Jones & Yarborough, 1985). However, recent research has shown that touch, like facial expression, is capable of communicating specific emotions (Hertenstein, Holmes, McCullough, & Keltner, 2009; Hertenstein, Keltner, App, Bulleit, & Jaskolka, 2006). In experiments that controlled for other sensory modalities, Hertenstein and his colleagues demonstrated not only that touch communicates emotional content to receivers but that observers can discern meanings associated with touch visually.

Persuasive Touch

Numerous studies have shown that when touch accompanies a persuasive request, compliance with the request increases (Andersen, 2008; Segrin, 1993). As we will learn shortly, there are considerable differences in touch across culture. However, the positive effects of touch on compliance seem to be cross-culturally robust. A study of tactile compliance gaining in France shows the same positive results as such compliance-gaining studies that were conducted in the United States, despite the fact that touch is more prevalent in France (Joule & Guéguen, 2007; Guéguen, 2002). Similarly, as in studies conducted in the United States, studies in France indicate that the individual making the request is evaluated more positively in the touch than in the no-touch condition (Erceau & Guéguen, 2007) and two touches are more effective than one in gaining compliance (Vaidis & Halimi-Falkowitz, 2008).

Functional Touch

Interpersonal touch is used functionally throughout the world. Barbers, hairdressers, dentists, nurses, shamen, coaches, surgeons, and a variety other jobholders engage in touch to perform vital human functions (Andersen, 2008; Montague, 1978). During such functional interactions normal rules of touch are often inapplicable, though in some traditional cultures this is not the case. Many Muslim women would not accept an examination from a male doctor unless a female doctor is not present and their husband consents to the examination (Naqib al-Misri & Keller, 1994).

Touch as Universal

In short, Centurions would note many salient similarities in tactile behavior throughout the world and some differences as well. This chapter examines these similarities and differences in touch but focuses primarily on differences among human cultures. Instead of simply noting where differences in touch exist among human societies, which produce a virtually infinite number of bicultural comparisons, this chapter focuses on the essential influences that produced differences among human cultures: climate, individualism/collectivism, gender orientation, and religion. In the following sections, both cross cultural variations in tactile behavior and their fundamental causes are discussed. The discussion starts with an examination of the substantial influence of climate on human tactile behavior.

CHANGES IN LATITUDE: CLIMATE AND TACTILE BEHAVIOR

The research on cultural tactile communication indicates that the most potent predictor of differences in touch is latitude, the distance from the equator (Albert & Ah Ha, 2004; Andersen et al., 2002; Andersen & Wang, 2006). Research suggests that regions generally called high-contact cultures (Hall, 1966; Patterson, 1983) include Arab/Islamic countries, Central and South America, Mediterranean countries, Southern and Eastern Europe, whereas low-contact cultures include Eastern Asia—particularly Northeast Asia, Northern Europe, and North America (Andersen, 2008; Andersen & Guerrero, 2008; Field, 1999; Hall, 1966; McDaniel & Andersen, 1998; Miller, Commons, & Gutheil, 2006; Montagu & Matson, 1979; Patterson, 1983; Shuter, 1976, 1977; Sussman & Rosenfeld, 1982).

Studies have shown that the Mediterranean region has particularly high levels of interpersonal touch. Any tourist can readily observe that in countries like Italy and Greece, touch is substantially higher than most places in the world. One study of intercultural touch showed that residents of Italy, a Mediterranean culture, displayed more interpersonal touch, particularly male–male touch than residents of Germany or the United States (Shuter, 1977). Another study that compared touch between citizens in England, the Netherlands, and France found no significant differences, but was hampered by the infrequency of touch, which occurred in only 9% of the interactions, as well as the lack of any southern French in the French sample (Remland, Jones, & Brinkman, 1991). In a study of adolescent behavior in fast-food restaurants in the United States versus France, Field (1999) reported significantly more stroking, hugging, and kissing among French adolescents than American adolescents. These differences between Northern European versus Mediterranean cultures and their derivative cultures were noted by Scheflen (1974) and Montagu and Matson (1979) who report that British and German people display less tactile contact than Eastern European Jews, Italians, French, Spanish, Cubans, and other people from other Latin American cultures. In a more recent study, hugs and kisses were deemed as more appropriate by therapists in Brazil than in the United States (Miller et al., 2006) consistent with both the Mediterranean origins and the equatorial location of Brazil compared to the United States. Several accounts show that tactile miscommunication is common between people from Arab culture and American culture (Almaney & Alwan, 1982; Cohen, 1987; Hall, 1966). People from Arab/Islamic cultures perceive Americans as aloof and "distant" because of their lack of tactile and olfactory communication; Arabs are often perceived as "pushy" and invasive because of their close proxemic distances and high levels of touch. In short, cultures that are more southerly, particularly those originating in the Middle East and Mediterranean, have much higher levels of day-to-day tactile contact than those in other parts of the world.

Even within a given country, northerners avoid touch and southerners tend to be much more tactilely oriented; any observant traveler witnesses more touch in Southern Italy, than in Northern Italy or Southern France compared to Northern France. Pennebaker, Rime, and Blankenship (1996) discovered that throughout the world northerners are less emotionally expressive than Southerners. More specifically, with regard to touch, in a study of 40 sites throughout the United States, Andersen, Lustig, and Andersen (1987, 1990) found that touch avoidance was significantly related to latitude with northerly sites displaying most touch avoidance. The data were collected from introductory communication classes at 40 large state universities preselected to represent all regions of the United States. Touch was significantly higher at southern universities in the United States than northern ones. For example, the four schools reported the highest levels of opposite sex touch avoidance were (in order): (1) Temple University, (2) University of New Hampshire, (3) University of Wisconsin, Milwaukee, and (4) University of Nebraska, Lincoln, all of which are northern colleges. The four schools with the lowest level of opposite-sex touch avoidance were (in order): (1) University of Utah, (2) San Diego State University, (3) Arizona State University, and (4) University of Georgia, of which three of four are southern colleges.

There are several possible explanations for the decreased tactile contact in the north versus the south: (1) decreased skin sensitivity, (2) neuroendocrine processes and biochemical changes, (3) less outdoor activity and sociability, (4) reduced skin availability, and (5) selective immigration to similar climatic regions.

First, climate may produce changes in the sensitivity of the skin and perhaps the entire human nervous system. Over 250 years ago, Montesquieu (1748/1989) observed that people in warmer climates are much more sensual and conscious of personal sensations, whereas northerners were less sensitive to internal feelings, less passionate, and less tactile. He suggested that in warm countries skin is more relaxed and nerve endings are more responsive to sensation. There is no doubt that cold can numb the skin though no studies could be located that show that this is a habitual reaction to chronic cold. However, research on haptic memory suggests that people will implicitly remember various kinds of haptic sensations and experiences (Kaas, Stoeckel, & Goebel, 2008) though it is unclear if these are habituated over time.

Second, neuroendocrine processes may be associated with the proclivity of southern people to touch more than northerners. Numerous studies have shown that increased sunlight is positively associated with happiness and negatively associated with depression, marital conflict, suicide, and aggression (Thorson & Kasworm, 1984). One possible mechanism for these associations is human neuroendocrine processes. The pineal gland is a neuroendocrine transducer that is light sensitive and regulates melatonin, oxytocin, and other hormones that affect virtually every organ of the body (Andersen et al., 1990; Sampson, 1975). It has long been known that sexual and gonadal functions are deregulated in the presence of sunshine through the pineal gland (Axelrod, 1975; Reiter, 1980; Wurtman, Axelrod, & Kelly, 1968). Depression, social withdrawal, and reduced human contact are characteristic of seasonal affective disorder, a common social and psychological problem in regions with little seasonal light (Rosenthal et al., 1986). In short, increased sunlight in lower latitudes may decrease inhibition and produce increased social interaction, including more interpersonal touch.

Third, sunnier weather may generate more social interaction as weather provides fewer obstacles to travel and communication. Winter weather at high latitude or high altitude does not facilitate outdoor travel to friends and neighbors and certainly limits outdoor social activity. This feature of cold climates was a greater obstacle for our ancestors who typically travelled on foot rather than by train, airplane, or car.

Fourth, considerable research suggests that southerners have fewer environmental and climatic challenges than northerners who are more serious and less affiliative because of the necessity of planning for inclement weather during the winter season. Pennebaker et al. (1996) maintain that in colder climates people spend more time dressing, storing food, and planning for winter, whereas in warmer climates people have more time and social access to one another year around. Northerly people are generally more serious, may be perceived as uptight, and tend to be more instrumental. Andersen et al. (1990) maintained:

> In Northern latitudes societies must be more structured, more ordered, more constrained, and more organized if the individuals are to survive harsh weather forces.... In contrast, Southern

latitudes may attract or produce a culture characterized by social extravagance and flamboyance that has no strong inclination to constrain or order their world. (p. 307)

Hofstede (2001) suggests that latitude leads to a chain of events beginning with the necessity of cultures from cold climates to plan and develop technology to survive in harsh environments. Indeed, Hofstede's extensive studies show that there is 0.68 correlation between latitude and gross national product, suggesting that cultures at higher latitudes may represent a region of the world where serious labor trumps gregarious social interaction. Hofstede's data also show a −0.83 correlation between latitude and population growth, suggesting the reproductive tactile interaction is more prevalent in sunnier climates, though a number of other factors are doubtlessly associated with this relationship.

Fourth, in warmer, sunnier climates more skin is available for tactile interaction. Andersen et al. (1990) claimed that the greater touch avoidance found in northerly regions "may be explained by the fact that southern regions allow less clothing, more skin exposure, and more tactile contact and may produce a more tactually or sexually oriented culture..." (p. 307). The sight of unclothed human skin may produce greater motivation to groom, stroke, or caress another individual. And certainly, the result of affiliative touch would be more gratifying when skin is available, than touch through layers of clothing in a northern winter. Although indoor heating may moderate this relationship, central heat is a luxury confined to highly developed countries. Even in the most affluent countries, indoor heat may be turned down for economic or ecological reasons.

Fifth, people often migrate to regions that resemble their homeland and establish their culture in the new region. For example Spanish and Portuguese immigrants were more likely to migrate to Latin American countries where the weather had greater similarity to their homeland. Likewise, the migration of Germans, Swedes, and Norwegians to the upper Midwest in the United States is an example of immigrants from a cooler climate, selecting a region with familiar, cool weather. The new culture of a region, thus, resembles the culture of the region's ancestors though climate may continue to exert an influence on its residents. As a result, people who had characteristics forged in northern climates maintained those characteristics in their new northerly residences. Similarly, settlement of peoples from sunny, southerly climates was maintained in their new adopted tropical homes.

TACTILE TRADITIONS: INDIVIDUALISM/COLLECTIVISM AND TOUCH

Another major determinant of the degree of touch in a culture is the individualism/collectivism of a culture. Individualism/collectivism is one of the most widely researched dimensions of intercultural behavior (Gudykunst & Lee, 2002; Gudykunst, Yoon, & Nishida, 1987; Hofstede, 2001). The prototypic individualist culture is the United States, though other Northern European-derived cultures such as Great Britain, Australia, New Zealand, Canada, and the Scandinavian countries are similarly individualistic (Hofstede, 2001).

The prototypic collectivist cultures are found in Asia such as Japan, Singapore, Taiwan, and Hong Kong, though many South American countries are similarly collectivistic. Similarly, several studies suggest that Mexican and Mexican-American cultures tend to show collectivistic traits that emphasize group and relational solidarity (Albert & Ah Ha, 2004; Andersen et al., 2002). Few studies exist on South American tactile behavior, and so most of the discussion of individualistic and collectivistic influences on tactile behavior will be based on Asian cultures. However, in his study of touch in Latin America, Shuter (1976) reported that "Columbians have a significantly lower mean contact score than do Costa Ricans or Panamanians...there is a progressive decline in the frequency on contact between interactants as one travels from Central to South America" (p. 50). This finding is consistent with the proposition that collectivistic countries are less tactile; Columbia is the second most collectivistic country in the world according to Hofstede (2001).

Collectivistic cultures emphasize the "we" identity rather than an "I" identity and tend to favor group orientation over individual orientation (Andersen et al., 2002). Also, collectivist cultures tend to think in terms of the whole rather than the individual (Nisbet, Peng, Choi, & Norenzayan, 2001). In collectivistic cultures, individual impulses to touch defer to the collective who may find touch unseemly and impolite, a departure from the shared norms that regulate individual impulses to preserve group harmony.

The most widely researched collectivistic region of the world is Asia. "China and other East Asian societies remain collectivist and oriented toward the group, whereas American and other European-influenced societies are more individualistic in orientation" (Nisbet et al., 2001, p. 395). Asian cultures, which have a highly collectivistic orientation, tend to be the least touch oriented of any of societies on earth, particularly in terms of public touch (Barnland, 1978; Jones, 1994;

McDaniel & Andersen, 1998). In their study of touch during departures from an international airport, McDaniel and Andersen indicate that the largest difference among the world's peoples is between Asians, who rarely touch in public, and virtually every other culture, which all manifest higher degrees of public touching than Asians. Among the citizens of 26 different nations observed by McDaniel and Andersen, the least touch was observed in citizens of the 10 Asian countries observed. Among Asians, consistent with the latitudinal explanation, Northeast Asians displayed the least touch, even less than Southeast Asians who also displayed low levels of public touch.

Why are Asian cultures so high in collectivism and so reticent about the display of public touch? Asia cultures are among the oldest, most homogeneous, and traditional cultures in the world. For centuries, even millennia, Asian societies have developed rules of conduct that have made life more harmonious for people in these cultures and simplified decision making. Multicultural places like the individualistic countries of United States and Australia have dozens of cultural streams and far fewer rules for traditional or harmonious behavior. Confucianism and other Asian philosophical and ethical traditions that emphasize decorum, rectitude, and prescribed social deportment (Joe, 1972) prevent Asians, influenced by these traditions, from engaging in touch, because it may be considered too uncouth and flamboyant for that culture (McDaniel &Andersen, 1998). Likewise, Buddhism with its emphasis on avoidance of unwholesome actions and promotion of positive acts may cause people to avoid touch since it may be perceived as sexual, overly familiar, or intrusively impolite. Some scholars have noted that Confucianism constitutes a virtual state religion, for at various times throughout history, Asian governments have sought to make Confucianism the official state ideology (Adler, 2006; Taylor & Arbuckle, 1995). Such efforts may have further inculcated Confucian values of decorum and decency upon Asian cultures inconsistent with public tactile presentations.

GENDER ORIENTATION: ASSUMPTIONS ABOUT GENDER, SEX, AND TACTILE BEHAVIOR

Abundant research shows that biological sex is a major factor throughout the world in the expression of tactile behavior. Across most societies, women touch other women the most, whereas men touch men the least; men are most avoidant of touch with other men (Andersen &

Leibowitz, 1978; Andersen, Lustig, & Andersen, 1987, 1990; Shuter, 1977). In opposite-sex dyads, men are somewhat more likely to touch women than women are to touch men, but research suggests that this relationship may reverse in marriage where women actually touch more. But how stable are these findings? Do they generalize to all cultures? In fact, these findings vary widely across the world depending on the gender orientation of the country.

Gender orientation is a close relative of biological sex. In most countries, women are more likely to be nurturant and men are more commonly assertive (Hofstede, 2001) even where there has been a conscious attempt to abolish these roles such as in Israeli Kibbutzim. But wide variations in gender roles exist across culture. Cultures differ extensively in their overall gender orientation, a variable called masculinity by Hofstede (2001) and gender by Andersen and associates (Andersen et al., 2002; Andersen & Wang, 2006). In fact, cultures range from highly masculine cultures such as Japan, Austria, Venezuela, Italy, Switzerland, and Mexico to more feminine or androgynous cultures such as Sweden, Norway, the Netherlands, Denmark, Costa Rica, and Yugoslavia, where there is less differentiation between roles of male and female. There are no matriarchal countries in the world, and so the countries identified variously by Hofstede as low in masculinity are actually androgynous since, in these cultures, men and women have many of the same rights and display more similar behavioral traits. Interestingly, it is the men across these cultures that vary the most. In feminine, or what I am calling androgynous cultures, it is the men's behavior that is most different.

Masculinity is a cultural label applied to a society in which social gender roles are clearly distinct: Men are supposed to be assertive, tough, and focused on material success; women are supposed to be modest, tender, and concerned with the quality of life. By contrast, femininity refers to societies in which social gender roles overlap: Both men and women are supposed to be modest, tender, and concerned with the quality of life. In masculine cultures, males tend to have the tactile prerogative, while women defer to or accept male tactile moves and decisions. In feminine cultures, such as Scandinavia, Costa Rica, Chile, and Portugal, male and female roles are much more equal and women can initiate touch nearly as often as men.

In addition, public affection, regardless of sex, is more prominent in feminine countries where comforting and nurturance is a cultural value. In Costa Rica, a feminine culture, Shuter (1976) observed much higher levels of cross-sex touching and embracing than in other countries.

RELIGIOUS INFLUENCES AND THE TACTILE TABOOS

Studies of touch avoidance within the United States' culture show that a person's religiosity is associated with approach or avoidance of tactile contact (Andersen & Leibowitz, 1978; Andersen et al., 1987). Across a number of samples, religion was associated with touch avoidance of both same-sex and opposite-sex interactants. Interestingly, the most touch-avoidant group in the United States was Protestants followed by Catholics, groups characterized by fundamentalist values or prescribed sex roles, respectively. Jewish people displayed less touch avoidance and people with no formal religious affiliation showed the lowest levels of touch avoidance. Similar findings have been reported by Montagu (1978) who suggested that religion, particularly fundamentalist Christian religions, discourage touch. He stated, "Two of the great achievements of Christianity have been to make a sin of tactual pleasures, and by the repression of sex to make it an obsession" (p. 249). Clearly, fundamentalist religions of many types tend to discourage tactile interaction.

Similarly, many Islamic cultures have rigidly proscribed gender roles such that women and men are expressly forbidden to touch one another outside of the marital context. These norms are based on the strongly held Muslim beliefs about purity and the closely followed taboos of Islamic culture (Van Meer, Veldhuis, & Schwerzel, 2008). Aristlotle placed touch among the most cherished and important senses, but by the middle ages, Islam, Christianity, and Judaism began to think of touch as base and animalistic (Jutte, 2008). Religions:

> forged a connection between the approving quotation of Aristotle and various places in the bible, thereby helping to ensure the mental association of touch with sinful behavior (voluptuousness and unrestrained sex drive) became widespread...haptical perceptions became a symbol of eroticism as such, to which poets and painters of not only the early modern age returned to time and time again. (Jutte, 2008, p. 6)

Of course, many scholars have suggested that religion is inherently patriarchal since its founders and leaders were men and its rules were designed for control, particularly of women (Bartkowski, 1997; Brown & Bohn, 1989; Reynaud, 2004). This critique of religion's roots is not difficult to accept. In Christianity, Islam, and Judaism, the sacred texts are written in a masculine voice with generic masculine pronouns, with god as male. Many religions have narrowly proscribed female tactile and sexual behavior and, at its extreme, have condoned genital mutilation of women to prevent tactile sexual sensation, a practice euphamistically referred to "female circumcision" (Boulware-Miller, 1985). It is noteworthy that people that hold strong religious views, particularly fundamentalist religious views, are least likely to touch and most likely to consider touch inappropriate and sinful, a legacy of the aforementioned religious traditions.

The Culture Controversy: A Caveat Regarding Racial and Ethnic Differences

When group differences in any behavior or cognition are observed, scholars are virtually certain to attribute them to culture. But other possibilities exist. Variations in tactile behavior could be due to climatic conditions, urban versus rural differences, geographic variation, the third rail of academic scholarship race. In the post-colonial, post-Nazi, post-apartheid era, scholarly discussions of racial differences are off limits to scholars, at least most of the time. However, no serious medical scholar would deny that Scandinavians are genetically predisposed to skin cancer, or the Ashkenazi Jews carry predispositions for Tay-Sachs, or that African Americans have an enhanced risk for sickle cell anemia. Nor are we in denial about the fact that Zulu or Dutch People are taller than Mong or Pygmies. Any serious track fan would have difficulty disputing that East Africans have a predisposition for long-distance running, usually turning the Boston Marathon into the Kenyan Invitational, or that people of West African heritage do considerably better in sprint events than most of us. However, when it comes to behavior, intelligence, or communicative differences, the conversation stops. This is neither scientifically ethical nor all that politically correct. It is time we had a real discussion about race and genetics, including a conversation about the fact that while all (wo)men are created equal, may be a wonderful political foundation, it is not all that true in terms of human behavior. Is it possible that Africans are genetically expressive or that Finns are biologically reticent? One conundrum of cultural differences is that they may not really be that cultural at all, but genetic relics of our biological heritage. Once we recognize real differences, it will be far easier to refute bogus racial beliefs and to recognize and even remediate genetic disadvantages. We need to have this conversation, however difficult it may be. One thing is for sure: We have no good science that proves that group differences in human behavior and communication are cultural and not genetic.

CONCLUSIONS

Cultures clearly vary in their tactile behavior and attitudes. Although these variations seem to be almost random across the globe, they can be explained, in part, by four fundamental forces. The first is latitude. Throughout the world there is a proclivity for increased touch to occur in regions closer to the equator. This may be due to greater sensitivity of the skin in warmer regions, neuroendocrine processes associated with light and subsequent affiliativeness and libidinousness, increased interpersonal contact among people in warmer latitudes, the greater availability of skin to touch in warmer regions, or voluntary migration of northern people to northern regions. Regardless, climate appears to be a powerful force in promoting more interpersonal warmth and immediacy, in general, and more tactile contact in particular in regions relatively closer to the equator.

The second force governing tactile behavior is collectivism, which is most predominant in Asia. Studies suggest that collectivist and Asian cultures engage in less interpersonal touch than individualistic and non-Asian cultures. This may be due to the maturity and homogeneity of these cultures that have adopted norms of appropriate behavior, including tactile norms across the millennia. It may also be due to the influence of Confucianism and Buddhism, philosophies that emphasize cooperation and the sublimation of individual impulses and behaviors to rules of comportment and decorum. Tactile behavior may be perceived in collectivistic cultures as intrusive, selfish, and immature, whereas in individualistic culture it may be perceived as an appropriate expression of warmth and affiliation.

Third, the gender orientation of a culture impacts tactile behavior. In more feminine cultures, touch is more symmetrical between the sexes and less likely to be the prerogative of men. Moreover, affiliative, friendly, and nurturant touch is more appropriate for both men and women in feminine cultures. In masculine cultures, the tactile behavior of men is more dominant, less affiliative, and not exceptionally nurturing. In feminine cultures, more androgynous patterns of tactile behavior are appropriate which permit men to use more feminine forms of touch in their tactile repertoire. Cultures with fundamentalist religious values tend to have the greatest number of proscriptions on tactile behavior, particularly female tactile behaviors.

Finally, religion has a major effect on tactile behavior. This chapter has summarized research of the rectitude and decorum or Confucian cultures. Likewise, it has been shown that fundamentalist religions of all stripes tend to restrict many forms of tactile behavior, particularly restricting the tactile freedom of women.

Although our understanding of culture patterns of tactile behavior has improved, some final caveats are in order. First, other dimensions of culture doubtlessly explain cultural differences in touch that are beyond the scope of this chapter. Second, in considering cultural differences in interpersonal touch, one should not discount the considerable similarities in tactile behavior that are often less visible background to the more obvious differences that constitute the foreground. Third, we should never discount the possibility of genetic and biological differences among groups that may constitute evolutionary group differences that appear as cultural differences. Finally, we should note that within each culture there are considerable individual differences in tactile behavior owing to innate dispositional factors, childrearing practices, family norms, religious prohibitions, and media models.

Cultural issues highlight the many paradoxes of touch. It is at once the most fundamental, intimate human sense, and the one about which there are substantial cultural, moral, legal, and political issues. Touch is at once intensely personal and one where collective cultural values are most likely to intervene. Indeed, if the world is becoming more homogenized or perhaps more dichotomized into the Islamic and non-Islamic world as Huntington (1993) suggested, it will be interesting to observe cultural trends in tactile behavior across the next centuries. It is up to future investigations to monitor the changing map of tactile behaviors across the cultures of the world.

REFERENCES

Adler, J. A. (2006, November). *Confucianism as religion/religious tradition/neither: Still hazy after all these years.* Paper presented at the annual meeting of the American Academy of Religion, Washington, DC.

Albert, R. D., & Ah Ha, I. (2004). Latino/Anglo-American differences in attributions to situations involving touch and silence. *International Journal of Intercultural Relations, 28,* 353–280.

Almaney, A. J., & Alwan, A. J. (1982). *Communicating with Arabs: A handbook for business executives.* Prospect Heights, IL: Waveland.

Andersen, P. A. (1985). Nonverbal immediacy in interpersonal communication. In A. W. Siegman & S. Feldstein (Eds.), *Multichannel integrations of nonverbal behavior* (pp. 1–36). Hillsdale, NJ: Erlbaum.

Andersen, P. A. (2008). *Nonverbal communication: Forms and functions.* Long Grove, IL: Waveland Press.

Andersen, P. A., & Guerrero, L. K. (1998). The bright side of relational communication. Interpersonal warmth as a social emotion. In P. A. Andersen & L. K. Guerrero (Eds.), *Handbook of communication and emotion* (pp. 305–331). San Diego, CA: Academic Press.

Andersen, P. A., & Guerrero, L. K. (2008). Haptic behavior in social interaction. In M. Grunwald (Ed), *Human haptic perception: Basics and applications* (pp. 155–163). Basel, Switzerland: Birkhauser.

Andersen, P. A., Guerrero, L. K., & Jones, S. M. (2006). Nonverbal intimacy. In V. Manusov & M. L. Patterson (Eds.), *The Sage handbook of nonverbal communication* (pp. 259–277). Thousand Oaks, CA: Sage.

Andersen, P. A., Hecht, M. L., Hoobler, G. D., & Smallwood, M. (2002). Nonverbal communication across cultures. In B. Gudykunst & B. Moody (Eds.), *Handbook of international and intercultural communication* (pp. 89–106). Thousand Oaks, CA: Sage.

Andersen, P. A., & Leibowitz, K. (1978). The development and nature of the construct touch avoidance. *Environmental Psychology and Nonverbal Behavior, 3*, 89–106.

Andersen, P. A., Lustig, M. W., & Andersen, J. F. (1987). Regional patterns of communication in the United States: A theoretical perspective. *Communication Monographs, 54*, 128–144.

Andersen, P. A., Lustig, M. W., & Andersen, J. F. (1990). Changes in latitude, changes in attitude: The relationship between climate and interpersonal communication predispositions. *Communication Quarterly, 38*, 291–311.

Andersen, P. A., & Wang, H. (2006). Unraveling cultural cues: Dimensions of nonverbal communication across cultures. In L. A. Samovar & R. Porter (Eds.), *Intercultural communication: A reader* (11th ed., pp. 250–266). Belmont, CA: Thompson/Wadsworth.

Axelrod, J. (1975). The pineal gland: A model to study the regulation of the B-adrenergic receptor. In D. B. Tower (Ed.), *The basic neurosciences*. New York, NY: Raven Press.

Barnland, D. C. (1978). Communication styles in two cultures: Japan and the United States. In A. Kendon, R. M. Harris, & M. R. Key (Eds.), *Organization of behavior in face to face interaction* (pp. 427–456). The Hague, Switzerland: Mouton.

Bartkowski, J. P. (1997). Debating patriarchy: Discursive dispute over spousal authority among evangelical family commentators. *Journal for the scientific study of religion, 36*, 393–410.

Boulware-Miller, K. (1985). Female circumcision: Challenges to the practice as a human rights violation. *Harvard Women's Rights Journal, 8*, 155–169.

Bowlby, J. (1969). *Attachment*. New York, NY: Basic Books.

Brown, D. E. (1991). *Human universals*. Philadelphia, PA: Temple University Press.

Brown, J. C., & Bohn, C. R. (1989). *Christianity, patriarchy and abuse: A feminist critique*. Cleveland, OH: Pilgrim Press.

Burgoon, J. K., Guerrero, L. K., & Floyd, K. (2010). *Nonverbal communication*. Boston, MA: Allyn & Bacon.

Cohen, R. (1987). Problems of intercultural communication in Egyptian-American diplomatic relations. *International Journal of Intercultural Relations, 11*, 29–47.

Erceau, D., & Guéguen, N. (2007). Tactile contact and the evaluation of the toucher. *Journal of Social Psychology, 147*, 441–444.

Field, T. (1999). American adolescents touch each other less and are more aggressive toward their peers as compared with French adolescents. *Adolescence, 34*, 753–758.

Field, T. (2001). *Touch*. Cambridge, MA: MIT Press.

Floyd, K. (1997). Communicating affection in dyadic relationships: An assessment of behaviors and expectancies. *Communication Quarterly, 45*, 68–80.

Floyd, K. (2000). Affectionate same sex touch: The influence of homophobia on observers' perceptions. *Journal of Social Psychology, 140,* 774–778.

Floyd, K. (2006). *Communicating affection: Interpersonal behavior and social context.* Cambridge, England: Cambridge University Press.

Floyd, K., Mikkleson, A. C., & Hesse, C. (2007). *The biology of human communication.* Florence, KY: Thompson Learning.

Gudykunst, W. B., & Lee, C. M. (2002). Cross-cultural communication theories. In B. Gudykunst & B. Moody (Eds.), *Handbook of international and intercultural communication* (pp. 25–50). Thousand Oaks, CA: Sage.

Gudykunst, W. B., Yoon, W. C., & Nishida, T. (1987). The influence of individual-collectivism on perceptions of communication in ingroup-outgroup relations. *Communication Monographs, 54,* 295–306.

Guerrero, L. K., Andersen, P. A., & Afifi, W. (2007). *Close encounters: Communication in relationships.* Thousand Oaks, CA: Sage.

Guéguen, N. (2002). Kind of touch, gender and compliance with a request. *Studia Psychologia, 44,* 167–172.

Hall, E. T. (1966). *The hidden dimension* (2nd ed.). Garden City, NY: Anchor/Doubleday.

Healthy People. (2010). Maternal, infant and child health. Retrieved from http://www.healthypeople.gov/Document/HTML/volume2/16MICH.html

Hertenstein, M. J., & Campos, J. J. (2001). Emotional regulation via maternal touch. *Infancy, 2,* 549–566.

Hertenstein, M. J., Holmes, R., McCullough, M., & Keltner, D. (2009). The communication of emotion via touch. *Emotion, 9,* 566–573.

Hertenstein, M. J., Keltner, D., App, B., Bulleit, B. A., & Jaskolka, A. R. (2006). Touch communicates distinct emotions. *Emotion, 6,* 528–533.

Hofstede, G. (2001). *Culture's consequences: Comparing values, behaviors, institutions and organizations across nations.* Thousand Oaks, CA: Sage.

Huntington, S. P. (1993). The clash of civilizations. *Foreign Affairs, 72,* 22–49.

Joe, W. J. (1972). *Traditional Korea: A cultural history.* Seoul, Korea: Chung An Press.

Jones, S. E. (1994). *The right touch: Understanding and using the language of physical contact.* Cresshill, NJ: Hampton Press.

Jones, S. E., & Yarbrough, E. (1985). A naturalistic study of the meanings of touch. *Communication Monographs, 52,* 19–56.

Joule, R. V., & Guéguen, N. (2007). Touch compliance and awareness of tactile contact. *Perceptual and Motor Skills, 103,* 581–588.

Jutte, R. (2008). Haptic perception: An historical approach. In M. Grunwald (Ed.), *Human haptic perception: Basics and applications* (pp. 3–13). Basel, Switzerland: Birkhauser.

Kaas, A. L., Stoeckel, M. C., & Goebel, R. (2008). The neural bases of haptic working memory. In M. Grunwald (Ed.). *Human haptic perception: Basics and applications* (pp. 113–129). Basel, Switzerland: Birkhauser.

Levine, S., & Stanton, M. E. (1990). The hormonal consequences of mother–infant contact. In K. Barnard & T. B. Brazelton (Eds.), *Touch: The foundation of experience* (pp. 165–194). Madison, CT: International Universities Press.

McDaniel, E. R., & Andersen, P. A. (1998). Intercultural variations in tactile communication. *Journal of Nonverbal Communication, 22,* 59–75.

Miller, P. M., Commons, M. L., & Gutheil, T. G. (2006). Clinicians' perception of boundaries in Brazil and the United States. *Journal of the American Academy of Psychiatry Law, 34,* 33–42.

Montagu, A. (1978). *Touching: The human significance of the skin* (2nd ed.). New York, NY: Harper & Row.
Montagu, A., & Matson, F. (1979). *The human connection*. New York, NY: McGraw-Hill.
Montesquieu, C. de S (1748/1989). *The spirit of the laws*. Cambridge, MA: Cambridge University Press.
Morhenn, V. B., Park, J. W., Piper, E., & Zak, P. J. (2008). Monetary sacrifice among strangers is mediated by endogenous oxytocin release after physical contact. *Evolution and Human Behavior, 29*, 375–383.
Morris, D. (1971). *Intimate behavior*. New York, NY: Random House.
Muir, D. W. (2002). Adult communication with infants through touch: The forgotten Sense. *Human Development, 45*, 95–99.
Naqib al-Misri, A. I., Keller, N. H. M. (1994). *Reliance of the traveler: A classic manual of Islamic sacred law*. Beltsville, MD: Amana Publications.
Nisbett, R. E., Peng, K., Choi, I., & Nerenzayan, A. (2001). Culture and systems of thought: Holistic versus analytic cognition. *Psychological Review, 108*, 291–310.
Patterson, M. L. (1983). *Nonverbal behavior: A functional perspective*. New York, NY: Springer Verlag.
Pennebaker, J. W., Rime, B., & Blankenship, V. E. (1996). Stereotypes of emotional expressiveness in Northerners and Southerners: A cross-cultural test of Montesquieu's Hypothesis. *Journal of Personality and Social Psychology, 70*, 372–380.
Prager, K. (1995). *The psychology of intimacy*. New York, NY: Guilford Press.
Reite, M. (1990). Touch, attachment, and health: Is there a relationship. In K. E. Barnard & T. B. Brazelton (Eds.), *Touch: The foundation of experience* (pp. 195–225). Madison, CT: International Universities Press.
Reiter, R. J. (1980). The pineal gland: A regulator of regulators. In J. M. Sprauge & A. N. Epstein (Eds.), *Progress in psychobiology and physiological psychology* (Vol. 9, pp. 323–356). New York, NY: Academic Press.
Remland, M., Jones, T. S., & Brinkman, H. (1991). Proxemic and haptic behavior in three European countries. *Journal of Nonverbal Behavior, 15*, 215–232.
Reynaud, E. (2004). Holy virility: The social construction of masculinity. In P. F. Murphy (Ed.), *Feminism and masculinities* (pp 136–150). Oxford, England: Oxford University Press.
Rosenthal, N. E., Carpenter, C. L., James, S. P., Parry, B. L., Rogers, S. L., & Wehr, T. A. (1986). Seasonal affective disorder in children and adolescents. *American Journal of Psychiatry, 143*, 356–358.
Sampson, P. H. (1975). Behavior and pineal functioning. In M. D. Altschule (Ed.), *Frontiers of pineal physiology* (pp. 204–222). Cambridge, MA: MIT Press.
Scheflen, A. E. (1974). *How behavior means*. Garden City, NY: Anchor.
Segrin, C. (1993). The effects of nonverbal behavior on outcomes of compliance-gaining attempts. *Communication Studies, 44*, 169–187.
Shuter, R. (1976). Proxemics and tactility in Latin America. *Journal of Communication, 26*, 46–52.
Shuter, R. (1977). A field study of nonverbal communication in Germany, Italy and the United States. *Communication Monographs, 4*, 298–305.
Sussman, N. M., & Rosenfeld, H. M. (1982). Influence of culture, language, and sex on conversational distance. *Journal of Personality and Social Psychology, 42*, 66–74.

Taylor, R., & Arbuckle, G. (1995). Confucianism. *Journal of Asian Studies, 54,* 387–394.
Thayer, S. (1986). History and strategies of research on social touch. *Journal of Nonverbal Behavior, 10,* 12–28.
Thorson, J. A., & Kasworm, C. (1984). Sunshine and suicide: Possible influences of climate on behavior. *Death Education, 8,* 125–136.
Vaidis, D. C. F., & Halimi-Falkowicz, S. G. M. (2008). Increases in compliance with a request: Two touches are more effective than one. *Psychological Reports, 103,* 88–92.
Van Meer, J. P., Veldhuis, G. J., & Schwerzel, J. (2008, April). *Bridging the culture gap: A cultural framework as a basis for cultural training.* Paper presented at the RTO Human Factors and Medicine Panel (HFM) Symposium held in Copenhagen, Denmark.
Wurtman, R. J., Axelrod, J., & Kelly, D. E. (1968). *The pineal.* New York, NY: Academic Press.

V

The Relevance of Touch for Development and Health

15

Maternal Touch and the Developing Infant

RUTH FELDMAN

Touch is the most basic mammalian maternal behavior. As soon as an infant is born, mammalian mothers begin to engage in the species-typical repertoire of maternal behavior, and these postpartum behaviors consist primarily of close physical proximity and the provision of maternal touch. Being such a widespread mammalian behavior, early maternal touch must carry important implications for survival and adaptation and contribute to the growth and development of the young. Moreover, this postpartum maternal repertoire must be supported by a unique neurobiological system of parenting that includes the functioning of specific genetic markers, brain circuitry, hormonal expression, autonomic response, and the epigenetic programming of stress and affiliation genes. Maternal touch patterns are among the most evolutionarily conserved behaviors and, as such, there is marked consistency in the genetic, neuroendocrine, and brain circuitry between humans and other mammals. Of particular interest is the feedback loop that begins with maternal touch and contact; continues with the effects of contact on organizing the infant's physiology and behavior and establishing attachment-related cues; and culminates in the effects of these organized infant social and exploratory behaviors on sensitizing maternal and infant's bonding-related physiology [e.g., the oxytocin (OT) response], thereby forming the unique mother–infant bond (Feldman, 2011). Such consistency in the role of maternal touch between humans and other mammals renders research in animal models particularly useful for understanding the biological underpinnings of early touch and contact and their effect on shaping the infant's capacity for social affiliation and stress modulation throughout life.

Not only are maternal touch and contact central to our evolutionarily based biology, maternal-infant physical closeness and the mother's affectionate touch are central components of the human cultural heritage. Throughout human history and across cultural communities, images of maternal-infant physical proximity—in sculptures, drawings, carvings, and ink paints—are deeply rooted in our collective unconscious and serve as the primary symbol for the human capacity to love. Maternal touch, therefore, is not just one more thing mothers do: It is the basic channel for the expression of parenting and serves as the bedrock of the individual's future capacity to provide love and nourishment to future attachment relationships. Attachment relationships, in turn—at least according to some perspectives—provide the motivating force that guides human development and defines the apex of the human condition (Bowlby, 1969; Feldman, 2011; Winnicott, 1956).

This chapter presents research conducted at our lab for over a decade on two important areas of maternal touch: its role as a central component in the repertoire of maternal behavior and the impact of an intervention called "Kangaroo Care (KC)" or skin-to-skin contact. In the first section, studies that address the expression of early touch and contact by human mothers, the biological substrates of touch in parenting behavior, and the contribution of early touch and contact to infant development across childhood and into adolescence will be discussed. In the second section, results from a longitudinal follow-up of premature infants who received the KC intervention will be presented, including the impact of KC on the preterm infant's self-regulatory competencies, neuromaturation, and physiological regulation, as well as on maternal outcomes and the parent–child relationship.

Overall, our empirical studies in humans follow two lines of research in animal models. The first is the elegant empirical program of Hofer and colleagues (1995), which demonstrated, in over 40 years of systematic research, that the mother's proximity and physical presence contain a set of biobehavioral provisions, such as maternal body heat, nursing, smell, or tactile contact—and that each provision regulates a specific physiological system in the pup, including the biological clock, heart rhythms, thermoregulation, or attention and exploration. By careful separation and systematic manipulation of each component of the maternal presence, the researchers were able to chart direct links between specific maternal provisions and the infant's biobehavioral maturation. This conceptual frame guided our research on the KC intervention and its sequelae. Premature birth and the ensuing separation between mother and child was conceptualized as a "natural experiment" for the effects of maternal bodily contact on infant development during a period of early and persistent maternal absence. Our intervention was based on the assumption that the provision of maternal proximity during this period of early and persistent deprivation would contribute to the maturation of the infant's physiological support systems that provide the basis for higher-order functions, such as exploration, attention, socialization, and behavior control. We expected similar effects following the KC intervention as those observed in other mammals following handling during periods of deprivation.

The second influence on our research on the effects of maternal touch as a more active and ubiquitous component of the maternal postpartum repertoire is the empirical work of Meaney and colleagues (Champagne, 2008; Meaney, 2001). In a series of creative and seminal studies, these researches showed that "licking and grooming," the typical touch behavior of parturient rat mothers, was transmitted from mother to daughter through mechanisms of social experience rather than through genetics and that crossfostering studies showed that higher licking and grooming was associated with higher OT receptor densities in brain areas central for the expression of parenting, including the paraventricular nucleus of the hypothalamus, the lateral septum, and the bed nucleus of the stria terminalis. Finally, these studies demonstrate that early maternal licking-and-grooming behaviors shape the infant's stress management systems through epigenetic influences and that the adult's capacity to handle stress is formed early in life through such patterns of maternal touch. Adapted to human research, these studies suggest that the human infant's susceptibility to stress and ultimate skill at regulating aversive life circumstances may have their roots in the mother's early tactile contact. Overall, this perspective underscores the role of early experience—particularly as related to touch and contact—in shaping the neurobiological system that supports the human capacity for social affiliation.

Finally, it is important to note that, although both continuous maternal proximity and active forms of touch are central components of the mother's early repertoire that provide essential environmental inputs for physiological and behavioral regulation, there are wide differences between cultures in patterns of parental touch. As will be discussed below, some cultures promote more ongoing physical contact between mother and infant whereas others engage more in active forms of touch. Such differences reflect wide cultural variations in the philosophical meaning systems that shape parenting, in the cultural perceptions on the nature of the self and its relation to the social world, and in the degree of separation between mother and child each culture considers acceptable during the first months of life (Feldman & Masalha, 2010; Tronick, 1995).

TOUCH AS A CENTRAL COMPONENT OF THE MATERNAL REPERTOIRE

Early Maternal Touch and Its Contribution to Infant Development

Immediately after the birth of a human infant, mothers begin to engage in typical maternal behaviors which in our species include holding the infant in a cradling position, gazing at the infant's face and body, expressing positive affect, emitting "motherese" (high-pitched vocalizations), and providing affectionate touch. The combination of these behaviors can be described as the "maternal postpartum repertoire" (Feldman, 2011). Affectionate touch, the human analogue to the "licking-and-grooming" behaviors of rat mothers, is the most prevalent active behavior in the maternal constellation, apart from social gaze at the infant's face and body, which provides the framework for social relatedness. These two behaviors—social gaze and affectionate touch—often co-occur and establish the basis for interpersonal mutuality between mother and infant in the first days after birth. Mothers use the maternal behavior constellation in general, and affectionate touch in particular, in concordance with the infant's social signals and adapt the provision of maternal behavior to the newborn's scant moments of attention. We found that during social interactions, newborns maintain social gaze for ~10% of the time, yet mothers provide nearly 70% of their maternal behavior during these moments of infant alertness. Such contingency provides infants their first experience of coordination between their own state and the responsive behavior of the social environment (Feldman & Eidelman, 2007). Further, the provision of maternal postpartum behavior and affectionate touch forms the basis for the development of a synchronous relationship between mother and child. The amount of maternal postpartum behaviors shaped the degree of mother–infant synchrony and level of maternal affectionate touch at 3 months. The mother's postpartum behavior also predicted the level of father–infant synchrony and paternal touch, pointing to the importance of early touch in setting the framework for the infant's engagement in multiple attachment relationships across infancy (Feldman & Eidelman, 2007).

Touch in the early neonatal period contributes to the infant's neurobehavioral, cognitive, and social–emotional growth. For instance, we found that the provision of breast milk in premature infants was associated with an increase in maternal postpartum behavior in general and was especially conducive for increasing maternal affectionate touch, which is generally low among mothers of premature infants. Infants who received more breast milk showed higher neurobehavioral maturation on the Neonatal Behavior Assessment Scale (Brazelton, 1973) and showed better cognitive development at 6 months. The effects of breast milk on development was thought to stem from two sources—a direct path that involves the effects of the specific proteins, enzymes, micronutrients, lipids, and long-chain polyunsaturated fatty acids included in breast milk which are critical for the growth and development of premature infants (Heird, 2001) and the indirect effect of increasing maternal affectionate contact, which in turn contributes to more optimal outcomes. Each of these paths was found to be uniquely predictive of cognitive development across infancy (Feldman & Eidelman, 2003b). Similarly, following infants at multiple time points across the first year, it was found that more maternal postpartum behavior, including affectionate touch, set the trajectory of maternal behavior on a more optimal path, and mothers who provided more postpartum touch were more sensitive and reciprocal at 3, 6, and 12 months. Using structural analysis, the latent factor of maternal sensitivity, measured from birth to 1 year, was found to predict better cognitive development and more complex symbolic play (Feldman, Eidelman, & Rotenberg, 2004).

At around 3 months of age, infants begin to engage in synchronous face-to-face interactions with their parents and such exchanges involve the coordination of nonverbal social signals in the different modalities, including gaze, touch, affective expression, and vocalizations. Touch synchrony—the coordination of the parent's affectionate touch with the parent and child's social gaze—becomes an important component of early interactions by which touch is integrated into the parent–infant mutually responsive system (Feldman, 2007). The experience of touch synchrony and missynchrony—moments in which mother provides stimulatory touch while the infant gaze averts and signals a need to rest—are related to physiological support systems that index the stress response, such as cortisol and respiratory sinus arrhythmia (RSA; Feldman, Singer, & Zagoory, 2010), and contribute to the development of brain circuits that support the development of social engagement (Johnson et al., 2005). Indeed, touch synchrony at 3 months with both mother and father was related to behavior adaptation at 2 years as assessed by lower externalizing and internalizing symptoms (Feldman & Eidelman, 2004), possibly because the integration of affectionate contact into the synchronous exchange helps orient the infant to the social world and its rules of conduct. Finally, touch synchrony between mother and infant at 3 months was found to predict the child's level of empathy at 5 years, as measured by the child's empathic understanding of the other's perspective during conflict discussion with the mother, empathic responding to a "painful" expression of the experimenter, and prosocial solutions to moral dilemmas that involve assistance to another person at a cost for the self. It is thus possible that the integration of affectionate touch into a mutually responsive early social system helps regulate the child and, further, that personal social signals become interwoven into a meaningful interpersonal experience that prepares the child for responsible engagement in the social world.

During the first year of life, maternal touch patterns undergo significant development. In a study that followed patterns of maternal touch at 3, 6, 9, and 12 months, infants were videotaped in caregiving and play sessions. Caregiving sessions were microcoded for nine patterns of maternal touch that were aggregated into three constructs—affectionate touch, stimulatory touch, and instrumental touch—while play sessions were coded for maternal sensitivity and dyadic reciprocity. Both maternal affectionate and stimulatory touch decreased markedly after the first 6 months of life, hand in hand with the significant increase in dyadic reciprocity (Ferber, Feldman, & Makhoul, 2008). Possibly, the affectionate touch patterns that define the maternal postpartum repertoire play a significant role as central components of the maternal style during the first 6 months of parenting. After that stage, with the development of infant mobility, intentionality, shared attention, and intersubjectivity, other forms of mutuality gradually take central stage and affectionate contact, although remaining an important component of close relationships throughout life, may no longer be the most prevalent maternal behavior.

Finally, maternal affectionate touch is one among several codes that compose the Mother Sensitivity construct in our global coding system for the analysis of parent–child interactions (Coding Interactive Behavior, or CIB; Feldman, 1998). Conceptually, this inclusion suggests that affectionate touch is one among several components that shape the maternal sensitive style, which serves as the cornerstone of infant social–emotional growth (Bowlby, 1969), but also that it does not stand alone. The specific components of the sensitive style undergo developmental changes, but its suitability and adaptiveness to the child's needs and signals remain. Mother sensitivity measured in the first 6 months, including affectionate touch, was found to predict cognitive development from 6 months to 5 years (Feldman & Eidelman, 2009), social competence with peers in kindergarten (Feldman & Masalha, 2010), lower behavior problems in the preschool years (Feldman & Masalha, 2007), better emotional adjustment in adolescence, and lower depression in adolescence (Feldman, 2010). Maternal sensitivity is also an individually stable construct and mothers who were sensitive at 3 months continued to be the same in adolescence (Feldman, 2010), indicating that early affectionate touch is integrated into the mother's stable and predictable style that supports growth throughout childhood and adolescence.

Variability in Parent–Infant Touch Patterns

Differences between maternal and paternal touch. Although both mothers and fathers provide affectionate touch to their infants and, by 3 months of age, engage in touch synchrony, there are differences in the typical patterns of maternal and paternal touch in both humans and biparental mammals. While mammalian mothers in species such as rats, lambs, and primates engage in grooming and contact forms of touch, fathers in biparental species provide stimulatory contact, tend to carry the infants in space, and encourage exploratory behavior (Mastripieri, Hoffman, Anderson, Carter, & Higley, 2009; Ziegler, 2000). Human fathers tend to engage in rough-and-tumble play, manipulate the infant's extremities, throw the infant in space, and encourage exploration (Lamb, 1977). Similarly, synchronous interactions between mothers and fathers differ in their temporal pattern. Mother–child interactions typically contain face-to-face exchanges between mother and child, involve rhythmic oscillations between low and medium arousal, and contain one peak of high positive arousal that is framed by a social gaze (Feldman, 2003). Father–child interactions, on the other hand, are quick; include several high peaks of positive arousal that appear at random, such as when father throws the child in air or plays with the child's extremities in a highly arousing manner; and focus on exploring the environment rather than the partner's face (Feldman, 2003). It is possible that infants need to experience interactions that are rhythmic, social, and predictable as well as those that are quick, unpredictable, and oriented to the outside world for optimal social–emotional growth. As will be discussed later, these maternal and paternal touch patterns are differentially related to the oxytocinergic system that supports bond formation in humans and mammals.

Dyadic and triadic touch. Triadic family interactions provide infants their first opportunity to engage in a multiperson social system and predict the development of children's social competence in the peer group (Feldman & Masalha, 2010). In a study of mothers, fathers, and their first-born child at 4 months, we examined synchrony in triadic social behavior at the microlevel. We found that infants spent the same amount of time playing with mothers and fathers during family sessions and that mothers and fathers provided similar amounts of social behavior, including affectionate touch.

Cultural variability. Cultures vary widely in patterns of maternal touch and contact. In more traditional societies, mothers maintain full bodily contact for a major portion of the day and cosleep with the infant at night throughout the first months or even years of life (LeVine, 2002). Such continuous contact serves a soothing function and reduces infant distress. It also emphasizes the inseparability of mother and child and represents an underlying interdependent orientation that stresses the connectedness between members of the cultural group. In more individualistic societies, on the other hand, mothers engage in more active forms of touch and do not maintain continuous contact, reflecting an independent orientation to childrearing and the self (Markus & Kitayama, 1991).

Observing family interactions among Israeli and Palestinian parents and their 5-month-old firstborn child in their home ecology, we found that Palestinian families positioned themselves in a way that continuous contact was maintained between both parents and the infant, and among the spouses, but that this position did not allow for face-to-face interactions or the expression of active touch, mutual gazing, or covocalizations. The continuous contact indeed reduced the infant's negative emotionality, and Palestinian infants fussed and cried significantly less than Israeli infants. On the other hand, Israeli couples sat in a position that enabled face-to-face interactions between each member of the triad and provided more affectionate touch. Infants reached higher levels of both positive and negative arousal, as active forms of touch are physiologically more stimulating than passive contact. These patterns reflect a more independent cultural orientation, one that emphasizes autonomy and social relationship between separate individuals who coordinate their behavior with each other (Feldman, Masalha, & Alony, 2006; Feldman, Masalha, & Nadam, 2001). Deep-rooted cultural philosophies on the nature of the self and its developmental goals may be transmitted from parents to children in the first months of life during their first social encounters, being expressed primarily through variations in patterns of parental touch and contact.

Biological Correlates of Maternal Touch: Hormonal, Autonomic, and Brain Systems

Neuroendocrine pathways: OT, cortisol, and prolactin. Animal studies have implicated the neuropeptide OT in the process of bond formation in a range of mammalian species, yet its role in human attachment has received less attention (Carter & Keverne, 2002; Insel & Young, 2001). In mammals, maternal touch has been closely linked with the expression of OT both centrally (in the brain) and peripherally, and our recent research points to the involvement of early parental touch in the expression of OT in humans. In a longitudinal study assessing OT across pregnancy and the postpartum, we assessed plasma OT from women at three time points: first trimester, last trimester, and first postpartum month. OT levels were highly stable among individuals and showed no mean-level change, and OT at the first trimester predicted the amount of maternal postpartum behavior, including gaze at infant face, positive affect, "motherese" vocalization, and affectionate touch. These data suggest a "priming" effect for OT across pregnancy for the emergence of the species-specific maternal repertoire in human mothers, similar to its role in other mammals (Feldman, Weller, Zagoory-Sharon, & Levine, 2007). Cortisol was also assayed from the maternal blood at early pregnancy, later pregnancy, and the postpartum. In contrast to OT, higher cortisol levels among mothers were related to the amount of maternal instrumental–functional touch they used (i.e., performing a task such as wiping the child's mouth or picking the infant up from a chair) rather than on touch that expressed love and affection. This finding points to an association between higher levels of stress in mothers and lower levels of the growth-promoting affectionate touch style. In a second study on OT and bond formation in mothers and fathers, 160 new parents (80 couples) were seen twice, in the first postpartum month and again at 6 months after the birth of the first child. At both time points, parents' plasma OT was assayed. Parents also were videotaped interacting with their infants in various contexts and were interviewed regarding their attachment to the infant. Contrary to our expectations, fathers and mothers had comparable levels of OT at both time points and baseline levels of OT were highly individually stable in both mothers and fathers. Most interestingly, husband and wife's OT levels were inter-related, suggesting a mutual influence of neuroendorcine pathways, or "endocrine fit," between partners. OT levels in the first postpartum weeks were related to the parent-specific behavioral repertoire. While maternal OT was related to the mother's affectionate contact, paternal OT correlated with stimulatory contact and father's encouragement of exploration, suggesting that the parent-typical behavioral repertoire is linked in some way to OT expression (Gordon, Zagoory-Sharon, Leckman, & Feldman, 2010a).

In a recent study, we examined whether the OT response in human parents is consistent with those observed in mammals. One hundred and twelve mothers and fathers engaged in a 15-minute play-and-contact session with their infants; OT was assessed before and after play. Similar to the findings from Meaney and colleagues (Francis, Champagne, & Meaney, 2000), which showed that natural variations in maternal licking and grooming were related to systematic differences in brain OT, we found that OT increased after the play interaction among mothers who provided a high level of affectionate touch (more than 67% of the time) but did not increase among mothers who provided a low level of affectionate touch. Among fathers, OT increased in those who provided high levels of stimulatory contact but not in those who provided minimal contact, similar to the findings for biparental fathers (Feldman, Gordon, et al., 2010). Thus, the parent-typical forms of touch—affectionate in mothers and stimulatory in fathers—seem to be associated with both baseline OT and with OT release following parent–infant contact.

Two additional studies highlight the associations between OT and parental touch. In the first, salivary OT was sampled from parents (mothers and fathers) and their 6-month-old infants before and after a session of parent–infant interaction. Results are the first to demonstrate not only measurable and consistent OT levels in infants, but a crossgeneration transmission of the OT response between human parents and their infants. Parent and infant's OT were correlated at both the pre- and post-interaction assessment and when parent–child interaction was characterized by a higher level of synchrony, including the integration of parental affectionate touch matched with parent and child's social gaze and a greater increase in both parent and child's OT was observed after the interaction (Feldman, Gordon, & Zagoory-Sharon, 2010).

Finally, we assessed the relation between maternal and paternal plasma OT and touch during triadic family interactions among parents and their 6-month-old firstborn child. Higher triadic synchrony, defined as moments of coordination between physical proximity and affectionate touch between the parents as well as between parent and infant while both parent and child are synchronizing their social gaze, was predicted by both maternal and paternal OT. Among mothers, triadic synchrony was also independently related to lower levels of CT. Results highlight the role of OT in the early formation of the family unit at the transition to parenthood. These findings further demonstrate the importance of the oxytocinergic system and touch among family members for the formation of the family unit during the transition to parenthood (Gordon, Zagoory-Sharon, Leckman, & Feldman, 2010b).

The effect of maternal touch on the infant's stress response during simulated maternal deprivation was assessed among two groups of mothers and their 6-month-old infants. In the first group, infants were assessed in the typical still-face paradigm, in which mother and infant interact for 3 minutes, mother then maintains a still-face for 2 minutes, and mother and infant finally resume play for 2 minutes. Cortisol was measured at baseline, reactivity, and recovery. In the second group, mothers maintained tactile contact during the still-face episode of the procedure. When maternal unavailability during the still-face episode was accompanied by maternal touch, infants showed a more attenuated stress response and returned to baseline levels more rapidly, while the stress response in the still-face-without-touch group was significantly higher and cortisol further increased, rather than decreased, at recovery. Thus, maternal touch appears to contribute to two elements that are considered central to resilience in mammals: attenuating the magnitude of the stress response and enabling a quick recovery to baseline states following stress (Feldman, Singer, & Zagoory, 2010). Similar findings for cortisol and stress emerged in a 10-year follow-up of the KC intervention and will be briefly described later. Other hormones involved in mediating rewards in humans and mammals, such as opioids, as well as hormones associated with hormones related to parenting are related to parental touch. Recently, we found correlations between OT and prolactin in new fathers and correlations between prolactin and the father's encouragement of toy exploration during interaction with the infant (Gordon, Zagoory-Sharon, Leckman, & Feldman, 2010c). Similarly, hormones associated with the regulation of hunger and satiety, such as cholecystokinin (CCK), have also been associated with touch and contact in mammals (Weller & Feldman, 2003). In a recent study, we found associations between parental OT and CCK in a sample of new parents, suggesting that the formation of the parent–infant bond involves inputs from reward pathways and brainstem-mediated homeostatic systems that combine to create the selective and enduring parent–infant bond (Feldman, 2011).

Autonomic response: RSA and the vagal brake. RSA, or cardiac vagal tone, measures the respiratory component in heart-rate variability and is thought to index the regulatory influences of the parasympathetic nervous system on the behaving organism and to provide a biomarker of the individual's emotion regulatory skills. Higher baseline vagal tone has been associated with better regulatory capacities and more optimal social engagement (Porges, 2003). The vagal brake—the degree of change in vagal tone in response to stressful situations—indicates the degree of stress the system experiences and the capacity of the system to mobilize sufficient energies to respond to environmental challenges.

Maternal postpartum affectionate touch, affect synchrony at 3 months, and affectionate touch at 3 months among mothers and fathers were predicted by the infant's baseline vagal tone in the neonatal period (Feldman & Eidelman, 2007). These findings indicate that the infant's biological dispositions toward social engagement and emotion regulation play a role in eliciting the parental response, particularly touch patterns. Similarly, the development of vagal tone throughout the gestational period in premature infants was related to the degree of mother–infant synchrony at 3 months (Feldman, 2006).

In the aforementioned study of simulated maternal deprivation—that is, using the still-face with and without touch—infant vagal tone was measured during baseline, reactivity and recovery. Similar to the findings for cortisol, maternal touch during the still-face episode decreased the magnitude of the change in vagal tone and the autonomic response returned quickly to baseline. This finding points to the multidimensional effects of maternal touch on attenuating the infant's stress response during moments of maternal unavailability (Feldman, Singer, et al., 2010).

Brain circuitry for parenting and touch: Functional magnetic resonance imaging studies. Animal studies and the emerging functional magnetic resonance imaging (fMRI) literature in humans have identified key brain areas that are central for parenting which include the hypothalamus, thalamus, anterior cingulate cortex, septal region, midbrain, and medial preoptic area—regions identified on the basis of knockout models and lesion studies in rodents (Swain, Lorberbaum, Kose, & Strathearn, 2007). Research from our group assessing the brain response of parents to infant stimuli, particularly pictures and cries, has validated these areas as central to the neurobiology of human attachment (Swain et al., 2004a, 2004b; Swain, Leckman, et al., 2007).

Two recent studies highlighted maternal touch in relation to these key parenting brain areas. The first assessed the effects of breastfeeding, associated with increased physical contact and affectionate touch, on brain activations and maternal sensitivity. Two groups of breastfeeding and formula-feeding mothers were scanned during the first postpartum month and again at 3–4 months postpartum, and mother–infant interactions were videotaped. Breastfeeding mothers showed greater activations in response to their infants' cries, including the bilateral thalamus, periaqueductal gray, globus pallidus, putamen, caudate, right amygdala, left anterior cingulate gyrus, and prefrontal cortex. Greater activations in these areas, in turn, predicted higher maternal sensitivity at 3 months, suggesting a link between breastfeeding, maternal contact, and the reorganization of the maternal brain in preparation for motherhood (Kim, Feldman, Leckman, Mayes, & Swain, 2011).

Similar findings emerged from a very recent study in which mothers observed themselves interacting with their infant while functional connectivity analysis assessed the mother's brain response during moments of affectionate touch. In response to their own affectionate touch of the infant, mothers of 4- to 6-month-old infants showed the expected activations in primary and secondary somatosensory cortices and in premotor and motor cortices. However, activations in the parenting network were detected *specifically during moments of affectionate touch*; activated areas included the left and right globus pallidus, putamen, posterior cingulate cortex, left and right insula, uncus, parahippocampal gyrus, and the right amygdale. Similar to the findings for infant stimuli, the prefrontal cortex also showed higher activations when mothers observed interactions that included affectionate touch between themselves and their infants (Atzil, Hendler, & Feldman, 2010).These new data suggest that the specific maternal brain circuitry responds as a cluster to the most primary mammalian maternal behavior—the provision of the species-specific form of touch.

Maternal Touch and Developmental Psychopathology

The most prevalent breeches in maternal-infant bonding are premature birth and maternal postpartum depression (PPD), each of which occurs in about 10–15% of the population in industrial societies (March of Dimes, 2006; Serretti, Olgiati, & Colombo, 2006). In both conditions, mothers have difficulty touching or making contact with their infants.

Premature birth. Prematurity involves disruption to the physical contact between mother and child during the child's postnatal hospitalization. This break in contact typically results in lower levels of maternal affectionate touch—and at times in increases in maternal instrumental, functional, and intrusive touch—even even after physical contact is resumed (Feldman, 2004). Aforementioned studies highlight the centrality of maternal touch for the infant's optimal growth. Reduced maternal touch, particularly in combination with the preterm infant's already compromised physiology, may place these infants at marked developmental risk (Weiss, 2005; Weiss, Wilson, & Morrison, 2004).

Several studies in our lab addressed touch patterns between parents and their premature infants. Both in the neonatal period and at 3 months of age, mothers and fathers of premature infants provided less affectionate touch to their infants than parents of full-term infants (Feldman & Eidelman, 2007). However, mothers of preterms varied in their ability to engage in affectionate touch. For instance, mothers who resolved the trauma of premature birth (i.e., were able to discuss the experience with openness, coherence, and richness; to utilize the assistance of the nursing staff during the hospitalization period; and to form specific plans for themselves and the infants after discharge) displayed more affectionate touch during interactions with their infants prior to discharge. Their infants, moreover, were more socially alert and less withdrawn (Keren, Feldman, Eidelman, Sirota, & Lester, 2003). Other research has shown that factors such as the parents' own adverse tactile experience as children and their satisfaction with the touch they experience as adults can influence the frequency with which they touch their preterm infant and the amount of affectionate touch they use (Weiss & Goebel, 2003). A mother's use of affectionate touch has been found to increase security of attachment among preterm infants and reduce their likelihood of developing emotional and behavioral problems as toddlers (Weiss, Wilson, Hertenstein, & Campos, 2000; Weiss, Wilson, St. Jonn Seed, & Paul, 2001).

Touch interventions for premature infants, in particular massage therapy, have been shown to improve the infant's state regulation and neuromaturation, reduce hospital stay, and accelerate motor development (Field, 1995). In a randomized control study of preterm massage, three groups were included: infants massaged by their mothers, infants massaged by trained nurses, and controls matched for demographic and medical conditions. While both massage groups showed a quicker weight gain (Ferber et al., 2002), mothers who massaged their own infants were more sensitive and provided more affectionate touch, and their infants showed higher social engagement during interactions at 3 months (Ferber et al., 2005).

Maternal PPD. Although PPD does not preclude maternal-infant physical contact, depressed mothers appear to avoid physical proximity and provide minimal levels of affectionate touch. In every sample we have observed—that is, in newborns, infants, toddlers, preschoolers, school-aged children, and adolescents of various cultures, backgrounds, and risk conditions—maternal depressive symptoms were negatively related with the amount of affectionate touch mothers used during infancy; depressed mothers often did not sit within the child's proximity and at later ages stayed outside the child's reach. In terms of the neuroendocrine basis of bonding, mothers with high depressive symptoms showed lower OT levels both at the first trimester of pregnancy and in the postpartum, suggesting that physiological support systems that prepare mothers for the expression of maternal behavior may be disrupted in PPD (Feldman, Weller, et al., 2007). Assessing maternal brain activations, mothers who reported high depressive symptoms and low care from their own mothers during childhood showed reduced activation on fMRI in key parenting brain areas, findings which point to the crossgeneration transmission of maladaptive parenting and its effects on the neurobiology of parenting (Kim et al., 2010).

In a longitudinal study of maternal PPD, a community cohort of more than 2,000 women was recruited in the second postpartum day to complete measures of depression and anxiety. Of these women, those who were consistently depressed across the first year and were diagnosed as suffering from a major depressive disorder when the infant was 9 months old were compared with women who were diagnosed with anxiety disorders and with matched controls. Of the three groups, depressed mothers showed the lowest levels of sensitivity and lower levels of touch synchrony than other groups; their infants, in turn, showed high cortisol reactivity to stress (Feldman et al., 2009). These findings accord with animal literature which suggests that maternal contact, handling, and touch shape the infant's stress management systems throughout life (Weller & Feldman, 2003). Follow-up of this cohort at 5 years of age currently shows that depressed mothers have lower levels of OT and their husbands—consistent with the "endocrine fit" hypothesis between cohabitating couples—similarly had lower OT levels as compared to control mothers and fathers. During interactions with their infant, depressed mothers showed less warmth, affectionate touch, and reciprocal interactions; they also preferred to sit out of the child's reach, highlighting specific difficulties in the domain of physical intimacy among depressed mothers. Children of clinically depressed mothers at 5 years, in turn, demonstrated higher levels of behavior problems, lower neurocognitive skills, and diminished capacity for empathy.

Our work suggests that infants of depressed mothers tend to show highly withdrawn behavior, presenting similar difficulties with physical proximity and touch as those shown by their mothers. Such withdrawal could be an early risk indicator for the development of depression in children and for potential touch aversion. In a study assessing withdrawal behavior in infants referred to a community-based mental health clinic, it was found that referred infants received higher withdrawal scores than nonreferred infants matched for demographic conditions and that maternal depressive symptoms, combined with reduced maternal sensitivity and reciprocity, predicted a clinical diagnosis on the infant withdrawal scale (Dollberg, Feldman, Keren, & Gudeney, 2006). Such findings point to the links between an infant's tendency to avoid touch and the risk for future psychopathology.

Feeding disorders and failure to thrive. The associations between maternal deprivation and children's growth restriction and nonorganic failure to thrive have been proposed since the early work of Spitz (1946) with World War II orphans. We examined the specific links between touch patterns and feeding problems among three groups of 9- to 34-month-old infants: children diagnosed with feeding disorders, children diagnosed with other primary disorders, and case-matched controls. Patterns of maternal and child touch and physical proximity were microcoded. Mothers of children with feeding disorders provided lower levels of touch in all categories, including affectionate, proprioceptive, and unintentional touch, and positioned their children out of arms' reach. In parallel, children with feeding disorders displayed less affectionate touch, more negative touch, and more rejection of the mother's contact. These children were also more withdrawn during feeding and play interactions, and the feeding sessions were less efficacious and more chaotic; in addition, children were less able to complete the meal (Feldman, Keren, Gross-Rozval, & Tyano, 2004).

Similar results emerged from a 1-year follow-up on the precursors of feeding disorders among low-risk premature infants, who are at a higher risk for feeding difficulties than infants born at term. Mother–infant feeding and nonfeeding interactions were observed prior to discharge, and feeding difficulties were assessed at 1 year through maternal interview and feeding observations. Infants whose mothers provided more affectionate touch in the neonatal intensive care unit (NICU) were more engaged during feeding and less withdrawn at 1 year, and the feeding sessions were characterized by higher independence and more efficacy. These children also exhibited fewer feeding problems at 1 year (Silberstein et al., 2009).

Taken together, the findings presented in this section demonstrate that in humans, similar to other mammals, maternal affectionate touch and physical contact are essential components of the maternal repertoire during the first months of life and contribute to the consolidation of the maternal sensitive style and the infant's ultimate growth. The findings also suggest that maternal touch involves a distinct neurobiological system, expressed in specific brain circuitry, hormonal markers, and autonomic response. These systems support the development of a healthy bond between mother and child and are disrupted in cases of psychopathology. Better understanding of these biological underpinnings may help uncover specific risks to infant development under a variety of risk conditions and lead to the construction of more specific interventions.

MATERNAL PHYSICAL CONTACT IN INFANCY UNDER CONDITIONS OF MATERNAL SEPARATION: THE KC INTERVENTION AND ITS LONG-TERM OUTCOME

Prematurity is a condition that involves both immaturity of physiological systems and maternal separation. Premature birth truncates the normal development of neurological systems that are responsible for the regulation of basic physiological processes, such as the biological clock, feeding, thermoregulation, stress management, attention, and social relationships (Feldman, 2004). Birth alters the developmental course of brain maturation and, since even the most optimal incubator conditions cannot mimic the intrauterine environment, delays the maturation of physiological regulators. As a result, premature infants often exhibit difficulties in the development of physiological and behavioral regulation in infancy. During later childhood and adolescence, children born prematurely often show higher levels of conduct disorders, more attention and hyperactivity problems, lower frustration tolerance, and poorer social skills (Allin et al., 2001; Malatesta, Grigoryev, Lamb, Albin, & Culver, 1986; McCormick, Workman-Daniels, & Brooks-Gunn, 1996; Ruff, 1986; Sigman, Cohen, Beckwith, & Parmelee, 1986; Thoman, Denenberg, Sievel, Zeidner, & Becker, 1981).

The KC Intervention

Similar to many other natural forms of therapy, the KC intervention emerged out of necessity. Confronted with a shortage of incubators in Bogota, Colombia, the medical staff used parents as natural incubators. Infants remained physically attached to the mother around the clock until they matured and were able to maintain their own body heat in the external environment, and fathers and other family members often participated in the KC intervention for parts of the day. A series of randomized clinical trials in Colombia showed that the "kangaroo mother intervention" was safe in caring for low birth-weight premature infants and did not increase mortality or morbidity rates as compared to infants cared for by standard incubator care (Charpak, Ruiz, de Calume, & Charpak, 1997; Sloan, Camacho, Rojas, & Stern, 1994). Over the last 15 years, the KC intervention has become a standard care option for parents in industrialized countries. Once the infants' medical condition stabilizes, infants are placed naked (wearing a diaper and sometimes a cap) on the parent's chest in the "kangaroo" position while still being attached to the monitoring devices. Parents are thus able to experience full body contact with their infant, an experience that improves their sense of efficacy and the bonding with the child (Affonso, Bosque, Wahlberg & Brady, 1993).

Most studies on the benefits of the KC intervention have assessed short-term outcomes measured during the hospitalization period, including an improvement in infant state, increase in nursing rates and maternal lactation, and improvement in the mother's mood and sense of parenting. However, authors have criticized these early studies on the basis of less-than-rigorous methodology, reliance on parental report, lack of observation of parent–infant interaction, and lack of longitudinal follow-up of the treated versus not treated infants (Charpak et al., 1997). Recently, however, several follow-up studies comparing infants receiving KC in the neonatal period with controls have been reported. Here, we describe our longitudinal research, which is among the most comprehensive follow-ups of the KC intervention. We suggest that, in addition to assessing the practical benefits of Kangaroo contact on preterm development, the KC intervention provides a unique experimental paradigm for addressing key theoretical issues in a human model. These issues include the short- and long-term effects of maternal separation, the positive impact of touch and contact on self-regulatory systems, the role of early experience in infant development, and the effects of minor variations in maternal bonding on later growth. Below we address these issues by looking at the impact of mother–infant contact on four domains: (1) infant self-regulation (infant arousal, attention, and emotion), (2) infant neuromaturation and physiological regulation, (3) maternal well-being and mood, and (4) parent–child relationships.

The Longitudinal KC Project: Long-Term Effects on Mother and Child

The Israeli longitudinal KC Project followed 146 low birth-weight premature infants and their families born in the Jerusalem and Tel-Aviv areas in Israel. All infants in the study were born with a birth weight below 1,750 g and a gestational age (GA) of 33 weeks or less to two-parent families of middle-class background. Seventy-three infants received KC for at least 1 hour per day for a period of at least 2 weeks and 73 cased-matched infants served as controls, matched for gender, birthweight, GA, degree of medical risk, and family demographic (including maternal and paternal age, education, and birth order). KC was provided by mothers, as fathers were not willing to commit to providing an hour a day for at least 14 consecutive days, which we required from mothers. No differences between groups were found on Apgar 1 and 5 scores, the ratio of vaginal to Cesarean delivery, and the family's social support network. The KC was targeted to a period when the infant was still incubated, and full maternal-infant bodily contact was precluded for medical reasons. Infants and their parents were seen at pre-kangaroo baseline (controls were observed at 32 weeks GA, matched to the mean age of KC initiation), at term age, and at 3 and 6 months corrected age. A subsample ($N = 70$) was observed at 12 and 24 months and at 5 years. Recently, we completed a comprehensive assessment of the majority of the sample ($N = 115$) at 10 years.

The pre-kangaroo and term observations took place in the hospital, the 3-month observation was conducted in the family home, and the 6-month assessment took place in a developmental laboratory, to allow for the assessment of infant behavior in different settings and contexts. The 1-, 2-, 5-, and 10-year assessments took place in a university laboratory. At 10 years, infants also received an actigraph that measured their sleep patterns over five consecutive nights. Multiple outcome measures were collected, including physiological measures; standard cognitive and neurocognitive tests; tests of attention and perception; mother–child, father–child, and family interactions in age-appropriate tasks and contexts; and parental interviews and self-reports. Overall, the findings demonstrate that the Kangaroo intervention has a beneficial multidimensional impact on child development that lasts across the first decade of life.

Infant self-regulation. Since the work of Hofer (1995) on maternal proximity, maternal physical contact has been shown to facilitate the development of regulatory functions in animal models. The earlier studies in Bogota, Colombia, first noted that the Kangaroo method had a stabilizing effect on the infant's physiological systems (Fischer, Sontheimer, Scheffer, Bauer, & Linderkamp, 1998; Ludington & Golant, 1993), contributed to thermoregulation, and improved oxygenation (Acolet, Sleath, & Whitelaw, 1989; Bauer, Sontheimer, Fischer, & Linderkamp, 1996; Bier et al., 1996; Bosque, Brady, Affonso, & Wahlberg, 1995; Fohe, Dropf, & Avenarius, 2000; Ludington-Hoe & Swinth, 1996; Tornhage,

Stude, Lindberg, & Serenius, 1998). Similarly, KC reduced infant crying (Michelsson, Christenson, Rothganger, & Winberg, 1996) and beta-endorphin levels (Mooncey, Giannakoulopoulos, Glober, Acolet, & Modi, 1997), pointing to the effects of KC on attenuating the stress response. KC has also been shown to contribute to state regulation, increasing both quiet sleep (Gale, Frank, & Lund, 1993) and alert states (Gale & Vandenberg, 1998), and to improve growth rates (Kambarami, Chidede, & Kowo, 1998)—findings that highlight the positive impact of skin-to-skin contact on growth and maturation. A review summing 25 years since the introduction of the Kangaroo Mother Intervention showed that, overall, the intervention was not only safe but helped improve the infant's regulatory capacities in the neonatal period and had a positive impact on the mother–infant and family relationship in later infancy (Charpak et al., 2005).

In light of the role of maternal contact in organizing the biological clock, we examined sleep-wake cyclicity patterns in the KC and control infants. Four hours of infant state were observed at pre-kangaroo and again at term age. As the sleep-wake cycle of newborns lasts between 60 and 70 minutes, this period enabled the detection of several sleep-wake cycles. States were defined according to Brazelton (1973) and included quiet sleep, active sleep, sleep-wake transition, unfocused alertness, alert wakefulness, and cry. A coder sat at the infant's bedside and marked infant state for each 10-second epoch. The distribution of states across the 4-hour period was examined and sleep-wake cyclicity was measured with spectral analysis, with higher amplitudes indicating better organization of the biological clock. No differences were found at the pre-kangaroo observation. At term age, infants who received KC showed longer periods of quiet sleep and alert wakefulness and shorter periods of active sleep; their sleep-wake cycle was also more organized. The consolidation of the sleep-wake cycle is required for the later fine-tuning of the arousal system and its regulation into micopatterns of activity and rest, observed in tasks such as attention shifting, arousal modulation, and attention maintenance (Feldman, Weller, Sirota, & Eidelman, 2002). As suggested, more organized sleep-wake cyclicity indicates a more mature balance between the reactive and regulatory aspects of the state system, which provides the global framework for experience, growth, and learning in the neonatal period (Brazelton, 1990).

At 3 months corrected age, infants' arousal modulation and emotion regulation was assessed as follows: infants were presented with 17 stimuli that increased in the magnitude of intrusiveness from a simple unimodel stimulus (light, soft sound) to multimodal, high-impact stimuli (a car flashing lights and making loud noises approaching the infant). Each stimulus was presented for 10 seconds with a 20-second break between stimuli. Infants who received skin-to-skin contact showed a higher "threshold" to negative emotionality and they were able to tolerate more aversive stimuli before crying. Similarly, the KC infants showed a better modulation of arousal to stimulus onset and offset. The ability to shift between optimal reactivity during information intake and to utilize the period of stimulus offset for rest and processing is an index of an efficient, task-specific and mature information processing system (Feldman & Mayes, 1999); findings suggest that KC impacted the infants' emotion regulation and arousal modulation capacities. The findings also highlight the role of maternal proximity in forming a barrier to outside stimulation and for increasing the threshold to negative reactivity, central components of the infant's emotion regulation capacities (Feldman, Weller, et al., 2002).

At 6 months corrected age, infant's exploratory behavior was assessed during a mother–infant exploration session. Infants in the KC group showed more sustained exploration, spent more time jointly manipulating the toy with their mother, and had longer periods of shared attention in which mother and child jointly attended to the toy (Feldman, Weller, et al., 2002).

The capacities to engage in sustained exploration and to enter into a process of shared attention precede the development of social–cognitive abilities that emerge toward the end of the first year.

At 1 year, infants who received KC were better able to manage separation distress. At the end of the visit, mothers were asked to leave the room and the infant remained with a stranger for several minutes. The child's behavior, affect, distress, and ability to maintain exploration were microcoded. Continuous with these infants' capacity to tolerate more distress at 3 months, KC infants showed less distress and were better able to maintain exploration of the environment during maternal absence.

Similar long-term effects were noted at 2 and 5 years. At 2 years, infants in the Kangaroo group showed better executive functions, measured with a delayed-response paradigm that taps the child's ability to suppress a dominant response after a delay. At 5 years, KC children showed better performance on the NEPSY, a neurocognitive test of executive functions that examines auditory and visual processing, and behavioral control.

Preliminary results from the 10-year assessment of 115 children are consistent with the findings across infancy and childhood. At both 5 and 10 years, general IQ no longer distinguished the group as it did across the first 2 years of life. However, the NEPSY test of executive capacities showed group differences at both 5 and 10 years, suggesting that as children grow, the benefits of early maternal contact become more specifically linked with regulatory skills and less with general intelligence. Possibly, the early differences between groups were influenced by the benefits to attention and frustration tolerance that are much more related to indices of mental development in infancy than in later years.

Infant neuromaturation and physiological regulation. The developmental theory of Gottlieb (1991) suggests that sensory development occurs sequentially, and during the first postnatal period, infants should receive significantly more stimulation to the primary senses—touch and proprioception—than to the secondary senses—vision and audition. Typical Western NICU conditions, however, reverse this order and bombard infants with continuous light and nonstop noise, which their immature systems cannot ward off (Als, 1991). Animal research has indicated that such conditions carry irreversible effects on neuromaturation, including permanent damage to the biological clock and information-processing capacities (Hao & Rivkees, 1999; Sleigh & Lickliter, 1998). Exposure to excessive pain also results in permanent structural and functional disruptions to brain maturation (Grunau, 2002).

Interestingly, intervention programs that attempt to address lack of appropriate stimulation, such as massage, rhythmic stimulation, or minimal handling to filter overwhelming stimulation, improve neuromaturation in terms of physical growth, motor maturity, and physiological organization in premature infants (Feldman & Eidelman, 1998). Thus, providing components of the maternal presence during a sensitive period for neurodevelopment (Schore, 2001; Tucker, 1992) and brain–behavior relationships can have a lasting impact on the physiological support systems that modulate arousal and manage stress throughout life (Laviola & Terranova, 1998). Indeed, Ludington-Hoe and Swinth (1996) suggested that skin-to-skin contact contributes to maturation in each of the five neurobehavioral systems that are compromised by premature birth, including autonomic, motor, state, attention–interaction, and self-regulation. KC also appears to buffer the experience of pain by functioning as an analgesic during painful medical procedures (Gray, Watt, & Blass, 2000) and assists in recovery after heart surgery (Gazzolo, Masetti, & Meli, 2000).

Several physiological systems that index neuromaturation, such as better stress reactivity and improved arousal regulation, were tested in our longitudinal study. The effect of KC on the maturation of the autonomic nervous system was operationalized by cardiac vagal tone (Porges, 1996), which has been used as a physiological marker of the infant's emotion regulation capacities. In premature infants, lower vagal tone is observed due to the immaturity of neurological systems. Vagal tone has also been associated with the degree of medical risk (DiPietro & Porges, 1991) and the resting vagal tone at term age was found to predict infant development up to 6 years of age (Doussard-Roosevelt, McClenny, & Porges, 2001). Thus, it is clear that interventions that can impact on the maturation of vagal tone are likely to have an important impact on the infant's neurodevelopmental maturation.

We measured vagal tone at pre-kangaroo baseline and at 37 weeks GA. The vagal tone index was extracted from 10 minutes of ECG recording according to a system developed by Porges. Although vagal maturation during this period was observed for all infants, those receiving KC showed a higher vagal tone at 37 weeks GA, indicating a quicker maturation of the autonomic nervous system (Feldman & Eidelman, 2003a). The findings suggest that kangaroo contact accelerates the neuromaturation rate during a period of rapid brain development as measured by objective physiological indices. Such findings point to the pervasive impact of maternal contact during periods of early separation.

Resting vagal tone in the neonatal period appears to shape the development of self-regulatory capacities throughout childhood (Feldman, 2009). We found that neonatal vagal tone was related to emotion regulation in the first year, attention regulation in the second year, and self-regulation skills at age five, including the capacity for self-restraint, lower levels of externalizing and internalizing symptoms, and better executive control. At 10 years, we measured vagal tone again in response to an emotional (inter-adult anger) and cognitive challenge. Consistent with previous research (El-Sheik, 2001) and with the findings demonstrated for maternal touch in infancy (Feldman, Singer, et al., 2010), children who received KC in infancy showed more optimal functioning of the autonomic nervous system, as observed in higher baseline vagal tone and a larger vagal brake in response to challenge.

Neuromaturation in the neonatal period was also tested with the Neonatal Behavior Assessment Scale (Brazelton, 1973). Following KC, infants scored higher on the orientation and habituation clusters. Poor orientation has been associated with stress reactivity and negative emotionality (Auerbach et al., 1999; Spangler & Scheubeck, 1993) and disrupted habituation is observed in conditions such as prenatal exposure to cocaine (Mayes, Granger, Frank, Schottenfeld, & Bornstein, 1993). Our findings are consistent with a Japanese study which showed higher orientation following KC (Ohgi et al., 2002). These findings point to the role of maternal contact in organizing infant orientation to the environment, possibly leading to more mature neurodevelopmental profiles throughout childhood.

Two other physiological systems were assessed at 10 years—sleep quality using actigraphs and functioning of the hypthalamic-pituitary-adrenal axis indexed by cortisol baseline and reactivity. At 10 years, the sleep of infants who received KC in infancy was less disrupted: there were fewer bouts of wakefulness, each bout lasted for a shorter duration, and the latency to falling asleep was quicker. In terms of cortisol reactivity, early maternal contact decreased the magnitude of the stress response and afforded quicker return to baseline, the two components of resilience.

The 10-year longitudinal results suggest that, similar to mammals, early maternal contact has a lifelong effect on physiological regulation and stress management systems. It is possible that the amazing long-term effects of a relatively short, inexpensive intervention relate to the immediate effects of the Kangaroo intervention on organizing the autonomic response, the stress management system, and the biological clock. Better organization of these systems during the early sensitive period possibly sets the trajectory of infant development on a more optimal path that continues in the same way across development.

Maternal well-being and mood. In addition to improving the infant's condition, KC has been shown to improve the mother's well-being and depression following premature birth. Dombrowski, Anderson, Santori, and Burkhammer (2001) have applied the KC intervention successfully with women who suffered PPD, based on the idea that physical contact has been associated with more positive maternal feeling toward the infant. KC mothers have reported more positive feelings toward their infants, lower parental stress, and better sense of the parenting role (Affonso et al., 1993; Neu, 1999). It was suggested that KC may help reverse some of the negative effects of premature birth on the mother, such as her identity as a competent parent, and the guilt and anxiety that typically accompany premature birth (Brooten et al., 1988). In addition, KC was found to contribute to maternal well-being in developing countries. Reports from Zimbabwe (Kambarami, Chidede, & Kowo, 1999) and Papua New Guinea (McMaster & Vince, 2000), among others, describe the positive effects of KC on maternal and infant well-being. These findings highlight the KC intervention as a natural, cost-free intervention, which does not require long training or sophisticated methodologies but carries a significant benefit to the infant and the mother–infant dyad.

In our research, similar effects of kangaroo contact on maternal mood were observed. Upon discharge, maternal PPD was lower among KC mothers, and an interaction effect of group and medical risk indicated that KC improved maternal mood to a greater extent among those with low-risk premature infants, who were able to provide KC in the few days after birth (Feldman, Eidelman, Sirota, & Weller, 2002). At term age, mothers also perceived their infants as less different than the average full-term neonate, and at 6 months KC mothers reported lower separation anxiety. These findings are significant since mothers of premature infants often suffer higher levels of anxiety and depression (Brooten et al., 1988) and perceive their infant as very different from the normal healthy child (Levy-Shiff, Sharir, & Mogilner, 1989). Thus, it appears that KC mothers were better prepared for the maternal role.

However, by ages 1, 2, and 5 years, no differences in maternal mood, a sense of well-being, parenting stress, or efficacy in the parenting role were observed among our groups. Similarly, we found no differences from the recent follow-up at 10 years. However, since PPD was associated with lower levels of mother–infant reciprocity, lower maternal touch, and reduced sensitivity across the first 10 years and because PPD exerts a long-term negative effect on children's cognitive, social, and emotional growth (Goodman & Gotlib, 1999), the improvement in the mother's postpartum mood following KC may have had an indirect effect on the child's social development and the ongoing mother–child relationship.

Parent–child relationships. Premature birth disrupts the development of maternal-infant bonding for reasons related to both maternal separation and infant dysregulation. Premature infants have difficulties maintaining visual attention during play (Eckerman, Hsu, Molitor, Leung, & Goldstein, 1999) and their emotional expressions are often unclear (Malatesta et al., 1986), making it harder for mothers to read the child's social signals. Preterm infants are also prone to negative emotionality and less able to modulate arousal, making the interactions less rewarding to the parent.

In our longitudinal study, mother–child interactions were conducted at every assessment and often involved several tasks and contexts. At the 3-month assessment, we conducted a home visit and observed father–infant and family interactions as well.

Upon discharge, mother–infant interactions were observed in the NICU and microcoded for the maternal behavior constellation. As expected, KC had its most notable effect on the mother's touch patterns, with mothers in the KC group showing more affectionate touch to their infants. Mothers were also more adaptive to infant signals and the infants were more alert during social interactions (Feldman, Eidelman, et al., 2002), indicating that the mother–infant dyad was off to a better start following the KC intervention.

At the 3- and 6-month assessments, more positive interactions between KC mothers and their infants continued. Global coding of mother–infant interactions with the CIB (Feldman, 1998) revealed that KC mothers were more sensitive and less intrusive, that infants were more socially engaged and less negative, and that the level of dyadic reciprocity between mother and child was higher compared to controls (Feldman, Weller, Eidelman, & Sirota, 2003). The improvements in relational pattern were observed on the dimensions that were reported as compromised by premature birth, such as reduced maternal sensitivity and intrusiveness, lower maternal-child reciprocity, and lower infant involvement. These more optimal interactions at 3 and 6 months predicted higher scores on the Mental Development Index of the Bayley Scales of Infant Development (Bayley, 1993) at 6, 12, and 24 months among the KC infants.

At 1 and 2 years, toddlers who received KC were more involved and socially alert during interactions, and the dyadic interactions were more reciprocal. These findings point to a persistent effect of early contact on better behavior organization and socialization across infancy. Significant findings on the same factors emerged at the 10-year assessment. At 10 years, children engaged in two interactions with their mothers that were coded with the childhood version of the CIB. The first was a positive interaction in which parent and child planned a "fun day" together and the second was a conflict interaction. Children who received KC in infancy showed higher social engagement, and the reciprocity between mother and child was higher.

These long-term findings suggest that early Kangaroo contact has lasting impact on children's social–emotional development and their capacity to engage in a synchronous relationship with their mother. The effects may be due to the fact that mother and child continue to mutually influence each other across development. Thus, a more socially responsive child elicits more synchronous interactions, and mother–child reciprocity, in turn, contributes to the development of child social engagement.

At 3 months, we also assessed father–child and family interaction patterns at a home visit. Father–child interactions in the KC group were more optimal in terms of higher paternal sensitivity, lower paternal intrusiveness, and higher father–child reciprocity. Although fathers did not engage in KC, the increase in infant regulation and sociability following KC may have contributed to the father's sensitive involvement. It is also possible that fathers adopted the more sensitive interaction of the Kangaroo mothers (Feldman, Weller, et al., 2003). Although the mechanisms for this improvement are not fully understood, a more positive atmosphere between mother and child may facilitate a better home atmosphere and more optimal fathering.

Triadic interactions between mother, father, and child were conducted at 3 months and microcoded for gaze and affect of each family member, proximity position between each two members, and touch patterns between each two family members (mother–infant, father–infant, and mother–father). The family atmosphere as a whole was globally coded on the dimension of coherence (the level of harmony, reciprocity, and unity in the triad) and intrusiveness (the degree to which members interfered with each other's communications). Families in the Kangaroo groups showed better functioning on both the microanalytic and global assessments. KC infants showed lower levels of gaze aversion and less negative affect, and both mothers and fathers affectionately touched their infants more often during triadic interactions. In addition, triadic interactions of KC families were described as more harmonious and less intrusive. Family processes, which are dynamic and multidimensional, are sensitive to changes in each family member, and these individual changes lead to better organization, harmony, and coherence in the triad following intervention (Fivas-Depeursinge & Corboz-Warnery, 1999). Thus, KC seems to have an impact on a large array of developmental processes, which extend beyond the mother–infant dyad and much beyond the neonatal period. The early improvements in infant self-regulation and in early mothering carry a positive effect on fathering and family processes, as well as the child's later cognition, learning, and social adaptation.

CONCLUSION

Touch and contact are the primary components of every loving relationship. Receiving touch and contact immediately after birth help the human infant organize orientation to the social world and function adaptively within society. Human mothers, similar to other mammalian mothers, are genetically programmed to provide the species-typical form of affectionate touch and physical contact to their infants immediately after birth. Such patterns of touch and contact are supported by specific physiological systems that include genetic, hormonal, and brain markers. Prematurity provides a natural experiment in assessing the effects of structured maternal-infant contact during a period of early and persistent maternal deprivation, on the infant's physiological maturation, regulatory function, and social relationships. The lasting effects of early skin-to-skin contact on the functioning of a variety of physiological and social systems across the first decade of life indicate that the provision of touch and proximity during this sensitive early period may have a lifelong impact on the infant's self-regulation, social relatedness, and capacity to handle stress and frustration. The provision of early contact also enables children to develop reciprocal relationships with their attachment partners and, consistent with the findings for OT in animals, to hopefully engage in loving relationships with their partners and provide more optimal parenting in the next generation.

REFERENCES

Acolet, D., Sleath, K., & Whitelaw, A. (1989). Oxygenation, heart rate and temperature in very low birth infants during skin-to-skin contact with their mothers. *Acta Paediatrica Scandinavica, 78,* 189–193.

Affonso, D., Bosque, E., Wahlberg, V., & Brady, J. P. (1993). Reconciliation and healing for mothers through skin-to-skin contact provided in an American tertiary level intensive care nursery. *Neonatal Network, 12,* 25–32.

Allin, M., Matsumoto, H., Santhouse, A. M., Nosarti, C., AlAsady, M. H., Stewart, A. L., ...Murray, R. M. (2001). Cognitive and motor function and the size of the cerebellum in adolescents born very pre-term. *Brain, 124,* 60–66.

Als, H. (1991). Neurobehavioral organization of the newborn: Opportunity for assessment and intervention. *NIDA Research Monograph, 114,* 106–116.

Atzil, S., Hendler, T., & Feldman, R. (2010, June). *Maternal brain and mother-infant synchrony.* Presented at the international conference for Human Brain Mapping, Barcelona, Spain.

Auerbach, J., Geller, B., Lezer, S., Shinewell, E., Belmaker, R. H, Levin, J., & Ebstein, R. (1999). Dopamine D4 receptor (D4DR) and serotonin transporter promoter (5-HTTLPR) plymorphisms in the determination of temperament in 2-month-old infants. *Molecular Psychiatry, 4,* 369–373.

Bauer, J., Sontheimer, D., Fischer, C., & Linderkamp, O. (1996). Metabolic rate and energy balance in very low birth weight infants during kangaroo holding by their mothers and fathers. *Journal of Pediatrics, 129,* 608–611.

Bayley, N. (1993). *Bayley Scales of Infant Development: Administering and Scoring manual.* New York, NY: Psychological Corporation.

Bier, J. A., Ferguson, A. E., Morales, Y., Liebling, J. A., Archer, D., Oh, W., & Vohr, B. R. (1996). Comparison of skin-to-skin contact with standard contact in low-birth-weight infants who are breast-fed. *Archives of Pediatrics and Adolescent Medicine, 150,* 1265–1269.

Bosque, E. M., Brady, J. P., Affonso, D. D., & Wahlberg, V. (1995). Physiologic measures of kangaroo versus incubator care in a tertiary-level nursery. *Journal of Obstetric, Gynecologic, and Neonatal Nursing, 24,* 219–226.

Bowlby, J. (1969). *Attachment and Loss. Vol.1: Attachment.* New York, NY: Basic Books.

Brazelton, T. B. (1973). *Neonatal Behavioral Assessment Scale.* Philadelphia, PA: J. B. Lippincott.

Brazelton, T. B. (1990). Saving the bathwater. *Child Development, 61,* 1661–1671.

Brooten, D., Gennaro, S., Brown, L., Butts, P., Gibbons, A., Bakewill-Sachs, S., ... Kumar, S. P. (1988). Anxiety, depression, and hostility in mothers of preterm infants. *Nursing Research, 37*, 213–216.

Carter, S. C., & Keverne, E. B. (2002). The neurobiology of social affiliation and pair bonding. *Hormones, Brain and Behavior, 1*, 299–339.

Champagne, F. A. (2008). Epigenetic mechanisms and the transgenerational effects of maternal care. *Frontiers in Neuroendocrinology, 29*, 386–397.

Charpak, N., Ruiz, J. G., de Calume, Z. F., & Charpak, Y. (1997). Kangaroo mother versus "traditional" care for newborn infants ≤ 2000 grams. A randomized, controlled trial. *Pediatrics, 100*, 682–688.

Charpak, N., Ruiz, J. G., Zupan, J., Cattaneo, A., Figueroa, Z., Tessier, R., ... Worka, B. (2005). Kangaroo mother care: 25 years after. *Acta Paediatrica, 94*, 514–522.

DiPietro, J. A., & Porges, S. W. (1991). Vagal responsiveness to gavage feeding as an index of preterm status. *Pediatric Research, 29*, 231–236.

Dollberg, D., Feldman, R., Keren, M., & Gudeney, A. (2006). Sustained withdrawal behavior in clinic-referred and non-referred infants. *Infant Mental Health Journal, 27*, 292–309.

Dombrowski, M. A., Anderson, G. C., Santori, C., & Burkhammer, M. (2001). Kangaroo (skin-to-skin) care with a postpartum woman who felt depressed. *American Journal of Maternal and Child Nursing, 26*, 214–216.

Doussard-Roosevelt, J. A., McClenny, B. D., Porges, S. W. (2001). Neonatal cardiac vagal tone and school-age developmental outcome in very low birth weight infants. *Developmental Psychobiology, 38*, 56–66.

Eckerman, C. O., Hsu, H. C., Molitor, A., Leung, E. H., & Goldstein, R. F. (1999). Infant arousal in an en-face exchange with a new partner: Effects of prematurity and perinatal biological risk. *Developmental Psychology, 35*, 282–293.

El-Sheik, M. (2001). Parental drinking problems and children's adjustment: Vagal regulation and emotional reactivity as pathways and moderators of risk. *Journal of Abnormal Psychology, 110*, 499–515.

Feldman, R. (1998). *Coding Interactive Behavior (CIB) Manual*. Unpublished Manual. Bar-Ilan University.

Feldman, R. (2003). Infant-mother and infant-father synchrony: The coregulation of positive arousal. *Infant Mental Health Journal, 24*, 1–23.

Feldman, R. (2004). Mother-infant skin-to-skin contact and the development of emotion regulation. In S. P. Shohov (Ed.), *Advances in psychology research* (Vol. 27, pp. 113–131). Hauppauge, NY: Nova Science.

Feldman, R. (2006). From biological rhythms to social rhythms: Physiological precursors of mother-infant synchrony. *Developmental Psychology, 42*, 175–188.

Feldman, R. (2007). Parent-infant synchrony and the construction of shared timing; physiological precursors, developmental outcomes, and risk conditions. *Journal of Child Psychology and Psychiatry, 48*, 329–354.

Feldman, R. (2009). The development of regulatory functions from birth to five years: Insights from premature infants. *Child Development, 80*, 544–561.

Feldman, R. (2010). The relational basis of adolescent adjustment: Trajectories of mother-child interactive behaviors from infancy to adolescence shape adolescents' adaptation. *Attachment and Human Development, 12*, 173–192.

Feldman, R. (2011). Parent-infant synchrony: A bio-behavioral model of mutual influences in the formation of social affiliation. *Monographs of the Society for Research in Child Development*. In press.

Feldman, R., & Eidelman, A. I. (1998). Intervention methods for premature infants: How and do they affect development. *Clinics in Perinatology, 25,* 613–626.

Feldman, R., & Eidelman, A. I. (2003a). Mother-infant skin-to-skin contact (Kangaroo Care) accelerates autonomic and neurobehavioral maturation in premature infants. *Developmental Medicine and Child Neurology, 45,* 274–280.

Feldman, R., & Eidelman, A. I. (2003b). Direct and indirect effects of maternal milk on the neurobehavioral and cognitive development of premature infants. *Developmental Psychobiology, 43,*1–12.

Feldman, R., & Eidelman, A. I. (2004). Parent-infant synchrony and the social-emotional development of triplets. *Developmental Psychology, 40,* 1133–1147.

Feldman, R., & Eidelman, A. I. (2007). Maternal postpartum behavior and the emergence of parent-infant synchrony in preterm and full-term infants: The role of neonatal vagal tone. *Developmental Psychobiology, 49,* 290–302.

Feldman, R., & Eidelman, A. I. (2009). Biological and environmental initial conditions shape the trajectories of cognitive and social-emotional development across the first five years of life. *Developmental Science, 12,* 194–200.

Feldman, R., Eidelman, A. I., & Rotenberg, N. (2004). Parenting stress, infant emotion regulation, maternal sensitivity, and the cognitive development of triplets: A model for parent and child influences in a unique ecology. *Child Development, 75,* 1774–1791.

Feldman, R., Eidelman, A. I., Sirota, L., & Weller, A. (2002). Comparison of skin-to-skin (Kangaroo) and traditional care: Parenting outcomes and preterm infant development. *Pediatrics, 110,* 16–26.

Feldman, R., Gordon, I., Schneiderman, I., Weisman, O., & Zagoory-Sharon, O. (2010). Natural variations in maternal and paternal care are associated with systematic changes in oxytocin following parent-infant contact. *Psychoneuroendocrinology, 35,* 1133–1141.

Feldman, R., Gordon, I., & Zagoory-Sharon, O. (2010). The cross-generation transmission of oxytocin in humans. *Hormones & Behavior,* Jun 15. [Epub ahead of print]

Feldman, R., Granat, A., Pariente, C., Kanety, H., Kuint, J., & Gilboa-Schechtman, E. (2009). Maternal depression and anxiety across the postpartum year and infant social engagement, fear regulation, and stress reactivity. *Journal of the American Academy of Child and Adolescent Psychiatry, 48,* 919–927.

Feldman, R., Keren, M., Gross-Rozval, O., & Tyano, S. (2004). Mother and child's touch patterns in infant feeding disorders: Relation to maternal, child, and environmental factors. *Journal of the American Academy of Child and Adolescent Psychiatry, 43,* 1089–1097.

Feldman, R., & Masalha, S. (2007). The role of culture in moderating the links between early ecological risk and young children's adaptation. *Development and Psychopathology, 19,* 1–21.

Feldman, R., & Masalha, S. (2010). Parent-child and triadic antecedents of children's social competence: Cultural specificity, shared process. *Developmental Psychology, 46,* 455–467.

Feldman, R., Masalha, S., & Alony, D. (2006). Micro-regulatory patterns of family interactions: Cultural pathways to toddlers' self-regulation. *Journal of Family Psychology, 20,* 614–623.

Feldman, R., Masalha, S., & Nadam, R. (2001). Cultural perspective on work and family: Dual-earner Israeli-Jewish and Arab families at the transition to parenthood. *Journal of Family Psychology, 15,* 492–509.

Feldman, R., & Mayes, L. C. (1999). The rhythmic organization of infant attention during habituation is related to infants' information processing. *Infant Behavior and Development, 22,* 37–49.

Feldman, R., Singer, M., & Zagoory, O. (2010). Touch attenuates infants' physiological reactivity to stress. *Developmental Science, 13,* 271–278.

Feldman, R., Weller, A., Eidelman, A. I., & Sirota, L. (2003). Testing a family intervention hypothesis: The contribution of mother-infant skin-to-skin contact (Kangaroo Care) to family interaction and touch. *Journal of Family Psychology, 17,* 94–107.

Feldman, R., Weller, A., Sirota, L., & Eidelman, A. I. (2002). Skin-to-skin contact (Kangaroo Care) promotes self-regulation in premature infants: Sleep-wake cyclicity, arousal modulation, and sustained exploration. *Developmental Psychology, 38,* 194–207.

Feldman, R., Weller, A., Zagoory-Sharon, O., & Levine, R. (2007). Evidence for a neuroendocrinological foundation of human affiliation: Plasma oxytocin levels across pregnancy and the postpartum predict maternal-infant bonding. *Psychological Science, 18,* 965–970.

Ferber, G. S., Feldman, R., Kohelet, D., Kuint, J., Dolberg. S., Arbel, E., & Welder, A. (2005). *Infant Behavior and Development, 28,* 74–81.

Ferber, S. G., Feldman, R., & Makhoul, R. I. (2008). The development of maternal touch across the first year of life. *Early Human Development, 84,* 363–370.

Ferber, S. G., Kuint, J., Weller, A., Dolberg, S., Feldman, R., Arbel, E., & Kohelet, D. (2002). Massage therapy by mothers and trained professionals enhances weight gain in preterm infants. *Early Human Development, 67,* 37–45

Field, T. (1995). Massage therapy for infants and children. *Journal of Developmental and Behavioral Pediatrics, 16,* 105–111.

Fischer, C. B., Sontheimer, D., Scheffer, F., Bauer, J., & Linderkamp, O. (1998). Cardiorespiratory stability of premature boys and girls during kangaroo care. *Early Human Development, 52,* 145–153.

Fivas-Depeursinge, E., & Corboz-Warnery, A. (1999). *The primary triangle.* New York, NY: Basic Books.

Fohe, K., Dropf, S., & Avenarius, S (2000). Skin-to-skin contact improves gas exchange in premature infants. *Journal of Perinatology, 20,* 311–315.

Francis, D. D., Champagne, F. C., & Meaney, M. J. (2000). Variations in maternal behaviour are associated with differences in oxytocin receptor levels in the rat. *Journal of Neuroendocrinology, 12,* 1145–1148.

Gale, G., Frank, L., & Lund, C. (1993). Skin-to-skin (kangaroo) holding of the incubated premature infant. *Neonatal Network, 12,* 49–57.

Gale, G., & Vandenberg, K. A. (1998). Kangaroo care. *Neonatal Network, 17,* 69–71.

Gazzolo, D., Masetti, P., & Meli, M. (2000). Kangaroo care improves post-extubation cardiorespiratory parameters in infants after open heart surgery. *Acta Paediatrica Scandinavica, 89,* 728–729.

Goodman, S. H., & Gotlib, I. H. (1999). Risk for psychopathology in the children of depressed mothers: A developmental model for understanding mechanisms of transmission. *Psychological Review, 106,* 458–90.

Gordon, I., Zagoory-Sharon, O., Leckman, J. F., & Feldman, R. (2010a). Oxytocin and the development of parenting in humans. *Biological Psychiatry, 68,* 377–382

Gordon, I., Zagoory-Sharon, O., Leckman, J. F., & Feldman, R. (2010b). Oxytocin, cortisol, and triadic family interactions. *Physiology and Behavior, 101,* 679–684.

Gordon, I., Zagoory-Sharon, O., Leckman, J. F., & Feldman, R. (2010c). Prolactin, oxytocin, and the development of paternal behavior across the first six months of fatherhood. *Hormones & Behavior, 58*, 513–518.

Gottlieb, G. (1991). Experiential canalization of behavioral development: Theory. *Developmental Psychology, 27*, 4–13.

Gray, L., Watt, L., & Blass, E. (2000). Skin-to-skin contact is analgesic in healthy newborn. *Pediatrics, 105*, e14–e24.

Grunau, R. (2002). Early pain in preterm infants. A model of long-term effects. *Clinics in Perinatology, 29*, 373–394.

Hao, H., & Rivkees, S. A. (1999). The biological clock of very premature primate infants is responsive to light. *Proceedings of the National Academy of Sciences of the United States of America, 96*, 2426–2429.

Heird, W. C. (2001). The role of polyunsaturated fatty acids in term and preterm infants and breastfeeding mothers. *Pediatric Clinics of North America, 48*, 173–188.

Hofer, M. A. (1995). Hidden regulators: Implications for a new understanding of attachment, separation, and loss. In S. Golberg, R. Muir, & J. Kerr (Eds.), *Attachment theory: Social, developmental, and clinical perspectives* (pp. 203–230). Hillsdale, NJ: Analytic Press.

Insel, T. R., & Young L. J. (2001). The neurobiology of attachment. *Nature Neuroscience, 2*, 129–136.

Johnson, M. H., Griffin, R., Csibra, G., Halit, H., Farroni, T., de Haan, M., … Richards, J. E. (2005). The emergence of the social brain network: Evidence from typical and atypical development. *Development and Psychopathology, 17*, 599–619.

Kambarami, R. A., Chidede, O., & Kowo, D. T. (1998). Kangaroo care versus incubator care in the management of well preterm infants—A pilot study. *Annals of Tropical Paediatrics, 18*, 81–86.

Kambarami, R. A., Chidede, O., & Kowo, D. T. (1999). Kangaroo care for well low birth weight infants at Harare Central hospital Maternity Unit-Zimbabwe. *Central African Journal of Medicine, 45*, 56–59.

Keren, M., Feldman, R., Eidelman, A. I., Sirota, L., & Lester, B. (2003). Clinical interview for high-risk parents of premature infants (CLIP): Relations to mother-infant interaction. *Infant Mental Health Journal, 24*, 93–110.

Kim, P., Feldman, R., Leckman, J. F., Mayes, L. C., & Swain, J. E. (2011). Breastfeeding, mothers' brain activation to own infants stimuli, and maternal sensitivity. *Journal of Child Psychology and Psychiatry*. In press.

Kim, P., Leckman, J. F., Mayes, L. C., Newman, M. A., Feldman, R., & Swain, J. E. (2010). Perceived quality of maternal care in childhood and structure and function of new mothers' brain. *Developmental Science, 13*, 662–673.

Lamb, M. E. (1977). A re-examination of the infant social world. *Human Development, 20*, 65–85.

Laviola, G., & Terranova, M. L. (1998). The developmental psychobiology of behavioral plasticity in mice: The role of social experiences in the family unit. *Neuroscience Biobehavioral Review, 23*, 197–213.

LeVine, R. A. (2002). Contexts and culture in psychological research. *New Directions for Child Development, 96*, 101–106.

Levy-Shiff, R., Sharir, H., & Mogilner, M. B. (1989). Mother- and father-preterm infant relationship in the hospital preterm nursery. *Child Development, 60*, 93–102.

Ludington, S. M., & Golant, S. K. (1993). *Kangaroo care: The best you can do for your preterm infant.* New York, NY: Bantum Press.
Ludington-Hoe, S. M., & Swinth, J. Y. (1996). Developmental aspects of kangaroo care. *Journal of Obstetric, Gynecologic, and Neonatal Nursing, 25,* 691–703.
Maestripieri, D., Hoffman, C. L., Anderson, G. M., Carter, C. S., & Higley, J. D. (2009). Mother-infant interactions in free-ranging rhesus macaques: Relationships between physiological and behavioral variables. *Physiology and Behavior, 96,* 613–619.
Malatesta, C. Z., Grigoryev, P., Lamb, C., Albin, M., & Culver, C. (1986). Emotion socialization and expressive development in preterm and full-term infants. *Child Development, 57,* 316–330.
March of Dimes. (2006). Peristats: Your online source for perinatal statistics. http://www.marchofdimes.com/peristats
Markus, H. R., & Kitayama, S. (1991). Culture and the self: Implications for cognition, emotion, and motivation. *Psychological Review, 98,* 224–253.
Mayes, L. C., Granger, R. H., Frank, M. A., Schottenfeld, R., & Bornstein, M. H. (1993). Neurobehavioral profiles of neonates exposed to cocaine prenatally. *Pediatrics, 91,* 778–783.
McCormick, M. C., Workman-Daniels, K., & Brooks-Gunn, J. (1996). The behavioral and emotional well-being of school-age children with different birth weight. *Pediatrics, 97,* 18–25.
McMaster, P., & Vince, J. D. (2000). Outcome of neonatal care in Port Moresby, Papua New Guinea: A 19-year review. *Journal of Tropical Pediatrics, 46,* 57–61.
Meaney, M. J. (2001). Maternal care, gene expression, and the transmission of individual differences in stress reactivity across generations. *Annual Review of Neuroscience, 24,* 1161–1192.
Michelsson, K., Christenson, K., Rothganger, H., & Winberg, J. (1996). Crying in separated and non-separated newborns: Sounds spectrographic analysis. *Acta Paediatrica Scandinavica, 85,* 471–475.
Mooncey, S., Giannakoulopoulos, X., Glober, V., Acolet, D., & Modi, N. (1997). The effect of mother-infant skin-to-skin contact on plasma cortisol and beta endorphin concentration in preterm infants. *Infant Behavior and Development, 20,* 553–557.
Neu, M. (1999). Parents' perception of skin-to-skin care with their preterm infants requiring assisted ventilation. *Journal of Obstetric, Gynecologic, and Neonatal Nursing, 28,* 157–164.
Ohgi, S., Fukud, M., Moriuchi, H., Kusumoto, T., Akiyama, T., Nugent, J. K., ... Saitoh, H. (2002). Comparison of kangaroo care and standard care: Behavioral organization, development, and temperament in healthy, low-birth-weight infants through 1 year. *Journal of Perinatology, 22,* 374–379.
Porges, S. W. (1996). Physiological regulation in high-risk infants: A model for assessment and potential intervention. *Development and Psychopathology, 8,* 143–145.
Porges, S. W. (2003). Social engagement and attachment: A phylogenetic perspective. *Annals of the New York Academy of Sciences, 1008,* 31–47.
Ruff, H. A. (1986). Attention and organization of behavior in high-risk infants. *Journal of Developmental and Behavioral Pediatrics, 7,* 298–301.
Schore, A. N. (2001). Effects of a secure attachment relationship on right brain development, affect regulation, and infant mental health. *Infant Mental Health Journal, 22,* 7–66.

Serretti, A., Olgiati, P., & Colombo, C. (2006). Influence of postpartum onset on the course of mood disorders. *BMC Psychiatry, 6,* 4.

Sigman, M., Cohen, S. E., Beckwith, L., & Parmelee, A. H. (1986). Infant attention in relation to intellectual abilities in childhood. *Developmental Psychology, 22,* 788–792.

Silberstein, D., Geva, R., Feldman, R., Gardner, J. M., Karmel, B. Z., Rozen, H., & Kuint, J. (2009). The transition to oral feeding in low-risk premature infants: Relation to infant neurobehavioral functioning and mother-infant feeding interaction. *Early Human Development, 85,* 157–162.

Sleigh, M. J., & Lickliter, R. (1998). Timing of presentation of prenatal auditory stimulation alters auditory and visual responsiveness in bobwhite quail chicks (*Colinus virginianus*). *Journal of Comparative Psychology, 112,* 153–160.

Sloan, N., Camacho, L. W., Rojas, E. P., & Stern, C. (1994). Kangaroo mother method: Randomised controlled trial of an alternative method of care for stabilized low-birth weight infants. *Lancet, 344,* 782–785.

Spangler, G., & Scheubeck, R. (1993). Behavioral organization in newborns and its relation to adrenocortical and cardiac activity. *Child Development, 64,* 622–633.

Spitz, R. (1946). Anaclitic depression. *Psychoanalytic Study of the Child, 2,* 313–342.

Swain, J. E., Leckman, J. F., Mayes, L. C., Feldman, R., Constable, R. T., & Schultz, R. T. (2004a). Neural substrates of human parent-infant attachment in the postpartum. *Biological Psychiatry, 55,* 153S.

Swain J. E., Leckman, J. F., Mayes, L. C., Feldman, R., Constable, R. T., & Schultz, R. T. (2004b). Brain circuitry of human parent-infant attachment in the postpartum. *Neuroimage, 22,* S27.

Swain, J. E., Leckman, J. F., Mayes, L. C., Feldman, R., Hoyt, E., Kang, H.,... Schultz, R. T. (2007). *Baby cry and picture stimuli activate parent brains according to gender, experience, psychology and dyadic relationship.* Paper presented at the Society for Neuroscience, San Diego, CA.

Swain, J. E., Lorberbaum, J. P., Kose, S., & Strathearn, L. (2007). Brain basis of early parent-infant interactions: Psychology, physiology, and in vivo functional neuroimaging studies. *Journal of Child Psychology and Psychiatry, 48,* 262–287.

Thoman, E. B., Denenberg, V. H., Sievel, J., Zeidner, L. P., & Becker, P. (1981). State organization in neonate: Developmental inconsistency indicates risk for developmental dysfunction. *Neuropediatrics, 12,* 45–54.

Tornhage, C. J., Stude, E., Lindberg, T., & Serenius, F. (1998). First week kangaroo care in sick very preterm infants. *Acta Paediatrica, 88,* 1402–1404.

Tronick, E. Z. (1995). Touch in mother-infant interaction. In T. M. Field (Ed.), *Touch in early development* (pp. 53–65). Mahwah, NJ: Erlbaum.

Tucker, D. M. (1992). Developing emotions and cortical networks. In M. R. Gunnar & C. A. Nelson (Eds.), *Developmental behavioral neuroscience: The Minnesota Symposia on Child Psychology* (Vol. 24, pp. 75–128). Hillsdale, NJ: Erlbaum.

Weiss, S. (2005). Haptic perception and the psychosocial functioning of preterm, low birth weight infants. *Infant Behavior and Development, 28,* 329–359.

Weiss, S., & Goebel, P. (2003). Parents' touch of their preterm infants and its relationship to their state of mind regarding touch. *Journal of Prenatal and Perinatal Psychology, 17,* 185–202.

Weiss, S., Wilson, P., Hertenstein, M., & Campos, R. (2000). The tactile context of a mother's caregiving: Implications for attachment of low birth weight infants. *Infant Behavior and Development, 23,* 91–111.

Weiss, S., Wilson, P., & Morrison, D. (2004). Maternal tactile stimulation and the neurodevelopment of low birth weight infants. *Infancy, 5*, 85–107.

Weiss, S., Wilson, P., St. Jonn Seed, M., & Paul, S. (2001). Early tactile experience of low birth weight children: Links to later mental health and social adaptation. *Infant and Child Development, 10*, 93–115.

Weller, A., & Feldman, R. (2003). Emotion regulation and touch in infants: The role of cholecystokinin and opioids. *Peptides, 24*, 779–788.

Winnicott, D. W. (1956). *Collected papers: Through pediatrics to psychoanalysis.* New York, NY: Basic Books.

Ziegler, T. E. (2000). Hormones associated with non-maternal infant care: A review of mammalian and avian studies. *Folia Primatologica, 71*, 6–21.

16

Tactile Dysfunction in Neurodevelopmental Disorders

CARISSA J. CASCIO

The importance of tactile sensation in early human development is indisputable. Nearly every aspect of human development, from motor to communication to social skills, is affected by the sense of touch. Touch is the first sense to develop in utero (Montagu & Adubato, 1978), with responses to light stroking beginning to emerge at only 8 weeks' gestational age. Minutes after birth, infants depend on tactile input to the mouth that elicits rooting and sucking reflexes for nursing (Muir, 2002). Along with other sensory signals, tactile input from maternal contact during feeding and cuddling provides an ongoing association of caregivers with comfort and nourishment. This association is central in the development of bonding and secure attachment (Main & Stadtman 1981; Myers, 1984; Weiss, Wilson, Hertenstein, & Campos, 2000), laying the foundation for healthy social behaviors later in development.

Accurate tactile and proprioceptive sensation is critical for the development of motor skills during childhood, with somesthetic touch being particularly important for fine motor development during the first few years of life (Weiss, Wilson, & Morrison, 2004). Tactile feedback from mechanoreceptors in the skin and joints critically guides the online modulation of gross motor functions, such as walking, and fine motor functions, such as grasping.

While the role of touch in motor and social development is relatively intuitive and straightforward, it may be less obvious that the sense of touch is also highly relevant to the development of communication skills. Touch is more developed than other senses at birth (Montagu, 1986) and is a primary mode of communication in the first year of life, serving as a precursor to verbal communication (Dunbar, 1996). In addition to this ontogenetic primacy of touch for social communication in the early development of the individual, touch is also believed to have phylogenetic primacy for communication (Hertenstein, Verkamp, Kerestes, & Homes, 2006). Nonverbal communication, such as tactile interactions during grooming behaviors, preceded verbal communication in the evolutionary history of primate development. Dunbar (1996) suggests that only as hominids evolved to form larger groups and forage in larger territories did the need for a distal modality of communication emerge, selecting for gestures and the vocalizations that led to verbal communication. Thus, human reliance on tactile nonverbal communication is rooted in our evolutionary history.

Taken together, such observations indicate that touch plays a crucial role in the early development of social, motor, and communication (verbal and nonverbal) skills. It is these basic skills that are the most commonly impacted by neurodevelopmental disorders (NDDs).

NEURODEVELOPMENTAL DISORDERS

The term "neurodevelopmental disorder" encompasses a broad range of conditions that manifest in early childhood, and for which known or presumed aberrations in nervous system function give rise to behavioral, emotional, motor, or cognitive differences. A practical basic taxonomy divides this broad group of disorders into two types: (1) disorders with known (often single gene) genetic or chromosomal etiology, and (2) disorders with complex or unknown genetic etiology (Tager-Flusberg, 1999). In this chapter, studies of tactile dysfunction for these two groups are reviewed, as well as for those in a third, associated category: disorders with known environmental etiologies in pre/perinatal development or in early infancy. It should be noted that the studies reviewed in this chapter do not represent an exhaustive list of all NDDs, but primarily those for which multiple, peer-reviewed studies of tactile perception and/or somatosensory function were located. The chapter concludes with a review of tactile-based approaches to treatment of NDDs and suggestions for future directions in research.

Disorders With Known Genetic or Chromosomal Etiologies

In many cases, NDDs derive from known aberrations in a single gene, a small group of genes, or a chromosome. Often these genetic and chromosomal mechanisms have been studied extensively in human and animal models, and consequently their effects are relatively well understood.

Down syndrome. Down syndrome is a chromosomal condition that arises from an extra copy of chromosome 21. This aberration is not inherited but results from a failure of chromosomal pairs to separate properly during cell division in gamete cells. Down syndrome presents with a characteristic profile including hypotonia, distinguishing facial features, heart defects, and mild to moderate cognitive impairment. The presence of low muscle tone and motor coordination difficulties, as well as fine motor impairments, has prompted several studies of somatosensory perception in this population.

Experimental studies of tactile perception in Down syndrome reveal deficits in somatic localization of touch, in graphesthesia (identification of a letter or form traced on the skin), and in stereognosis (identification of a shape or form using only the tactile sense; Brandt, 1996). The specificity of the stereognosis deficit to the tactile system is unclear, as some studies found similar visual shape recognition deficits and others did not. All studies, however, have ruled out cognitive interference either by utilizing multiple control groups matched on mental and chronological age or by demonstrating that the task was performed adequately in the visual domain and thus instructions were understood. A study by Lewis and Bryant (1982) illustrated that children with Down syndrome are less likely to tactually explore materials and to coordinate touch with vision in the exploration of surfaces, compared to typically developing children of the same mental age.

In addition to these behavioral tests of somatosensory perception, several electroencephalographic (EEG) studies recording somatosensory-evoked potentials (SEPs) have been performed in samples of children with Down syndrome. SEPs are electrical signals recorded from the scalp in response to repeated electrical stimulation of a peripheral somatosensory nerve—typically the median nerve—that innervates the thumb and first two digits. Electrical stimulation provides a more reliable and robust response than mechanical stimulation and is noninvasive and safe for use with infants (Tombini et al., 2009). An additional benefit of using SEPs in young and cognitively impaired individuals is that brain response can be measured in the absence of any overt behavioral response. It also provides a measure of nerve conduction velocity in infants, young children, and individuals with intellectual disability, which is often interpreted as an index of generalized neural processing speed. This processing speed is reflected in the latency of observed waveforms, while the amplitude of the waveform is generally associated with the magnitude of neural activity (often interpreted as the number or coherence of active neurons).

The results of such studies suggest that children with Down syndrome exhibit slower conduction velocity (Chen & Fang, 2005; Ferri, Del Gracco, Elia, Musumeci, & Stefanini, 1996; Kakigi, Shibasaki, & Ikeda, 1989) and that the cortical responses to somatosensory stimulation are larger in amplitude (Ferri et al., 1996; Kakigi et al., 1989) and wider in topographic distribution across the scalp (Kakigi & Shibasaki, 1993) than in control samples. The origin of these abnormal responses is still unknown; however, the hypothesis that associated hypothyroidism contributed to impaired nerve conduction was refuted in a study of thyroxine-treated infants by van Trotsenburg and colleagues (2006). These neural differences in somatosensory processing may underlie the problems with discriminative aspects of touch noted earlier for children with Down syndrome and also contribute to the motor difficulties seen in this population.

Prader–Willi syndrome. Prader–Willi syndrome (PWS) is a rare genetic condition arising from the deletion or lack of expression of a set of genes on the paternal copy of chromosome 15. PWS presents with characteristic features including hyperphagia and obesity, hypogonadism, and hypotonia, which is particularly prominent in infancy. Most individuals with PWS exhibit mild to moderate intellectual disability. The presence of very low muscle tone in addition to exceptionally high tolerance for painful stimuli (Priano et al., 2009) suggests impairment in somatosensory perception. Brandt and Rosen (1998) investigated stereognosis and median nerve conduction velocity in a small sample of children with PWS and found no differences from the norm. However, they did report reduced signal amplitude from the median nerve, possibly reflecting a reduction in the number of sensory afferent fibers in this nerve. A study of a larger sample of adults with PWS assessed peripheral and central nervous system sources of impaired tactile perception using a combination of psychophysical sensory threshold testing, peripheral nerve conduction velocities, and SEPs (Priano et al., 2009). They replicated the finding of normal peripheral nerve conduction and extended it to brainstem and cortical SEPs, reporting psychophysical evidence of abnormally high thermal and pain thresholds for individuals with PWS. A strength of this study was a comparison group of obese adults, helping to rule out somatosensory abnormalities that could result from metabolic factors. The results suggested that altered pain perception in PWS is not attributable to peripheral, brainstem, or cortical sources, but investigators did not rule out possible involvement of the dorsal root ganglion in the spinal cord. Replication of these results, as well as more comprehensive investigation of possible cortical or brainstem contributors using functional magnetic resonance imaging, will help to clarify the neural basis of high pain tolerance and its potential relationship to other somatosensory factors in PWS.

Angelman syndrome. The maternal counterpart to the PWS paternally inherited deletion on chromosome 15 gives rise to Angelman syndrome (AS). Individuals with AS exhibit severe intellectual and developmental delay; speech impairment; frequent laughing or smiling; and motor symptoms, including ataxia, tremor, hand flapping, or uncontrolled movements of the limbs. Associated features include increased sensitivity to heat (Williams et al., 2005) and other potentially sensory-based fascinations, such as with water or "crinkly" materials (e.g., paper, plastic; Williams et al., 2005). A systematic study of sensory processing patterns in AS was conducted by Walz and Baranek (2006), using a parental report measure. Among the findings were hyporesponsiveness to tactile and vestibular input, which may elicit the sensation seeking associated with certain textures and other tactile experience that was noted by Williams and colleagues regarding patients with AS. The deletion on chromosome 15 that occurs in AS includes genes that code for gamma-aminobutyric acid (GABA) receptor subunits on GABA-A receptors. The GABAergic system is important for cortical inhibitory neurotransmission, which plays an important role in cortical sensory processing mechanisms, such as lateral inhibition and oscillatory patterns that affect sensory gating. Effects on this system are related to aberrant somatosensory responses in AS (Egawa et al., 2008). Further study is needed to clarify the role of the GABA system in hyper/hypo-responsiveness to tactile input in AS, as well as whether reduced registration of tactile input contributes to the sensory-seeking behaviors seen in this population.

Rett syndrome. Rett syndrome is not an inherited disorder but usually results from a spontaneous mutation in a gene on the X chromosome. Because it is a sex-linked mutation, it is almost always seen in girls; males with the mutation on their single X chromosome typically do not survive gestation. Rett syndrome is classified as a pervasive developmental disorder by *DSM-IV-TR* (American Psychiatric Association, 2000) and shares some features with autism. Individuals with Rett syndrome present with typical development in the first year of life, followed by a regressive loss of language and motor abilities. Prominent features include characteristic repetitive hand mannerisms such as hand wringing; these typically replace more purposeful hand movements that had begun to develop but then disappear.

Intellectual disability is also typical, as are gastrointestinal problems and seizures.

In 1991, Yoshikawa, Kaga, Suzuki, Sakuragawa, and Arima reported abnormally large amplitude SEPs in younger children with Rett syndrome; however, they noted that older children with the syndrome exhibited normal amplitudes. This developmental difference within the Rett syndrome group was attributed to cortical hyperexcitability that subsides with age. Kimura, Nomura, and Segawa (1992) also noted developmental changes in shorter-latency SEPs. In younger children, latencies were normal but in older children latencies of brainstem and spinal SEPs were increased, suggesting a degenerative process. Taken together, these results suggest that early in the development of the syndrome, somatosensory signals travel at a normal speed into the brain and produce abnormally large cortical responses. Later in development, signals are slower to reach the brain, but the cortex shows a normal amplitude of response. These changes in the strength and timing of the cortical response suggest that abnormalities of somatosensory processing may be attributable to an amplification or gating problem in the thalamus where modulatory activity on sensory signals filters their impact on sensory cortex.

Fragile X syndrome. Fragile X syndrome (FXS) is another X-linked genetic disorder that arises from a mutation of the FMR1 gene on the X chromosome. The protein (FMRP) that this gene encodes plays an important role in neural development. Symptoms of FXS include mild intellectual disability, characteristic facial features such as large ears and an elongated forehead, low muscle tone, hyperactivity, and hypersensitivity to sensory stimuli. Several studies have investigated sensory hypersensitivity in FXS with a focus on tactile sensitivity. Baranek and colleagues (2008) conducted a longitudinal study of sensory processing in FXS using convergent observational and parent-report measures. Their findings suggested that both hyper- and hyporesponsiveness to sensory stimuli increase with age and development in the first 5 years of life, including tactile sensitivity. In addition, tactile defensiveness, an aversion to tactile sensation and experience, was one of five factors found to distinguish boys with FXS from boys with other developmental disabilities (Lachiewicz, Spiridigliozzi, Gullion, & Ransford, 1994) and is a prominent enough feature to be commonly used prospectively to help identify males at risk for FXS (Butler et al., 1991; Hagerman, Amiri, & Cronister, 1991).

Ferri et al. (1996) report abnormally large (giant) SEPs over frontal and parietal areas of children who have FXS, with aberrant distributions that are more heavily weighted toward frontal electrodes than in children without FXS. Giant SEPs are associated with cortical hyperexcitability, and this finding was replicated in a case study of a boy with FXS (Musumeci, Elia, Ferri, Scuderi, & Del Gracco, 1994). This hyperexcitability of somatosensory response is consistent with the increased levels of tactile defensiveness observed for individuals with FXS. These differences at the cortical level may be downstream from more peripherally driven response differences to sensory stimuli. For instance, electrodermal response has been used as an index of peripheral sympathetic nervous system arousal when exposed to sensory stimulation. Miller and colleagues (1999) noted increased skin conductance responses in children with FXS to stimuli in all sensory modalities, including tactile.

Because it is associated with a predictable mutation on a single gene, animal models of FXS have been useful in understanding more about the neurobiology of the disorder. In strains of mice that are missing the FMR1 gene, profound effects have been seen in the organization of somatosensory cortex. FMR1 has a role in the development of sensory cortical circuits (Bureau, Shepard, & Svoboda, 2008). For example, the gene influences FMRP's control of GABA-releasing interneurons (Selby, Zhang, & Sun, 2007) that are intrinsic to the functioning of cortical circuits and the normal maturation of dendritic spines in somatosensory cortex (Galvez & Greenough, 2005). These processes are impaired in FXS. However, compensatory environmental sensory exposure can rescue both cortical and behavioral effects of these impairments in mice with the Fragile X mutation. With enrichment of the sensory environment, layer 5 pyramidal neuron dendritic arborization is rescued in sensory cortex, as are habituation and sensory exploration behaviors (Restivo et al., 2005).

Disorders With Complex or Unknown Genetic Etiologies

Many NDDs are known by increased familial risk to be heritable to some degree, but, unlike those above, cannot be traced to a single gene or chromosome. For these disorders, more research is necessary to determine the full array of genetic contributors to the disorder, and these genetic factors are likely to act in concert to confer a susceptibility that then interacts with environmental factors to produce the full syndrome. By virtue of their relatively unknown biological origins, these disorders are typically identified clinically, based solely on behavioral features. Examples of these NDDs include autism spectrum disorders (ASDs), disorders of linguistic and scholastic skills development, and attention-deficit hyperactivity disorder (ADHD).

Autism Spectrum Disorders. ASDs, also known as pervasive developmental disorders, are conditions that develop during childhood and affect complex behaviors such as communication and social interaction. Autistic disorder is the most commonly diagnosed variant in this group and is defined by impairment in a triad of behavioral areas. For a diagnosis of autism, a child must exhibit qualitative impairment in social interaction, communication, and restricted and/or repetitive patterns of behavior. These symptoms must also show onset before the age of 3 years. These symptoms are sometimes accompanied by intellectual disability, although a wide range of cognitive functioning is seen in autism. A diagnosis of PDD-NOS is typically given to a child who shows similar impairments but in an atypical or milder manner, or for whom the age of onset of symptoms is not before the age of 3 years. Asperger's syndrome generally refers to children with social impairments and repetitive behaviors, but who do not exhibit a significant delay in language or cognitive development.

Many individuals with ASD exhibit unusual responses to sensory stimuli, with tactile defensiveness being a very common symptom. Several studies have investigated basic somatosensory processing in ASDs. Parent questionnaires that address sensory processing generally provide evidence that tactile defensiveness is more common in autism than in typical development (Tomchek & Dunn, 2007) or in other developmental disabilities, although rates may be similar to, or even lower than, those in FXS (Rogers, Hepburn, & Wehner, 2003). The relation between tactile defensiveness and the full complement of core features of autism remains unclear, but Baranek, Foster and Berkson (1997), also using parent questionnaires, reported that tactile defensiveness was significantly associated with certain kinds of rigid and stereotyped behaviors in autism and other developmental disabilities.

Unusual responses to tactile stimulation in ASD are not limited to tactile defensiveness. Tactile seeking behaviors are often noted, such as repetitive rubbing of certain textures or surfaces, and an affinity for deep pressure input such as intense hugging or squeezing (Grandin, 2000). Experimental studies also provide evidence of uniquely pleasurable responses to certain tactile stimuli (Pernon, Pry, & Baghdadli, 2007).

The range of unusual emotional responses to tactile stimuli has prompted the investigation of tactile thresholds in individuals with ASD using classical psychophysical approaches. Assessment of threshold identifies the amount of physical stimulation or degree of change in tactile stimulation that is perceptible to an individual. In individuals who show tactile defensiveness, a higher degree of sensitivity to tactile stimulation (i.e., lower thresholds) would be predicted, while individuals who seem to seek out additional tactile input or react positively to touch might be expected to be less sensitive (i.e., higher thresholds).

The presence of lower thresholds, thus enhanced sensitivity to sensory stimuli, has been found in several studies among people with autism (for review see Mottron, Dawson, Soulières, Hubert, & Burack, 2006). This sensitivity has largely, although not entirely (O'Riordan & Passetti, 2006), been noted in the tactile system. Blakemore and colleagues (2006) investigated this possibility in adults with Asperger's syndrome and found that they had greater sensitivity to high-frequency (but not low frequency) vibration when measured at the fingertip, a site often chosen for psychophysical experiments because of its dense innervation by mechanoreceptors. This result was interpreted as a putative difference in mechanoreceptor afferent function, as high- and low-frequency vibrations are signalled by different types of mechanoreceptors (Pacinian and Meissner's corpuscles, respectively). Both types of mechanoreceptor convey signals through large myelinated afferents (A-fibers), while unmyelinated afferents (C-fibers) convey primarily pain and temperature information (although see below for a description of C-touch afferents, which constitute an exception to this general rule). A subsequent study failed to replicate high-frequency vibrotactile threshold differences at the fingertip in children with ASDs (Güçlü, Tanidir, Mukaddes, & Unal, 2007), but this study was limited by a small sample size, which may have reduced power to detect group differences. The authors of this study did, however, note significant correlations between tactile and affective responses of children identified through parent questionnaires, suggesting that aberrant responses to tactile stimulation may arise from emotional or even cognitive mechanisms rather than from differences in physiological response of the somatosensory system.

This interpretation is supported in part by a study from Cascio and colleagues (2008) in which adults with autism were tested on a variety of psychophysical tasks including both the palmar surface and the dorsal forearm. In addition to extending tactile psychophysics beyond the fingertip, an advantage of testing the forearm site is its innervation by C-touch afferents (Olausson et al., 2002). These afferents are believed to constitute a unique system for conveying affective touch signals that are central to mother–infant bonding and early social communication (McGlone, Vallbo, Olausson, Loken, & Wessberg, 2007). In this study, a lower threshold for low-frequency vibration was noted at the forearm site, but not at the palmar surface which has no innervation by C-touch afferents. In addition, greater sensitivity was observed for painful thermal stimuli, while there were no group differences in thresholds for innocuous thermal stimuli. Test–retest data from two sessions suggested that while the pain thresholds for the control group stayed relatively constant, pain sensitivity in the autism group was significantly lower at the second session than at the first. These data together support the idea that either a top–down emotional regulatory mechanism, an affective mechanism that includes C-touch afferents, or a combination of these two contributes to altered tactile sensitivity in autism, rather than solely a neurophysiological mechanism restricted to class A afferent subtypes. While psychophysical studies of discriminative touch processing in ASD have yielded mixed results, the emotional aspects of touch are more consistently reported to be affected in ASD (Cascio et al., 2008; Güçlü et al., 2007).

While several studies of touch response have emphasized potential roles of different peripheral afferent populations, others have been driven by cortical models of ASD. Tommerdahl, Tannan, Cascio, Baranek, and Whitsel (2007) tested adults with autism on a vibrotactile localization paradigm with an adapting stimulus. The presence of a preliminary adapting stimulus has been shown to improve tactile localization and is thought to do so via a spatial tuning mechanism in somatosensory cortex that depends on GABA-mediated inhibition of neighboring cortical minicolumns. This inhibition of surrounding cortex under extended stimulation may sharpen the signal by limiting it to a localized area of cortex. The investigators noted that individuals with autism exhibited greater sensitivity to touch during baseline performance than the control group, a finding predicted by other studies demonstrating enhanced tactile perception in individuals with autism. Interestingly, the group with autism did not exhibit the improvement in the presence of the adapting stimulus that was observed for the control group.

The picture of somatosensory processing in ASD is a complex one that will require considerable additional study. The co-occurrence of tactile hyperresponsiveness/defensiveness and hyporesponsiveness/touch seeking presents a challenge to experimental study. Current evidence suggests that touch with an emotional basis is more affected than discriminative touch, and differences in discriminative ability tend to fall on the side of enhanced tactile perception in ASD. There is also burgeoning evidence that organization of somatosensory cortex is aberrant in this group of NDDs. For instance, magnetoencephalography (MEG) of somatosensory cortex in individuals with autism has shown an unusual organization of somatotopic maps representing the body surface in the brain (Coskun et al., 2009),

Disorders affecting linguistic and scholastic skills development. Some NDDs specifically affect language abilities or isolated scholastic skills such as math and reading. Among these, developmental dyslexia has been well-studied from a basic sensory processing perspective. Developmental dyslexia is defined as failure to achieve reading ability commensurate with general intellectual ability, educational opportunities, and motivation. There is evidence in the visual and auditory systems that reading impairments in dyslexia are secondary to a generalized sensory impairment for rapidly changing or transient stimuli (Eden et al., 1996; Hairston, Burdette, Flowers, Wood, & Wallace, 2005). This has been extended to the somatosensory system, which includes channels that are specifically tuned to process transient, dynamic stimuli.

Adults with dyslexia show impairments in judging the simultaneity of a series of tactile stimuli (Laasonen, Service, & Virsu, 2001, 2002), have elevated detection thresholds for certain frequencies of vibration (Stoodley, Talcott, Carter, Witton, & Stein, 2000), and are impaired at discriminating the duration of a tactile stimulus (Cascio, Morris, & Sathian, 2002). In contrast, Grant, Zangaladze, Thiagarajah, and Sathian (1999) reported impairment in discrimination of the orientation of a grating impressed statically onto the skin, a task used to index tactile spatial processing (Johnson & Phillips, 1981). However, Grant and colleagues (1999) reported only a trend toward impairment in discrimination of texture differences by actively scanning gratings varying in ridge width, a task thought to involve temporal information (Cascio & Sathian, 2001). Moore, Brown, Markee, Theberge, and Zvi (1999) demonstrated impaired localization of tactile stimulation in individuals with dyslexia. Using somatosensory-evoked magnetic fields, Renvall, Lehtonen, and Hari (2005) demonstrated that the response recovery in somatosensory cortex is impeded in dyslexia, leading to smaller responses to successive stimuli in a sequence. This is in keeping with the notion of a temporal processing deficit that extends to the tactile system.

Evidence for decreased interhemispheric transfer of tactile signals has been found in both individuals with developmental language disorder (Fabbro, Libera, & Tavano, 2002) and dyslexia (Moore et al., 1999), although Davidson, Leslie, and Sarron (1990) found no group differences in interhemispheric transfer time in children with reading disability. A study by Soltesz, Szuchs, Dekany, Markus, and Csepe (2007) also demonstrated that stereognosis is compromised in developmental dyscalculia, an analogous disorder that exclusively affects mathematical skills. Thus, the combined evidence suggests that even for linguistic and scholastic skills that typically do not rely on touch, individuals with impairments of scholastic skills experience tactile stimuli differently than individuals without these impairments. This supports the idea that dyslexia and other neurobiologically driven scholastic problems may arise from more generalized sensory processing problems.

Attention-deficit hyperactivity disorder. A subset of NDDs primarily affects motor or executive behaviors, although social, communicative, or scholastic dysfunction may be secondary characteristics. One example is ADHD, which is characterized by impulsiveness, hyperactivity, and inattention. Parush, Sohmer, Steinberg, and Kaitz (1997) tested a sample of children with ADHD and found that their tactile thresholds were normal, but that they showed perceptual and cortical (measured by SEP) differences for suprathreshold tactile stimuli. Cortical responses were characterized by increased amplitude of late components of the SEP waveform. An increased incidence of tactile defensiveness was also noted in this sample. Later, these researchers confirmed that children with ADHD who experienced tactile defensiveness had significantly larger SEP amplitudes over central electrodes than either controls or ADHD children without tactile defensiveness (Parush, Sohmer, Steinberg, & Kaitz, 2007). However, a study by Ghanizadeh (2008) failed to find differences between ADHD subtypes when assessing tactile function using a checklist. Bröring, Rommelse, Sergeant, and Scherder (2008) found that girls with ADHD tended to show higher levels of tactile defensiveness than boys with ADHD, suggesting that girls may be more at risk for tactile dysfunction. Reynolds and Lane (2009) found that sensory over-responsivity in ADHD confers a greater risk for comorbid anxiety. A possible genetic basis of altered somatosensory perception in ADHD was discovered by Scherder, Romelse, Bröring, Faraone, and Sergeant (2008) who found similar impairments in children with ADHD and their unaffected siblings. These investigators also found no association between tactile impairments in ADHD and pain tolerance, supporting clear distinctions in these somatosensory domains.

In brain-based studies, primary and secondary somatosensory cortical responses to electrical stimulation of the median nerve were measured with MEG from adults with ADHD (Dockstader et al., 2008). Investigators found altered patterns of synchronization and desynchronization of cortical rhythms in the ADHD group. Using a similar paradigm, this group investigated cortical oscillations of the magnetoencephalographic response to unpredictable median nerve stimulation (Dockstader, Gaetz, Cheyne, & Tannock, 2009). These rhythms are believed to represent a mechanism for linking perception and action, a link that may be compromised in ADHD. The ADHD group showed lower oscillatory activity relative to controls, suggesting a deficit in the perception-to-action system. Finally, a structural brain study using

CHAPTER 16 NEURODEVELOPMENTAL DISORDERS 421

voxel-based morphometry, conducted by Carmona et al. (2005), demonstrated reduced gray matter in a variety of brain regions including somatosensory cortex in ADHD. These atypicalities of cortical structure and function related to somatosensory processing are likely the neural underpinnings of tactile defensiveness and decreased tactile discriminative abilities (Parush et al., 1997) in ADHD. However, more research must be done to replicate both neural and behavioral findings.

Disorders Arising From Early Environmental Factors

Some NDDs are known to be primarily environmental in etiology. These conditions often arise as a result of prenatal, perinatal, or early environmental factors that impact the nervous system. In this section, tactile dysfunction is addressed for three examples in this category: cerebral palsy (CP), fetal alcohol syndrome (FAS), and children who experience early sensory deprivation.

Cerebral palsy. One of the most common examples of NDD that arises from environmental factors is CP, which is actually an umbrella term to describe a group of disorders that are characterized by impaired motor abilities and are nonprogressive throughout development. The most common variant is spastic diplegia, which affects the lower extremities with hypertonia. Spastic hemiplegia (one side affected) or tetraplegia (all four limbs affected) are less common variants that are also characterized primarily by hypertonia. These variants of CP are caused by GABA deficiencies in the corticospinal tract or motor cortex. Ataxic and dyskinetic variants are more rare, the former arising from cerebellar damage and the latter from damage to the extrapyramidal motor system and basal ganglia. These neural systems can be damaged by intrauterine trauma such as maternal infection, exposure to teratogens, complications during labor and delivery, hypoxic brain injury, or other pre- or perinatal trauma.

There are ubiquitous reports of impaired discriminative tactile abilities in CP (see Clayton, Fleming, & Copley, 2003, for a comprehensive review). Wingert, Burton, Sinclair, Brunstrom, and Damiano (2008) found texture perception to be impaired in a CP sample relative to controls. Impaired stereognosis has been reported (Wingert et al., 2008), although this skill is likely to be particularly affected by motor impairments in manipulating objects (Dahlin, Komoto-Tufvesson, & Salgeback, 1998). Also impaired is finer-grained tactile spatial discrimination (Sanger & Kukke, 2007). In addition to discriminative ability, important information can also be obtained from affective responses to tactile stimuli. Curry and Exner (1988) postulated that the preference for hard versus soft objects was a manifestation of sensory-seeking behavior that resulted from decreased somatosensory awareness.

Neural studies of somatosensory processing in CP have provided insight into the basis for these sensory differences. Kulak, Sobaniec, Kuzia, and Bockowski (2006) noted altered SEPs in a CP group in response to somatosensory stimulation. Tomita and colleagues (2006) noted that the amplitude and topographic distribution of SEPs varies across subtypes of CP, which may reflect differential involvement of various sensorimotor systems. Investigation of sensory thalamocortical pathways in prematurely born children, using diffusion tensor imaging (Hoon et al., 2009), demonstrated significant relationships between tactile thresholds and the periventricular white matter injury that precipitated CP. This is important in light of the traditional understanding that motor, not sensory, tracts are the primary site of damage in CP (Wilke & Staudt, 2009) and highlights the inextricable link between somatosensory and motor systems. These results parallel other findings for high-risk infants which have shown that severe perinatal morbidity (such as white matter injury) predicts lower thresholds for reactivity to touch and more distress for infants when touched (Weiss & Wilson, 2006).

Fetal alcohol syndrome. Among the deleterious consequences of prenatal exposure to teratogenic substances is FAS, which results from chronic prenatal exposure to ethanol. FAS results in characteristic facial features; decreased growth; and delays in cognition, movement, and speech that arise from abnormal brain development. These effects continue to manifest as decreased IQ and impairments in executive function in adolescence and adulthood (Streissguth, Randels, & Smith, 1991). Dodge and colleagues (2009) reported that heavily or moderately exposed children show impairments in interhemispheric transfer of tactile information in a finger touch localization test. Children who were prenatally exposed to alcohol also have shown deficits in sensorimotor skills such as postural control (Roebuck, Simmons, Mattson, & Riley, 1998).

In nonhuman primate models of prenatal alcohol exposure, increased tactile defensiveness and reduced habituation to repeated tactile stimulation have been reported (Schneider et al., 2009), although stronger effects were obtained in conditions that included prenatal maternal stress. Rats exposed to prenatal alcohol exhibit dysmorphology in the somatosensory (barrel) cortex (Oladehin et al., 2007), which is at least partially mediated by a reduction in serotonin innervation

(Zhou, West, & Blake, 2005). Serotonin has a pivotal role in the development of sensory cortex, and these alterations are believed to give rise to sensorimotor deficits seen in FAS. Macaque monkeys similarly exposed to prenatal alcohol show significant decreases in neuron number in primary somatosensory cortex (Miller, 2007). The global deficits seen in FAS include tactile perceptual abilities that impact sensorimotor development; the evidence from animal models also suggests that affective responses to touch may be compromised by chronic prenatal alcohol exposure.

Early sensory deprivation. Sensory input early in infancy is critical to healthy development, and tactile input in the form of caregiver contact is a crucial component of this input. Natural experiments present themselves in cases of very premature or institutionalized infants who experience relatively little of this kind of tactile input in their neonatal environment. The effects of this lack of contact are deleterious and extend far beyond aberrations in sensory processing. Sensory integration, however, is clearly parametrically modulated by the length of time spent in such impoverished environments (Lin, Cermak, Coster, & Miller, 2005), resulting in diminished tactile discrimination abilities and heightened negative affective responses to tactile stimulation (Cermak & Daunhauer, 1997). This, in turn, impacts social and other behavioral development more broadly (Cermak & Groza, 2004).

Animal models allow the experimental investigation of touch deprivation in early development. Tactile deprivation in infant rats results in impaired active touch discriminative abilities (Carvell & Simons, 1996). As in humans, however, the effects of reduced contact early in infancy extend well beyond sensory abilities (Harlow & Harlow, 1962). Lack of tactile maternal contact (experimentally isolated from possible confounding variables such as deprivation of nourishment or heat) results in reduced levels of essential growth hormone gene expression (Schanberg, Ingledue, Lee, Hannun, & Batolome, 2003). Main and Stadtman (1981) found that lack of ventral–ventral contact early in infancy is associated with repetitive behaviors such as echolalia and stereotypies. The animal literature is replete with studies linking abnormal or absent early maternal touch to decreased cognitive abilities, novelty exploration, and attachment (Hertenstein et al., 2006).

Examples of the importance of early tactile contact from the animal literature have resulted in the exploration of touch-based interventions for isolated premature human infants, with dramatic success (Kuhn & Schanberg, 1998). Research has shown that preterm infants whose mothers touch their infants more frequently and who use touch that is more stimulating to the infant's nervous system have more advanced gross motor development and better visual-motor skills at 1 year of age (Weiss et al., 2004). Additional touch has been demonstrated to improve developmental outcomes in institutionalized infants as well (Casler, 1965). A meta-analysis of studies of infant massage efficacy suggests that interactions between mother and infant are significantly improved by regular touch (Underdown, Barlow, Chung, & Stewart-Brown, 2006). Such studies emphasize the important role of touch in early development and suggest that therapeutic approaches incorporating touch should continue to be used and developed in the treatment of premature infants. Research suggests that touch may be particularly important to the development of children born prematurely because of their underdeveloped nervous systems and their lack of exposure to normative tactile experiences that typically occur both in utero and during the neonatal period (Weiss, 2005).

USE OF TOUCH IN THERAPEUTIC INTERVENTIONS

As described earlier, therapeutic touch has been demonstrated to be highly effective in improving outcomes for very premature infants or infants with other perinatal obstacles to development. In older children, sensory-based interventions have become a prominent clinical focus for a variety of NDDs. Sensory integration therapy (SIT) addresses hypo- or hyperresponsiveness to sensory input using one-on-one play between the therapist and the child and is used frequently for children with ASD and disorders of scholastic skill acquisition. Activities in SIT typically involve a combination of sensory stimulation and movement or a sensory stimulus to which the child is asked to respond. The child is guided through these activities in a way that is both fun and challenging. Part of the theoretical basis for this kind of therapy is that there is a hierarchy within which different sensory systems fall, and proficiency in some systems are prerequisite to the proper development of others. This is often represented as a pyramid, with the tactile sense at the bottom, along with the vestibular and proprioceptive systems (Williams & Shellenberger, 1996). Thus tactile, proprioceptive, and vestibular sensation (i.e., proximal senses) are considered important for the proper development and integration of other senses as they are earliest to develop and provide a physical framework of the child's body in space and its boundaries upon which more distal senses such as vision and audition build. There have been conflicting reports as to the efficacy of SIT in various NDD populations (Baranek, 2002; Roberts, King-Thomas, & Boccia, 2007), although there is a consensus that the approach is understudied and more extensive and rigorous research is needed (Baranek, 2002; Schaaf & Miller, 2005).

Other therapeutic approaches that are specific to the tactile system include repetitive brushing of the skin and the use of deep pressure stimulation with weighted vests. The use of weighted vests is posited to improve attention and hyperactivity by modulating arousal levels. Reports from practitioners using this treatment were collected by Olson and Moulton (2004), who found that therapists did endorse improvements in attention after using the vests, although the potential for a self-selecting response bias among the therapists was acknowledged. A review conducted by Stephenson and Carter (2009) found little empirical evidence for the efficacy of weighted vests. Another controversial approach is the Wilbarger protocol, an intensive home treatment program in which deep pressure massage using a brush and gentle joint compression are administered by parents several times a day, often prescribed as part of a "sensory diet" (Wilbarger & Wilbarger, 1991). Enthusiastic anecdotal evidence describes gains in attention and improvements in sensory defensiveness, but very little empirical research has been conducted. A study by Kimball and colleagues (2007) measured salivary cortisol levels in four children before and after several administrations of the protocol and found that levels changed between pre- and post-test measurements. This preliminary evidence suggests that deep pressure stimulation affects arousal levels in these children.

The dearth of empirical research for these popular tactile therapeutic approaches highlights the importance of collaborative, translational research. Basic scientists with knowledge of neural and physiological responses and training in experimental design must join forces with clinicians and educators who have expertise in behavior and real-life applications. Such collaboration can either support these therapeutic approaches with a rigorous evidence base, or help to inform changes to these therapeutic approaches based on the evidence gathered from such translational work.

CONCLUSIONS

The work reviewed in this chapter reflects the central role of tactile processing in the development of social, communicative, and motor behavior. Disorders that affect neural development are associated with impairments in somatosensory discriminative abilities and affective responses to tactile stimulation, as measured by parent report, laboratory observation, and psychophysical approaches. The neural mechanisms underlying these differences are not well understood at this point, but a number of possible contributors have been discussed in the chapter. These include peripheral afferent pathology (particularly of the C-touch class of afferents), thalamocortical gating mechanisms in the flow of sensory information to primary somatosensory cortex, cortical structural patterns such as columnar organization and GABA-mediated inhibition of lateral cortical columns, rhythmic responses within sensory cortex, and top–down modulation of sensory cortical responses by prefrontal or other areas of cortex devoted to cognitive control.

NDDs that were previously attributed solely to motor system dysregulation, such as CP, are now being re-examined, and a prominent role for the somatosensory system has been demonstrated. Research suggests that the lack of tactile input for neonates has profound negative consequences not just for sensory processing but for development more generally. Therapeutic addition of tactile input for infants (through specific types of maternal touch, massage or kangaroo care) is showing promise in ameliorating these effects. Particularly for NDDs of complex or unknown genetic origin such as ADHD and autism, tactile-centered therapeutic approaches in older children may be effective in modulating arousal, attention, and sensory defensiveness. However, there is a substantial need for translational research both on the efficacy of these approaches and on their putative neural mechanisms.

A major challenge to progress in the field is the overlap between the phenotypic features of NDDs, which may arise from very different etiologies, and the disparate phenotypes that can arise from similar etiologies. Continued research at the levels of genetics, neural systems, and behavior is crucial if a clearer picture of the role of touch in NDDs is to emerge.

REFERENCES

American Psychiatric Association. (2000). Pervasive developmental disorders. *Diagnostic and statistical manual of mental disorders* (4th ed., pp. 69–84). Washington, DC: Author.

Baranek, G. T. (2002). Efficacy of sensory and motor interventions for children with autism. *Journal of Autism and Developmental Disorders, 32,* 397–422.

Baranek, G. T., Foster, L. G., & Berkson, G. (1997). Tactile defensiveness and stereotyped behaviors. *American Journal of Occupational Therapy, 51,* 91–95.

Baranek, G. T., Roberts, J. E., David, F. J., Sideris, J., Mirrett, P. L., Hatton, D. D., & Bailey, D. B. (2008). Developmental trajectories and correlates of sensory processing in young boys with fragile X syndrome. *Physical and Occupational Therapy in Pediatrics, 28,* 79–98.

Blakemore, S. J., Tavassoli, T., Calo, S., Thomas, R. M., Catmur, C., Frith, U., & Haggard, P. (2006). Tactile sensitivity in Asperger syndrome. *Brain and Cognition, 61,* 5–13.

Brandt, B. R. (1996). Impaired tactual perception in children with Down's syndrome. *Scandinavian Journal of Psychology, 37,* 312–316.

Brandt, B. R., & Rosen, I. (1998). Impaired peripheral somatosensory function in children of imprinted genes. *Acta Paediatrica, 423,* 55–57.

Bröring, T., Rommelse, N., Sergeant, J., & Scherder, E. (2008). Sex differences in tactile defensiveness in children with ADHD and their siblings. *Developmental Medicine and Child Neurology, 50,* 129–133.

Bureau, I., Shepherd, G.M., & Svoboda, K. (2008). Circuit and plasticity deficits in the developing somatosensory cortex of FMR1 knock-out mice. *Journal of Neuroscience, 28*(20), 5178–5188.

Butler, M. G., Allen, A., Haynes, J. L., Singh, D. N., Watson, M. S., & Breg, W. R. (1991). Anthropometric comparison of mentally retarded males with and without the fragile X syndrome. *American Journal of Medical Genetics, 38,* 260–268.

Carmona, S., Villarroya, O., Bielsa, A., Tremols, V., Soliva, J. C., Rovira, M., ... Bulbena, A. (2005). Global and regional grey matter reductions in ADHD: A voxel-based morphometric study. *Neuroscience Letters, 389,* 88–93.

Carvell, G. E., & Simons, D. J. (1996). Abnormal tactile experience early in life disrupts active touch. *Journal of Neuroscience, 16,* 2750–2757.

Cascio, C. J., McGlone, F., Folger, S., Tannan, V., Baranek, G., Pelphrey, K. A., & Essick, G. (2008). Tactile perception in adults with autism: a multidimensional psychophysical study. *Journal of Autism Development Disorders, 38,* 127–137.

Cascio, C. J., Morris, M. K., & Sathian, K. (2002). Impaired tactile perception in developmental dyslexia. *Society for Neuroscience Abstracts,* 154.11.

Cascio, C. J., & Sathian, K. (2001). Temporal cues contribute to tactile perception of roughness. *Journal of Neuroscience, 21,* 5289–5296.

Casler, L. (1965). The effects of extra tactile stimulation on a group of institutionalized infants. *Genetic Psychology Monographs, 71,* 137–75.

Cermak, S. A., & Daunhauer, L. A. (1997). Sensory processing in the post-institutionalized child. *American Journal of Occupational Therapy, 51,* 500–507.

Cermak, S. A., & Groza, V. (2004). Sensory processing problems in post-istitutionalized children: Implications for social work. *Child and Adolescent Social Work Journal, 15,* 5–37.

Chen, Y. J., & Fang, P. C. (2005). Sensory evoked potentials in infants with Down's Syndrome. *Acta Paediatrica, 94,* 1615–1618.

Clayton, K., Fleming, J. M., & Copley, J. (2003). Behavioral responses to tactile stimuli in children with cerebral palsy. *Physical and Occupational Therapy in Pediatrics, 23,* 43–62.

Coskun, M. A., Varghese, L., Reddoch, S., Castillo, E. M., Pearson, D. A., Loveland, K. A.,... Sheth, B. R. (2009). How somatic cortical maps differ in autistic and typical brains. *NeuroReport, 20,* 175–179.

Curry, J., & Exner, C. (1988). Comparison of tactile preferences in children with and without cerebral palsy. *American Journal of Occupational Therapy, 42,* 371–377.

Dahlin, L. B., Komoto-Tufvesson, Y., Salgeback, S. (1998). Surgery of the spastic hand in cerebral palsy: Improvements in stereognosis and hand function after surgery. *Journal of Hand Surgery, 23*, 334–339.

Davidson, R. J., Leslie, S. C., & Sarron, C. (1990). Reaction time measures of interhempisheric transfer time in reading disabled and normal children. *Neuopsychologia, 28*, 471–485.

Dockstader, C., Gaetz, W., Cheyne, D., & Tannock, R. (2009). Abnormal neural reactivity to unpredictable sensory events in attention-deficit/hyperactivity disorder. *Biological Psychiatry, 66*, 376–383.

Dockstader, C., Gaetz, W., Cheyne, D., Wang, F., Castellanos, F. X., & Tannock, R. (2008). MEG event-related desynchronization and synchronization deficits during basic somatosensory processing in individuals with ADHD. *Behavioral and Brain Functions, 4*, 1–13.

Dodge, N. C., Jacobson, J. L., Molteno, C. D., Meintjes, E. M., Bangalore, S., Diwadkar, V., . . . Jacobson, S. W. (2009). Prenatal alcohol exposure and interhemipsheric transfer of tactile information: Detroit and Cape Town findings. *Alcoholism: Clinical and Experimental Research, 33*, 1628–1637.

Dunbar, R. (1996). *Grooming, gossip, and the evolution of language.* Cambridge, MA: Harvard University Press.

Eden, G. F., Van Meter, J. W., Rumsey, J. M., Maisog, J. M., Woods, R. P., & Zeffiro, T. A. (1996). Abnormal processing of visual motion in dyslexia revealed by functional brain imaging. *Nature, 382*, 66–69.

Egawa, K., Asahina, N., Shiraishi, H., Kamada, K., Takeuchi, F., Nakane, S., ... Saitoh, S. (2008). Aberrant somatosensory evoked responses imply GABAergic dysfunction in Angelman syndrome. *NeuroImage, 39*, 593–599.

Fabbro, F., Libera, L., & Tavano, A. (2002). A callosal transfer defect in children with developmental language disorder. *Neuropsychologia, 40*, 1541–1546.

Ferri, R., Del Gracco, S., Elia, M., Musumeci, S. A., & Stefanini, M. C. (1996). Age and height dependent changes of amplitude and latency of somatosensory evoked potentials in children and young adults with Down's Syndrome. *Clinical Neurophysiology, 26*, 321–327.

Galvez, R., & Greenough, W. T. (2005). Sequence of abnormal dendritic spine development in primary somatosensory cortex of a mouse model of the fragile X mental retardation syndrome. *American Journal of Medical Genetics, 135*, 155–160.

Ghanizadeh, A. (2008). Tactile sensory dysfunction in children with ADHD. *Behavioral Neurology, 20*, 107–112.

Grandin, T. (2000). *An inside view of autism.* Fort Collins, CO: Colorado State University.

Grant, A. C., Zangaladze, A., Thiagarajah, M. C., & Sathian, K. (1999). Tactile perception in developmental dyslexia: a psychophysical study using gratings. *Neuropsychologia, 30*, 1201–1211.

Güçlü, B., Tanidir, C., Mukaddes, N. M., & Unal, F. (2007). Tactile sensitivity of normal and autistic children. *Somatosensory and Motor Research, 24*, 21–33.

Hagerman, R. J., Amiri, K., & Cronister, A. (1991). Fragile X checklist. *American Journal of Medical Genetics, 38*, 283–287.

Hairston, D. W., Burdette, J. H., Flowers, D. L., Wood, F. B., & Wallace, M. T. (2005). Altered temporal profile of visual-auditory multisensory interactions in dyslexia. *Experimental Brain Research, 166*, 474–480.

Harlow, H. F., & Harlow, M. K. (1962). The effect of rearing conditions on behavior. *Bulletin of the Menninger Clinic, 26*, 213–224.

Hertenstein, M. J., Verkamp, J. M., Kerestes, A. M., & Homes, R. M. (2006). The communicative function of touch in humans, nonhuman primates, and rats: a review and synthesis of the empirical research. *Genetic, Social and General Psychology Monographs, 132*, 5–94.

Hoon, A. H., Stashinko, E. E., Nage, L. M., Lin, D. D., Keller, J., Bastian, A., ... Johnston, M. V. (2009). Sensory and motor deficits in children with cerebral palsy born preterm correlate with diffusion tensor imaging abnormalities in thalmocortical pathways. *Developmental Medicine and Child Neurology, 51*, 697–704.

Johnson, K. O., & Phillips, J. R. (1981). Tactile spatial resolution. I. Two-point discrimination, gap detection, grating resolution, and letter recognition. *Journal of Neurophysiology, 46*, 1177–1192.

Kakigi, R., & Shibasaki, H. (1993). Scalp topography of somatosensory evoked potentials following median and posterior tibial nerve stimulation in Down's Syndrome. *Brain Topography, 5*, 253–261.

Kakigi, R., Shibasaki, H., & Ikeda, A. (1989). Pain-related somatosensory evoked potentials following CO laser stimulation in man. *Electroencephalography and Clinical Neurophysiology, 74*, 139–146.

Kimball, J. G., Lynch, K. M., Stewart, K. C., Williams. N. E., Thomas, M. A., & Atwood, K. D. (2007). Using salivary cortisol to measure the effects of a Wilbarger protocol based procedure on sympathetic arousal: A pilot study. *American Journal of Occupational Therapy, 61*, 406–413.

Kimura, K., Nomura, Y., & Segawa, M. (1992). Middle and short latency somatosensory evoked potentials in the Rett syndrome: chronological changes of cortical and subcortical involvements. *Brain Development, 14*, 37–42.

Kuhn, C. M., & Schanberg, S. M. (1998). Responses to maternal separation: mechanisms and mediators. *International Journal of Developmental Neuroscience, 16*, 261–270.

Kulak, W., Sobaniec, W., Kuzia, S. J., & Bockowski, L. (2006). Neurphysiologic and neuroimaging studies of brain plasticity in children with spastic cerebral palsy. *Experimental Neurology, 198*, 4–11.

Laasonen, M., Service, E., & Virsu, V. (2001). Temporal order and processing acuity of visual, auditory, and tactile perception in developmentally dyslexic young adults. *Cognitive, Affective, and Behavioral Neuroscience, 1*, 394–410.

Laasonen, M., Service, E., & Virsu, V. (2002). Crossmodal temporal order and processing acuity in developmentally dyslexic young adults. *Brain and Language, 80*, 340–354.

Lachiewicz, A. M., Spiridigliozzi, G. A., Gullion, C. M., & Ransford, S. N. (1994). Aberrant behaviors in boys with fragile X syndrome. *American Journal on Mental Retardation, 98*, 567–579.

Lewis, V. A., & Bryant, P. E. (1982) Touch and vision in normal and Down's syndrome babies. *Perception, 11*, 691–701.

Lin, S. H., Cermak, S., Coster, W. J., & Miller, L. (2005). The relation between length of institutionalization and sensory integration in children adopted from Eastern Europe. *American Journal of Occupational Therapy, 59*, 139–147.

Main, M., & Stadtman, J. (1981). Infant response to rejection of physical contact by the mother: Aggression, avoidance, and conflict. *Journal of the American Academy of Child Psychiatry, 20*, 292–307.

McGlone, F., Vallbo, A. B., Olausson, H., Loken, L. S., & Wessberg, J. (2007). Discriminative touch and emotional touch. *Canadian Journal of Experimental Psychology, 61*, 171–183.

Miller, L. J., McIntosh, D. N., McGrath, J., Shyu, V., Lampe, M., Taylor, A. K., ... Hagerman, R. J. (1999). Electrodermanl responses to sensory stimuli in individuals with fragile X syndrome: a preliminary report. *American Journal of Medical Genetics, 83*, 268–279.

Miller, M. W. (2007). Exposure to ethanol during gastrulation alters somatosensory-motor cortices and the underlying white matter in the macaque. *Cerebral Cortex, 17*, 2961–2971.

Montagu, A. (1986). *Touching: The human significance of the skin.* New York: Perennial Library.

Montagu, A., & Adubato, S. A. (1978). *Touching: The human significance of the skin.* New York: Harper and Row.

Moore, L. H., Brown, W. S., Markee, T. E., Theberge, D. C., & Zvi, J. C. (1999). Callosal transfer of finger localization information in phonologically dyslexic adults. *Cortex, 32*, 311–322.

Mottron, L., Dawson, M., Soulières, I., Hubert, B., & Burack, J. (2006). Enhanced perceptual functioning in autism: An update, and eight principles of autistic perception. *Journal of Autism and Developmental Disorders, 36*, 27–43.

Muir, D. W. (2002). Adult communications with infants through touch: The forgotten sense. *Human Development, 45*, 95–99.

Musumeci, S. A., Elia, M., Ferri, R., Scuderi, C., & Del Gracco, S. (1994). Evoked spikes and giant somatosensory evoked potentials in a patient with fragile X syndrome. *The Italian Journal of Neurological Sciences, 15*, 365–368.

Myers, B. J. (1984). Mother-infant bonding: the status of the critical-period hypothesis. *Developmental Review, 4*, 240–274.

Oladehin, A., Margaret, C. P., Maier, S. E., Li, C. X., Jan, T. A., Chappell, T. D., & Waters, R. S. (2007). Early postnatal alcohol exposure reduced the size of vibrissal barrel field in rat somatosensory cortex but did not disrupt barrel field organization. *Alcohol, 41*, 253–261.

Olausson, H., Lamarre, Y., Backlund, H., Morin, C., Wallin, B. G., Starck, G., ... Bushnell, M. C. (2002). Unmyelinated tactile afferents singal touch and project to insular cortex. *Nature Neuroscience, 5*, 900–904.

Olson, L. J., & Moulton, H. J. (2004). Use of weighted vests in pediatric occupational therapy practice. *Physical and Occupational Therapy in Pediatrics, 24*, 45–60.

O'Riordan, M., & Passetti, F. (2006). Discrimination in autism within different sensory modalities. *Journal of Autism and Developmental Disorders, 36*, 665–675.

Parush, S., Sohmer, H., Steinberg, A., & Kaitz, M. (1997). Somatosensory functioning in children with attention deficit hyperactivity disorder. *Developmental Medicine and Child Neurology, 39*, 464–468.

Parush, S., Sohmer, H., Steinberg, A., & Kaitz, M. (2007). Somatosensory function in boys with ADHD and tactile defensiveness. *Physiology and Behavior, 90*, 553–558.

Pernon, E., Pry, R., & Baghdadli, A. (2007). Autism: Tactile perception and emotion. *Journal of Intellectual Disability Research, 51*, 580–587.

Priano, L., Miscio, G., Grungi, G., Milano, E., Baudo, S., Selliti, L., ... Mauro, A. (2009). On the origin of sensory impairment and altered pain perception in Prader-Willi syndrome: A neurophysiological study. *European Journal of Pain, 13*, 829–835.

Renvall, H., Lehtonen, R., & Hari, R. (2005). Abnormal response recovery in the right somatosensory cortex of dyslexic adults. *Cerebral Cortex, 15*, 507–513.

Restivo, L., Ferrari, F., Passino, E., Sgobio, C., Bock, J., Oostra, B. A., ... Ammassari-Teule, M. (2005). Enriched environment promotes behavioral and morphological recovery in a mouse model for the fragile X syndrome. *Proceedings of the National Academy of Sciences, 102*, 11557–11562.

Reynolds, S., & Lane, S. J. (2009). Sensory overresponsivity in and anxiety in children with ADHD. *American Journal of Occupational Therapy, 63*, 433–440.

Roberts, J. E., King-Thomas, L., & Boccia, M. L. (2007). Behavioral indexes of efficacy sensory integration therapy. *American Journal of Occupational Therapy, 61*, 555–562.

Roebuck, T. M., Simmons, R. W., Mattson, S. N., & Riley, E. P. (1998). Prenatal exposure to alcohol affects the ability to maintain postural balance. *Alcoholism, Clinical and Experimental Research, 22*, 252–258.

Rogers, S. J., Hepburn, S., & Wehner, E. (2003). Parent reports of sensory symptoms in toddlers with autism and those with other developmental disorders. *Journal of Autism and Developmental Disorders, 33*, 631–642.

Sanger, T. D., & Kukke, S. N. (2007). Abnormalities of tactile sensory function in children with dystonic and diplegic cerebral palsy. *Journal of Child Neurology, 22*, 289–293.

Schaaf, R. C., & Miller, L. J. (2005). Occupational therapy using a sensory integrative approach for children with developmental disabilities. *Mental Retardation and Developmental Disabilities Research Review, 11*, 143–148.

Schanberg, S. M., Ingledue, V. F., Lee, J. Y., Hannun, Y. A., & Batolome, J. V. (2003). PKC alpha mediates maternal touch regulation of growth-related gene expression in infant rats. *Neuropsychopharmacology, 28*, 1026–1030.

Scherder, E. J. A., Rommelse, N. N. J., Bröring, T., Faraone, S. V., & Sergeant, J. A. (2008). Somatosensory functioning and experienced pain in ADHD families: A pilot study. *European Journal of Paediatric Neurology, 12*, 461–469.

Schneider, M. L., Moore, C. F., Larson, J. A., Barr, C. S., Dejesus, O. T., & Roberts, A. D. (2009). Timing of moderate level prenatal alcohol exposure influences gene expression of sensory processing behavior in rhesus monkeys. *Frontiers in Integrative Neuroscience, 3*, 30.

Selby, L., Zhang, C., & Sun, Q. (2007). Major defects in neocortical GABAergic inhibitory circuits in mice lacking the fragile X mental retardation protein. *Neuroscience Letters, 412*, 227–232.

Soltesz, F., Szucs, D., Dekany, J., Markus, A., & Csepe, V. (2007). A combined event related potential and neuropsychological investigation of developmental dyscalculia. *Neuroscience Letters, 417*, 181–186.

Stephenson, J., & Carter, M. (2009). The use of weighted vests with children with autism spectrum disorders and other disabilities. *Journal of Autism and Developmental Disorders, 39*, 105–114.

Stoodley, C. J., Talcott, J. B., Carter, E. L., Witton, C., & Stein, J. F. (2000). Selective deficits in vibrotactile sensitivity in dyslexic readers. *Neuroscience Letters, 295*, 13–16.

Streissguth, A. P., Randels, S. P., & Smith, D. F. (1991). A test-retest study of intelligence in patients with fetal alcohol syndrome: Implications for care. *Journal of the American Academy of Child and Adolescent Psychiatry, 30*, 584–587.

Tager-Flusberg, H. (1999). *Neurodevelopmental disorders*. Cambridge, MA: MIT Press.

Tombini, M., Pasqualetti, P., Rizzo, C., Zappasodi, F., Dinatale, A., Seminara, M.,...Agostino, R. (2009). Extrauterine maturation of somatosensory pathways in preterm infants: A somatosensory evoked potential study. *Clinical Neurophysiology, 120,* 783–789.

Tomchek, S. D., & Dunn, W. (2007). Sensory processing in children with and without autism: A comparative study using the Short Sensory Profile. *The American Journal of Occupational Therapy, 61,* 190–200.

Tomita, Y., Fukuda, C., Kafo, Y., Maegaki,Y., Shiota, S., & Amisaki, T. (2006). Topographic MN-SSEPs (N18, N20, and N30) might characterize underlying CNS involvements in representative types of cerebral palsy. *Brain and Development, 28,* 653–659.

Tommerdahl, M., Tannan, V., Cascio, C. J., Baranek, G. T., & Whitsel, B. L. (2007). Vibrotactile adaptation fails to enhance spatial localization in adults with autism. *Brain Research, 1154,* 116–123.

Underdown, A., Barlow, J., Chung, V., & Stewart-Brown, S. (2006). Massage intervention for promoting mental and physical health in infants aged under six months. Cochrane Database, *Systematic Reviews,* 18:CD005038.

Van Trotsenburg, A. S. P., Smit, B. J., Koelman, J. H. T. M., Dekker-van der Sloot, M., Ridder, J. C. D., Tijssen, J. G. P.,...Vulsma, T. (2006). Median nerve conduction velocity and central conduction time measured with somatosensory evoked potentials in thyroxine-treated infants with Down's Syndrome. *Pediatrics, 118,* 825–832.

Walz, N. C., & Baranek, G. T. (2006). Sensory processing patterns in persons with Angelman syndrome. *The American Journal of Occupational Therapy, 60,* 472–479.

Weiss, S. (2005). Haptic perception and the psychosocial functioning of premature, low birth weight children. *Infant Behavior and Development, 28,* 329–359.

Weiss, S., & Wilson, P. (2006). Origins of tactile vulnerability in high risk infants. *Advances in Neonatal Care, 6,* 25–36.

Weiss, S. J., Wilson, P., Hertenstein, M. J., & Campos, R. G. (2000). The tactile context of a mother's caregiving: Implications for attachment of low birth weight infants. *Infant Behavior and Development, 23,* 91–111.

Weiss, S. J., Wilson, P., & Morrison, D. (2004). Maternal tactile stimulation and the neurodevelopment of low birth weight infants. *Infancy, 5,* 85–107.

Wilbarger, P., & Wilbarger, J. (1991). *Sensory defensiveness in children ages 2–12: An intervention guide for parents and other caretakers.* Santa Barbara, CA: Avanti Educational Programs.

Wilke, M., & Staudt, M. (2009). Does damage to somatosensory circuits underlie motor impairment in cerebral palsy. *Developmental Medicine and Child Neurology, 51,* 686–687.

Williams, C. A., Beaudet, A. L., Clayton-Smith, J., Knoll, J. H., Kyllermann, M., Laan, L. A.,...Wagstaff, J. (2005). Angleman Syndrome 2005: Updated consensus for diagnostic criteria. *American Journal of Medical Genetics, 140,* 413–418.

Williams, M. S., & Shellenberger, S. (1996). *"How does your engine run?" A leader's guide to the alert program for self-regulation.* Albuquerque, NM: TherapyWorks.

Wingert, J. R., Burton, H., Sinclair, R. J., Brunstrom, J. E., & Damiano, D. L. (2008). Tactile sensory abilities in cerebral palsy: Deficits in roughness and object discrimination. *Developmental Medicine and Child Neurology, 50,* 832–838.

Yoshikawa, H., Kaga, M., Suzuki, H., Sakuragawa, N., & Arima, M. (1991). Giant somatosensory evoked potentials in the Rett syndrome. *Brain Development, 13*, 36–39.

Zhou, F. C., West, J. R., & Blake, C. A. (2005). General discussion at the fetal alcohol syndrome symposium. *Experimental Biology and Medicine, 230*, 407–412.

17

Touch in People Who Are Visually Impaired

MORTON A. HELLER AND ANNE McCLURE WALK

*B*lind people are just like the rest of us: they just can't see. However, visual impairment has substantial consequences for an individual's life and his/her interaction with the world. It impacts pattern perception, mobility and spatial orientation, and educational opportunities. Although blindness can clearly alter a person's social and economic well being, this chapter will focus on touch perception in people who are blind or have very low vision (VLV). It will not discuss mobility or the social consequences of blindness, since those are properly the subjects of other chapters.

There are a number of important reasons for research interest in the consequences of visual impairment for touch perception. People who are congenitally blind (CB) and born without sight must rely on touch for much of their pattern perception. Because they lack visual experience and visual imagery, an examination of "pure touch," without any visual contamination is possible. This fascination with touch in the CB individual is due to a desire for experimental control. If a researcher blindfolds a sighted person, the memory of visual imagery still remains. Consequently, the effects of blindfolding are not comparable to acquired or congenital blindness. Millar (2008) has argued that touch can provide substitute information for a lack of sight in blindness. There is considerable empirical data in support of this position (see Heller & Ballesteros, 2006).

MYTHS AND REALITY

One common misconception is that blind people invariably compensate for their lack of sight with reliance on touch, and an increased ability in that sense. The sensory compensation hypothesis seems compelling, but the evidence is contradictory in this area (see Heller & Ballesteros, 2006). While some blind individuals have exceptional tactile skills, others do not (Dulin & Hatwell, 2006). The experimental evidence bearing on this idea will be discussed later in this chapter. Clearly, visual experience can matter and may play a role in the final outcome. People who are late blind (LB) or have VLV may benefit from early sight. Individuals with VLV may have large object perception and residual light perception. Many of these VLV people refer to themselves as blind, use a long cane for mobility, and read Braille. They are likely to have minimal or no pattern perception. If they can see the location of a strong light source, this can help with mobility.

One caveat in this area is that development of perception in touch in blind people proceeds at a different rate than in vision in the sighted (see Hatwell, 1985). There are educational lags as well, as many blind people graduate from high school when they are much older than their sighted counterparts. It takes longer to acquire information using the sense of touch. Also, the education of a visually impaired person is different from that of a sighted individual. It may involve considerable time devoted to mobility training, for example. Furthermore, this can come at the expense of time devoted to a number of academic subjects. There are other differences as well, which will be discussed as deemed appropriate.

PATTERN PERCEPTION

Many researchers have stressed the idea that pattern perception, using touch, is less adequate than in vision (e.g., Lederman et al., 1990). The argument stems from the observation that many forms take longer to explore using touch compared with vision. Thus, active exploration of forms using touch, or haptics, may often be sequential when forms or objects are large. This can impose a burden on memory for touch. However, one can make the identical argument for vision. If one looks at a very large building, for example, one may need to look at sections of it sequentially. The important point is that vision is suited to pattern perception on a much larger scale than when using haptics. One cannot feel the skyline of a large city, but it is possible to feel a model of a skyline, if that were available. The differences that appear between vision and touch may be differences in scale, rather than in nature.

The idea that touch is slow and cumbersome may derive, in part, from the observation of blindfolded sighted subjects in the laboratory. While undergraduate students are convenient participants in research projects, they are relatively unskilled in the use of touch for pattern perception. They are generally much slower than blind subjects in many pattern perception tasks (see Heller & Ballesteros, 2006). It may be a mistake to attempt to generalize from poor and slow performance by blindfolded sighted subjects to haptics in blind people. For example, there is clear evidence that blind individuals show better performance in a variety of tasks (Sathian, 2000). Thus, it is difficult to assume deficiencies in touch when much of the evidence derives from blindfolded sighted persons with poor haptic skills.

PICTURES TO TOUCH

Many researchers have assumed that an understanding of pictures may be very difficult for the sense of touch. For example, some researchers have argued that it may be hard to express depth relations in tangible pictures (e.g., Holmes, Hughes, & Jansson, 1998; Jansson & Holmes, 2003). Thus, one would not expect people, who are born without sight, to understand perspective. However, this assumes that linear perspective is solely a visual phenomenon (e.g., Arditi, Holtzman, & Kosslyn, 1988). Arditi et al. (1988) found that CB people did not seem to use perspective in their mental imagery. Unlike the illusion of converging diagonals that one sees when looking at railroad tracks, when feeling a 3D rectangle, the receding outside edges do not normally feel as if they converge in the distance. On this interpretation, perspective distortion is a form of illusory misperception that characterizes vision, but not touch. However, Kennedy and Juricevic (2006) have claimed that perspective in drawings involves the laws of direction, and direction is meaningful for touch as well as vision. Note, however, that sighted people need to learn to draw in perspective. Untutored drawing may not be all that good, as any art instructor can attest. Moreover, perspective effects can induce illusions in sighted individuals.

There are other reasons to expect difficulties for blind people in the interpretation or production of tangible drawings. One argument is that drawings are not ecologically valid for touch (e.g., Lederman, Klatzky, Chataway, & Summers, 1990). On this theoretical point of view, touch has evolved to cope with objects and their material properties, such as hardness, softness, texture, and so forth. Lederman et al. (1990) have argued that visual mediation is needed when one feels a picture. Blindfolded sighted individuals routinely report using visual imagery when they feel pictures. In that respect, there are certainly empirical reports that it may be difficult for blindfolded sighted (Lederman et al., 1990) or blind people to name tangible pictures that they feel (e.g., Heller, 1989). Therefore, visual experience, combined with haptic skills, may help the LB, since they did better than the sighted or CB in naming tangible pictures (Heller, 1989).

It is important to point out that naming is a coarse measure of perceptual functioning, and likely taps higher level cognitive processing. One can certainly recognize a person, yet forget his/her name. Moreover, if one were to view a picture of an unfamiliar object, it is unlikely that the perceiver will name it correctly. We do not assume that a very young child cannot see a cat properly, because the child calls the cat a "doggy."

There is little doubt that categorical and linguistic information play an important role in naming failures when naïve CB people first attempt to identify tangible raised-line pictures (see Heller, Calcaterra, Burson, & Tyler, 1996). Most of these individuals have had little or no experience with drawing or the recognition of drawings. However, perceptual recognition of pictures can be very high in a matching task (Heller, Brackett, & Scroggs, 2002). Moreover, the recognition of tactile pictures is superior when categorical information is provided (Heller, Calcaterra, & Burson, et al., 1996). Heller et al. asked blindfolded and blind people to name tangible pictures. Performance was excellent when participants were given categorical information. For example, it was easy for blindfolded participants to select the picture of say, an apple, from three pictures of "fruit." Also, it greatly helped participants identify tangible pictures when they were told the major category to which a picture belonged. Thus, it was much easier to verbally identify a tangible picture of a table when told first that it is a type of furniture. These results suggest that many reported naming failures in haptic picture identification and low performance in the CB may be related to a lack of access to categorical information, rather than perceptual failures, per se.

Heller, Brackett, Scroggs, Allen, and Green (2001) found that CB individuals understood the Piagetian water-level problem. The task was intended to determine if visual experience were necessary to understand the physical concept that water levels stay horizontal when water is in a tilted container (see Figure 17.1). Piaget asked children to anticipate the water level in a tilted container, and then asked them to draw the water level as they looked at water in a tilted container (Piaget & Inhelder, 1956).

The Heller et al. (2001) haptic experiment required groups of CB, LB, participants with VLV, and blindfolded sighted individuals to feel raised-line pictures of tilted jars drawn at four angles: $-60°$, $-30°$, $30°$, and $60°$. On each trial, the subjects were exposed to four raised-line

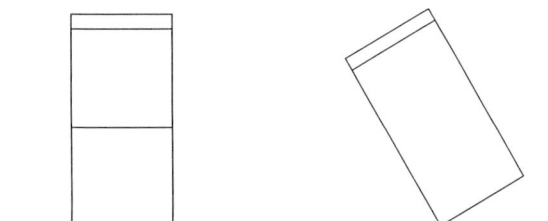

FIGURE 17.1 Shows a model raised-line jar with a horizontal water level. The drawing of the jar on the right was used in an earlier study where participants had to draw in the water line while blindfolded, using a raised-line drawing kit. Adapted with permission from "Perception of the horizontal and vertical in tangible displays: Minimal gender differences," by M. A. Heller, J. A. Calcaterra, S. L. Green, & S. L. Barnette, 1999, *Perception, 28*, 387–394. Copyright 1999 by Pion Publishers.

pictures of the jars at one of these angles. Only one of the jars had the correct depiction of the water level, and the task was to indicate which one was correct. The best performance was shown by the participants with VLV (about 98% correct), but lower accuracy was found for the CB and the blindfolded sighted participants. Performance of the CB and blindfolded sighted participants was comparable. Clearly, visual experience and visual imagery are not needed for understanding the task. There is little doubt that experience with pictures can be helpful, but this experience could occur in the haptic modality.

Vision is not needed to discriminate figure from ground in the embedded figures task. This task is analogous to a camouflage situation, where it may be difficult to see a figure against a complex background. Heller et al. (2003) asked groups of CB, LB, VLV, and blindfolded sighted subjects to try to locate target figures in simple and complex backgrounds. The VLV participants had high levels of performance. It was interesting that they did almost as well as an additional group of sighted participants using vision. While touch is slower than vision, it may accomplish many of the same things, but on a smaller scale. The performance of the CB and blindfolded sighted subjects was similar, again indicating that visual experience is not needed to segregate figure from ground in raised-line pictures.

What then of the frequently expressed idea that linear perspective is a problem for people who are CB? Initially, this may be the case for naïve CB individuals without any experience with drawing. However, Heller, Kennedy, and Joyner (1995) found that some blind participants used aspects of perspective when making drawings of a model house. Heller, Calcaterra, Tyler, and Burson (1996) asked CB, LB, people with

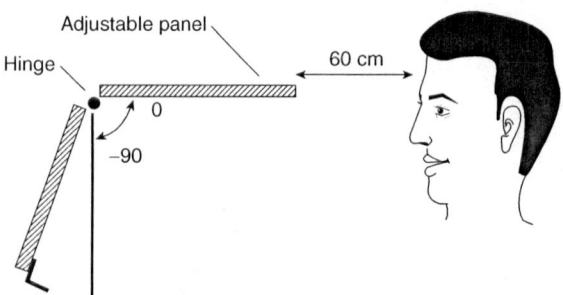

FIGURE 17.2 This shows the board used to test the understanding of perspective in people who are congenitally blind. The board is shown in a horizontal orientation, where the image is a very narrow rectangle. Adapted with permission from "Production and interpretation of perspective drawings by blind and sighted people," by M. A. Heller, J. A. Calcaterra, L. A. Tyler, & L. L. Burson, 1996, *Perception, 25,* 321–334. Copyright 1996 by Pion Publishers.

VLV, and blindfolded participants to feel a board at a number of angles and then make raised-line pictures of the board to "show the slant" (see Figure 17.2). The board was either upright or slanted at −67.5°, −45°, −22.5°, or horizontal. When upright, the image would be a rectangle. The visual image changed to foreshortened views as the board was tilted, that is, a rectangular surface prompted an image that was considerably shorter when at a slant than when upright. The CB participants did not show any differences in the heights of their drawings when the board was tilted. Their spontaneous drawings indicated a lack of any appreciation of linear perspective. The others produced drawings that varied in height as a function of angle, and this indicates the role of visual imagery and prior experience with pictures in their interpretation of tangible drawings. However, this experience need not be visual. In a subsequent experiment, the participants were exposed to the tangible pictures in Figure 17.3. They were told that the drawings indicated how the board would look to a sighted person. Then they felt the board at the different angles, and their task was to indicate which picture corresponded to the board at a slant. The results showed that while the performance of late-blind subjects was higher than the CB and blindfolded sighted participants, the differences between the groups were not statistically significant. The results indicate that while visual experience is helpful, it is obviously not necessary. Haptic experience may successfully substitute for visual experience.

Other research has yielded results that are consistent with the idea that CB people can understand perspective drawings of complex objects and very complicated views of a model house (Heller, Brackett,

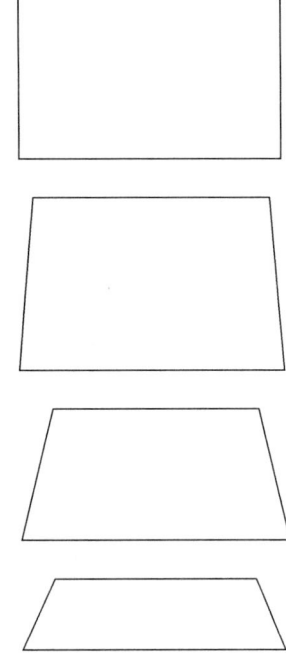

FIGURE 17.3 This figure illustrates the raised-line drawings used in the experiment on linear perspective. The figure shows the perspective drawings of the panel at −67.5°, −45°, −22.5°, and horizontal. The drawing of the vertical panel is at the top. Adapted with permission from "Production and interpretation of perspective drawings by blind and sighted people," by M. A. Heller, J. A. Calcaterra, L. A. Tyler, & L. L. Burson, 1996, *Perception*, 25, 321–334. Copyright 1996 by Pion Publishers.

Scroggs, et al., 2002; Heller et al., 2009). CB persons are able to adopt the viewpoint of another individual in a haptic analog of the Piagetian three-mountain task (Heller & Kennedy, 1990). Thus, prior visual experience is not needed to permit an individual to go beyond egocentrism and understand the viewpoint of another person.

Linear perspective may be comprehensible to blind people, but perhaps not without some experience with pictures (see Heller, 1989; Heller & Ballesteros, 2006; Heller, Brackett, Scroggs, et al., 2002; Heller et al., 2009). A number of CB individuals made very revealing comments when first exposed to perspective drawings. For example, one person remarked, after feeling an object that included as square shape (Heller, Brackett, Scroggs, et al.), "Oh, so you sighted people don't feel it as square." She was referring to the perspective distortion that existed in a raised-line drawing of the square surface. In a more recent study, a number of CB individuals said that they thought that it was "funny" that the experimenter referred to elevation when describing the vantage point of drawings of a model house. They did not realize that in the context of this experiment perspective depends upon elevation of a vantage point. It was also curious that a CB participant thought that sighted people should be able to see around the sides of objects, because of their peripheral vision. These examples illustrate the lack of familiarity with the rules of depiction that is found with people who are CB. They may have difficulty understanding just what is "visible," when an experiment demands this of them. In earlier research (Heller, Brackett, Scroggs, et al.), for example, one CB participant asked if a sighted person could see anything beyond the closest plane of the frontal view of a hexagonal solid. Thus, he did not know if he should include the receding visible surfaces in his drawings, since he had no idea about what would be visible in a drawing of this object. His initial thought was that sighted people would only see the closest surface, namely a rectangle with the long parts at the side, and the short sides at the top of the hexagonal solid. He did not realize that he should have been able to see three of the surfaces in a frontal view.

Complex perspective raised-line drawings are comprehensible to blind people, including pictures that depict elevated three-quarter views. Heller et al. (2009) found that CB subjects were able to correctly interpret elevated views of a model house, when the views were frontal, but also when they were elevated from a corner. Somewhat lower performance by the CB was found when tasks were more difficult and the task required them to discriminate between different amounts of elevation. However, the outcome indicated similar accuracy, in most instances, between the CB and blindfolded participants, with generally faster performance by the blind subjects. It was concluded that drawings might have considerable potential utility for people who are visually impaired, and even for those who are blinded from birth and lack visual experience.

ILLUSIONS IN TOUCH AND BLINDNESS

For quite some time, many researchers have been interested in haptic illusions. Of particular significance are the ways in which haptic illusions are both similar to and different from comparable visual illusions, and how they come to exist in CB individuals, who purportedly have no experience with perspective. A number of researchers assume that illusions are the result of mistaken perception of depth (Fisher, 1970) and inaccurate perception of depth/size constancy in drawings (Gregory, 1963). One might assume that since CB individuals have no experience with visual depth perception, most of the illusions that are common in vision would cease to exist in touch. However, these presumably "visual" illusions occur in touch and in people who are blind from birth.

The horizontal–vertical illusion and the Muller-Lyer illusion have both appeared in CB samples. Heller and Joyner (1993) had CB, LB, and blindfolded sighted subjects explore raised-line drawings of inverted T or L shapes. They found that when making size judgments about the horizontal and vertical extents, LB and sighted subjects acted similarly; the illusion existed haptically in the inverted T shapes, but not in the L shapes. CB subjects, on the other hand, showed the illusion with both types of stimuli. However, a later study showed no differences across the groups; CB, LB, and blindfolded sighted participants all showed the illusion for both inverted T and L shapes (Heller, Brackett, Wilson, Yoneyama, & Boyer, 2002). Thus, the results indicate some differences between spatial processing in the CB and other participants.

Traditionally, the horizontal–vertical illusion using inverted T shapes has been partially attributed to bisection, which may be true in both vision and touch. It is thought that people judge a bisected line as shorter than a continuous line. This may explain the stronger illusion seen using inverted T shapes rather than L shapes in the previous study.

However, both studies showed that the illusion was stronger in the larger stimuli (where the lines measured 10.16 cm) than in the smaller stimuli (where the lines measured 2.54 cm). This may be an indication of another factor at play: radial tangential scanning. In other words, the illusion may be due to the proprioceptive information. Namely, it was due to input from the movement in the arm rather than to the actual haptic coding of the stimuli. Further evidence for this comes from Heller, Calcaterra, Burson, and Green (1997). They demonstrated that subjects are more likely to use scanning strategies that employ the entire arm when exploring large stimuli, but are likely to use only movement of the finger and wrist when exploring small stimuli. They also showed that subjects treated bisected and continuous lines in the same way, when the lines did not comprise the configuration of an inverted T. This indicates that bisection cannot be the sole explanation of the existence of the horizontal–vertical illusion in touch. It seems that radial tangential scanning also plays a crucial role.

The Mueller-Lyer illusion has also been shown to exist in CB individuals. In this illusion, two horizontal or two vertical lines, equal in length, appear different sizes depending on whether wings are inward of the end of the line (wings-in stimuli) or outward of the end (wings-out stimuli). Heller, Brackett, Wilson, Yoneyama, Boyer, and Steffen (2002) found that the presence of the Mueller-Lyer illusion was unaffected by visual experience. A traditional explanation for the visual Mueller-Lyer illusion is that people are responding to global size, rather than line length. This hypothesis would predict that participants would be more accurate in estimates of the length of a stimulus that had plain (vertical) ends, if it matched the global size of the wings in and wings out stimuli. This was not found to be the case in touch. Participants underestimated wings in stimuli even when they were matched in global size to the stimuli with plain ends, which was inconsistent with the global size explanation of the illusion.

An alternative, more likely explanation is the confusion hypothesis. This hypothesis proposes that participants misjudge the lengths of the lines because they cannot feel where the line ends and the wings begin. This may be a result of sensory inhibition or confusion. If participants do not possess the tactile acuity to feel exactly where the line ends and the wing begins, it is unlikely that they will accurately estimate the length of the straight line. This hypothesis can be used to explain both the overestimation of the wings-out stimuli as well as underestimation of the wings-in stimuli compared to plain-ended stimuli of equal global size.

It should be noted that this particular illusion is very sensitive to the manner of exploration employed (Heller et al., 2005). For example, the illusion is attenuated when tracing with two index fingers is used, and barely exists when participants use two hands to explore the stimuli. This may be because the body can more easily be engaged as a frame of reference when two hands are used.

One geometrical illusion that does not exist in touch or blind people is the Ponzo illusion. It consists of two horizontal lines, equal in length, which are placed at varying heights between two converging lines, like in a picture of railroad tracks receding into the distance. In vision, the higher line, which is closer in proximity to the converging lines, appears larger (Heller, Hasselbring, Wilson, Shanley, & Yoneyama, 2004). It is thought that this illusion exists in vision because of perspective cues; the top line appears to be further in the distance, and so it is assumed to be larger. Thus, one possible explanation for the lack of its existence in touch is the lack of visual experience that blind people have with perceptual encoding. However, blindfolded sighted participants, as well as those who were CB, also did not show the illusion (Heller et al., 2004). Similar results with a very different methodology were reported by Casla, Blanco, and Travieso (1999). An alternative explanation is that, in the study reported, participants felt the stimuli sequentially. The presence of the Ponzo illusion may be dependent on experiencing the entire array simultaneously, as in vision. Misapplied size constancy scaling may then play a role in the induction of the illusion.

Many illusions that exist in vision have also been shown to exist in touch and in CB samples. For example, the haptic horizontal–vertical illusion occurs with curves in blindfolded sighted and in CB individuals (Heller et al., 2008). Most of the traditional explanations for the visual illusions deal with visual perspective and would therefore indicate a need for previous visual experience in order for the illusion to exist in touch. However, recent work has shown that the haptic illusions may be due to alternative explanations, typically involving the impact of scanning and movement patterns. If one does not adopt optimal methods for feeling illusory patterns, then misperception is likely. However, there are clearly instances where illusions may be overcome with optimal exploration strategies, namely the use of multiple fingers of both hands (e.g., Heller et al., 2005). Thus, while the illusions may occur in both the senses of vision and touch, and occur in blind people, causal factors may not always be identical.

MAPS

Maps may be very useful for blind people, but they pose a number of challenges. Some of the difficulties in tangible maps are similar to those in maps that are viewed, but some are unique to the sense of touch. Use of a map of any sort requires that the individual understand the relationship between himself/herself and the map, and the relationship between the map and larger space in the world. Mobility derived from map use also depends on successful orientation in the environment. Directions in the map need to be related to directions in the world. Spatial frames of reference need to be understood, namely the horizontal and vertical if people are to understand the cardinal directions of north, south, east and west. There can be difficulties derived from the original perception of the map itself. If maps are too small, then they tax the acuity of the skin, and touch is subject to reduced spatial acuity compared to vision. If a map is too large, it can be difficult to get an overview, because the map must be explored sequentially. This places a severe burden on memory.

Rossano and Warren (1989) have pointed out that if a map is misaligned with respect to the environment, then it is difficult to make use of it for directional judgments. They asked visually impaired participants to point to locations in space, but they had to get spatial information from very simple tangible maps. Errors were large, but larger when the maps were misaligned, that is, straight ahead on the map did not correspond to straight ahead in the environment. Moreover, differences between sighted and blind subjects appeared that were attributed to visual experience with object rotations. Scale can also be a problem for blind people. For example, one visually impaired individual told

M. Heller that she found it very difficult to use maps because of the radical change in scale from the map to larger scale space.

Tangible maps are certainly useful to many blind people. However, there are large individual differences in map-reading skills in people who are visually impaired, just as there are in sighted individuals. It is difficult to come to any clear generalizations about task difficulty for blind people and touch, given this variability.

BRAILLE

Braille is a useful written method of communication for people who are visually impaired (Foulke, 1982; Millar, 1997). It is an abstract code in which the letters of the alphabet are represented by varying patterns and numbers of small raised dots within a two by three matrix. The dot locations in these six loci are a matrix including two across and three vertically, with vertical size limited to just about 6 mm. The small size of Braille configurations adds to the difficulty of learning and reading Braille. Furthermore, it is very rare to ever find a sighted person who is able to read Braille text with any proficiency using the sense of touch. While these sighted persons may exist, the authors of this chapter have never met such an individual. For example, Heller (1993) compared the reading skills of blind individuals who were frequent readers of Braille, with sighted subjects. The sighted participants had the Braille code visible, but could not see the embossed two-letter Braille words they felt. The number of words correct for the sighted and blind participants (out of 25) were 7.1 and 25, respectively. It was not surprising that the blind subjects excelled. However, the task was exceptionally difficult for sighted individuals. The sighted participants had great difficulty discriminating which dots belonged to which Braille characters, owing to the very small size of the dots and minimal spacing between the characters in normal Braille.

There is little doubt about the importance and value of Braille, yet it is a dying skill. It is important to learn to read in childhood, whether the modality is in vision or touch. However, most people who lose their sight do so much later in life, at a time when tactile acuity diminishes and the impact of visual loss is difficult to cope with. If one loses sight at 50, it is very unlikely that the affected individual will devote the time needed to learn to read with his/her fingers. If visual loss occurs at 30 because of diabetic retinopathy, the same holds true, with the added complication of neuropathy and greatly reduced tactile sensitivity.

Skilled readers of Braille are likely to have learned to read in early childhood, and generally use the index fingers of both hands to scan text. Most use the right hand to read and the left as a locator in the text, and to find the next line of Braille (see Millar, 1997, 2008, for a more detailed discussion). Novice readers tend to repeatedly trace over a single character, as if to try to ascertain the global shape. Fast reading requires smooth, uninterrupted lateral scanning, and this vertical "scrubbing," that is vertical tracing, slows reading. Moreover, slow readers often stray from the line of text (Foulke, 1982). Millar has argued that both hands are normally used for reading in the skilled reader, but they alternate, with the right hand reading the line of Braille and the left locating the next line and beginning reading that line after the right has finished with the prior line. A similar description was provided by Foulke (1982). According to Foulke, slow readers use a single finger to read, and if two are used, then they simply scan together. Proficient readers start reading with the left index finger, and then switch to the right index finger by the middle of the line of text. They then use the left index finger to find the start of the next line of Braille. Thus, the left index finger starts the reading of each line of text.

Earlier literature looked at laterality effects, with very mixed results. There have been reports of better performance by the left hand, presumably due to better pattern perception in the right hemisphere (Heller, Rogers, & Perrry, 1990). While the right hemisphere has advantages for spatial tasks, the left is verbal. Therefore, it is not surprising that the results in the literature are mixed, since reading has spatial and verbal components (Millar, 2008).

Braille characters are defined by orientation, much as letters are in print. Thus, Braille characters corresponding to a B and C differ in orientation; both contain two dots, but they are vertical in the letter B and horizontal in the C. It is not surprising that Braille character recognition was degraded by tilt (Heller, 1992, 1993). Large orientation effects were found in sighted and in blind subjects. However, blind and sighted participants reported using different strategies when attempting to compensate for slant. Sighted individuals said that they imagined the patterns moving as they mentally rotated them, but CB individuals did not report this sort of imaginal process. In a later experiment Heller, Calcaterra, Green, and Lima (1999) compared LB, CB, and sighted subjects on Braille characters that were upright, left–right reversed, or a +180° rotation. The sighted subjects had much more difficulty than the blind individuals with the left–right reversals, and the LB participants were not affected at all by these reversals. Both groups of blind participants performed better than the sighted participants. The results were interpreted as showing that visual experience is hardly necessary for coping with changes in orientation. In fact, it is probably experience that matters, and this experience need not be visual. Note that blind individuals who are Braille readers are practiced with left–right reversals, since they must compensate for this when writing using a Braille slate. The Braille slate is a portable pocket device for embossing Braille dots. It includes a template with openings that correspond to the 2 by 3 possible positions of Braille dots. However, the person using the slate must use it with Braille paper upside-down to push in the dots with a stylus, and then turn the paper over, right to left, to reveal the raised dots. Thus, blind persons are practiced with left–right reversals if they use a Braille slate.

NEW TECHNOLOGY

New technology has had the potential to provide considerable assistance to people who are visually impaired. Blind individuals who can read Braille have been able to make good use of Braille displays that provide instant refreshable tangible output from their computers. Currently, individuals are likely to use Braille displays with a single line of refreshable Braille with home computers or laptops, but very expensive full-page Braille displays exist. Also, screen readers allow blind people to read the contents of word processors without a Braille display.

The recent advances in virtual touch hold considerable promise for communicating useful information to blind individuals. These devices use motors to provide force-feedback and constraints against manual manipulations. This permits the devices to simulate shapes, texture, weight, and other important properties of real objects. A very interesting device that is still under development provides 3D haptic shape information about sculptures to an individual sitting at a computer terminal (Jansson, Bergamasco, & Frisoli, 2003). The device uses an exoskeleton system to provide haptic simulations derived from movement of the hand/arm. One difficulty in some virtual touch devices is that they may depend on a single point source of resistance to simulate a shape. This is very limiting, and similar to using a single finger to feel a large 3D object. Multiple fingers work much better than a single finger for this purpose (Jansson & Monaci, 2004). The restriction of an observer to a single finger places a substantial load on memory. However, work is underway to use multiple virtual touch devices to enhance haptic perception (Munoz Sevilla, 2006).

A further problem is that it can be difficult to understand complex objects using virtual touch without any visual guidance of the hand (Jansson, 2002). Totally blind individuals are unable to see their hands and could have considerable difficulty making effective use of virtual touch. However, just as virtual touch has numerous potential applications for the education of sighted individuals, it may also hold promise for people who are blind or have VLV.

AGING

The senses become less acute as we age, and this also occurs in touch. Stevens, Foulke, and Patterson (1996) studied tactile sensitivity in a relatively large number of blind and age-matched sighted adults. The measure of acuity was the two-point threshold. Acuity declined in both groups at a comparable rate of about 1% per year. The practical implications of this bear on reading Braille, where the raised dots are very closely spaced. Enlarging the display is not an option for previously printed Braille material. In addition, the authors found a positive correlation between Braille reading rates and tactile acuity.

Visual declines also occur in aging, and the majority of blind people lose their sight when much older, due to the increased frequency of cataracts and macular degeneration as a function of age (Klein, 1991; Stevens, Foulke, & Patterson, 1996). These visual losses occur at a time in life when it would be more difficult to acquire necessary skills with the sense of touch.

The results of the study of Stevens, Foulke, and Patterson (1996) also bear on the previously mentioned sensory compensation hypothesis. Blind participants had better spatial acuity on their reading finger, and this advantage was maintained throughout (also see Van Boven, Hamilton, Kaufman, Keenan, & Pascual-Leone, 2000; Sathian, 2000). However, their increased acuity compared with the sighted did not appear on the lip, a skin location that is as sensitive as the fingertip, but not normally used for reading Braille.

CONCLUSIONS

A large number of studies show advantages for blind participants with prior visual experience. These studies show faster and more accurate performance in a wide range of tasks for LB and VLV participants compared with the sighted. In some cases, there was clear evidence of better tactile acuity in the blind (e.g., Sathian, 2000; Stevens, Foulke, & Patterson, 1996). Blind participants with visual experience did better in picture matching (Heller, Brackett, Scroggs, et al., 2002), tangible picture recognition (Heller, 1989), and a host of other tasks (see Heller & Ballesteros, 2006).

How can we explain the advantages that have been found for the LB and VLV participants? These individuals benefit from increased tactile skill and acuity, owing to experience in using the hands for pattern perception. In addition, this is combined with prior visual experience and visual imagery. People who are blind from birth may respond with greater speed than the typical blindfolded sighted participant, but performance was often comparable as measured by accuracy.

It is very difficult to separate the effects of visual experience from visual imagery. People who are LB or have VLV benefit from both of these effects. In addition, people with remaining residual vision may also perform better if they are not blindfolded. This could occur if they are able to see their hands, even if they cannot see objects that they touch.

Comparisons between blind and sighted individuals should be undertaken with the understanding that there could be a wealth of differences between these groups of participants that have nothing to do with the variables of interest. Researchers generally assume that the only important differences between subject groups involves visual experience or visual imagery. However, there are other variables that may be extremely important. It is an oversimplification to assume that the only important differences between samples of subjects entail visual experience, since their experience, age of onset of blindness, and education may vary tremendously. Consequently, these experiential differences may not derive from visual sensory experience, and may have little to do with vision, per se.

Furthermore, many blind people have had little or no experience with haptic pictures (Dulin & Hatwell, 2006). Their sole contact with 2D pattern perception may be limited to Braille and perhaps tangible maps. It is certainly difficult to acquire a number of mathematical and other concepts without access to tangible graphics. Unfortunately, this is the experiential background of many blind persons.

Much of the older research literature on congenital blindness involved people who were blinded in incubators by retinopathy of prematurity (ROP). Excessive oxygen while in an incubator can damage the retina along with the brain. Insufficient oxygen can damage the lungs and lead to an early death. It is difficult to know how to interpret this older literature, and especially difficult to know whether the results from people with ROP will generalize to other CB individuals.

It is important to use tasks that are "fair" when attempting to evaluate the possible effects of visual experience or visual imagery. Similarly, it may be questionable to test groups of individuals with very different educational experience, and not control for this. Also, differential familiarity with stimuli obviously matters and complicates group comparisons.

It is common to read research reports where blindfolded sighted participants are referred to as "normal." This reference is a misnomer. Blindfolded sighted individuals are very unskilled in the use of touch for pattern perception, and their performance may further suffer owing to the withdrawal of visual guidance from blindfolding (see Heller, 1993). It would be easy to come to mistaken conclusions about the potential of touch or of blind individuals from the typical, very convenient blindfolded sighted research participant.

Blind people can make good use of graphics and tactile illustrations may enhance their educational experience in important ways. The fact that instruction in drawing may assist them is not surprising and should be expected. The use of tactile illustrations for blind individuals should be encouraged, and may hold considerable utility for communication about patterns, objects, and space.

In summary, blindness is a relatively rare disorder early in life, but becomes much more common in the aged. The blindfolded sighted person using touch is typically much slower than blind individuals, and often less accurate than the LB or those with minimal residual vision. Of course, this depends on age of onset of blindness. A number of illusions of extent occur in touch, namely the horizontal–vertical and Mueller-Lyer illusions. However, illusions that depend on perspective cues, such as the Ponzi, are not found in touch. Many researchers are interested in haptic applications in blind people, especially virtual touch, maps, and Braille. Unfortunately, fewer people have become proficient in Braille, largely because of the prevalence of late onset blindness. Skilled older readers of Braille may maintain their advantages in tactile spatial acuity into old age, but one can generally expect declines in tactile acuity as one ages. The latest developments in haptic pictures, force-feedback, virtual touch, and computer technology have great potential to provide practical assistance to blind individuals.

REFERENCES

Arditi, A., Holtzman, J. D., & Kosslyn, S. M. (1988). Mental imagery and sensory experience in congenital blindness. *Neuropsychologia, 26*, 1–12.

Casla, M., Blanco, F., & Travieso, D. (1999). Haptic perception of geometric illusions by persons who are totally congenitally blind. *Journal of Visual Impairment and Blindness, 93,* 583–588.

Dulin, D., & Hatwell, Y. (2006). The effects of visual experience and training in raised-line materials on the mental spatial imagery of blind persons. *Journal of Visual Impairment and Blindness, 100,* 414–424.

Fisher, G. H. (1970). An experimental and theoretical appraisal of the perspective and size-constancy theories of illusions. *Quarterly Journal of Experimental Psychology, 22,* 631–652.

Foulke, E. (1982). Reading Braille. In W. Schiff & E. Foulke (Eds.). *Tactual perception: A sourcebook* (pp. 168–208). Cambridge, UK: Cambridge University Press.

Gregory, R. L. (1963). Distortions of visual space as inappropriate constancy scaling. *Nature, 199,* 678–680.

Hatwell, Y. (1985). *Piagetian reasoning and the blind.* New York, NY: American Foundation for the Blind Press.

Heller, M. A. (1989). Picture and pattern perception in the sighted and blind: The advantage of the late blind. *Perception, 18,* 379–389.

Heller, M. A. (1992). The effect of orientation on tactual Braille recognition: Optimal "touching positions." *Perception & Psychophysics, 51,* 549–556.

Heller, M. A. (1993). Influence of visual guidance on Braille recognition: Low lighting also helps touch. *Perception & Psychophysics, 54,* 675–681.

Heller, M. A., & Ballesteros, S. (Eds.). (2006). *Touch and blindness: Psychology and neuroscience.* Mahwah, NJ: Lawrence Erlbaum Associates.

Heller, M. A., Brackett, D. D., & Scroggs, E. (2002). Tangible picture matching in people who are visually impaired. *Journal of Visual Impairment and Blindness, 96,* 349–353.

Heller, M. A., Brackett, D. D., Scroggs, E., Allen, A. C., & Green, S. (2001). Haptic perception of the horizontal by blind and low vision individuals. *Perception, 30,* 601–610.

Heller, M. A., Brackett, D. D., Scroggs, E., Steffen, H., Heatherly, K., & Salik, S. (2002). Tangible pictures: Viewpoint effects and linear perspective in visually impaired people. *Perception, 31,* 747–769.

Heller, M. A., Brackett, D. D., Wilson, K., Yoneyama, K., & Boyer, A. (2002). Visual experience and the haptic horizontal-vertical illusion. *British Journal of Visual Impairment, 20,* 105–109.

Heller, M. A., Brackett, D. D., Wilson, K, Yoneyama, K., Boyer, A., & Steffen, H. (2002). The Haptic Muller-Lyer illusion in sighted and blind people. *Perception, 31,* 1263–1274.

Heller, M. A., Calcaterra, J. A., Burson, L. L., & Tyler, L. A. (1996). Tactual picture identification by blind and sighted people: Effects of providing categorical information. *Perception & Psychophysics, 58,* 310–323.

Heller, M. A., Calcaterra, J. A., Green, S. L., & Barnette, S. L. (1999). Perception of the horizontal and vertical in tangible displays: Minimal gender differences. *Perception, 28,* 387–394.

Heller, M. A., Calcaterra, J., Green, S., & Lima, F. (1999). The effect of orientation on Braille recognition in persons who are sighted and blind. *Journal of Visual Impairment and Blindness, 93,* 416–419.

Heller, M. A., Calcaterra, J. A., Tyler, L. A., & Burson, L. L. (1996). Production and interpretation of perspective drawings by blind and sighted people. *Perception, 25,* 321–334.

Heller, M. A., Calcaterra, J. A., Burson, L. L., & Green, S. L. (1997). The tactual horizontal-vertical illusion depends on radial motion of the entire arm. *Perception & Psychophysics, 59,* 1297–1331.

Heller, M. A., Hasselbring, K., Wilson, K., Shanley, M., & Yoneyama, K. (2004). Haptic illusions in the sighted and blind. In S. Ballesteros and M. A. Heller (Eds.). *Touch, blindness and neuroscience* (pp. 135–144). Madrid, Spain: UNED Press.

Heller, M. A., & Joyner, T. D. (1993). Mechanisms in the tactile horizontal/vertical illusion: Evidence from sighted and blind subjects. *Perception & Psychophysics, 53,* 422–428.

Heller, M. A., Kappers, A. M., McCarthy, M., Clark, A., Riddle, T., Fulkerson, E., ... Russler, K. (2008). The effects of curvature on haptic judgments of extent in sighted and blind people. *Perception, 37,* 816–840.

Heller, M. A., & Kennedy, J. M. (1990). Perspective taking, pictures and the blind. *Perception & Psychophysics, 48,* 459–466.

Heller, M. A., Kennedy, J. M., & Joyner, T. D. (1995). Production and interpretation of pictures of houses by blind people. *Perception, 24,* 1049–1058.

Heller, M. A., McCarthy, M., Schultz, J., Greene, J., Shanley, M., Clark, A., ... Prociuk, J. (2005). The influence of exploration mode, orientation and configuration on the haptic Mueller-Lyer illusion. *Perception, 34,* 1475–1500.

Heller, M. A., Riddle, T., Fulkerson, E., Wemple, L., Kranz, C., Guthrie, S., & Klaus, P. (2009). The influence of viewpoint and surface detail in blind and sighted people when matching pictures to complex objects. *Perception, 38,* 1234–1250.

Heller, M. A., Rogers, G. J., & Perry, C. L. (1990). Tactile pattern recognition with the Optacon: Superior performance with active touch and the left hand. *Neuropsychologia, 28,* 1003–1006.

Heller, M. A., Wilson, K., Steffen, H., Yoneyama, K. & Brackett, D. D. (2003). Superior haptic perceptual selectivity in late-blind and very-low-vision subjects. *Perception, 32,* 499–511.

Holmes, E., Hughes, B., & Jansson, G. (1998). Haptic perception of texture gradients. *Perception, 27,* 993–1008.

Jansson, G. (2002). Perceiving complex virtual scenes without visual guidance. In M. L. McLaughlin, J. Hespanha, & G. Sukhatme (Eds.), *Touch in virtual environments* (pp. 169–179). Upper Saddle River, NJ: Prentice Hall.

Jansson, G., Bergamasco, M., & Frisoli, A. (2003). A new option for the visually impaired to experience 3D art at museums: Manual exploration of virtual copies. *Visual Impairment Research, 5,* 1–12.

Jansson, G., & Holmes, E. (2003). Can we read depth in tactile pictures? In E. Axel & N. Levent (Eds.). *Art beyond sight: A resource guide to art, creativity and visual impairment* (pp. 1146–1156). New York, NY: American Foundation for the Blind Press.

Jansson, G., & Monaci, L. (2004). Haptic identification of objects with different numbers of fingers. In S. Ballesteros & M. A. Heller (Eds.), Touch, blindness and neuroscience (pp. 209–219). Madrid, Spain: UNED Press.

Kennedy, J. M., & Juricevic, I. (2006). Form, projection and pictures for the blind. In M.A. Heller & S. Ballesteros (Eds.) *Touch and blindness: Psychology and Neuroscience* (pp. 73–93). Mahwah, NJ: Lawrence Erlbaum Associates.

Klein, R. (1991). Age-related eye disease, visual impairment, and driving in the elderly. *Human Factors, 33*, 521–525.

Lederman, S. J., Klatzky, R. L., Chataway, C., & Summers, C. D. (1990). Visual mediation and the haptic recognition of two-dimensional pictures of common objects. *Perception & Psychophysics, 47*, 54–64.

Millar, S. (1997). *Reading by touch*. London, UK: Routledge.

Millar, S. (2008). *Space and sense*. New York, NY: Psychology Press.

Munoz Sevilla, J. A. (2006). Tactile virtual reality: A new method applied to haptic exploration. In M. A. Heller & S. Ballesteros (Eds.), *Touch and blindness: Psychology and neuroscience* (pp. 121–136). Mahwah, NJ: Lawrence Erlbaum Associates.

Piaget, J., & Inhelder, B. (1956). *The child's conception of space*. London, UK: Routledge and Kegan Paul.

Rossano, M. J., & Warren, D. H. (1989). The importance of alignment in blind subjects. Use of tactual maps. *Perception, 18*, 805–816.

Sathian, K. (2000). Practice makes perfect: Sharper tactile perception in the blind. *Neurology, 54*, 2203–2204.

Stevens, J. C., Foulke, E., & Patterson, M. Q. (1996). Tactile acuity, aging and Braille reading in long-term blindness. *Journal of Experimental Psychology: Applied, 2*, 91–106.

Van Boven, R. W., Hamilton, R. H., Kaufman, T., Keenan, J. P., & Pascual-Leone, A. (2000). Tactile spatial resolution in blind Braille readers. *Neurology, 2*, 230–234.

18

Massage Therapy: A Review of Recent Research

TIFFANY FIELD

Massage therapy has been practiced since before recorded time, as evidenced by cave drawings in many places. Research on massage therapy, however, is relatively recent. Until this study, our reviews of the literature have featured mostly research from our own lab (Field, 1998; Field, Diego, & Hernandez-Reif, 2007). Fortunately, the field has grown so that this review on the last several years of massage therapy studies represents several different research groups.

Massage therapy has been used primarily to treat pain, although it is increasingly used for other problems, including job stress, depression, autoimmune conditions like asthma, dermatitis, and diabetes and immune conditions, most especially cancer (see Field, Diego, Hernandez-Reif, Deeds, & Figuereido, 2006, for a review).The current review briefly summarizes massage therapy research on preterm infant growth, on attention disorders like autism, on decreasing depression, on reducing pain, and on enhancing immune function. These topics represent the research published over the last several years. In addition, research is presented on moderate pressure as the critical massage therapy variable as well as potential underlying mechanisms for the massage therapy effects.

PRETERM INFANT MASSAGE

In a series of studies, underlying mechanisms for massage therapy effects on preterm infant weight gain were explored. In one of the first of these studies, preterm infant weight gain following massage therapy was related to increased vagal activity and gastric motility, which may have contributed to more efficient food absorption (Diego, Field, Hernandez-Reif, Deeds, Ascencio, & Begert, 2007). In a subsequent study, preterm neonates were randomly assigned to a moderate pressure massage group for three 15-minute periods per day for 5 days or a control group who received standard nursery care without massage therapy (Field, Diego, et al., 2008). During the 5-day treatment period, the massaged preterm infants showed greater increases in: (1) weight gain; (2) serum levels of insulin; and (3) serum levels of IGF-1 (see Figure 18.1). Increased weight gain was significantly correlated with insulin and IGF-1 levels. Thus, these data suggest that weight gain was related to increased serum insulin and IGF-1 levels following massage therapy. IGF-1 levels have also been increased in the cortex of preterm infants and newborns following massage (Guzzetta et al., 2009).

Another potential mechanism underlying the growth effects of massage is the increase in temperature noted in preterm infants during massage therapy. In this study, temperature was monitored in preterm infants randomly assigned to a control or moderate pressure massage group (Diego, Field, & Hernandez-Reif, 2008). A greater increase in temperature was noted in the preterm infants receiving massage therapy, even though the incubator portholes remained open during the 15-minute massage therapy session which could have let in lower temperature air and contributed to lower body temperature.

Another group explored the potential underlying mechanism of reduced energy expenditure in preterm neonates receiving massage (Lahat, Mimouni, Ashbel, & Dollberg, 2007). The same massage treatment as used in our preterm infant studies was also provided in this study. Metabolic measurements were performed by direct calorimetry using a metabolic cart. Energy expenditure was significantly lower in the massaged infants after the 5-day massage therapy period than

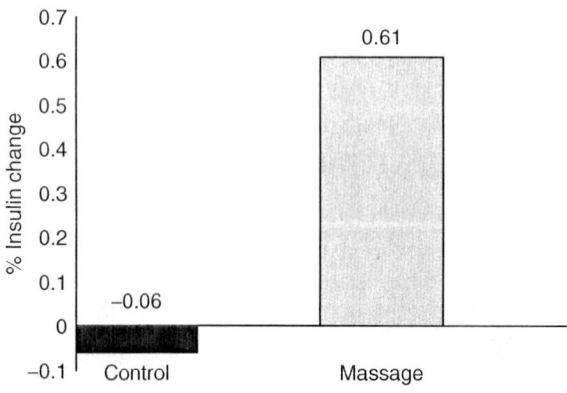

FIGURE 18.1 Percentage (%) insulin change following preterm infant massage.

after the period without massage. This decreased energy expenditure may in part be responsible for the enhanced growth associated with massage therapy.

Preterm infants receiving moderate pressure massage also show fewer stress behaviors, as was noted in two studies by our group. In the first study, the moderate versus light pressure massage group gained significantly more weight per day, and during the behavior observations, the moderate pressure massage group showed significantly lower increases in (1) active sleep; (2) fussing; (3) crying; (4) movement; and (5) stress behavior (hiccupping) (Field et al., 2006). They also showed a smaller decrease in deep sleep, a greater decrease in heart rate, and a greater increase in vagal activity.

In the second study, preterm infants residing in the neonatal intensive care unit were randomly assigned to a massage therapy or to a control group (Hernandez-Reif, Diego, & Field, 2007). The preterm infants in the massage therapy group received three 15-minute massages each day for 5 consecutive days, using the usual preterm massage procedure consisting of moderate pressure stroking of the head, shoulders, back, arms and legs, and kinesthetic exercises, including flexion and extension of the limbs. Preterm infants receiving the massage therapy showed fewer stress behaviors and less activity from the first to the last day of the study. The findings suggest that massage has pacifying or stress-reducing effects on preterm infants, which is noteworthy given that they experience numerous stressors during their hospitalization.

This, in turn, may explain improved immune function in preterm neonates. In a study in which mothers massaged their infants on the face and limbs as well as passively exercised their upper and lower limbs four times a day, the incidence of delayed-onset sepsis was significantly lower in the intervention group (Mendes & Procianoy, 2008). The massage group also had a shorter hospital stay by 7 days. In a study on full-term infants, the group receiving the massage had 50% less risk of diarrhea and other illnesses (Jump, Fargo, & Akers, 2006).

MASSAGE THERAPY ENHANCES ATTENTIVENESS

Increased vagal activity is also a reliable indicator of attentiveness. Stimulation of the vagus (the 10th cranial nerve) is critical for attentiveness. The vagus nerve has a branch to the heart and effectively slows heart rate (Porges, 2001). The vagus nerve may be responsible for mediating the effects of massage therapy on attentiveness. In many studies, increased vagal activity has been accompanied by decreased heart rate and blood pressure (see Field & Diego, 2008, for a review). Increased attentiveness is typically associated with decreased heart rate. For example, in a study on adults being assessed for EEG patterns associated with massage therapy, moderate pressure massage versus light pressure massage was associated with enhanced attentiveness, including slower heart rate and EEG patterns that accompany attentiveness (Diego, Field, Sanders, & Hernandez-Reif, 2004).

Enhanced attentiveness has also been demonstrated in children with autism following a massage therapy program (Silva, Schalock, Ayers, Bunse, & Budden, 2009). In this study, trainers worked with children 20 times over a 5-month period, and parents gave their children a daily massage (Silva et al., 2009). Improvement was evaluated in two settings, at preschool by teachers (blind to the group assignment) and by parents at home. Teacher evaluations suggested that the treated children showed greater improvement on social and language skills and a decrease in autistic behaviors as compared with the wait-list control children. These findings were confirmed by parent data indicating that the gains had generalized across contexts.

MASSAGE THERAPY DECREASES DEPRESSION

The sensitivity and responsivity of mothers during interactions with their infants and the responsiveness of infants have been significantly improved by massage therapy in both nondepressed and depressed mothers and their infants (Lee, 2006). Similarly, positive effects have been noted in depressed mothers and their infants following a period of the mothers giving the massages (O'Higgins, St. James Roberts, & Glover, 2008). These studies highlight the fact that the massager also benefits simply from giving the massages. This would not be surprising given that pressure receptors are stimulated in the hands of the person providing the massage, and the stimulation of pressure receptors appears to be critical for massage therapy effects (Diego et al., 2004).

In a study we conducted, prenatal depression was reduced by moderate pressure massage (Field, Figueiredo, et al., 2008). Prenatally depressed women were randomly assigned to a control group or a group who received massage twice weekly from their partners from 20 weeks' gestation until the end of pregnancy. Self-reported leg pain, back pain, depression, anxiety, and anger decreased more for the massaged pregnant women than for the control group women. In addition, the partners who massaged the pregnant women versus the control group partners reported less depressed mood, anxiety, and anger

TABLE 18.1 Percentage (%) decrease in cortisol in massage therapy studies in several conditions

	Cortisol	
	Urine (%)	Saliva (%)
Anorexia	–	↓10
Asthma	–	↓37
Bulimia	↓32	↓29
Burn	–	↓20
Chronic fatigue	↓41	↓32
Dancers	–	↓35
Depressed infants	↓53	↓33
Depressed mothers	↓28	↓28
Fibromyaligia	–	↓6
Grandparents	↓28	–
HIV Adults	↓45	–
Hypertension	↓23	↓19
Job Stress	↓24	–
Juvenile rheum arthritis	↓31	↓27
Post traumatic stress	↓30	↓11
Psychiatric-Ch & Adol	↓9	↓34
Sex abuse	↓31	↓25

Dashes indicate the absence of urine or saliva assays for the study.

across the course of the massage therapy period. Finally, scores on a relationship questionnaire improved more for both the women and the partners in the massage group.

Several studies have shown reduced cortisol associated with depression following massage therapy, averaging a 31% decrease in cortisol across studies from our lab (see Field, Hernandez-Reif, Diego, Schanberg, & Kuhn, 2005, for a review; see Table 18.1). This is consistent with decreases noted by others, including a 37% decrease by one group (Bost & Wallis, 2006) and a 38% decrease by another group (Lawler & Cameron, 2006). In another study, a significant decrease was noted in depression, anxiety, heart rate, and cortisol following massage (Garner et al., 2008).

MASSAGE THERAPY REDUCES PAIN

In cancer patients, massage has been notably effective for both immediate pain reduction and mood enhancement (Kutner et al., 2008). In this study, adults with advanced cancer who were experiencing moderate-to-severe pain and who were enrolled in hospice received 30-minute massages or simple-touch sessions over a 2-week period. Massage was more effective for both immediate pain and mood. In a review on massage therapy and cancer care, the authors noted that some large cancer centers in the United States have started to integrate massage therapy into their programs based on the positive effects of massage on cancer pain (Russell, Sumler, Beinhorn, & Frenkel, 2008).

The massage therapy studies on pain in our lab have resulted in reduced pain in all chronic pain conditions from lower back pain in pregnancy to labor pain, back pain, migraine headaches, fibromyalgia, and juvenile rheumatoid arthritis (see Field et al., 2006, for a review). In a study on migraine headaches, the participants, who were randomly assigned to massage or control conditions, completed daily assessments of migraine headaches and sleep patterns for 13 weeks (Lawler & Cameron, 2006). The massage participants had a lower migraine frequency and better sleep quality during the intervention weeks and the 3 follow-up weeks. Immediately after the massage sessions, decreases were noted in state anxiety, heart rate, and cortisol.

In a study on osteoarthritis of the knee, participants were assigned either to a treatment (twice weekly massage sessions) or to a control group (delayed intervention). The group receiving massage therapy reported reduced pain and stiffness and showed increased range of motion and time to walk in seconds (Perlman, Sabina, Williams, Njike, & Katz, 2006).

Massage therapy has also been provided for children and adolescents at pediatric pain clinics (Suresh, Wang, Porfyris, Kamasinski-Sol, & Steninhorn, 2008). After the therapy sessions, the children and adolescents reported significantly lower levels of pain, discomfort and depressed mood. In a similar study on postoperative pain management, back massages resulted in decreased pain intensity and unpleasantness as well as lower anxiety levels (Mitchinson et al., 2007). In at least two recent studies, musculoskeletal conditions improved significantly following massage therapy. In one study, the symptoms decreased, and physical and mental scores improved (Hamre et al., 2007), and in the other study, 23% of the participants experienced fewer symptoms (Cambron, Dexheimer, & Swenson, 2007).

Although most of the massage therapy studies have been conducted on patients in clinical settings, some laboratory research has also been performed to determine its effects on pain. For example, one group studied the effects of massage on mechanical hyperalgesia (pressure pain thresholds) and perceived pain using delayed onset muscle soreness as a model for myalgia (Frey Law et al., 2008). The participants were assigned to a deep-tissue massage group, a superficial touch group or a no-treatment control group. Exercises were then performed to induce delayed onset muscle soreness. The deep massage decreased pain by 48% during the muscle stretch.

The mechanism most frequently used to explain massage therapy effects on pain syndromes is the "Gate theory" (see Field et al., 2006, for a review). According to that theory, pain stimulates shorter and less myelinated (or less insulated) nerve fibers than pressure that stimulates more insulated and longer nerve fibers. Thus, the message from the pressure stimulation reaches the brain prior to the pain message and "closes the gate" to the pain stimulus. This metaphor for the electrical and chemical changes that likely occur has been commonly used to explain the effect of grabbing your crazy bone when it has been bumped.

Another theory that is commonly referenced is the deep sleep theory. In deep sleep, less substance P is emitted and therefore less pain occurs because substance P causes pain. We directly tested the "enhanced deep sleep leading to less substance P" theory in our study on fibromyalgia (Field et al., 2002). Following a period of massage therapy, more time was spent in deep sleep, and lower levels of substance P were noted in the saliva samples taken (see Figure 18.2).

Still another theory is that less pain results from increased levels of serotonin, serotonin being the body's natural antipain chemical (Field et al., 2002). Serotonin also decreases cortisol and depression, which are also important effects of massage therapy. And, serotonin is also noted to decrease substance P and other pain-causing chemicals, highlighting the complex interaction between massage therapy's effects on biochemistry.

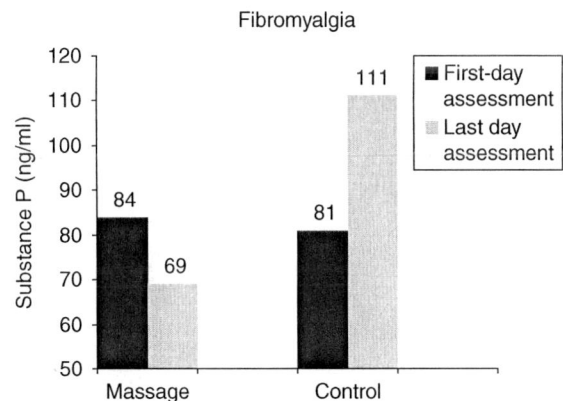

FIGURE 18.2 Substance P decrease following massage therapy of individuals with fibromyalgia.

MASSAGE THERAPY ENHANCES IMMUNE FUNCTION

Children with cancer have been noted to benefit from massage therapy (Post-White et al., 2009). After four weekly massage sessions alternating with four weekly quiet-time control sessions, massage was more effective at reducing heart rate and anxiety levels in the children. The parents conducted the massages, and they also reported experiencing less anxiety following the sessions.

In several studies, natural killer (NK) cells and NK cell activity have increased following massage therapy (Field et al., 2006). This finding suggests that both the clinical condition and immune function would improve following massage therapy given that NK cells, as the front line of the immune system, ward off viral cells, bacterial cells, and cancer cells. In our studies on breast cancer, NK cells and NK cell cytotoxicity (activity) increased, suggesting improved immune function (Hernandez-Reif et al., 2004, 2005; see Figure 18.3). The clinical condition of these women would be expected to improve inasmuch as NK cells are known to destroy tumor cells (Brittenden, Heys, Ross, & Eremin, 1996). Stimulation of pressure receptors during massage therapy might be the underlying mechanism for the increased NK cells mediated by increased vagal tone and decreased cortisol (noted to kill NK cells) (Diego et al., 2004).

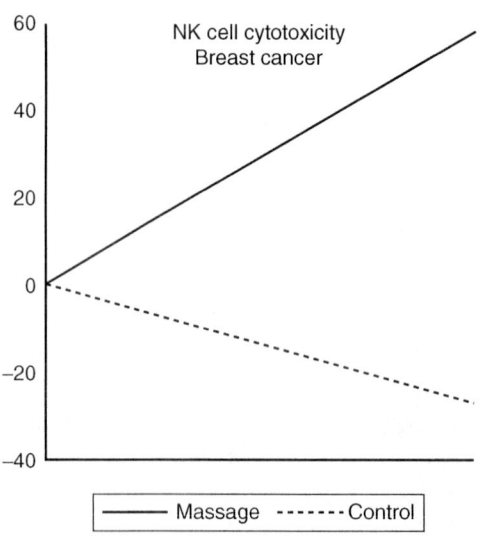

FIGURE 18.3 Increase in natural killer cell cytotoxicity (activity) following massage therapy of individuals with breast cancer.

In a study on healthy individuals, massage therapy decreased cortisol and increased the number of circulating lymphocytes (CD 25+, CD 56+, and CD 4+). It also reduced the levels of inflammatory cytokines (IL-4, 5, 10, and 13) leading to enhanced immune function (Rapaport, Schettler, & Bresee, 2010).

Individuals with HIV have also benefited from massage. For example, in one study Dominican HIV+ children were randomized to receive either massage treatment or a control/friendly visit twice weekly for 12 weeks (Shor-Posner et al., 2006). Significantly more children in the control group exhibited a decline in CD4 cells (the cells that are killed by the virus). A significant increase in CD4+ cells was observed over the 12-week trial in the older massaged children, while a significant increase in NK cells was shown in the younger massaged children.

MODERATE PRESSURE IS NECESSARY

Moderate pressure seems to be necessary for massage therapy to be effective (Diego et al., 2004). Our findings that moderate versus light pressure massage is effective suggests involvement of pressure receptors. Animal studies also indicate that pressure receptor stimulation activates the vagus (Pauk, Kuhn, Field, & Schanberg, 1986; Schanberg & Field, 1987). Further, at least three studies we conducted comparing light pressure to moderate pressure massage showed that lower heart rate and less central nervous system arousal was associated with moderate pressure massage (see Field & Diego, 2008, for a review; see Table 18.2).

TABLE 18.2 Decrease in arousal related to decreased heart rate, EEG relaxation pattern (increased delta and decreased alpha and beta waves), and shift to left frontal EEG activation in adults following massage therapy session

	Moderate Pressure Massage	
Arousal	Pre	Post
↓ Heart rate	78	72
↑ Delta	3.36	3.49
↓ Alpha	3.15	2.82
↓ Beta	2.41	2.20
EEG Activ.	−0.32	0.00

MASSAGE INCREASES VAGAL ACTIVITY

Vagal activity increases immediately after massage therapy sessions and across repeated sessions of massage therapy (Diego, Field, & Hernandez-Reif, 2007). In these studies, significant increases in vagal activity occurred following massage therapy. This likely happens by the stimulation of pressure receptors that are innervated by vagal afferent fibers, which ultimately project to the limbic system including hypothalamic structures involved in autonomic nervous system regulation and cortisol secretion.

These pathways are supported by several lines of evidence. First, anatomical studies indicate that baroreceptors, and to a lesser extent, mechanoreceptors under the skin (i.e., Pacinian corpuscles) are innervated by vagal afferent fibers projecting to the vagal nucleus of the solitary tract, the predominant source of afferent inputs to the efferent neurons of the nucleus ambiguous and the dorsal motor nucleus of the vagus (Kandel, Schwartz, & Jessell, 2000). Second, functional studies indicate that electrical vagal stimulation results in reduced cortisol responses in depressed patients (O'Keane, Dinan, Scott, & Corcoran, 2005). Third, as already noted, we have recently shown that moderate pressure massage (but not light pressure massage) elicits a significant increase in vagal activity in both infants and adults (see Field & Diego, 2008, for a review). Fourth, data collected across several studies by our group and others indicate that massage therapy decreases heart rate (Diego et al., 2004; Kaye et al., 2008; Kubsch, Neveau, & Vandertie, 2000), lowers blood pressure (Ahles et al., 1999; Hernandez-Reif, Field, Diego, & Largie, 2002; Kubsch et al., 2000), and reduces cortisol levels (see Field et al., 2005, for a review; Kim, Cho, Woo, & Kim, 2001). And fifth, an fMRI study revealed that massage therapy increased cerebral blood flow across several brain regions involved in depression and stress regulation, including the amygdala and the hypothalamus (Ouchi et al., 2006), suggesting that massage therapy involves hypothalamic regulation of autonomic nervous system activity, cortisol secretion, and limbic activity associated with emotion regulation.

VAGAL ACTIVITY IS INVERSELY RELATED TO CORTISOL

Inverse relationships between vagal activity and cortisol levels have also been reported (Thayer & Sternberg, 2006). In addition, psychological stressors that reduce vagal activity have been noted to increase cortisol (Spangler, 1997). Increased vagal activity results in a slowing of physiology (decreased heart rate and blood pressure) and downregulation of cortisol (Porges, 2001). Others have interpreted this relationship as vagal activity playing an inhibitory role in the regulation of allostatic systems (Thayer & Sternberg, 2006). As Thayer and Sternberg noted, the prefrontal cortex and amygdala are important central nervous system structures linked to the regulation of emotion and allostatic systems including hypothalamic pituitary adrenal axis function.

SUMMARY

This review briefly summarizes recent empirical research on the behavioral, physiological and biochemical effects of massage therapy including decreased heart rate, blood pressure and cortisol. These effects have been noted in many conditions, following moderate pressure massage, and they appear to be mediated by the stimulation of pressure receptors and increased vagal activity. Increased serotonin and decreased substance P may explain its pain-alleviating effects. Positive shifts in frontal EEG also accompany moderate pressure massage along with increased attentiveness, decreased depression, and enhanced immune function including increased NK cells, making massage therapy one of the most effective forms of touch.

ACKNOWLEDGMENTS

This research was supported by a merit award (MH46586), NIH grants (AT00370 and HD056036) and Senior Research Scientist Awards (MH00331 and AT001585) and a March of Dimes Grant (12-FYO3–48) to Tiffany Field and funding from Johnson & Johnson Pediatric Institute to the Touch Research Institutes.

REFERENCES

Ahles, T. A., Tope, D. M., Pinkson, B., Walch, S., Hann, D., Whedon, M., ... Silberfarb PM. (1999). Massage therapy for patients undergoing autologous bone marrow transplantation. *The Journal of Pain and Symptom Management, 18,* 157–163.

Bost, N., & Wallis, M. (2006). The effectiveness of a15 minute weekly massage in reducing physical and psychological stress in nurses. *The Australian Journal of Advanced Nursing, 23,* 28–33.

Brittenden, J., Heys, S., Ross, J., & Eremin, O. (1996). Natural killer cells and cancer. *American Cancer Society, 77,* 1226–1243.

Cambron, J. A., Dexheimer, J., Coe, P., & Swenson, R. (2007). Side effects of massage therapy: A cross sectional study of 100 clients. *Journal of Alternative & Complementary Medicine, 13,* 793–796.

Diego, M., Field, T., & Hernandez-Reif, M. (2007). Preterm infant massage consistently increases vagal activity and gastric mobility. *Acta Paediatrica, 96,* 1588–1591.

Diego, M., Field, T., & Hernandez-Reif, M. (2008). Temperature increases in preterm infants during massage therapy. *Infant Behavior and Development, 31,* 149–152.

Diego, M. A., Field, T., Sanders, C., & Hernandez-Reif, M. (2004). Massage therapy of moderate and light pressure and vibrator effects on EEG and heart rate. *International Journal of Neuroscience, 114,* 31–45.

Field, T. (1998). Massage therapy effects. *American Psychologist, 53,* 1270–1281.

Field, T., & Diego, M. (2008). Vagal activity, early growth and emotional development. *Infant Behavior and Development, 31,* 361–373.

Field, T., Diego, M., Cullen, C., Hernandez-Reif, M., Sunshine, W., & Douglas, S. (2002). Fibromyalgia pain and substance P decrease and sleep improves after massage therapy. *Journal of Clinical Rheumatology, 8,* 72–76.

Field, T., Diego, M. & Hernandez-Reif, M. (2007). Massage therapy research. *Developmental Review, 27,* 75–89.

Field, T., Diego, M., Hernandez-Reif, M., Deeds, O., & Figuereido, B. (2006). Moderate versus light pressure massage therapy leads to greater weight gain in preterm infants. *Infant Behavior and Development, 29,* 574–578.

Field, T., Diego, M., Hernandez-Reif, M., Dieter, J. N., Kumar, A. M., Schanberg, S., & Kuhn, C. (2008). Insulin and-like growth factor-1 increased in preterm neonates following massage therapy. *Journal of Developmental & Behavioral Pediatrics, 29,* 463–466.

Field, T., Figueiredo, B., Hernandez-Reif, M., Diego, M., Deeds, O., & Ascencio, A. (2008). Massage therapy reduces pain in pregnant women, alleviates prenatal depression in both parents and improves their relationships. *Journal of Bodywork and Movement Therapies, 12,* 146–150.

Field, T., Hernandez-Reif, M., Diego, M., Schanberg, S., & Kuhn, C. (2005). Cortisol decreases and serotonin and dopamine increase following massage therapy. *International Journal of Neuroscience, 115,* 1397–1413.

Frey Law, L. A., Evens, S., Knudtson, J., Nus, S., Scholl, K., & Sluka, K. A. (2008). Massage reduces pain perception and hyperalgesia in experimental muscle pain: A randomized, controlled trial. *Journal of Pain, 9,* 714–721.

Garner, B., Phillips, L. J., Schmidt, H. M., Markulev, C., O'Connor, J., Wood, S. J., ... McGorry, P. D. (2008). Pilot study evaluating the effects of massage therapy on stress, anxiety and aggression in young adult psychiatric inpatient unit. *Australian and New Zealand Journal of Psychiatry, 42,* 414–422.

Guzzetta, A., Baldini, S., Bancale, A., Baroncelli, L., Ciucci, F., Ghirri, P., ... Maffei, L. (2009). Massage accelerates brain development and the maturation of visual function. *The Journal of Neuroscience, 29,* 6042–6051.

Hamre, H. J., Witt, C. M., Glockmann, A., Ziegler, R., Willich, S. N., & Kiene, H. (2007). Rhythmical massage therapy in chronic disease: A 4 year prospective cohort study. *Journal of Alternative & Complementary Medicine, 13,* 635–642.

Hernandez-Reif, M., Diego, M., & Field, T. (2007). Preterm infants show reduced stress behaviors and activity after 5 days of massage therapy. *Infant Behavior and Development, 30,* 557–561.

Hernandez-Reif, M., Field, T., Diego, M., & Largie, S. (2002). Weight perception by newborns of depressed versus non-depressed mothers. *Infant Behavior and Development, 24,* 305–316.

Hernandez-Reif, M., Field, T., Ironson, G., Beutler, J., Vera, Y., Hurley, J.,...Fraser, M. (2005). Natural killer cells and lymphocytes are increased in women with breast cancer following massage therapy. *International Journal of Neuroscience, 115,* 495–510.

Hernandez-Reif, M., Ironson, G., Field, T., Katz, G., Diego, M., Weiss, S.,...Burman, I. (2004). Breast cancer patients have improved immune functions following massage therapy. *Journal of Psychosomatic Research, 57,* 45–52.

Jump, V. K., Fargo, J. D., & Akers, J. F. (2006). Impact of massage therapy on health outcomes among orphaned infants in Ecuador: Results of a randomized clinical trial. *Family & Community Health, 29,* 314–319.

Kandel, E., Schwartz, J. H., & Jessell, T. M. (2000). *Principles of neural science* (4th ed). New York, NY: McGraw-Hill.

Kaye, A. D., Kaye, A. J., Swinford, J., Baluch, A., Bawcom, B. A., Lambert, T. J., & Hoover J. M. (2008). The effects of deep-tissue massage therapy on blood pressure and heart rate. *Journal of Alternative and Complementary Medicine, 14,* 125–128.

Kim, M. S., Cho, K. S., Woo, H., & Kim, J. H. (2001). Effects of hand massage on anxiety in cataract surgery using local anesthesia. *Journal of Cataract and Refractive Surgery, 27,* 884–890.

Kubsch, S. M., Neveau, T., & Vandertie, K. (2000). Effect of cutaneous stimulation on pain reduction in emergency department patients. *Complementary Therapies in Nursing and Midwifery, 6,* 25–32.

Kutner, J. S., Smith, M. C., Corbin, L., Hemphill, L., Benton, K., Mellis, B. K., ...Fairclough, D. L. (2008). Massage therapy versus simple touch to improve pain and mood in patients with advanced cancer: A randomized trial. *Annals of Internal Medicine, 149,* 138.

Lahat, S., Mimouni, F. B., Ashbel, G., & Dollberg, S. (2007). Energy expenditure in growing preterm infants receiving massage therapy. *Journal of the American College of Nutrition, 26,* 356–359.

Lawler, S. P., & Cameron, L. D. (2006). A randomized, controlled trial of massage therapy as a treatment for migraine. *Annals of Behavioral Medicine, 32,* 50–59.

Lee, H. K. (2006). The effects of infant massage on weight, height, and mother-infant interaction. *Taehan Kanho Hakhoe Chi, 36,* 1331–1339.

Mendes, E. W., & Procianoy, R. S. (2008). Massage therapy reduces hospital stay and occurrence of late-onset sepsis in very preterm neonates. *Journal of Perinatology, 28,* 815–820.

Mitchinson, A. R., Kim, H. M., Rosenberg, J. M., Geisser, M., Kirsh, M., Cikrit, D., & Hinshaw, D. B. (2007). Acute postoperative pain management using massage as an adjuvant therapy: A randomized trial. *Archives of Surgery, 142,* 1158–1167.

O'Higgins, M., St. James Roberts, I., & Glover, V. (2008). Postnatal depression and mother and infant outcomes after infant massage. *Journal of Affective Disorders, 109,* 189–192.

O'Keane, V., Dinan, T. G., Scott, L., & Corcoran, C. (2005). Changes in hypothalamic-pituitary-adrenal axis measures after vagus nerve stimulation therapy in chronic depression. *Biological Psychiatry, 58,* 963–968.

Ouchi, Y., Kanno, T., Okada, H,. Yoshikawa, E., Shinke, T., Nagasawa, S., . . . Doi, H. (2006). Changes in cerebral blood flow under the prone condition with and without massage. *Neuroscience Letters, 407,* 131–135.

Pauk, J., Kuhn, C., Field, T., & Schanberg, S. (1986). Positive effects of tactile versus kinesthetic or vestibular stimulation on neuroendocrine and ODC activity in maternally-deprived rat pups. *Life Sciences, 39,* 2081–2087.

Perlman, A. L., Sabina, A., Williams, A. L., Njike, V. Y., & Katz, D. L. (2006). Massage therapy for osteoarthritis of the knee: A randomized controlled trial. *Archives of Internal Medicine, 166,* 2533–2538.

Porges, S. W. (2001). The polyvagal theory: Phylogenetic substrates of a social nervous system. *Psychoneuroendocrinology, 23,* 837–861.

Post-White, J., Fitzgerald, M., Savik, K., Hooke, M. C., Hannahan, A. B., & Sencer, S. F. (2009). Massage therapy for children with cancer. *Journal of Pediatric Oncology Nursing, 26,* 16–28.

Rapaport, M., Schettler, P., & Bresee, C. (2010). A preliminary study of the effects of a single session of Swedish massage on hypothalamic pituitary adrenal and immune function in normal individuals. *The Journal of Alternative and Complementary Medicine, 16,* 1079–1088.

Russell, N. C., Sumler, S. S., Beinhorn, C. M., & Frenkel, M. A. (2008). Role of massage therapy in cancer care. *Journal of Alternative and Complementary Medicine, 14,* 209–214.

Schanberg, S., & Field, T. (1987). Sensory deprivation stress and supplemental stimulation in the rat pup and preterm human neonate. *Child Development, 58,* 1431–1447.

Shor-Posner, G., Hernandez-Reif, M., Miguez, M. J., Fletcher, M., Quintero, N., Baez, J., . . . Zhang G. (2006). Impact of a massage therapy clinical trial on immune status in young Dominican children infected with HIV-1. *Journal of Alternative & Complementary Medicine, 12,* 511–516.

Silva, L. M., Schalock, M., Ayers, R., Bunse, C., & Budden, S. (2009). Qigong massage treatment for sensory and self-regulation problems in young children with autism: A randomized controlled trial. *The American Journal of Occupational Therapy, 63,* 423–432.

Spangler, G. (1997). Psychological and physiological responses during an exam and their relation to personality characteristics. *Psychoneuroendocrinology, 22,* 423–441.

Suresh, S., Wang, S., Porfyris, S., Kamasinski-Sol, R., & Steninhorn, D. M. (2008). Massage therapy in outpatient pediatric chronic pain patients: Do they facilitate significant reductions in levels of distress, pain, tension, discomfort, and mood alterations? *Paediatric Anaesthesia, 18,* 884–887.

Thayer, J. F., & Sternberg, E. (2006). Beyond heart rate variability: Vagal regulation of allostatic systems. *Annals of the New York Academy of Sciences, 1088,* 361–372.

19

Haptic Feedback: Technology and Medical Applications

ALLISON M. OKAMURA

*H*aptic feedback technology is used to provide artificial touch sensations to humans. Haptic feedback in a virtual environment attempts to make the user feel as if he or she is touching a real environment. Similarly, haptic feedback to a human operating a remote robot (teleoperation) or wearing an artificial limb (prosthesis) seeks to give the user a sense of "telepresence," such that the user feels he or she is touching an environment directly rather than through a mechanism. Another purpose of haptic-feedback technology is to generate arbitrary touch experiences, which may not normally occur, or even be physically realizable, during interaction with the natural world. Such systems are useful for psychology or neuroscience experiments, entertainment, and enhancement of human–machine performance.

A haptic-feedback system typically consists of a haptic device and its control (together known as a *haptic interface*) and *haptic rendering*, which is a means to define the desired touch sensation to be generated (Figure 19.1). Examples of haptic rendering mechanisms include a computer processing a virtual environment, a computer handling communication with a remote robot for teleoperation, and a mobile phone operating system deciding the characteristics of a vibration to display based on the identity of an incoming caller.

The design of haptic-feedback systems is informed by both an understanding of the human sense of touch and engineering concepts from the fields of robotics and virtual reality. In general, haptic feedback can include both tactile and force (kinesthetic) aspects of touch. This is most natural, because a realistic touch experience for a human user typically involves feeling touch sensations through the skin as well as forces through muscles and joints. Although an ideal haptic-feedback system includes both "force feedback" and "tactile feedback,"

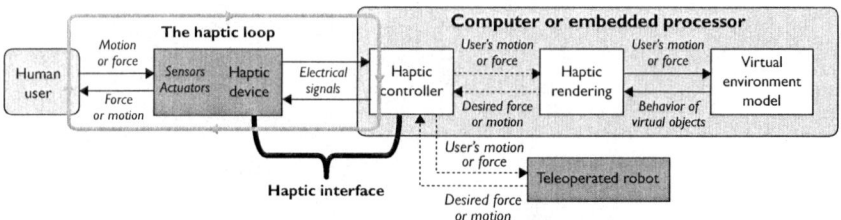

FIGURE 19.1 Block diagram of a haptic feedback system. The human user applies motion or force to the haptic device, whose behavior is governed by its own dynamics and signals from a haptic controller. The controller, renderer, and virtual environment model reside in a computer or embedded processor. Alternatively, in a teleoperation scenario, the controller can communicate with a remote robot.

these aspects are typically considered separately for engineering design purposes.

When designing haptic displays, we must consider the capabilities and limitations of human touch. At a low level, this allows us to engineer haptic interfaces that provide the necessary stimulation to generate a sensation in the user, but are not overdesigned so as to display minute stimuli that the human might not be able to perceive. Similarly, stimuli that are too strong may be rejected by human users as not useful, uncomfortable, or even painful. At a higher level, the design of the haptic system (which also includes haptic rendering) must consider what form of haptic interaction will generate a desired perception for the user. This often requires new research; haptics engineers and scientists will hypothesize that a particular haptic system will generate a specific percept, and then test that hypothesis. This may happen directly or indirectly, since the explicit goal of the haptic feedback may be to enhance performance of a task rather than perception.

After the relevant characteristics of human touch are defined and specifications for the haptic interaction are created, engineering development involves the design or selection of hardware (a haptic device), including relevant sensor and actuator technology. Training in the field of mechatronics, the combination of mechanical and electrical engineering, is usually needed to develop such devices. Alternatively, many commercial haptic (primarily force-feedback) devices exist with varying capabilities and corresponding costs. Examples of such devices will be provided in the next section. The haptic interface is completed when a control system is developed to cause the hardware to generate the desired mechanical stimuli. Finally, haptic rendering is usually accomplished through software written to compute a force or motion that will result in the desired percept or human–machine performance.

CHAPTER 19   HAPTIC FEEDBACK   **471**

Although the concept of haptic feedback is straightforward, there exist many technical challenges in creating useful systems. These include the lack of a complete understanding of the human sensing and motor control capabilities, practical limitations in the design and performance of hardware, and imperfect models used for control and rendering. Consider the goal of displaying an artificially generated surface texture, say, that of corduroy, to a human operator. First, the haptic system designer would want to know how humans sense that texture—what receptors are involved, how sensory signals are processed in the brain to generate the "corduroy" percept, and how that percept changes depending on the characteristics of exploration. Second, the designer needs to develop mechatronic hardware and control that generates the appropriate mechanical stimuli to activate the same sensory signals in the human operator. Or if the designer is very clever, he or she might be able to create "haptic illusions" (Hayward & MacLean, 2008), in which simpler devices are used to generate the desired percept without recreating the low-level stimuli. The haptic device should allow unfettered movement of the human user, and simultaneously track the user's input, such as motion or force. Third, the designer must develop a haptic rendering scheme in which the user's input is mapped to the appropriate stimuli. This is especially challenging when the mapping requires very accurate models of the physical world, and when computational power is restricted. Finally, haptic-feedback technology is most compelling when combined with corresponding visual and/or auditory displays. Interesting perceptual effects (often for the purpose of scientific inquiry) can also be achieved when these displays provide conflicting information (e.g., Srinivasan, Beauregard, & Brock, 1996).

This chapter provides an introduction to the science and engineering concepts behind haptic-feedback technology and illustrates several uses of haptic feedback in medical applications.

FORCE-FEEDBACK SYSTEMS

This section describes the engineering design of interfaces and rendering for force feedback. Portions of this section delve into equations characterizing the dynamics and control of haptic devices. While such a detailed treatment is not necessary to understand the general operation of a haptic device, this analysis demonstrates how dynamic and control properties can significantly affect the performance of a haptic device when used to generate stimuli. Naturally, it is important for scientists and end-users in medicine to understand the performance properties and fundamental limitations of haptic interfaces used as scientific or medical tools.

The Haptic Loop

Haptic interfaces are the combination of a haptic device and computer control of that device. In a typical *haptic loop* (Figure 19.1), sensors are used to determine human input (typically motion or force), a computer determines the haptic feedback to be provided to the human, and a haptic interface is used to physically generate the touch sensations. Usually the sensing mechanism is integrated into the design of the haptic device. After one pass through the haptic loop, the user will typically react, consciously or subconsciously (and sometimes unavoidably due to the physics of the interaction), and the user input motion or force will change. Then, the haptic loop repeats.

In force-feedback systems, the haptic loop is typically repeated 500 to 1,000 times per second. This is necessary for two reasons: First, a fast update rate prevents the user from noticing the discrete changes in system output. Our extreme sensitivity to discontinuities in touch, such as force "steps," requires a faster update rate than that of video displays. Second, force-feedback systems can be unstable if too much time passes between the execution of one output command and the next. Such instability can be felt as a slight buzzing by the user, or gross oscillations that could be dangerous in certain applications. Stability depends on many factors, including the desired fidelity of the haptic rendering and the passive mechanical properties and active behaviors of the user.

Force Interfaces

Kinesthetic, or force-feedback, systems seek to display forces to a human operator, typically through a robot manipulandum grasped by or attached to the hand. Although the human will feel distributed tactile sensations through the manipulandum, this is only a design consideration in terms of the shape of the robot's end-effector. Common end-effectors include a stylus (grasped by the user with multiple fingers) or a thimble (typically for the index finger).

Impedance and admittance. Force-feedback interfaces can be categorized as being of the *impedance type* or *admittance type*. An impedance-type system allows the user to move the robot freely in space, and senses that motion. Desired forces are computed corresponding to that motion, and the device's motors and linkages are used to generate those forces. Ideally, impedance-type haptic devices are completely *back-drivable*, so that when the desired force is zero, the user can move without feeling any force. In practice, the user will always feel some forces resulting from the inherent physical dynamics of the device—typically the inertia and friction. Lowering such undesirable inherent dynamic forces while maintaining a rigid structure that can transmit desired virtual forces is a major concern in the development of force-feedback devices. In addition, impedance-type devices use force-source actuators. That is, the actuator is a transducer that takes in an electrical signal and generates a force (or torque) output. An example of a typical impedance-type force-feedback device, the Phantom Omni (SensAble Technologies, Inc.) is shown in Figure 19.2.

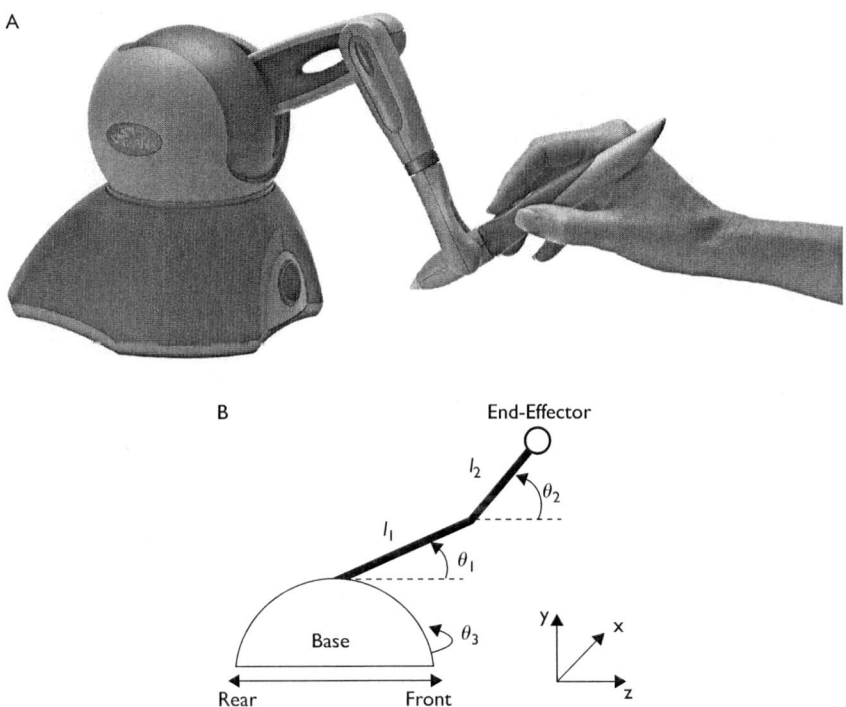

FIGURE 19.2 (A) A commercially available impedance-type force-feedback device, the Phantom Omni (© Copyright SensAble Technologies, Inc.). Printed with permission from SensAble Technologies, Inc. (B) Schematic of the device kinematics. The configuration shown is not possible due to joint limits, but is used to define a set of typical joint variables.

Admittance-type systems directly measure the force input of the human user, then control the haptic device to move proportionally to that force. Admittance-type systems use mechanisms that are less back-drivable than those of impedance-type systems. When the user applies a force to the end-effector, the robot can remain stationary or "admit" to the user's input so that it allows a constrained movement. The actuator is a velocity source, so that an electrical input signal generates a motion, rather than force, output. Such force-based systems can theoretically display the same motion-force relationships as impedance systems, but with a different causality in the control structure. An example of a typical admittance-type force-feedback device, the HapticMASTER (MOOG FCS, Inc.) is shown in Figure 19.3.

Because of their movement accuracy and precision, admittance-type systems are popular in scientific applications such as psychology and neuroscience experiments. However, the need for force sensing increases cost significantly—so for commercial applications, impedance-type systems are more common. In addition, admittance-type systems can effectively display (or resist) larger forces than impedance systems. Accordingly, admittance robots will have heftier, stronger linkages to transmit that force.

Force-feedback device kinematics. The forward kinematics of a haptic device, or more generally for any robot, describe a mathematical

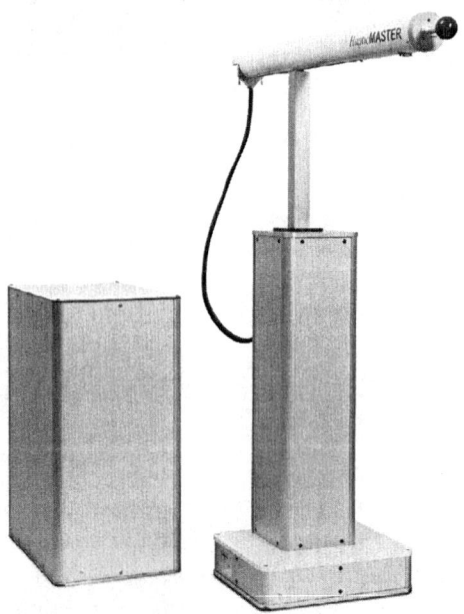

FIGURE 19.3 A commercially available admittance-type force-feedback device, the Haptics-Master (© Copyright MOOG). Printed with permission from MOOG.

mapping from joint space and to the Cartesian workspace. This mapping can be nonlinear and involve multiple equations when the device has multiple degrees of freedom. For example, the Phantom Omni (Figure 19.2) has three degrees of freedom: two that move the arm in a vertical plane, and one to rotate the base, which effectively rotates that plane. Although the Omni mechanism has many more joints than degrees of freedom, they are connected by links such that only three joint variables need to be defined to fully describe the position of the end-effector in Cartesian space. Using geometry, one can develop the forward kinematics function

$$x = f(\theta) \tag{1}$$

where $x = [x \; y \; z]^T$ is a vector describing the end-effector Cartesian position, and $\theta = [\theta_1 \; \theta_2 \; \theta_3]^T$ is a vector describing three independent joint positions. The function also uses constants that depend on link lengths and shape. Using the forward kinematics, sensors at the joints may be used to compute the position of the end effector. Usually this calculation can be performed very accurately; joint position sensors such as optical encoders are used to give haptic devices such as the Phantom Omni position resolution on the order of 10 μm. The main errors in forward kinematics arise from the assumption that the "rigid" links of the robot do not physically deform—this is accurate unless very large forces are applied.

In addition, the forward kinematics can be differentiated with respect to time to develop a relationship between joint velocities and end-effector velocities. These are linearly related by a Jacobian matrix, J:

$$\frac{dx}{dt} = J \frac{d\theta}{dt} \tag{2}$$

Thus, if joint position measurements can be numerically differentiated with respect to time (using a series of joint position measurements) to obtain joint velocities, the instantaneous end-effector velocity can be computed. The most significant potential error in this calculation is in the measurement or computation of $d\theta/dt$, especially when the device is moving very slowly.

Generating forces. For an impedance-type force-feedback interface, we will use haptic rendering to determine the force to be displayed to the human user. Haptic rendering will be described in the next section; we now concern ourselves with the problem of generating these known, desired forces using the haptic device. The desired force is usually defined in the Cartesian workspace as a vector, which for the Phantom Omni would be $f = [f_x\ f_y\ f_z]^T$. However, to generate that force using the actuators (in this case, direct-current motors) attached to joints of the Phantom Omni, we must determine the torques applied by the actuators. The Jacobian matrix used in the differential forward kinematics can also be used to relate joint torques and end-effector forces as follows:

$$\tau_{actuators} = J^T f \qquad (3)$$

where $\tau_{actuators} = [\tau_1\ \tau_2\ \tau_3]^T$ is a vector of the joint torques corresponding to actuators the three joint positions described earlier, and J^T is the transpose of the Jacobian matrix.

Ideally, to control an impedance-type haptic device to display a particular force, one would only need to program Equation 3 into the haptic interface control software, so that the actuators of the haptic device generate the appropriate torques to match the desired end-effector force. This is often done when the force being displayed does not need to be perfectly accurate. However, what the user actually feels is not just f, but also forces arising from the dynamics of the robot. Physically, the torques computed from Equation 3 must be transmitted from the actuators to the end-effector through links and joints, which inherently have some mass and friction. A general matrix equation of motion written in joint space that includes such terms is

$$M(\theta)\frac{d^2\theta}{dt} + C\left(\theta, \frac{d\theta}{dt}\right) + N(\theta) = \tau_{actuators} + \tau_{user} = \tau_{actuators} + J^T f_{user} \qquad (4)$$

where M is the inertia matrix, C is a vector of velocity-dependent terms such as Coriolis, centripetal and friction torques, and N is a vector of position-dependent terms due to effects as stiffness and gravity. The "external" loads are given on the right-hand side of the equation, where $\tau_{actuators}$ is the vector of actuator torques computed from Equation 3 and $\tau_{user} = J^T f_{user}$ is the vector of user torques applied. We use the Jacobian to bring f_{user} into this equation, because the user actually applies a force to the end-effector. This quantity is also the force that the user feels. Solving for f_{user} in Equation 3 shows that the user feels not only $\tau_{actuators}$, but also the inherent dynamic properties of the system described on the left-hand side of the equation. Additional control techniques would be needed to effectively cancel out undesired dynamic forces and achieve $\tau_{user} = -\tau_{actuators}$. In practice, most impedance-type haptic devices are carefully designed to have low inertia and friction, no stiffness, and balancing mechanisms to remove the effects of gravity. The most obvious dynamic force felt by the user is that from inertia, which occurs when the user accelerates quickly—but the small physical workspace of many impedance haptic devices prevents very high accelerations.

Generating motions. For admittance-type haptic systems, the user input is force and the output is a desired motion. The relationship between applied force and desired motion is determined by a haptic rendering algorithm, but the control of the haptic interface must generate an actual motion that approximates the desired motion. This can be accomplished using a number of control methods, and we will focus on the proportional-integral-derivative (PID) control. PID control seeks to minimize the error between two variables (in this case, motion variables x_{actual} and $x_{desired}$) by generating actuator forces or torques that bring the difference, or error, between these variables to zero. The proportional (P) term reacts to the current error, the integral (I) term reacts based on the sum of recent errors, and the derivative (D) term reacts based on the rate of change of error. For $e = x_{desired} - x_{actual}$,

$$f_{actuators} = J^{-T}\tau_{actuators} = K_p e(t) + K_i \int_0^t e(\tau)d\tau + K_d \frac{de(t)}{dt} \quad (5)$$

where K_p, K_i, and K_d and the proportional, integral, and derivative, gains, respectively. The ability of this controller to make the haptic system reach the desired configuration depends on the dynamics of the robot, the strength of the actuators and mechanical transmission, and the corresponding ability of the system to reject the "external" disturbance of the user pushing physically on the device.

Haptic Rendering

Haptic rendering computes the desired force or motion to be displayed to the user, based on the user's input. In this section we will assume the motion-to-force causality of impedance-type haptic systems, but the opposite causality can usually be computed very similarly for admittance-type systems.

Virtual environments. In virtual environments, the relationship between the user's input motion and the haptic device's output force is only limited by the performance of the haptic system and the designer's imagination. But in most practical applications, the goal of the virtual environment is to simulate a real environment, so rendering consists of simulating the real physics.

We define the haptic interaction point (HIP) as the location of the user in the virtual environment. This corresponds to a location on the physical haptic device where the forces are to be displayed. For a haptic device such as the Phantom Omni, the [x y z] position of the HIP in the virtual world is usually a linearly scaled version of the [x y z] position of the Phantom end-effector in the real world. A typical virtual environment contains immoveable objects like walls and moveable objects like balls. Consider the example given in Figure 19.4, in which the HIP at various points in time is represented by a series of open circles, and there is a solid, vertical wall to the right. The plane of the wall is perpendicular to the page.

The first step in haptic rendering, called *collision detection*, determines whether the HIP is contacting any of the virtual objects. This can be a simple geometric calculation. For the situation illustrated in Figure 19.4, we ask: Is the x-component of the HIP position greater than x_{wall}? If so, contact has occurred. For very complex virtual environments, which may include surfaces consisting of thousands of polygons, parallel computing or optimization may be needed to accurately detect collisions at desirable haptic loop rates.

The second step in haptic rendering is the force computation. If collision has occurred, an interaction force must be generated. The virtual wall is the building block of most virtual environments (even polygonal meshes are essentially a collection of very small walls), and the interaction with the wall is usually computed using a spring model (or Hooke's Law):

$$f = kx \qquad (5)$$

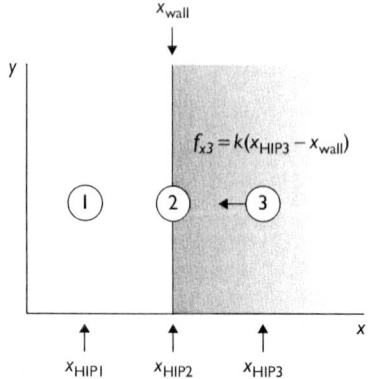

FIGURE 19.4 Haptic rendering of a vertical virtual wall with position x_{wall} and stiffness k. The haptic interaction point (HIP) is shown in three x positions, x_{HIP1}, x_{HIP2}, and x_{HIP3}, all with the same y position. Because $x_{HIP3} > x_{wall}$, collision is detected and a corresponding force in the x-direction is computed.

where x is the vector penetration of the HIP into the virtual wall, f is the desired vector force to be displayed to the user, and k is a scalar stiffness that is greater than zero. Note that for the example given in Figure 19.4, the x vector has an x-value that is the x-component of the HIP minus the x-coordinate of the wall, and the y- and z-values are zero if the wall is a frictionless surface. In general, the virtual wall could have any orientation; geometric calculations are needed to compute the appropriate penetration and force vectors. In addition, the force computation could include terms that describe damping, nonlinear friction (e.g., Coulomb friction), and inertia, and the virtual environment can also separately simulate the dynamics of moving objects even when the user is not touching them.

Teleoperation. Teleoperation, the control of remote robots, can be used to accomplish tasks that are too remote, small-scale, or hazardous for direct human manipulation. In teleoperation systems, the operator manipulates a "master" input device (for our purposes, a haptic device), and a "slave" robot follows the input. Typically the slave robot will follow the master with a variant of the basic PID control law described earlier. Teleoperation is particularly advantageous in unstructured environments, where autonomous robotic systems cannot be used due to the limitations of artificial intelligence, sensor data interpretation, and environment modeling. Another important advantage of teleoperation over direct manipulation is the position scaling gain, which allows master motions to be mapped to smaller slave motions, thereby improving user accuracy. The goal of haptic technology in teleoperation is to provide "transparency," in which the human operator does not feel as if he is operating a remote mechanism, but rather that his own hands are contacting the remote environment.

Rendering in teleoperation consists of determining the force to be displayed to the operator based on the slave's interaction with the environment. Teleoperator force feedback can be achieved with or without the use of force sensors. A slave-tracking controller can be applied to the master actuators, providing haptic feedback to the human operator through a technique known as "position-position" or "position exchange" teleoperation. This amounts to a force estimation technique in which the difference between the desired and actual position of the slave robot (where the desired position is that of the master manipulator) is an indication of force being applied to the environment. However, the fidelity of such systems is limited since there are dynamic forces present in most robots that are difficult to account for and could mask relatively minute forces from interacting with the remote environment. Alternatively, force can be directly measured using sensors on the slave robot, although the environment may place constraints on size, geometry, cost, biocompatibility, and sterilizability.

During teleoperation, cameras are typically used to produce a rich visual scene of the remote environment, which the operator views on a monitor, or through a viewing console. These images can be augmented in real time with overlaid artificial graphics that enhance the operator's sensory experience and can display either sensed or estimated forces. This sensory transduction is a form of sensory substitution, which we will call graphical force feedback. This allows the user to visualize the applied forces, although the force is not felt using his or her hands or arms. In an exploration task, it may be advantageous to provide a graphical display about the measured dynamic properties of the environment instead of the force applied by the robot.

TACTILE-FEEDBACK SYSTEMS

While force-feedback systems may stimulate cutaneous receptors simply by virtue of the user grasping the robot manipulandum, the tactile sensation in such situations is not directly controlled. In contrast, tactile-feedback systems are designed to convey force, contact, and shape information to the skin. Typical tactile display systems provide little kinesthetic sensation. They are usually designed for very specific purposes, such as the transmission of contact events, contact location, slip/shear, texture, and local shape. This approach is logical because each type of cutaneous receptor has its own set of properties (e.g., frequency response, receptive field, spatial distribution) and can be associated with specific sensed parameters (e.g., local skin curvature, skin stretch, and vibration).

As described in the "corduroy" example in the introduction to this chapter, the development of tactile-feedback systems that render realistic contact with the skin is very challenging. To accurately create a desired local shape and pressure distribution on the fingertip, a dense array of actuators is usually required—such systems are currently only practical in scientific research. Most devices aimed at tactile perception have not yet been used in commercial applications, with the notable exceptions of Braille displays for the blind and vibration feedback for entertainment and simple user interfaces. Due to the wide variety of tactile-feedback systems, there is no underlying theory that captures the design goals and behavior for all systems. Thus, this section is organized into the main types of tactile displays and their primary design considerations.

Local Shape

The goal of local shape tactile feedback is to display spatially distributed information to the skin. In many designs, the tactile device is very literal—it attempts to mimic the shape of the surface a real environment so that, when finger comes in contact with the tactile device, it feels like the desired surface. Local shape is most commonly displayed using arrays of pins that move normal to the skin. A layer of elastic material can cover the pins to provide smooth contact with the skin. Other systems move individual contacts laterally rather than up and down, and others are arrays of electro-cutaneous elements in which electrodes pass small levels of current through the skin. Psychophysical and perceptual experiments, involving design parameters such as number of pins, spacing, and amplitude, are used to optimize the performance of these devices. Various actuator technologies are used to create tactile arrays, including piezoelectric, shape-memory alloy (SMA), electromagnetic, pneumatic, electro-rheological, micro-electromechanical system (MEMS), and electro-tactile.

We will first consider an example of a complex, costly tactile-feedback system designed for neuroscience and psychophysical experiments. Killebrew et al. (2007) developed a tactile stimulator with 400 independently controlled pins fit into a 1 cm^2 area. This system can present arbitrary spatiotemporal stimuli to the skin at a rate of 20 Hz. The actuation unit for this system, consisting of a large rack of motors connected to the pins by wires, is much too bulky for commercial applications. But as the highest-resolution tactile-feedback system built to date, it can be used for scientific research and to evaluate potential designs and rendering algorithms for lower-resolution displays. On the other end of the spectrum is a desktop tactile display system by Wagner, Lederman, and Howe (2004) that fits 36 pins into a 1 cm^2 area, as shown in Figure 19.5. This device uses low-cost, commercially available servomotors and can move the pins individually at up to 25 Hz (depending on the amount of pin deflection). In addition, tactile-feedback systems have used *lateral* pin motion to stretch the skin in a way that generates a perception of local shape. Hayward and Cruz-Hernandez (2000) first introduced this concept, and the most recent version of their design is a 60-element array in an approximately 1 cm^2 area. (The consistency of the area covered by tactile displays is due to the desire for reasonable coverage of the finger pad). The force of the individual pins moving laterally provides sufficient skin pad motion/stretch to excite mechanoreceptors.

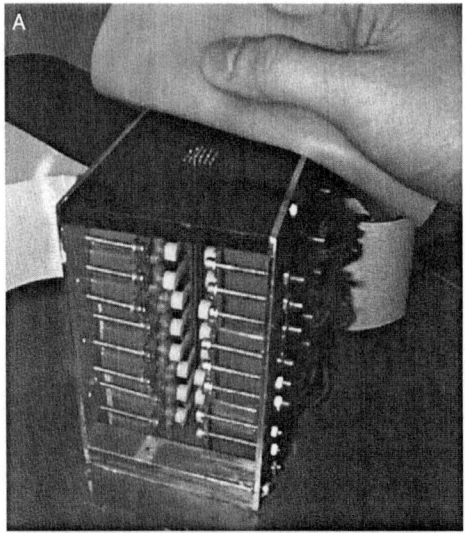

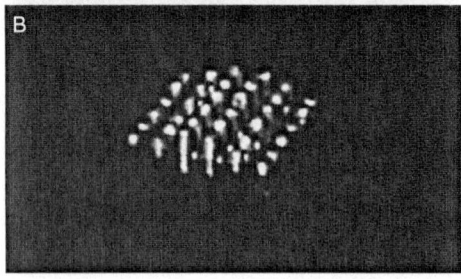

FIGURE 19.5 (A) A 36-pin tactile display designed for desktop use. (B) A close-up of the 6 × 6 display, simulating a sine wave profile. Images courtesy of Robert D. Howe. Printed with permission.

Contact Motion

Contact motion tactile-feedback systems attempt to display the motion of a single area of contact relative to the skin (usually on a finger). Arrays of pins, discussed in the previous section, can be used to display motion of a contact point or contact patch. However, here we will focus on devices that are specialized for the display of contact location and motion.

We begin with basic contact location display. A particularly compelling design is a system that uses a cylinder that rolls over the surface of the finger, changing the contact location as it moves (Provancher, Cutkosky, Kuchenbecker, & Niemeyer, 2005). The single tactile element is normally held away from the skin, but comes into contact when the operator pushes on a virtual object through the use of push-pull wires that allow the actuators to be mounted far away from the hand. The tactile-feedback mechanism can be integrated with a force-feedback device to provide a combination of force and tactile information to the operator. Experiments with this system have shown human operators perform object manipulation better in a virtual environment when contact location is displayed.

The sensation of slip, or movement of the contact patch, is also important for manipulation. Some systems have been created expressly for slip display that use cylinders (Johnson & Phillips, 1998) or balls (Webster, Murphy, Verner, & Okamura, 2005) that rotate under the fingertip, as shown in Figure 19.6. Experiments have shown that knowledge of slip improves task performance in a virtual environment.

A combination of slip and lack of slip, controlled by changing friction properties of the surface of the tactile display, generates

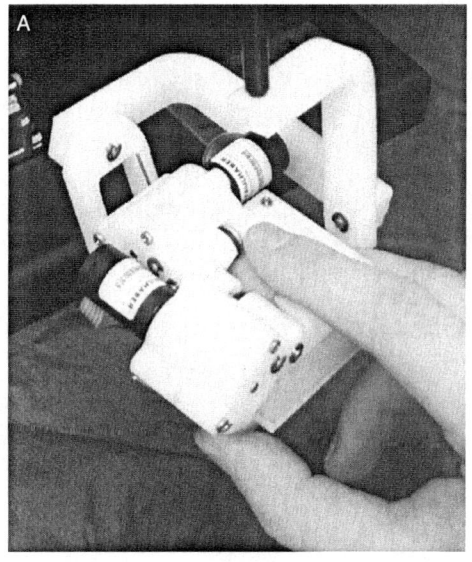

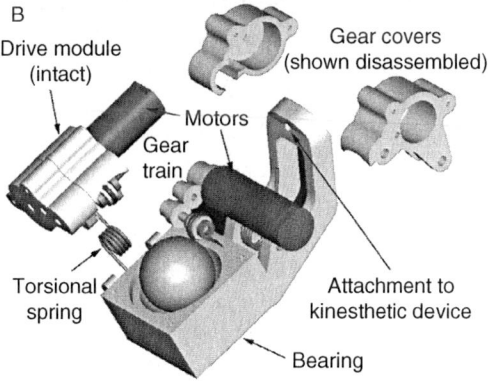

FIGURE 19.6 (A) A tactile slip display, shown integrated with a kinesthetic feedback device. (B) Slip is displayed through a ball, whose rotation is controlled by two motors. Reprinted with permission from "A novel two-dimensional tactile slip display: Design, kinematics and perceptual experiment," by R. J. Webster, T. E. Murphy, L. N. Verner, and A. M. Okamura, 2005, *Association for Computing Machinery Transactions on Applied Perception, 2*, 150–165. Copyright 2005 by Association for Computing Machinery, Inc.

very compelling sensations in a small package (Winfield, Glassmire, Colgate, & Peshkin, 2007). In this system, friction properties between the human finger and plate are varied by vibrating the plate at ultrasonic frequencies. Using measurements of the position and velocity of the finger, the friction of the entire plate can be modified to indirectly display different shear forces to the user. A key feature of this mechanism is that the user must move laterally over the surface to feel a (friction) force, which makes the display behave like a real, passive surface.

Vibration

Vibration feedback is the most practical means for providing tactile sensation, due to the simplicity of actuation and lack of necessary directionality. It can be used to convey events, such as making and breaking contact, display spatial patterns, or simply encode more abstract information. Popular vibrating actuators include voice-coil motors (such as those used in loudspeakers) and piezoelectric materials (which deflect a small amount with applied voltage). In addition, the conventional motors used in high-fidelity force-feedback displays can be used to add vibration feedback to force feedback at the end effector.

Impact or contact events are significantly enhanced with vibration feedback. In force feedback devices, the force of contact with a virtual wall grows as penetration increases, as described by Equation 5. This rendering, especially when the stiffness is limited for stability reasons, lacks the crispness of interaction with real hard objects. Thus, vibrations can be generated by the motors of a force-feedback device or an add-on vibrating actuator at the instant the HIP comes into contact with a virtual wall (Figure 19.7). This approach has been shown to add significant realism to virtual environments (Kuchenbecker, Fiene, & Niemeyer, 2006; Okamura, Dennerlein, & Cutkosky, 2001). A familiar example of this effect is the vibration displayed by a video game controller when a virtual car runs into a wall or a virtual racquet hits a virtual tennis ball.

Vibrations can also provide the user with information about physical interaction phenomena with vibratory signals, such as roughness and texture patterns. In teleoperation, sensors such as accelerometers located on the slave robot can acquire vibration signals, which are then relayed though a vibrating element on the master haptic device. It has been shown that users can identify the roughness of remote environments through vibration feedback alone (Kontarinis & Howe, 1995).

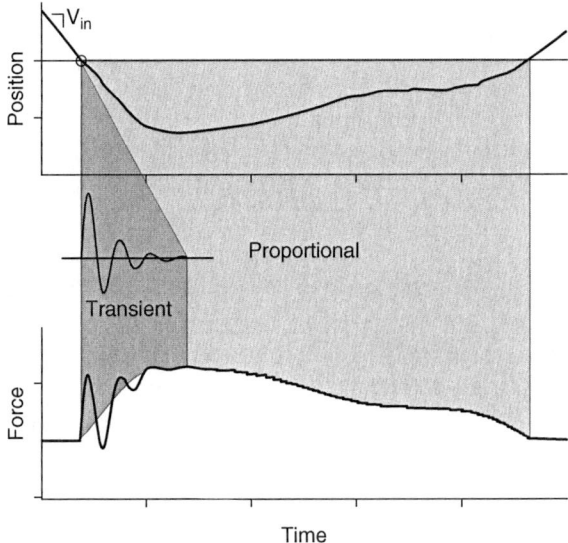

FIGURE 19.7 Open-loop vibration signals, superimposed on penetration-based feedback forces, improve the realism of hard surfaces in virtual and teleoperated environments. Reprinted with permission from "Improving contact realism through event-based haptic feedback," by K. J. Kuchenbecker, J. Fiene, and G. Niemeyer, 2006, *IEEE Transactions on Visualization and Computer Graphics, 12*, 219–230. Copyright 2006 by Institute of Electrical & Electronics Engineers (© IEEE 2006).

Abstract information can also be conveyed using vibrations, provided that users can learn to recognize the signals. The vibration of a mobile phone to signal an incoming call is a simple example; researchers are developing more sophisticated vibration-based "haptic icons" that display a greater variety of information (Chan, MacLean, & McGrenere, 2008). The primary design goal here is that vibrations representing different types of information are easily distinguishable, so the signals must be strong and clear. Human vibration sensitivity ranges from DC to over 1 kHz, with peak sensitivity around 250 Hz, and commercial *vibrotactile* actuators have been specifically designed for this purpose.

MEDICAL APPLICATIONS

Some of the most promising applications of haptic technology are in the medical domain. These include surgery, surgical simulation, and rehabilitation.

Surgery

In traditional open surgery, a surgeon can use the proprioceptive and cutaneous senses to determine the amount of force being applied to patient, as well as integrate haptic information to form dynamic models of tissue. However, in manual minimally invasive surgery (MIS), surgeons use a long-shafted instrument that eliminates tactile cues and masks force cues. The lack of significant haptic feedback in MIS may lead to increased intra-operative injury. While teleoperated robot-assisted minimally invasive surgery (RMIS) presents numerous benefits, including enhanced dexterity and visualization, it eliminates all natural haptic feedback because the surgeon no longer holds the surgical instrument. This has been a major complaint of surgeons using RMIS systems (Westebring-van der Putten, Goossens, Jakimowicz, & Dankelman, 2008).

Force feedback in surgery. There are several approaches to providing force feedback in RMIS, following the methods for general teleoperators described earlier. Most research systems measure or estimate the forces applied to the patient by the surgical instrument, and provide resolved forces to the hand via a force-feedback device. However, conventional force sensors are of limited applicability in surgery, which places severe constraints on size, geometry, cost, biocompatibility, and sterilizability. Some researchers have been able to implement practical force-sensing systems by designing specialized force-sensing instruments (Kuebler, Seibold, & Hirzinger, 2005; Zemiti, Morel, Ortmaier, & Bonnet, 2007), as shown in Figure 19.8. Using position-position control, the forces applied to the patient can be estimated without using

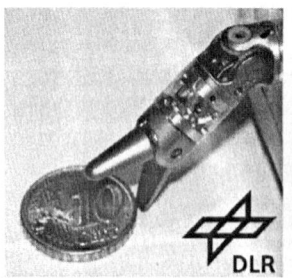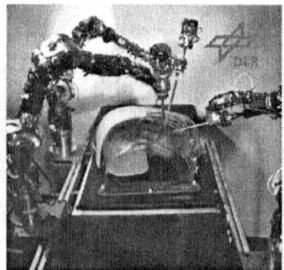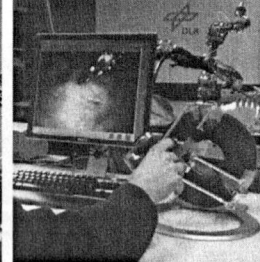

FIGURE 19.8 An experimental teleoperated robotic surgery system with haptic feedback. The system includes force-sensing instruments, robotic arms, and a master haptic device commercially available from Force Dimension, Inc. Images courtesy of DLR Institut für Robotik und Mechatronik. Printed with permission.

force sensors. For patient-side robots designed with low inertia and friction, the difference between the desired and actual position of the patient-side robot is an indication of the level of force applied to the environment (Mahvash & Okamura, 2007).

The most fundamental limitation to force feedback for general teleoperators is that it is not possible to achieve "transparency," in which the exact environment properties are replayed to the human operator. Such transparency would require perfect models of robot dynamics, no time delays (any processing or communication results in some delay), and perfect environment force sensing or estimation. If the controller gains (e.g., of a PID controller) are set too high, the effects of small errors and delays in the system can cause uncontrollable oscillations, or instability, in a force-feedback teleoperator. An alternative to direct force feedback is sensory substitution, for example, audio and graphics (Kitagawa, Dokko, Okamura, & Yuh, 2005). Because visual observation of how the tissue responds to instrument motions is essential to surgical performance, sensory substitution should not obstruct the surgeon's view of the patient through the endoscopic camera (Reiley et al., 2008).

Recent results have demonstrated the utility of force feedback in surgery on artificial tissue models. Several studies (e.g., Wagner & Howe, 2007) found that force feedback reduced unintentional injuries, but extended operating time. Graphical displays of force information results in superior performance to no force feedback (Reiley et al., 2008), but direct force feedback to the surgeon's hand is even better (Gwilliam et al., 2009). This may depend on the task; for grasping, providing both vision and force feedback was better for characterizing tissues than vision or force feedback alone (Tholey, Desai, & Castellanos, 2005).

Tactile feedback in surgery. In some surgical procedures, which surgeons have performed for decades using hand-held instruments, tactile information such as contact location and pressure distribution may not be needed. However, tactile feedback is important for exploration tasks such palpation, which is used to identify tissue mechanical properties (Gwilliam et al., 2009).

As described earlier, numerous tactile-feedback mechanisms exist; for teleoperation, corresponding tactile sensors are also required. Etlaib and Hewit (2003) provide a review of tactile sensing technology for RMIS, describing sensors for detecting local mechanical properties of tissue such as compliance, viscosity, and surface texture (all indications of the tissue health) and sensors for data to be directly fed back to the surgeon, such as pressure distribution or deformation. Tactile-feedback devices use this data to create the perception that the surgeon's fingertip is directly contacting the patient. The development of array-type tactile devices for RMIS is challenging due to constraints in size and weight. The display must be attached to the surgeon's finger or mounted at the end-effector of the master robot, without impeding the surgeon's motion. Pin displays developed for MIS and RMIS have been actuated using shape-memory alloys (Howe, Peine, Kontarinis, & Son, 1995), micromotors (Ottermo, Stavdahl, & Johansen, 2005), and pneumatic systems (Culjat et al., 2008; Moy, Wagner, & Fearing, 2000). One study combining kinesthetic and tactile displays shows that maintaining an appropriate force is necessary for the surgeon to use spatially distributed force information from a tactile sensor (Feller, Lau, Wagner, Perrin, & Howe, 2004).

Surgical Simulation

A wide variety of medical procedures, both for diagnosis and therapy, require significant manual skill. Historically, trainees have been practiced on cadavers, animals, mannequins, and (under supervision from an experienced clinician) patients. Computer-based surgical simulation provides an efficient, safe, and ethical method for training clinicians by emphasizing the user's real-time interaction with medical instruments, surgical techniques, and realistic organ models. For maximum effectiveness, a simulator should provide haptic feedback to the user that mimics that present in real surgery (Bholat, Haluck, Murray, Gorman, & Krummel, 1999). It is hypothesized that haptic-feedback medical simulators will: (1) reduce the risk to patients, (2) allow trainees to practice with unusual medical conditions, (3) provide objective feedback based on data acquired during training, and (4) allow for more or more efficient training time, with less effort on the part of human instructors.

Numerous haptic medical simulators have been developed, for procedures ranging from needle insertion (for drawing blood) to colonoscopy to minimally invasive surgery. Most effective haptic simulators have several common features:

- A realistic manual interface. The trainee grasps a haptic device whose end-effector appears to be a real medical instrument.
- A graphical virtual environment that displays images similar to what a clinician would encounter in a real medical procedure. For example, this could be an X-ray-like image for an angioplasty simulator or a realistic "camera view" of the liver for a laparoscopic surgery. The instrument-tissue interaction, including tissue deformation, should appear realistic.

- Haptic feedback (typically force feedback) that is similar to what the clinician would feel in a real procedure.
- A means to collect and display performance data. This allows the trainee to evaluate progress. In addition, the simulator may provide views not typically available during real clinical procedures, to help the trainee understand the procedure better.

Researchers have demonstrated that some commercial and research simulators are effective in developing minimally invasive surgery skills (Basdogan, De, Kim, Muniyandi, & Srinivasan, 2004). In particular, haptic feedback seems to be effective when provided in early training (Strom et al., 2006). Surveys of simulator designs and simulator evaluation methods include (Liu, Tendick, Cleary, & Kaufmann, 2003; Satava, 2001). As an example of a complete haptic-feedback simulator, consider the system used for hysteroscopy training in Figure 19.9 (Harders et al., 2006). This simulator provides realistic visualization and haptic feedback in real time, and incorporates continuum

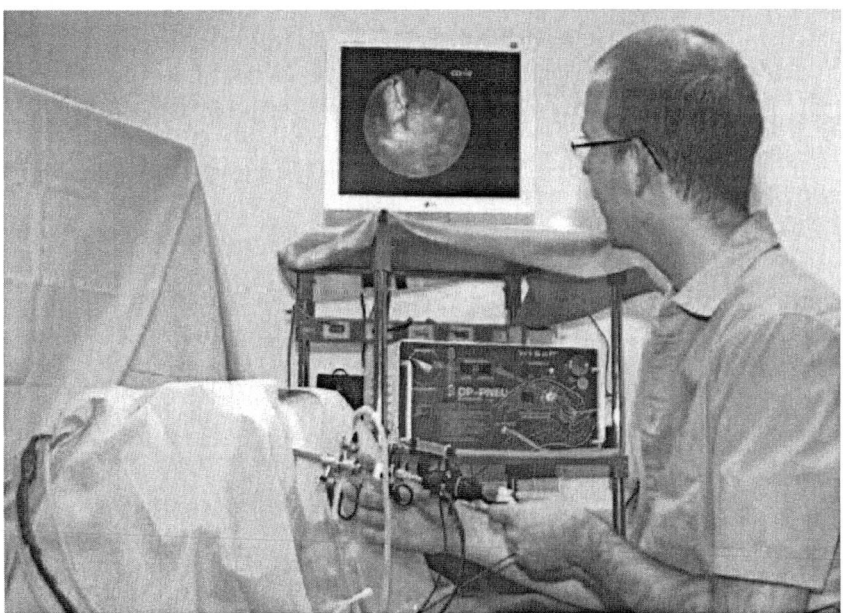

FIGURE 19.9 An example surgical simulator with haptic feedback: Hysteroscopy training simulation environment. Reprinted with permission from "Highly-realistic, immersive training environment for hysteroscopy, by M. Harders, M. Bajka, U. Spaelter, S. Tuchschmidi, H. Bleuler, and G. Szekely, 2006, *Proceedings of Medicine Meets Virtual Reality, 119*, 176–181. Copyright by from IOS Press (© IOS Press 2006).

mechanics-based tool-tissue interaction modeling. The uterus model is anatomically detailed and populated with material properties based of measurements of real tissues. The system requires parallel computing capability for real-time haptic feedback and uses a custom-built force feedback device that fits under the patient mannequin and has an appropriate workspace for the procedure.

Simulator technology is rapidly improving in areas such as haptic device performance and accuracy of soft-tissue modeling. However, it is not yet understood what simulation components lead to improved performance of medical procedures and, most importantly, patient outcomes. In addition, the costs of haptic technology are still high, so most clinical training laboratories use simulators that do not incorporate haptic feedback.

Rehabilitation

Haptic feedback also plays a role in noninvasive therapies, rehabilitation in particular. The touch interaction between patients and therapists is recreated and improved upon by rehabilitation robots. In addition, basic studies on brain function and movement disorders are enabled by haptic-feedback technology.

Rehabilitation robotics. Rehabilitation robotics involves the use of automatically controlled mechanisms to provide therapy and assistance to humans with disabilities (Van der Loos, 1995). The user population for these systems includes any person with a physical or mental impairment that substantially limits one or more of the major life activities. Rehabilitation robots represent a powerful tool for understanding the mechanisms of movement disorders because they allow researchers to manipulate mechanical features of movement in a way not possible by human intervention. This approach can then be translated to treatment by providing compensation to augment performance, or improve neuromotor learning.

There are two main ways in which rehabilitation robots may be interfaced through a subject: through a single contact area such as a joystick (usually the hand for upper-extremity robots), or through multiple contact areas such as an exoskeleton. The former allows Cartesian space force/torque application, and the latter joint space torque application. Most existing systems have fixed bases, so that the user does not need to support the weight of the device. While both upper-extremity

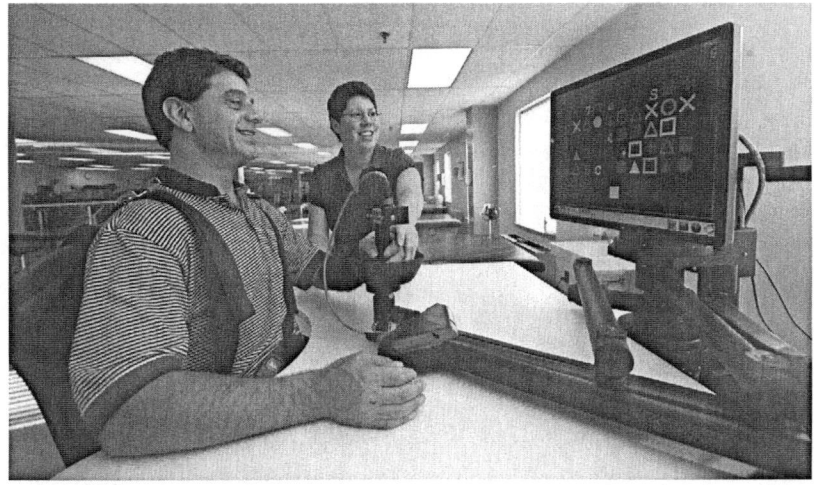

FIGURE 19.10 A commercially available impedance-controlled rehabilitation robot that provides force feedback to the user. The InMotion 2.0 Shoulder Robot (© Interactive Motion Technologies) is based upon the MIT-MANUS (Aisen et al., 1997). Printed with permission from Interactive Motion Technologies, Inc., Watertown, MA, USA.

systems and locomotor training/gait orthoses can use haptic feedback, we will focus here on upper-extremity systems due to their similarity to the types of haptic systems discussed earlier in this chapter. Several Cartesian upper-extremity fixed-base robots that have undergone clinical trial testing. For example, the MIT-MANUS is a two-joint robot arm that is grasped at the endpoint by the subject, as shown in Figure 19.10 (Aisen, Krebs, Hogan, McDowell, & Volpe, 1997; Fasoli, Krebs, Stein, Frontera, & Hogan, 2003). It is a two-degree-of-freedom impedance-type haptic device that can apply forces to the operator (in this case, a patient) using the approaches described earlier in this chapter.

Assessment and therapy methods using haptics. As an alternative to human-only therapy, a robot has several advantages for intervention: (1) after set up, the robot can provide consistent, lengthy therapy without tiring; (2) using sensors, the robot can acquire data to provide an objective quantification of recovery; and (3) the robot can implement therapy exercises not possible by a human therapist. All of these features are important, but the latter two are most relevant to haptics—data acquisition for modeling human motor function, and novel implementation of training and assistance methods.

Ideally, a rehabilitation robot would be able to provide many different forms of mechanical input, such as assisting, resisting, perturbing, and stretching, based the subject's real-time response. Most rehabilitation robots have been designed to use assisting or resisting forces to achieve desired motion. Some common assistance methods include (1) passive motion, in which the robot moves the subject through a desired pattern, (2) active assistance, in which a subject-initiated movement is subsequently guided by the robot, (3) active constraint, or force channel, which allows only subject motion toward a target, and (4) mirror image, in which the less impaired arm motion is measured and used to guide motion of the more impaired arm (Lum, Burgar, Shor, Majmundar, & Van der Loos, 2002). Resistance to motion is achieved by a control law that increases forces opposing the subject's desired motion with speed and/or proximity to the target, such as a linear damping field (Stein et al., 2004). Related to resistance training, feedback distortion can also be used in isometric and isotonic conditions to alter a subject's perception of therapeutic exercises (Brewer, Fagan, Klatzky, & Matsuoka, 2005). Other work has exploited the after-effect of training forces (i.e., adaptation) that magnify original errors (Emken & Reinkensmeyer, 2005; Patton, Phillips-Stoykov, Stojakovich, & Mussa-Ivaldi, 2005). With the capability to record motions and forces automatically, robotic systems can provide objective data to quantify how specific deficits change during training (Van der Loos, 1995), as well as identify the mechanism of the deficit (Smith & Shadmehr, 2005).

Most work in upper-limb extremity therapy has emphasized retraining movement ability for individuals who have had neurologic injury, such as a cerebral stroke or spinal cord injury. For example, the MIT-MANUS system benefits both acute and chronic stroke subjects using different types of therapy (assisting and resisting motion; Aisen et al., 1997; Fasoli et al., 2003). These studies show improved recovery, but have not yet elucidated the relationship between external mechanical forces and neural plasticity. Positive clinical results have also been obtained from other systems such as the Bi-Manu-Track (Hesse et al., 2005; Reinkensmeyer, Emken, & Cramer, 2004). Individuals receiving robotic therapy improved over those receiving electrical stimulation of the wrist extensor muscles by 15 points on the "Fugl-Meyer" score for upper-extremity movement ability (gains with other devices ranged between 0 and 5 points).

Neuroscience researchers have also used robots to study neurologic impairments. For example, Patton et al. (2005) found that error-enhancing robot therapy improves reaching in stroke subjects more than control strategies that assist movement. Interestingly, the virtual environments presented to the human subjects in such studies are usually not representative of real, physical dynamics. Force fields such as velocity-dependent "curl" fields (in which the direction of the force vector applied to the user is dependent on the user's speed) are used to create an environment that is completely new to all subjects. This enables study of the subjects learning to make reaching movements in a novel environment. Finally, we note that robotic/haptic devices can also be used to estimate human arm dynamics. Since some movement therapies depend on the actual arm dynamics, the ability to estimate patient-specific dynamic properties is important.

The two main challenges to demonstration of significant gains with rehabilitation robots are (1) the design of optimal movement tasks and mechanical inputs and (2) the design and manufacture of inexpensive, safe, practical robotic systems.

Haptic feedback for prosthetics. Presentation of haptic information to the wearer of a prosthesis, particularly the upper limb or hand, is another active area of research. Targeted reinnervation, which involves moving intact nerves from the residual limb to intact muscles elsewhere, causes sensations at the new location to be perceived as sensations coming from the missing limb (Kuiken, Marasco, Lock, Harden, & Dewald, 2007). Sensations have also been evoked by stimulating peripheral nerves in the residual limb (Dhillon & Horch, 2005). More commonly, methods of sensory substitution are being developed in which the sensory information from the prosthesis is mapped onto another intact sensory modality. Force information has been successfully provided to users via electrical stimulation and tactile displays (Kaczmarek, 2000), as well as vibrotactile feedback (Cipriani, Zaccone, Micera, & Carrozza, 2008). Proprioceptive information about hand configuration or elbow angle has been provided via vibrotactile and skin stretch feedback (Bark, Wheeler, Premakumar, & Cutkosky, 2008). Due to confounding factors, such as the noisiness of electromyography control, it has thus far been difficult to precisely characterize the effectiveness of artificial haptic feedback in prosthesis use.

PROGRESS AND FUTURE DIRECTIONS

Haptic technology, which is used to provide compelling touch "artificial" sensations to human operators, draws from the fields of mechatronics, robotics, control theory, neuroscience, and psychology. Haptic interfaces enhance or direct the user experience in both virtual and teleoperated environments, in applications ranging from entertainment to medical interventions.

The major challenges in haptic technology development can be categorized in terms of engineering research and development and human science. On the engineering side, we desire haptic devices that are smaller, lighter and more robust, as well as able to present stronger or higher-fidelity stimuli. This will require advances in sensing, actuation and transmission, materials, and mechanical and kinematic design. In addition, improved control theory and dynamic models are needed predict and solve problems related to stability and transparency of haptic interfaces in both virtual and teleoperated environments. New haptic device designs will be driven by an increased understanding of human sensing and motor control capabilities. In particular, models of human perception that can predict "haptic illusions" (Hayward & MacLean, 2008) will enable the development of clever haptic mechanisms that exploit human sensing limitations with simpler hardware requirements.

Medical applications are a major driving force in current haptic technology research. In surgery, the need for haptic feedback in many types of interventions has been supported by the results of human factors experiments. However, practical constraints of cost, geometry, and biocompatibility hinder the inclusion of haptic feedback, particularly as an addition to an existing robot-assisted surgery system. New surgical system designs that consider haptic feedback at a fundamental design stage are needed. Improvements in surgical simulation will be made through increasingly physically accurate and computationally efficient models of instrument-tissue interaction, coupled with haptic interfaces that feel dynamically equivalent to traditional surgical tools. Similarly, rehabilitation science will be improved through better control of haptic interfaces that apply motions or force to a control or patient subject. Once more appropriate strategies for rehabilitation are identified, patients will benefit from low-cost, wearable haptic interfaces (or orthotics/exoskeletons) that can be used for training or assistance outside the clinic. Haptic feedback for prosthetics will grow in importance, commensurate with the increasing complexity of prosthetic hands and improvements to direct brain control being developed in advanced prosthetics research projects. While the current focus in haptics for prosthetics is sensory substitution, developing techniques in peripheral nerve and cortical stimulation should enable more natural touch feedback.

ACKNOWLEDGMENTS

The author thanks Amy Blank, Netta Gurari, Blake Hannaford, and Tomonori Yamamoto for their contributions to this article.

REFERENCES

Aisen, M. L., Krebs, H. I., Hogan, N., McDowell, F., & Volpe, B. (1997). The effect of robot-assisted therapy and rehabilitative training on motor recovery following stroke. *Archives of Neurology, 54,* 443–446.

Bark, K., Wheeler, J. W., Premakumar, S., & Cutkosky, M. R. (2008). Comparison of skin stretch and vibrotactile stimulation for feedback of proprioceptive information. *Proceedings of IEEE Symposium on Haptic Interfaces for Virtual Environments and Teleoperator Systems, 71*–78.

Basdogan, C., De, S., Kim, J., Muniyandi, M., & Srinivasan, M. A. (2004). Haptics in minimally invasive surgical simulation and training, *IEEE Computer Graphics and Applications, 24,* 56–64.

Bholat, O. S., Haluck, R. S., Murray, W. B., Gorman, P. G., & Krummel, T. M. (1999). Tactile feedback is present during minimally invasive surgery. *Journal of the American College of Surgeons, 189,* 349–355.

Brewer, B. R., Fagan, M., Klatzky, R., & Matsuoka, Y. (2005). Perceptual limits for a robotic rehabilitation environment using visual feedback distortion. *IEEE Transactions on Neural Systems and Rehabilitation Engineering, 13,* 1–11.

Chan, A., MacLean, K. E., & McGrenere, J. (2008). Designing haptic icons to support collaborative turn-taking. *International Journal of Human-Computer Studies, 66,* 333–355.

Cipriani, C., Zaccone, F., Micera, S., & Carrozza, M. C. (2008). On the shared control of an EMG-controlled prosthetic hand: Analysis of user-prosthesis interaction. *IEEE Transactions on Robotics, 24,* 170–184.

Culjat, M. O., King, C. H., Franco, M. L., Bisley, J. W., Dutson, E., & Grundfest, W. S. (2008). Pneumatic balloon actuators for tactile feedback in robotic surgery. *Industrial Robot, 35,* 449–455.

Dhillon, G. S., & Horch, K. W. (2005). Direct neural sensory feedback and control of a prosthetic arm. *IEEE Transactions on Neural Systems and Rehabilitation Engineering, 13,* 468–472.

Emken, J., & Reinkensmeyer, D. (2005). Robot enhanced motor learning: Accelerating internal model formation during locomotion by transient dynamic amplification. *IEEE Transactions on Neural Systems and Rehabilitation Engineering, 13,* 33–39.

Etlaib, M. E. H., & Hewit, J. R. (2003). Tactile sensing technology for minimal access surgery—A review. *Mechatronics, 13,* 116–117.

Fasoli, S., Krebs, H., Stein, J., Frontera, W., & Hogan, N. (2003). Effects of robotic therapy on motor impairment and recovery in chronic stroke. *Archives of Physical Medicine and Rehabilitation, 84,* 477–482.

Feller, R. L., Lau, C. K. L., Wagner C. R., Perrin, D. P., & Howe, R. D. (2004). The effect of force feedback on remote palpation. *Proceedings of IEEE International Conference on Robotics and Automation,* 782–788.

Gwilliam, J., Mahvash, M., Vagvolgyi, B., Vacharat, A., Yuh, D., & Okamura, A. M. (2009). Effects of haptic and graphical force feedback for teleoperated palpation. *Proceedings of IEEE International Conference on Robotics and Automation,* 677–682.

Harders, M., Bajka, M., Spaelter, U., Tuchschmidi, S., Bleuler, H., & Szekely, G. (2006). Highly-realistic, immersive training environment for hysteroscopy. *Proceedings of Medicine Meets Virtual Reality, 119,* 176–181.

Hayward, V., & Cruz-Hernandez, M. (2000). Tactile display device using distributed lateral skin stretch. *Proceedings of IEEE Symposium on Haptic Interfaces for Virtual Environments and Teleoperation Systems*, 1309–1314.

Hayward, V., & MacLean, K. E. (2008). A brief taxonomy of tactile illusions and demonstrations that can be done in a hardware store. *Brain Research Bulletin, 75*, 742–752.

Hesse, S., Werner, C., Pohl, M., Rueckriem, S., Mehrholz, J., & Lingnau, M. L. (2005). Computerized arm training improves the motor control of the severely affected arm after stroke: A single-blinded randomized trial in two centers. *Stroke, 36*, 1960–1966.

Howe, R. D., Peine, W. J., Kontarinis, D. A., & Son, J. S. (1995). Remote palpation technology. *IEEE Engineering in Medicine and Biology, 14*, 318–323.

Johnson, K. O., & Phillips, J. R. (1998). A rotating drum stimulator for scanned embossed patterns and textures across the skin. *Journal of Neuroscience Methods, 22*, 221–231.

Kaczmarek, K. A. (2000). Sensory augmentation and substitution. In J. D. Bronzino (Ed.), *CRC handbook of biomedical engineering* (143.1–143.10). Boca Raton, FL: CRC Press.

Killebrew, J. H., Bensmaia, S. J., Dammann, J. F., Denchev, P., Hsiao, S. S., Craig, J. C., & Johnson, K. O. (2007). A dense array stimulator to generate arbitrary spatio-temporal tactile stimuli. *Journal of Neuroscience Methods, 161*, 62–74.

Kitagawa, M., Dokko, D., Okamura, A. M., & Yuh, D. D. (2005). Effect of sensory substitution on suture manipulation forces for robotic surgical systems. *Journal of Thoracic and Cardiovascular Surgery, 129*, 151–158.

Kontarinis, D. A., & Howe, R. D. (1995). Tactile display of vibratory information in teleoperation and virtual environments. *Presence, 4*, 387–402.

Kuchenbecker, K. J., Fiene, J., & Niemeyer, G. (2006). Improving contact realism through event-based haptic feedback. *IEEE Transactions on Visualization and Computer Graphics, 12*, 219–230.

Kuebler, B., Seibold, U., & Hirzinger, G. (2005). Development of actuated and sensor integrated forceps for minimally invasive robotic surgery. *International Journal of Medical Robotics and Computer Assisted Surgery, 1*, 96–107.

Kuiken, T. A., Marasco, P. D., Lock, B. A., Harden, R. N., & Dewald, J. P. A. (2007). Redirection of cutaneous sensation from the hand to the chest skin of human amputees with targeted reinnervation. *Proceedings of the National Academy of Sciences, 104*, 20061–20066.

Liu, A., Tendick, F., Cleary, K., & Kaufmann, C. (2003). A survey of surgical simulation: Applications, technology, and education. *Presence, 12*, 599–614.

Lum, P. S., Burgar, C. G., Shor, P. C., Majmundar, M., & Van der Loos, M. (2002). Robot-assisted movement training compared with conventional therapy techniques for the rehabilitation of upper limb motor function following stroke. *Archives of Physical Medicine and Rehabilitation, 83*, 952–959.

Mahvash, M., & Okamura, A. M. (2007). Friction compensation for enhancing transparency of a teleoperator with compliant transmission. *IEEE Transactions on Robotics, 23*, 1240–1246.

Moy, G., Wagner, C., & Fearing, R. S. (2000). A compliant tactile display for teletaction. *Proceedings of IEEE International Conference on Robotics and Automation*, 3409–3415.

Okamura, A. M., Dennerlein, J. T., & Cutkosky, M. R. (2001). Reality-based models for vibration feedback in virtual environments. *ASME/IEEE Transactions on Mechatronics, 6*, 245–252.

Ottermo, M. V., Stavdahl, O., & Johansen, T. A. (2005). Electromechanical design of a miniature tactile shape display for minimally invasive surgery. *Proceedings of World Haptics Conference*, 561–562.

Patton, J. L., Phillips-Stoykov, M. E., Stojakovich, M., & Mussa-Ivaldi, F. A. (2005). Evaluation of robotic training forces that either enhance or reduce error in chronic hemiparetic stroke survivors. *Experimental Brain Research, 168*, 368–383.

Provancher, W. R., Cutkosky, M. R., Kuchenbecker K. J., & Niemeyer, G. (2005). Contact location display for haptic perception of curvature and object motion. *International Journal of Robotics Research, 24*, 691–702.

Reiley, C. E., Akinbiyi, T., Burschka, D., Chang, D. C., Okamura, A. M., & Yuh, D. D. (2008). Effects of visual force feedback on robot-assisted surgical task performance. *Journal of Thoracic and Cardiovascular Surgery, 135*, 196–202.

Reinkensmeyer, D., Emken, J., & Cramer, S. (2004). Robotics, motor learning, and neurologic recovery. *Annual Review of Biomedical Engineering, 6*, 497–525.

Satava, R. M. (2001). Accomplishments and challenges of surgical simulation. *Surgical Endoscopy, 15*, 232–241.

Smith, M. A., & Shadmehr, R. (2005). Intact ability to learn internal models of arm dynamics in Huntington's disease but not cerebellar degeneration. *Journal of Neurophysiology, 93*, 2809–2821.

Srinivasan, M. A., Beauregard, G. L., & Brock, D. L. (1996). The impact of visual information on the haptic perception of stiffness in virtual environments. *Proceedings of IEEE Symposium on Haptic Interfaces for Virtual Environment and Teleoperator Systems*, 555–559.

Stein, J., Krebs, H. I., Frontera, W. R., Fasoli, S., Hughes, R., & Hogan, N. (2004). Comparison of two techniques of robot-aided upper limb exercise training after stroke. *American Journal of Physical Medicine and Rehabilitation, 83*, 720 728.

Strom, P., Hedman, L., Sarna, L., Kjellin, A., Wredmark, T., & Fellander-Tsai, L. (2006). Early exposure to haptic feedback enhances performance in surgical simulator training: A prospective randomized crossover study in surgical residents. *Surgical Endoscopy, 20*, 1383–1388.

Tholey, G., Desai, J. P., & Castellanos, A. E. (2005). Force feedback plays a significant role in minimally invasive surgery—Results and analysis. *Annals of Surgery, 241*, 102–109.

Van der Loos, H. F. M. (1995). VA/Stanford rehabilitation robotics research and development program: Lessons learned in the application of robotics technology to the field of rehabilitation. *IEEE Transactions on Rehabilitation Engineering, 3*, 46–55.

Wagner, C. R., Lederman, S. J., & Howe, R. D. (2004). Design and performance of a tactile shape display using RC servomotors. *Haptics-e, 3*(4). Retrieved from http://www.haptics-e.org/Vol_03/he-v3n4.pdf

Wagner, C. R., & Howe, R. D. (2007). Force feedback benefit depends on experience in multiple degree of freedom robotic surgery task. *IEEE Transactions on Robotics, 23*, 1235–1240.

Webster, R. J., Murphy, T. E., Verner, L. N., & Okamura, A. M. (2005). A novel two-dimensional tactile slip display: Design, kinematics and perceptual experiment. *ACM Transactions on Applied Perception, 2,* 150–165.

Westebring-van der Putten, E. P., Goossens, R. H. M., Jakimowicz, J. J., & Dankelman, J. (2008). Haptics in minimally invasive surgery—A review. *Minimally Invasive Therapy and Allied Technologies, 17,* 3–16.

Winfield, L., Glassmire, J., Colgate, J. E., & Peshkin, M. (2007). T-PaD: Tactile pattern display through variable friction reduction. *Proceedings of World Haptics Conference,* 421–426.

Zemiti, N., Morel, G., Ortmaier, T., & Bonnet, N. (2007). Mechatronic design of a new robot for force control in minimally invasive surgery. *IEEE/ASME Transactions on Mechatronics, 12,* 143–153.

Index

A/ASP. *See* Adolescent/Adult SP (A/ASP)
Aβ afferents, 41
Abuse, 258–259, 262. *See also* Questionnaire
  measures with touch subscale, 256
Acid-sensing ion channels (ASIC), 52–53
  role in mechanotransduction, 74, 75
Active and passive accompaniment, 281
Actuator, 470, 473–474, 476–477. *See also* Force feedback systems; Tactile feedback system
  BCIs, 111
  in tactile feedback systems, 480
  vibration feedback and, 484
  vibrotactile, 484–485
Acuity, 449
  and dexterity, 106
  grid test, 72
  spatial, 445
  tactile, 87–88, 92, 97, 104
Aδ afferents, 39
Adequate stimulus, 123, 132
ADHD. *See* Attention-deficit hyperactivity disorder (ADHD)
Adolescents
  tactile behavior, 355
  touch measures in, 265
Adolescent/Adult SP (A/ASP), 227
Adult partners conflict, 260
Adult touch measures, 251
  Tie Sign Functions Scale, 252
  Tie Signs Coding Sheet, 252
  touch log record, 251–252
Affectionate touch, 376. *See also* Touch

communication index, 260–261
  measures, 256
Afferent fiber types, 123
Aging, 90, 449
aIPS. *See* Anterior intraparietal sulcus (aIPS)
Alabama parenting questionnaire, 256–257
Allodynia, 33, 39. *See also* Touch, hypersensitivity
Androgynous cultures. *See also* Feminine cultures
Angelman syndrome (AS), 413
Anger, 310
Anterior intraparietal sulcus (aIPS), 147, 152
  cortical map expansion, 92–93
  electrical noise stimulation, 94
  neuron loss, 91
  problems, 91
  sensory stimulation, 93
  skin elasticity, 15
  spatial discrimination with, 92
  tactile acuity, 91, 92
  tactile coactivation, 93
  tactile performance, 87, 90
Apocrine sweat/scent glands, 20
Arousal, 463
  conductance level, 233
  degree of, 232
  between mother and child, 379, 392
  reduction, 234, 316
  repetitive skin brushing, 425
AS. *See* Angelman syndrome (AS)
ASDs. *See* Autism spectrum disorders (ASDs)
ASH neuron, 64

499

ASIC. *See* Acid-sensing ion channels (ASIC)
Asperger's syndrome, 416
Atoh1 gene, 125
ATP receptor, 40–41
Attachment relationships, 374
Attentional manipulations, 196
Attention-deficit hyperactivity disorder (ADHD), 222, 415, 420–421
Autism spectrum disorders (ASDs), 415–418
  autistic disorder, 416
  mechanoreceptors, 417
  somatosensory processing, 418
  symptoms, 416
  tactile seeking behaviors, 416

Barrier function
  in epidermis, 11–12
  shunt pathways, 13
BAX cells, 78
Bayesian decision theory, 195–196
Bayesian priors, 195–196
BCI. *See* Brain–computer interface (BCI)
BDNF. *See* Brain-derived neurotrophic factor (BDNF)
Behavioral state, 274
Biobehavioral provisions, 374
Blind. *See* Congenitally blind (CB); Late blind (LB); Visual impaired
Blindfolded sighted individuals, 451
Blindness, 451
Blood oxygen level dependent (BOLD), 96
Body, 3
Body schema/image, 110, 197
BOLD. *See* Blood oxygen level dependent (BOLD)
Braille, 446–447, 448
Braille slate, 448
Brain
  neurons in, 161
  plasticity, 90–91
  reorganization, 94

SI position, 164
SII position, 164
Brain–computer interface (BCI), 111
Brain-derived neurotrophic factor (BDNF), 42
Buddhism, 360

C afferents, 38, 39
Caenorhabditis elegans. *See* also
    Drosophila melanogaster
  mechanosensitive channel, 67
  mechanotransduction features, 71
  membrane stretch model, 67
  response comparison, 74
  tether model, 67–68
  touch responses in, 63–64
  TRN monitoring, 74
Calcium, role in epidermis, 10
Capsaicin, 39
Cardiac vagal tone, 383
Caregiver touch, 274
  father–child relationship, 282–283
  fetal response, 275–276
  maternal touch, 276–282
Caregiver–Infant Touch Scale, 279
CB. *See* Congenitally blind (CB)
CCK. *See* Cholecystokinin (CCK)
CE. *See* Cornified envelope (CE)
Cellular components, 27, 66–67
Cerebral palsy (CP), 421–422
Childhood trauma questionnaire, 259
Children, 88–90
Cholecystokinin (CCK), 383
Circumcision, female, 363
Coding procedures, 261–262
Coercive discipline Scale, 262
Collectivism, 359
Collision detection, 478
Comforting touch. *See* Touch, nurturing
Comprehensive child maltreatment scales, 259
Conduction velocity, 123–124
Confucianism, 360
Confusion hypothesis, 444

Congenitally blind (CB), 435
  occipital cortex, 108
  perspective understanding in, 439–440
  size discrimination, 205
  tactile stimuli representation, 203
  tactile TOJ task, 208
Contact motion tactile feedback systems, 482
Continuum mechanics model, 127
Corneocytes, 7
Cornified envelope (CE), 11
Cortical map
  disintegration, 93
  expansion, 92
Cortical structural patterns, 426
CP. See Cerebral palsy (CP)
Criterion referenced test, 230
  congruency task, 197–203
Crossmodal, 189–210
  calibration, 205–206
  delayed matching to sample task, 205
  influences, 204–209
  integration, 204
  plasticity, 108–110
  transfer task, 204
Cross-sex relationships, 304
Culture/cultural, 317, 356
  American, 356, 362
  Arab/Islamic, 356, 362
  Asian, 359, 364
  collectivistic, 359-360, 364
  differences in, 354
  gender orientation of, 364
  highcontact, 355
  Latin American, 355
  Mediterranean, 355
  Polish, 338
  Southern latitudes, 358
  touch in, 359
  variability, 380
  Western, 310, 358
Cutaneous mechanoreceptive afferents
  neural coding, 132

PC afferents, 130–131
RA afferents, 128–130
SA1 afferents, 125–128
SA2 afferents, 131–132
types, 124–125
Cutaneous neuroendocrinology, 17–18
Cutaneous receptors, 124, 300. See also Sensory—system
Cutaneous touch, 254
Cytochrome P450 (CYP), 12
Cytokeratin, 9

D hair. See Down hair afferents (D hair)
Deafferentation, effect of, 94
Deep sleep theory, 461
Defensive response, 232
Degenerin/Epithelial Na^+ Channels (DEG/ENaC), 52–53
Demodex folliculorum, 21
Deprivation, 423
  maternal, 382, 384, 388
  persistent, 375
  sensory, 108
  stimulus effect, 360
  tactile, 264, 423
Dermatoglyphs, 13
Dermis, 5, 13. See also Epidermis; Skin, human
  cutaneous neuroendocrinology, 17–18
  functionality, 14
  innervation, 16–17
  skin elasticity, 15
  vascularization, 15–16
Desktop tactile display system, 481, 482
Desmosomes, 9
Development, 290, 291
  behavioral, 423
  brain, 395
  contributions to tactile performance, 88
  dermis, 13, 15, 18
  dyslexia, 419

Development (cont.)
  embryonic, 80
  hair follicle, 26
  haptic technology, 494
  of infants, 263
  lessons learned from, 77
  Meissner's corpuscles, 42
  mental, 398
  multisensory influences on touch, 204–209, 210
  postnatal, 78
  processes, 18
  Rett syndrome, 414
  Sebaceous gland, 21
  social–emotional, 398
  tactile acuity, 89
  touch and, 351, 409
  TRNs, 63, 64
Developmental theory, 394
Direct gating model, 47, 48
Directed attention hypothesis, 194
Discipline
  assessment of parent, 262
  Coercive Discipline Scale, 262
  Daily Discipline Interview, 256, 257
Distal senses, 424
Dome, 24
Dorsal columns, 35–36
Dorsal root ganglia (DRG), 59
  somatosensory neuron cell bodies, 60
Down hair afferents (D hair), 39
Down syndrome, 411–412
DRG. See Dorsal root ganglia (DRG)
Drosophila melanogaster, 68. See also *Caenorhabditis elegans*
  mechanotransduction features in, 71
  mutation identification, 69–70
  NOMPA proteins, 70
  NOMPB proteins, 71
  NOMPC proteins, 70
  sensory structures in, 68–69
  TRP channels, 70
Drosophila TRPA channel PAINLESS, 76

Dual-pathway theories, 150
Dual-tether model, 68
Duration index, 253
Dyadic parent–child interaction coding system, 257–258
Dyslexia, developmental, 419–420
Dysregulated function, 248

Eccrine glands sweat, 19–20
ECG. See Electrocardiogram (ECG)
ECM. See Extracellular matrix (ECM)
Ectoderm. See Epidermis
EDA. See Electrodermal activity (EDA)
EEG studies. See Electroencephalographic studies (EEG studies)
Elasticity, 15
Elderly
  acuity, 93
  brain volumes, 91
  high-level tactile performance, 91
  sensory stimulation, 93
  tactile function, 88
Electrocardiogram (ECG), 234
Electrodermal activity (EDA), 232–234
Electroencephalographic studies (EEG studies), 411
Emotions, 305–312, 353
  anger, 310
  basic, 308
  decoding accuracy, 309
  hedonics, 306–308
  love, 311
  negatively valenced, 311
  tactile behaviors, 310
Empiricism, 34
Endocrine
  endocrine fit, 381, 387
  neuroendocrine pathways, 380
  neuroendocrine process, 356
  neuroendocrine transducer, 357
  sebaceous glands, 21
  skin as, 17
Enhanced deep sleep leading to less substance P" theory, 461

cell differentiation and turnover, 9, 10
cells, 8
epidermal keratins, 9
Epidermis, 5, 6. *See also* Dermis; Skin, human
 calcium role, 10
 merkel cells, 8
 outer layer, 7, 8
 permeability barrier, 11–13
 single-layered periderm, 6–7
 skin protection, 8
 skin surface morphology, 13
 thickness, 12
Epidural ridges. *See* Intermediate ridges
Equifinality, 301
Equipotentiality, 301
Ethnicity/ethnic
 differences, 11, 21, 25, 363
 skin color and, 26
 touch behavior, 264
 variation, 13, 20
Extracellular matrix (ECM), 5
 dermis functionality, 14
Extracellular recording techniques, 62

Face-to-face touch coding system, 249
Failure to thrive, 388
FAS. *See* Fetal alcohol syndrome (FAS)
Father–child interactions, 282–283, 379. *See also* Maternal touch; Parent–child touch measures
FDs. *See* Feeding disorders (FDs)
Feeding disorders (FDs), 285, 388
Feminine cultures, 361, 364
Femininity, 361
Fetal alcohol syndrome (FAS), 422–423
Fibrils, anchoring, 14
Fibroblast, 14
Filaments, anchoring, 14
Fine motor functions, 409
Finger nail, 25–26

FITS. *See* Functions of infant touch scale (FITS)
Fluid-filled sacs, 131
fMRI. *See* Functional magnetic resonance imaging (fMRI)
Force
 computation, 478
 interfaces, 472
 rendering, 477–480
 admittance type, 474
 device kinematics, 474–475
Force feedback systems, 471, 472. *See also* Actuator; Haptic feedback; Tactile feedback system
 actuator, 473
 force interfaces, 472
 generating forces, 475–477
 generating motions, 477
 impedance type, 472–473
 limitation in, 487
 matrix equation of motion, 476
 in surgery, 486–487
Forward genetic screening, 60
Fragile X syndrome (FXS), 414–415
Frequency index, 253
Functional magnetic resonance imaging (fMRI), 144, 384
 functions examined, 248–249
Functions of infant touch scale (FITS), 248. *See also* Infant touch scale (ITS)
 11item version, 248
Functions of Touch Scale, 281
FXS. *See* Fragile X syndrome (FXS)

GA. *See* Gestational age (GA)
GABA. *See* Gamma aminobutyric acid (GABA)
GABAergic system, 413
Gamma aminobutyric acid (GABA), 413
Gastrulation, 6
Gate theory, 461
Gated ion channel, 65
Gating
 channel, 67
 direct, 48

Gating (cont.)
  indirect, 48, 49
  mechanism, 67, 426
  models, 47
  spring, 70, 76
Gender, 329
  effects, 312–313, 315
  orientation, 361
Generator potentials, 38
Genetic/genes
  gentle body touch, 64
  PWS, 412
  reverse genetics, 60
  touch stimuli transduction, 65
  touch-receptive neurons, 64
  touch-related genes, 63, 68, 77
Gestational age (GA), 391
Glabrous skin, 4, 24
Golgi tendon organ, 138
GOT. *See* Grating orientation task (GOT)
Graphesthesia, 411
Grating orientation task (GOT), 87, 89
  visual discrimination, 152
Grid test, 62, 63, 72
Gross motor functions, 409
Growth, 21
  emotional, 397
  hair, 22
  maternal touch, 385

Hair fiber, 24–25
Hair follicle, 21
  cell growth and death, 22
  epithelium, 23
  hormone production, 22
  immunological status, 22–23
  neuronal networks, 23–24
  skin types, 24
Halstead–Reitan neuropsychological test battery, 230–231
Hand-arm vibration syndrome (HAVS), 95
Haptic communication, 351
  emotional, 353
  functional touch, 354
  human infants, touch with, 352

human sexuality and touch, 353
persuasive touch, 354
tactile affection and intimacy, 352–353
touch as universal, 354–355
design of, 469–471
future of, 493–494
Haptic device, 478
Haptic feedback, 469, 470. *See also* Force feedback systems; Rehabilitation robotics; Tactile feedback system
  assessment and therapy through, 491
  haptic loop, 471, 472
  in noninvasive therapies, 490
  for prosthetics, 493
  rehabilitation robotics, 490
  surgical simulation, 488–490
Haptic illusions, 442, 494
  horizontal–vertical illusion, 443
  Mueller Lyer illusion, 443
Haptic interaction point (HIP), 478
Haptic interface, 469, 472
Haptic loop, 471, 472
Haptic perception, 162, 189
  crossmodal calibration, 205–206
  crossmodal task, 204, 205
  multisensory integration, 205, 206–207
  multisensory interactions, 204–205
  object representation in 3D, 171
  RFs in SI, 165–167
  somatosensory cortex, 163–165
  somatosensory periphery, 162–163
  spatial representation, 167–171
Haptic processing, 143
  aIPS, 147
  Brodmann Areas, 144
  dual pathway theories, 150
  group average SPM, 145, 147
  human cortical regions, 145, 149
  LOtv, 147
  macrogeometric and microgeometric properties, 143–144
  neuroimaging findings, 146

SI involvement, 148
SII, 144, 145, 146
visuo haptic convergence in, 150–153
Haptic rendering, 469, 478–479
HAVS. *See* Hand-arm vibration syndrome (HAVS)
Health
  mental, 259
  skin immune system, 27
Heart rate
  as touch response, 234–236
  variability, 234
Hedonics, 306–308
High-contact cultures, 355
Higher-order functions, 375
High-threshold mechanoreceptors (HTM), 39
HIP. *See* Haptic interaction point (HIP)
HIV patients and massage therapy, 463
Homunculus, 166
Horizontal–vertical illusion, 443
HTM. *See* High-threshold mechanoreceptors (HTM)
Hyperalgesia, 39
Hypersensitivity, 33
Hypothalamic–pituitary–adrenal axis, 18

I/TSP. *See* Infant/Toddler SP (I/TSP)
IA currents. *See* Intermediately adapting currents (IA currents)
Iav isoform. *See* Inactive isoform (Iav isoform)
IF. *See* Index finger (IF)
Illusion, 442
  confusion hypothesis, 444
  horizontal–vertical illusion, 443
  Mueller-Lyer illusion, 443–444
  Ponzo illusion, 444
Immunoglobulins, 27
Impedance-controlled rehabilitation robot, 491
Inactive isoform (Iav isoform), 50
Index finger (IF), 99
Indirect gating model, 48, 49

Individualism, 359
Individualist culture, 359
Infant
  high-impact stimuli, 392–393
  neuromaturation, 394
  self-regulation, 390
  sleep-wake cycle, 392
  touch, 283–286
  unimodel stimulus, 392
Infant touch scale (ITS), 246. *See also* Parent–child touch measures
  components, 246
  touch locations, 246
  touch type categories, 246
Infant/Toddler SP (I/TSP), 227
  functions, 248
Innate immune system mast cells, 24
Innervation, 16
  by C-touch afferents, 417
  targeted, 493
Insular cortex activations, 179
Intensity coding, 136, 137–138
Intermediate ridges, 125, 126
Intermediately adapting currents (IA currents), 73
Intermittent TBS (iTBS), 104
  shape selectivity in, 148
  visuo haptic convergence, 152–153
Interspike interval, 43
Intimacy, 303–305. *See also* Touch
Intrauterine trauma, 421
Invasive behavior, 341
IPS, 147, 152. *See also* Brain
iTBS. *See* Intermittent TBS (iTBS)
ITS. *See* Infant touch scale (ITS)

Joint afferents, 132, 138

Kangaroo Care (KC), 374
  infant neuromaturation, 394
  infant self regulation, 391–394
  intervention, 389–390
  maternal well-being and mood, 396–397
  parent–child relationships, 397–399
  physiological regulation

KC. *See* Kangaroo Care (KC)
Keratinocytes, 7, 46–47
Keratinohyalin, 7
Kinesthetic receptors, 300. *See also* Sensory—system

Labeled line system, 34
   for encoding information, 35
Laminae I/II, 36
Langerhans cells, 8
Late blind (LB), 436
   picture interpretation, 438
Lateral occipital complex (LOC), 146
Lateral occipital tactile visual area (LOtv), 146
LB. *See* Late blind (LB)
Light touch, 36, 230
Live tactile interaction body chart, 255
LOC. *See* Lateral occipital complex (LOC)
Local shape, 481
Location index, 253
Long term depression (LTD), 102
Long term potentiation (LTP), 102
LOtv. *See* Lateral occipital tactile visual area (LOtv)
Low contact cultures, 355
LTD. *See* Long term depression (LTD)
LTP. *See* Long term potentiation (LTP)
Luria–Nebraska neuropsychological battery, 230
   LOtv, 146

Macrogeometric properties, 143. *See also* Microgeometric properties
   LOC, 146
   macrogeometry selectivity, 148
   POC involvement, 147–148
   shape selective brain regions, 147
   vision and touch, 150
Magnetoencephalography (MEG), 418

Maltreatment. *See also* Questionnaire
   child, 258
   measures with a touch subscale, 256
Mammalian mechanosensory cells, 51
Mammalian somatosensory neurons, 60
Map, 445–446
Masculine cultures, 361
Masculinity, 361
Massage, preterm infant, 455–457
   energy expenditure reduction, 456
   growth effects, 456
   insulin change percentage, 456
   stress behavior reduction, 457
Massage therapy, 455–465
   attentiveness enhancement, 457–458
   cortisol reduction, 459
   depression reduction, 458
   effects of, 463
   immune enhancement, 462–463
   moderate pressure, 463
   pain reduction, 459–461
   serotonin, 461
   vagal activity after, 464–465
Maternal postpartum repertoire, 376. *See also* Maternal touch
Maternal sensitivity, 378–379
   autonomic response, 383–384
   biological correlates, 380
   brain circuitry, 384–385
   breast milk effects, 377
   cortisol levels, 381
   developmental psychopathology, 385
   early maternal touch, 376–379
   feeding disorders, 388–389
   functions of, 280–281
   in infancy, 389
   infant's stress response, 383–384
   KC intervention, 389–390
   longitudinal studies, 281–282

maternal behaviors, 373, 376, 386–388
Maternal touch, 276–279, 373, 374. *See also* Parent–child touch measures; Touch—infants and
  age related changes, 282
  mother sensitivity, 378
  negative touches, 280
  neuroendocrine pathways, 380–383
  parent–infant touch, 379, 285–286
  physical contact in infancy, 389
  positive touch, 280
  premature birth, 385–386
  research in animal models, 374
  SF procedure, 277–278
  touch patterns, 279–280
  touch synchrony, 377
Maximum likelihood estimation (MLE), 195
Mean field approach, 106
Measurement, 219–238. *See also* Parent–child touch measures; Parent–infant; Mother–child relationship
  adults, 221, 226–229, 237
  children, 220–233
  infants, 226, 227, 230, 237
mec genes, 64, 65–67
Mechanoreceptor potential (MRP), 69
Mechanoreceptors, 17, 24, 78
  low-threshold, 75
  mammalian, 78
  Meissner's corpuscles, 86–87
  somatosensory representation effect, 87, 88
  subsets, 72
  tactile acuity, 87
Mechanosensation, 52, 75
Mechanosensitivity, 77–78
Mechanotransduction, 47, 162
  approaches for mammalian gene identification, 77
  channels, 50
  cuticle of worm, 62
  direct gating model, 47, 48

extracellular recording techniques, 62
  features in *C. elegans* and *D. melanogaster*, 71
  grid test, 62, 63
  indirect gating model, 47, 48, 49
  ion channel expression, 78
  MEC gene homologs, 74, 75
  mechanosensitivity, 77–78
  model, 38
  patch clamp analysis, 61
  protein complex, 79
  role of mammalian homologs, 73–74
  skin nerve technique, 62
  stimulus response comparison, 74
  tether requirement, 78–79
  tethered model, 48–49
  TRP channels, 76–77
Medial occipital cortex (MOC), 149
Medulla, 24
MEG. *See* Magnetoencephalography (MEG)
Meissner's corpuscle, 16–17, 42, 129. *See also* Pacinian corpuscle
  density, 86–87
Melanocytes, 26
Melanogenesis process, 26–27
Memantine, 102
Membrane stretch model, 67
MEMS. *See* Micro electromechanical system (MEMS)
Mental health
  clinic, 257
  community controls, 259
  community-based, 387
Merkel cell–neurite complexes, 43
  functions, 43–44
  mechanosensory cell use, 44–45
  neurotrophins role, 44
  photoablation effect, 44
Merkel cells, 8, 125
Merkel's touch spots, 24
Mesoderm. *See* Dermis
Micro electromechanical system (MEMS), 481

Microgeometric properties, 143, 148. *See also* Macrogeometric properties
  area responsibilities, 148–149
  SI involvement, 148
  tactile/haptic texture selective regions, 149
Microneurography, 36, 37
Microtubule cells, 64
Minimally invasive surgery (MIS), 486
MLE. *See* Maximum likelihood estimation (MLE)
MOC. *See* Medial occipital cortex (MOC)
Modality appropriateness hypothesis, 194
Molecular processes of touch, 47–53, 59–80
Mother–child relationship, 275, 379. *See also* Maternal touch
Motherese, 376
Motion
  dynamic, 125
  haptic exploration, 175
  perception of direction, 175, 176–177
  perception of speed, 177
  RAs, 128, 130, 133, 134, 139
MRP. *See* Mechanoreceptor potential (MRP)
Mueller-Lyer illusion, 443–444
Multisensory body representations, 196–197
  crossmodal congruency task, 197–199
  multisensory interaction role, 203
  postural remapping, 200–201
  rubber hand experiment, 202–203
  tracking location of touch, 199–200
  ventral premotor cortex neurons, 201
  visual influences on perceived location, 197
Multisensory integration, 205, 206–207
Multisensory integrator, 195
Mus musculus, 60, 74

Muscle spindle afferents, 138
Myelinated somatosensory neurons. *See* Aβ afferents
Myelination, 16, 35

Naming as perceptual function, 438
Nanchung isoform (Nan isoform), 50
Natural killer (NK) cells, 462
  in massage therapy, 462–463
NaV channels. *See* Voltage gated Na⁺ channels (NaV channels)
NDDs. *See* Neurodevelopmental disorders (NDDs)
Negatively valenced emotions, 311
Neglect, 231, 264
Neonatal Behavior Assessment Scale, 377
Neonatal intensive care unit (NICU), 388
NEPSY, 393
Nerve fiber bundle, 24
Nerve growth factor (NGF), 78
Neural coding, 132
  cutaneous form perception, 134–136
  flutter and vibration perception, 132–133
  intensity coding, 136, 137–138
  motion detection, 133, 134
  roughness perception, 137
  texture perception, 134
Neurite ending, 129
Neurobiological system
  maternal touch, 388–389
  parenting, 373
Neuroderm, 6
Neurodevelopment
  disorders, 410
  infant's, 395
  maternal presence, 394
Neurodevelopmental disorders (NDDs), 410
  affecting skill development, 418–420
  from environmental factors, 421
  etiologies, 410, 415
  types, 410

Neuroendocrinology, cutaneous, 3
Neuroimaging, 101, 143, 146, 147, 171, 179
Neuromaturation, 394, 395
  ASH, 64
  direct iontuning curve, 176
  direction tuning curve, 176
  FLP, 65
  mechanoreceptive bristle shaft, 68
  myelinated, 35
  networks, 23
Neuron, 167
  in brain, 161
  orientation selectivity, 167–168, 169
  pyramidal, 415
  RA neuron, 37
  Raster plot, 168
  secondary, 36
Neurophysiology, 34, 37, 124, 128, 131–138
Neuropsychological
  battery, 226, 230
  measures, 225
Neurotransmitters, 18, 23
  hair follicle events, 22
  Merkel cell, 8, 43
Neurotrophins, 44
NGF. *See* Nerve growth factor (NGF)
NICU. *See* Neonatal intensive care unit (NICU)
No mechanoreceptor potential (NOMP), 69–71
  body politics, 330
  gender differences in, 329–330
Nociceptive responses, 178
  capsaicin, 39
  NaV channels, 40
Nociceptors
  ATP, 40–41
  RTX ablation, 39–40
  sensing ability, 40
  TRPV1, 39
NOMP. *See* No mechanoreceptor potential (NOMP)
Nonhairy skin. *See* Glabrous skin

Onychocytes, 25
Open-loop vibration signals, 485
Orientation discrimination, 205
Orientation effects. *See also* Braille
Orienting response, 232
Oxytocin (OT), 353, 373
  parental touch, 381–382

Pacinian corpuscle, 16, 41–42. *See also* Meissner's corpuscle
Pacinian corpuscle afferents (PC afferents), 125, 130–131, 168
  flutter and vibration perception, 132–133
  texture perception, 134
Pain, 178
  acute, 39
  characterization, 178–179
  hyperalgesia, 39
  neural coding distribution, 179
  sensation of, 36
  STT neurons, 178
Papillary ridges, 126
Parchment skin illusion, 190
Parent Behavior Inventory, 262
Parent–child conflict tactics scale, 256, 258
  FITS, 248–249
  infant touch scale, 246
Parent–child touch measures, 246. *See also* Mother–child relationship
  face to face touch coding system, 249
  recollections of early childhood touch scale, 249–250
  interactions. See Caregiver touch
  touch patterns, 379–380
Parent–infant. *See also* Mother–child relationship
  games, 277
  assessing environments, 258
  brain areas, 384
  care and abuse experience questionnaire, 258–259
  childhood trauma questionnaire, 259

Parent–infant (*cont.*)
 comprehensive child maltreatment scales, 259
 dyadic parent–child interaction coding system, 257–258
 harsh or negative, 256, 258
 neurobiological system of, 373, 375, 388
 parent–child conflict tactics scale, 258
Parenting. *See also* Mother–child relationship
 Alabama parenting questionnaire, 256–257
 trauma inventory, 259–260
Parieto occipital cortex (POC), 147
Patch clamp analysis, 61
Pathological pain. *See* Hyperalgesia
Pattern perception, 436–437. *See also* Braille
PC afferents. *See* Pacinian corpuscle afferents (PC afferents)
Perceptual learning, 98, 99
Perinatal morbidity, 422
Peripheral sensory neurons, 36
 Aδ afferents, 39
 C afferents, 38, 39
 keratinocytes, 46–47
 mechanotransduction model, 38
 microneurography, 36, 37
 nociceptors, 39–41
Peripheral somatosensory receptors. *See also* Skin, human; Touch
 Aβ afferents, 41
 RA afferents, 41–42
 reverse genetics, 37–38
 SA afferents, 43–46
 distortion, 437, 441
 linear, 440–442
 perceptual recognition, 437
 Ponzo illusion, 444
Perspective. *See also* Illusion
 complex, 442
PET. *See* Positron emission tomography (PET)
Phantom limb sensation, 94

Physical abuse subscale, 258
 alpha coefficient, 259
 test–retest reliability, 259
Physical assault scale, 258
Physical contact assessment, 224–225
Physical punishment scale, 258
Physiology/physiological
 electrophysiology, 69
 neurophysiology, 34
 oxytocin response, 373
 of skin, 27–28
Piagetian water level problem, 438–439
Picture, tangible, 437
 complex perspective, 442
 linear perspective, 440–442
 perceptual recognition, 437
Pigment (melanin)–producing cells, 8
Pilo Ruffini corpuscle, 24
Pineal gland, 357
Pinocchio illusion, 138
pINS. *See* Posterior insular cortex (pINS)
PKD. *See* Polycystic kidney disease (PKD)
Plasticity
 associated with body part loss, 94
 brain, 85
 intensified or reduced use effects, 95–96
 mean field approach, 106
 neural, 492
 perceptual learning, 98, 99
 physical activity effects, 97–98
 stimulation, 105–106
 tactile discrimination abilities, 105–106
 time scales, 99–100
 touch thresholds, 106
 training effects, 98, 99
POC. *See* Parieto occipital cortex (POC)
Polycystic kidney disease (PKD), 50, 51–52
Ponzo illusion, 444

Positron emission tomography
(PET), 147
Posterior insular cortex
(pINS), 145
Postpartum depression (PPD),
385, 386
Postural remapping, 200–201
PPD. *See* Postpartum depression
(PPD)
Prader–Willi syndrome (PWS),
412–413
Premature birth, 385–386, 389
Pressure, test of reactivity to, 230
Proportional integral derivative
control (PID control). 477
Proprioception, 138
Proprioceptive afferent, 123
 size and shape perception, 124
 types, 138
Proprioceptive touch, 254
Proteins, 10
 cytoskeletal, 49
 extracellular, 65
 immunoglobulins, 22, 27
 intracellular, 49
 MEC, 67
 mechanotransduction, 47, 50, 73
 nociceptive neurons, 39
 NOMPA and NOMPB, 70
 PKD, 52
 sensor, 8
 stomatin-like, 53
 structural, 11
 tethering, 48
 transduction, 71
Proximity, maternal, 374, 375,
386, 393
Psychological states, 345
Psychophysiology, 63, 101, 238
 assessment, 88
 studies, 132–133, 136, 174,
417–418, 481
Public goods game, 315
Punishment, 257
 measures with a touch subscale,
256, 263

scale, 258, 262
Purdue pegboard test, 89
Putative low threshold
mechanoreceptive neurons, 73
PVD neurons, 64
PWS. *See* Prader–Willi syndrome
(PWS)

Questionnaire
 Affectionate Communication
Index, 260
 Alabama Parenting, 256–257
 Assessing Environments, 258
 Childhood Experience of Care
and Abuse, 256, 258–259
 Childhood Trauma, 256, 259
 Coercive Discipline Scale, 262
 Comprehensive Child
Maltreatment Scales for
Adults, 259
 Conflict Tactics Scale, 258, 260
 Early Trauma Inventory,
259–260
 Parent, 221, 226, 416
 Parent Behavior Inventory, 262
 Parent-Child Conflict Tactics
Scale, 256, 258
 Physical Contact Assessment,
224–225
 Recollections of Early Childhood
Touch Scale, 249
 Recollections of Early Childhood
Touch Scale, 249
 relationship, 459
 retrospective, 246
 self-report, 221, 247, 252, 256
 Sensory Over-Responsivity
Inventory, 226
 Sensory Processing Measure,
226, 227
 Social Touch Questionnaire,
221, 225
 Tactile Somatosensory
Dysfunction Checklist, 221, 223
 TACTYPE, 223
 Teacher, 226

Questionnaire (*cont.*)
  Tie Signs Coding Sheet and Functions Measure, 247, 252
  Touch Avoidance Measure, 221, 224, 317
  Touch Inventory for Preschoolers, 220, 221
  Touch Inventory of Elementary School Aged Children, 221
  touch items, involving, 262

RA afferents. *See* Rapidly adapting afferents (RA afferents)
RA type I Aδ neurons (RAI Aδ neurons), 41. *See also* Microneurography
RAI Aδ neurons. *See* RA type I Aδ neurons (RAI Aδ neurons)
RAM. *See* Rapidly adapting Mechanoreceptor (RAM)
Rapidly adapting afferents (RA afferents), 41, 124–125, 128
  flutter and vibration perception, 132–133
  innervations, 130
  Meissner's corpuscle, 42, 129, 130
  motion detection, 133, 134
  neurite ending, 129
  Pacinian corpuscles, 41–42
  sensitivity, 130
  spatial representation, 129, 130
Rapidly adapting Mechanoreceptor (RAM), 72
Reactive touch types, 284
Reactivity
  behavioral, 221, 237
  cortisol, 396
  physiologic, 221, 237
  stress, 394, 395
  test of, 230
  to touch, 226, 422
Receptive field (RF), 128, 163, 165
  hypothetical neuron, 167
  in SI, 165–166
  somatosensory homunculus, 166
Receptor. *See also* Mechanoreceptor; Touch

ATP, 40
cutaneous, 144
ending, 132
GABA, 131, 413
G-protein-coupled, 40
Light Touch, 241
neurons, 74
neurotrophin, 42
nuclear, 10
OT, 375
P2X, 40
Pacinian, 16
sensory nerve, 5, 43
sheet, 171
Skin, 91, 161
thermal, 124
touch, 80
Trk, 42
TrkB, 44
TRPV, 50
TRPV1, 39
tyrosine kinase, 42
Rehabilitation robotics, 490, 492. *See also* Haptic feedback
  challenges, 493
  robot, 491
Religiosity, 362
Repetitive sensory stimulation, 108, 100–101
Repetitive TMS (rTMS), 104
Resiniferatoxin (RTX), 39
Retinopathy of prematurity (ROP), 450
Rett syndrome, 413–414
Reverse genetics, 37. *See also* Skin, human
Revised conflict tactics scale, 260
RF. *See* Receptive field (RF)
RMIS. *See* Robotassisted minimally invasive surgery (RMIS)
Robotassisted minimally invasive surgery (RMIS), 486
  illusion, 111
ROP. *See* Retinopathy of prematurity (ROP)
rTMS. *See* Repetitive TMS (rTMS)
RTX. *See* Resiniferatoxin (RTX)

Rubber hand
    experiment, 202–203
    endings, 46
Ruffini. *See* Pilo Ruffini corpuscle complex, 131

S. basale. *See* Stratum basale (S. basale)
S. germinativum. *See* Stratum basale (S. basale)
S. granulosum. *See* Stratum granulosum (S. granulosum)
SA afferents. *See* Slowly adapting afferents (SA afferents)
SA Aβ fibers type I (SAI), 43
SA Aβ fibers type II (SAII), 43
SA1 afferents. *See* Slowly adapting type 1 afferents (SA1 afferents)
SA2 afferents. *See* Slowly adapting type 2 afferents (SA2 afferents)
SAI. *See* SA Aβ fibers type I (SAI)
SAI afferents, 43
SAII. *See* SA Aβ fibers type II (SAII)
SAII afferents, 45–46
Salivary cortisol measure, 236–237
SAM. *See* Slowly adapting Mechanoreceptor (SAM)
Schwann cells, 16, 17, 42
SCR. *See* Skin conductance response (SCR)
Seasonal affective disorder, 357
Sebaceous glands, 21
Sebum, 13, 21
Secondary somatosensory cortex (SII), 101, 144
    curvature preference, 170
    selective responses, 169, 170
Self report
    measures, 246n
    method, 302
Self touch, 284
SensOR. *See* Sensory Over Responsivity Scale (SensOR)
Sensorimotor skills, 422
    continua, 172
    deprivation, 423–424
    modality, 34
    nerve receptors, 5
    processing measure, 227
Sensory
    blends, 28
    system, 274
    transduction, 480
Sensory deprivation, 108, 421, 423
    Bayesian decision theory, 195, 196
    MLE account, 194–195
    multisensory integrator, 195
Sensory dominance
    attentional manipulations, 196
Sensory ending structure, 61
Sensory Integration and Praxis Test (SIPT), 229
Sensory integration therapy (SIT), 424
Sensory Over Responsivity Scale (SensOR), 228
    SensOR assessment, 229
Sensory processing, 36, 143, 146, 226, 413
    in ASD, 418
    cortical, 91, 98, 413
    global measures of, 220
    measure.227
    of mechanical force, 42
    visual cortex, 109
Sensory Profiles (SPs), 227
SEP. *See* Spatial event plot (SEP)
SEPs. *See* Somatosensory evoked potentials (SEPs)
Serotonin, 423, 461
SESs. *See* Socioeconomic statuses (SESs)
Sexual abuse subscale, 259
SF. *See* Still-face (SF)
Shape-memory alloy (SMA), 481
Shunt pathways, 13
SI. *See* Somatosensory cortex (SI)
SII. *See* Secondary somatosensory cortex (SII)
Single-layered periderm, 6–7
Single-tether model, 67–68
SIPT. *See* Sensory Integration and Praxis Test (SIPT)
SIS. *See* Skin immune system (SIS)

SIT. *See* Sensory integration therapy (SIT)
Size discrimination, 205
   immune system, 27–28
   innervation, 16–17
   nerve technique, 62, 72–73
   pigmentation, 26–27
Skin, 3-29. *See also* Dermis; Epidermis; Touch
   advances in disciplines, 3
   eccrine sweat glands, 19–20
   elasticity, 15
   hair fiber, 24–25
   hair follicle, 21–24
   nail, 25–26
   sebaceous glands, 21
   surface morphology, 13
   structural examination, 3
   tactile rituals, 351
   tissue types, 5
   types, 24
   vascularization, 15–16
   in warm countries, 357
   wrinkling, 13
Skin appendages, 18. *See also* Skin, human
   apocrine sweat/scent glands, 20
Skin conductance response (SCR), 233
   characteristics, 6
   difference from other mammals, 4
   protection, 4
Skin immune system (SIS), 27
Sleep-wake cycle, 392
Slip, 483
Slit worm preparation, 66
Slowly adapting afferents (SA afferents), 41, 43
   Merkel cell–neurite complexes, 43–45
   Ruffini endings, 46
   SAI afferents, 43
   SAII afferents, 45–46
Slowly adapting mechanoreceptor (SAM), 72
Slowly adapting type 1 afferents (SA1 afferents), 125

Atoh1 gene, 125
continuum mechanics model, 127
cutaneous form and texture perception, 134–136, 137
innervation density, 128
macrogeometric property, 146
Merkel cells, 125
ridge types, 126–127
SEPs, 129
skin types, 126
surround suppression effect, 127–128
Slowly adapting type 2 afferents (SA2 afferents), 125, 131
   joint afferents, 132
   Ruffini complex, 131
   sensitivity, 132
SLP. *See* Stomatin like protein (SLP)
slp3. *See* Stomatin like protein 3 (slp3)
SMA. *See* Shape-memory alloy (SMA)
Social Touch Questionnaire (STQ), 225
Socioeconomic status (SES), 341
Somatic inputs diversity and importance, 124
Somatosensation, 35–36
Somatosensory cortex (SI), 95, 144, 163
   bold signals, 96
   hemodynamic responses in, 95, 96
   motion, 175–177
   position in brain, 164–165
   RFs, 165–167
   signal pathways, 165
   spatial form representation, 167–169
   temperature and pain representations, 177–179
   texture and vibration, 172–175
   ventral processing stream, 165
Somatosensory dysfunction checklist, 223
Somatosensory evoked potentials (SEPs), 411

Somatosensory pathways, 34–35
  sensation of pain, 36
  sensory modality, 34, 36
  somatosensation, 35–36
  mechanotransduction, 162
Somatosensory periphery
  mechanoreceptive afferents, 163
  spatial isomorphism, 163
  crossmodal plasticity, 108–110
Somatosensory plasticity
  changes in body schema and ownership, 110–111
Somatosensory processing, 422
Somatosensory system, 59, 419
  SCN9A mutation effect, 60
  touch sensation in mice, 71–72
Somesthetic system, 274. *See also* Sensory—system
Soothing, 248, 284
Spastic diplegia, 421. *See also* Cerebral palsy (CP)
Spastic hemiplegia, 421. *See also* Cerebral palsy (CP)
Spatial event plot (SEP), 134–135
Spatial isomorphism, 163
Spinal thalamic tract neurons (STT neurons), 178
SPM. *See* Statistical parametric map (SPM)
SPs. *See* Sensory Profiles (SPs)
Startle responses, 232
Statistical parametric map (SPM), 145
  confounding factors, 345
  homophobia, 346
  observational studies, 341–345
Status and touch, 341–346. *See also* Touch and gender
  beliefs and perceptions, 341
  relation to gender, 345
  winners and losers, 343–344
Still-face (SF), 277
  procedure, 246
  with touch periods, 279
Stimulation, passive
  exposure through coactivation, 100–103

  TMS, 104–105
Stimulation, *See also* Tactile stimulation
  plasticity, 105–106
  rehabilitation using, 107–108
Stimulus, 167
  isomorphic representation, 163
  parameters, 136
  shape, 146
  visual and haptic shape selective brain regions, 147
Stochastic resonance, 94
Stomatin-like protein (SLP), 53
Stomatin-like protein 3 (*slp3*), 75
STQ. *See* Social Touch Questionnaire (STQ)
Stratum basale (S. basale), 8
Stratum corneum (S. corneum), 4, 7, 11
Stratum granulosum (S. granulosum), 7
Stress response, 97
  cardiovascular, 236
  index, 377
  infant's, 382
Stressors, noxious, 3
Striking bodily illusions, 201
  following massage therapy, 461
STT neurons. *See* Spinal thalamic tract neurons (STT neurons)
Substance P
  in deep sleep, 461
Sulci. *See* Dermatoglyphs
Surgical simulator, 489
Surround suppression effect, 127–128
Sweat, 20
  in old age, 91, 92
  in professional pianists, 97

Tactile acuity, 87. *See also* Tactile coactivation
  development in children, 89
  cultures, 364
Tactile behavior, 259. *See also* Tactile traditions
  child's, 265
  variations in, 363

Tactile acuity (cont.)
  cortical reorganization, 101, 102
  linear correlation analysis, 101
  LTP and LTD, 102
  using memantine, 102
  repetitive sensory stimulation
    protocols, 100–101
  repetitive stimulation, 103
Tactile coactivation, 93. See also
    Tactile acuity
  changes of cortical maps, 101
  tactile learning protocols, 100
Tactile coding systems, 261
Tactile defensiveness, 220, 221
  ADHD, 420
  ASDs, 416
Tactile discrimination, 43
  behavioral tests of, 63
  human, 92
  thresholds, 96
  two-point, 101
Tactile dysfunction, 409
  neurodevelopmental
    disorders, 410
  therapeutic interventions,
    424–425
Tactile feedback system, 480
  contact motion, 482
  deskop, 481, 482
  local shape, 481
  slip, 483
  in surgery, 487–488
  vibration feedback, 484–485
Tactile hyperacuity task, 99
Tactile Interaction Index (TII),
    253–255
Tactile learning protocols, 100
Tactile object recognition
    scanning, 161
  olfactory contributions to, 191–192
  PWS, 412
Tactile perception, 220
  auditory contributions to, 190–191
  Tactile Somatosensory
    Dysfunction Checklist, 221, 223
  visual contributions to, 193–194
  of children, 88–90

  mechanoreceptor density and,
    86–88
  tactile haptic task performance, 86
  tactile perception dependence, 88
Tactile performance
  aging and, 90–94
Tactile sensation, 409
Tactile sensitivity
  aging, 449
  in autism, 418
  FXS, 414
  measures of sensory response, 226
  visual loss and, 446
Tactile somatosensory dysfunction
    checklist, 223
Tactile stimulation
  fetal response, 275
  habituation, 422
  health, 274
  on infant, 286
  neonatal grasping, 207
  passive, 98
  quality of, 282
  crossmodal delayed matching to
    sample task, 205
  external frame of reference,
    207, 208
  spatial orientation, 207
Tactile stimuli
  crossmodal congruency task,
    201–202
  using tactile TOJ task, 203, 208
  ventral premotor cortex
    neurons, 201
  visual orientation, 207–208
Tactile threshold, 416, 420, 422
Tactile traditions, 351
  cross cultural similarities, 351
  culture controversy, 363
  gender orientation, 360–361
  individualism/collectivism,
    359–360
  latitude, changes in, 355–358
  north vs. south, 356
  religious influences and tactile
    taboos, 362
  rituals, 351

tactile miscommunication, 356
Tactile Vulnerability Assessment (TVA), 237
TACTYPE, 223
TAM. *See* Touch Avoidance Measure (TAM)
TBS. *See* Theta burst stimulation (TBS)
Teleoperation, 479
Telepresence sense, 469
  neural coding distribution, 179
  perception, 178
  STT neuron sensitivity, 178
Temperature
  cortical area involvement, 179
Temporal order judgment (TOJ), 203
Tethered model, 48–49
  flutter range, 175
  PC afferent response, 174
  representation in SI, 173–174
Texture. *See also* Touch
  coarse textural features, 172
  vibrations, 172, 173
  vibratory frequency perception, 174
Thermal receptors, 124
Thermoreceptive afferents, 123
Thermoregulation, 22
Theta burst stimulation (TBS), 104
Three dimension (3D), 150
Tie Sign Functions Scale, 252–253
Tie Signs Coding Sheet, 252
TII. *See* Tactile Interaction Index (TII)
til A D. *See* Touch insensitive larva A D (til A D)
TIP. *See* Touch Inventory for Preschoolers (TIP)
TMS. *See* Transcranial magnetic stimulation (TMS)
TOJ. *See* Temporal order judgment (TOJ)
Touch, 28, 33, 283, 290, 299, 300, 303, 320, 351, 409. *See also* Touch locations
  active and passive accompaniment, 281
  and affect, 286

amount, 254
behavioral measure, 219, 231
characteristics, 263
cognitive context, 307–308
comforting, 254
contextual variables, 306
couples, between, 304–305
discriminative, 35, 36
diverse, 254
drawing validity, 437
and emotion regulation, 287–288
fetal response, 275–276
formalized, 302, 343
function, 248–249
harsh, 254
health professionals and patients, 250–251
infants and, 274, 286 287
intensity, 249, 253
interpersonal, 354
light touch, 36, 230
location, 199–200, 246, 249
maternal, 254, 285–286, 373
measures of response, 220, 221, 226
in motor and social development, 409
multiple response measurement, 237
negative, 280
nurturing, 254
painful, 39
patterns, 283–284
perception, 72, 109–110
physical contact assessment, 224–225
physiologic measurement, 231, 232, 236
plasticity modality specificity, 112
positive, 280
in preschool period, 288–289
primary function, 352
properties, 281, 286
qualities, 288
reactive types, 284
religiosity, 362
response to, 219, 337
role, 409–410

Touch (*cont.*)
  salivary cortisol measure, 236–237
  scale functions, 248–249
  self touch, 284
  sense of, 4, 86, 91
  sensory processing measure, 227
  sexual, 304, 307, 353
  soothing, 248, 284
  status and, 341, 345–346
  stimulating, 254
  stroking, 307
  synchrony and missynchrony, 377
  Touch Test, 223
  tracking location, 199–200
  types, 246, 251, 254, 282
  unintentional, 280
  and vision, 206
  beliefs, 332–333
  body parts and qualitative
    differences, 336–337
  experimental studies, 338, 339–340
  gender comparisons, 336
  homophobia, role of, 331
  men and women, asymmetry, 332,
    333–336
  men and women touch
    behavior's, 337
  observational studies, 333
  reactions to being touched,
    337–341
Touch and gender, 331–341
  attitudes, 331–332
  relation to status, 345–346
Touch avoidance, 316–317
  correlates, 317
  in northerly regions, 358
  religiosity, 362
  in United States, 356
Touch Avoidance Measure (TAM),
  224, 317
Touch avoidant people, 317, 362
Touch behavior, *See also* Tactile
  behavior
Touch communication, 273,
  299, 301
  and affect, 286
  approaches to study, 301 303

  caregiver touch, 274
  compliance, 313–316
  emotion and, 305
  future directions, 320
  individual differences, 316–318
  infants and, 274, 283, 285–286
  intimacy, 303–305
  liking, 312–313
  modalities, 318–319
  in preschool period, 288–289
Touch insensitive larva A D
  (til A D), 69
Touch Inventory for Preschoolers
  (TIP), 220, 222
  ITS, 246
  TII location index, 253
Touch measures, 245, 247, 261
  adult–adult touch, 251
  affectionate communication, 260
  coding procedures, 261–262
  conflict between adult
    partners, 260
  for elementary school aged
    children, 222
  facets of, 263–266
  future measurement, 262
  health professionals and patients,
    250–251
  parent–child touch, 246
  parenting practices, 256, 258
  for preschoolers, 220, 222
  questionnaires, 262
  recollections of early childhood
    touch scale, 249–250
  strengths in, 262–263
  structured measures, 245
  structured measures with touch
    subscale, 255, 256
  with touch subscale, 255, 256
  for use across populations, 253
Touch responsive neuron (TRN), 63
  gene requirement, 64–65
  microtubule cells, 64
  nonciliated, 64
Touch sensation, 61
  behavioral assay, 72
  gated current types, 73

gene requirement for touch
  stimuli, 65–67
gene requirement for TRNs, 64–65
genes involvement, 64, 69–71
mec genes, 64, 65–67
mechanotransduction features, 71
in mice, 71–72
models for responsive channels,
  67–68
psychophysical test uses, 63
response in C. elegans, 63–64
skin nerve technique, 72–73
slit worm preparation, 66
stimuli, 60
unc-86 genes, 64, 65
Touch Test, 223
Trace elements, 25
Transcranial direct current
  stimulation, 104
Transcranial magnetic stimulation
  (TMS), 85, 104–105, 109, 147
Transient receptor potential ankryin
  (TRPA), 50, 51
Transient receptor potential
  channels (TRP channels),
  49, 178
  DEG/ENaC, 52–53
  PKD, 51–52
  stomatin-like proteins, 53
  TRPA, 76–77
  TRPA1, 51
  TRPN1, 51
  TRPV, 50–51
Transient receptor potential
  channels (TRP channels), 70
Transient receptor potential
  mechanoreceptor potential
  (TRPN), 50, 51
Transient receptor potential
  melastatin (TRPM), 50
Transient receptor potential
  musolipin (TRPML), 50
Transient receptor potential
  vanilloid (TRPV), 50, 51
Transient receptor potential
  vanilloid 1 (TRPV1), 39, 47
Transparency, 479

Trauma
  Childhood Trauma
    Questionnaire, 256
  intrauterine, 421
  of premature birth, 386
  scale, 259
Trauma inventory, early, 259–260
TRN. *See* Touch responsive
  neuron (TRN)
TRP channels. *See* Transient receptor
  potential channels (TRP channels)
TRPA. *See* Transient receptor
  potential ankryin (TRPA)
TRPM. *See* Transient receptor
  potential melastatin (TRPM)
TRPML. *See* Transient receptor
  potential musolipin (TRPML)
TRPN. *See* Transient receptor
  potential mechanoreceptor
  potential (TRPN)
TRPV. *See* Transient receptor
  potential vanilloid (TRPV)
TRPV1. *See* Transient receptor
  potential vanilloid 1 (TRPV1)
TVA. *See* Tactile Vulnerability
  Assessment (TVA)
Two-point discrimination, 88

unc-86 gene, 64, 65
Uncoordinated like mutants (*uncl*
  mutants), 69
Uncoordinated mutants (*unc*
  mutants), 69
Unintentional touch, 280
Use dependent plasticity, 112
UV radiation (UVR), 3
  in massage therapy, 464

Vagal activity
  and cortisol levels, 464–465
Vagal tone, 383
  cardiac, 383, 394
  heart rate variability, 234
  infant's baseline, 384
  massage therapy, 235
  neurological system immaturity
    effect, 394–395

Vagal tone (*cont.*)
  NK cells, 462
  respiratory sinus arrhythmia, 234
  resting, 395
Varied touch. *See* Touch—diverse
Ventral premotor cortex
    neurons, 201
Ventral processing stream, 165
Ventrolateral posterior (VPL), 36
Very low vision (VLV), 435
  Piagetian water level problem, 439
Vestibular sensation, 424
Vestibular touch, 254
Vibration, 28, 72, 132, 484–485
  corduroy perception, 173
  fl utter, 133
  HAVS, 95
  human sensitivity, 485
  lamellar capsule, 42
  Light touch, 36
  open-loop, 485
  Pacinian corpuscle, 41
  PC Afferents, 130, 134
  RAs and PCs, 132,
  during scanning, 172
  sinusoidal, 174
  threshold detection, 133
Vibration feedback, 484–485
Vibratory frequency
  tactile perception of, 174
Vibroacoustic stimulation, 275
Virtual touch device, 448
Vision, 90, 109. *See also* Touch

Vision and touch, 150
  convergence sites, 153
  crossmodal transfer, 150, 151, 153
  neural convergence, 152
Visual agnosia, 152
Visual cortex, 109
Visual dominance effects, 194
  maps and, 445–446
  myth about, 435–436
  new technology for, 448
  pattern perception, 436–437
  perspective distortion, 437, 441
  perspective understanding in,
    439–440
  Piagetian water level problem, 439
  spatial acuity, 448
  visual decline, 449
Visual impaired, 435. *See also* Illusion
  linear perspective, 440–441
  in texture processing, 153–154
Visuo haptic convergence
  in shape processing, 150–153
VLV. *See* Very low vision (VLV)
Voltage gated Na⁺ channels (NaV
    channels), 40
von Frey test, 72
VPL. *See* Ventrolateral posterior (VPL)

Wide dynamic range neurons. *See*
    Spinal thalamic tract neurons
    (STT neurons)
Wilbarger protocol, 425
Writing motor behavior, 161